ORAL TOLERANCE
New Insights and Prospects
for Clinical Application

ANNALS OF THE NEW YORK ACADEMY OF SCIENCES
Volume 1029

ORAL TOLERANCE
New Insights and Prospects for Clinical Application

Edited by Howard L. Weiner, Lloyd Mayer, and Warren Strober

The New York Academy of Sciences
New York, New York
2004

Copyright © 2004 by the New York Academy of Sciences. All rights reserved. Under the provisions of the United States Copyright Act of 1976, individual readers of the Annals *are permitted to make fair use of the material in them for teaching or research. Permission is granted to quote from the* Annals *provided that the customary acknowledgment is made of the source. Material in the* Annals *may be republished only by permission of the Academy. Address inquiries to the Permissions Department (editorial@nyas.org) at the New York Academy of Sciences.*

Copying fees: *For each copy of an article made beyond the free copying permitted under Section 107 or 108 of the 1976 Copyright Act, a fee should be paid through the Copyright Clearance Center, Inc., 222 Rosewood Drive, Danvers, MA 01923 (www.copyright.com).*

♾ *The paper used in this publication meets the minimum requirements of the American National Standard for Information Sciences—Permanence of Paper for Printed Library Materials, ANSI Z39.48-1984.*

Library of Congress Cataloging-in-Publication Data

Oral tolerance : new insights and prospects for clinical application / edited by Howard L. Weiner, Lloyd Mayer, and Warren Strober.
   p. ; cm. — (Annals of the New York Academy of Sciences ; v. 1029)
  Includes bibliographical references and index.
  ISBN 1-57331-508-7 (cloth : alk. paper) — ISBN 1-57331-509-5 (pbk. : alk. paper)
  1. Immunological tolerance—Congresses. 2. Oral mucosa—Immunology—Congresses.
  [DNLM: 1. Immune Tolerance—physiology—Congresses. 2. Administration, Oral—Congresses. 3. Autoimmune Diseases—therapy—Congresses. 4. Disease Models, Animal—Congresses. QW 504 O634 2004] I. Weiner, Howard L. II. Mayer, Lloyd F. III. Strober, Warren. IV. Series.
  Q11.N5 vol. 1029
  [QR188.4]
  500 s—dc22
  [616.07
                    2004028017

GYAT/PCP
Printed in the United States of America
ISBN 1-57331-508-7 (cloth)
ISBN 1-57331-509-5 (paper)
ISSN 0077-8923

ANNALS OF THE NEW YORK ACADEMY OF SCIENCES

Volume 1029
December 2004

ORAL TOLERANCE
New Insights and Prospects for Clinical Application

Editors
HOWARD L. WEINER, LLOYD MAYER, AND WARREN STROBER

This volume is the result of a conference entitled **Oral Tolerance: Mechanisms and Applications,** presented by the New York Academy of Sciences, and held on October 23–26, 2003 in New York City.

CONTENTS

Preface. *By* LLOYD MAYER	xi
Oral Tolerance: Overview and Historical Perspectives. *By* ALLAN MCI. MOWAT, LUCY A. PARKER, HELEN BEACOCK-SHARP, OWAIN R. MILLINGTON, AND FERNANDO CHIRDO	1

Part I. Anatomy and Physiology

The Anatomy of Mucosal Immune Responses. *By* PAUL GARSIDE, OWAIN MILLINGTON, AND KAREN M. SMITH.	9
How the Gut Links Innate and Adaptive Immunity. *By* MARTIN RUMBO, PASCALE ANDERLE, ARNAUD DIDIERLAURENT, FRÉDÉRIC SIERRO, NATHALIE DEBARD, JEAN-CLAUDE SIRARD, DANIELA FINKE, AND JEAN-PIERRE KRAEHENBUHL.	16
Activation of a Unique Population of $CD8^+$ T Cells by Intestinal Epithelial Cells. *By* MATTHIEU ALLEZ, JENS BRIMNES, LING SHAO, IRIS DOTAN, ATSUSHI NAKAZAWA, AND LLOYD MAYER.	22
Compartmentalization of the Mucosal Immune Responses to Commensal Intestinal Bacteria. *By* ANDREW J. MACPHERSON AND THERESE UHR	36

Isolated Lymphoid Follicles Can Function as Sites for Induction of Mucosal
 Immune Responses. *By* ROBIN G. LORENZ AND RODNEY D. NEWBERRY ... 44

Anatomy and Physiology: Summary of Part I. *By* JIRI MESTECKY 58

Part II. Mechanisms of Oral Tolerance: Dendritic Cells

Involvement of Dendritic Cell Subsets in the Induction of Oral Tolerance and
 Immunity. *By* MARINA FLEETON, NIKHAT CONTRACTOR, FRANCISCO
 LEON, JIANPING HE, DENISE WETZEL, TERENCE DERMODY, AKIKO
 IWASAKI, AND BRIAN KELSALL.. 60

Intestinal Epithelial Cells Control Dendritic Cell Function. *By* MONICA
 RIMOLDI, MARCELLO CHIEPPA, MARISA VULCANO,
 PAOLA ALLAVENA, AND MARIA RESCIGNO 66

Uptake of Antigens from the Intestine by Dendritic Cells. *By* GORDON
 MACPHERSON, SIMON MILLING, ULF YRLID, LESLEY COUSINS, EMMA
 TURNBULL, FANG-PING HUANG....................................... 75

In Vivo Enhancement of Dendritic Cell Function. *BY* JANINE BILSBOROUGH
 AND JOANNE L. VINEY... 83

Regulation of Tolerance in the Respiratory Tract: TIM-1, Hygiene, and the
 Environment. *By* DALE T. UMETSU AND ROSEMARIE H. DEKRUYFF 88

Mechanisms of Oral Tolerance: Dendritic Cells—Summary of Part II. *By*
 TERRENCE A. BARRETT.. 94

Part III. Mechanisms of Oral Tolerance: Regulatory T Cells

CD4$^+$ CD25$^+$ Regulatory T Cell Selection. *By* ANDREW J. CATON, CRISTINA
 COZZO, JOSEPH LARKIN III, MELISSA A. LERMAN, ALINA BOESTEANU,
 AND MARTHA S. JORDAN 101

Insights into the Mechanism of Oral Tolerance Derived from the Study of
 Models of Mucosal Inflammation. *By* WARREN STROBER, IVAN FUSS,
 MONICA BOIRIVANT, AND ATSUSHI KITANI. 115

Immune Regulation in the Intestine: A Balancing Act between Effector and
 Regulatory T Cell Responses. *By* FIONA POWRIE 132

IL-10–Producing T Regulatory Type 1 Cells and Oral Tolerance. *By*
 MANUELA BATTAGLIA, CARMEN GIANFRANI, SILVIA GREGORI,
 AND MARIA-GRAZIA RONCAROLO. 142

Natural Killer T Cells in Mucosal Homeostasis. *By* ARTHUR KASER,
 EDWARD E.S. NIEUWENHUIS, WARREN STROBER, LLOYD MAYER,
 IVAN FUSS, SEAN COLGAN, AND RICHARD S. BLUMBERG 154

Mechanisms of Oral Tolerance: Regulatory T Cells—Summary of Part III.
 Moderators: CATHRYN NAGLER-ANDERSON AND WARREN STROBER 169

Part IV. *In Vivo* Effectors

Regulation of Autoreactive T Cell Function by Oral Tolerance to Self-
 Antigens. *By* CAROLINE C. WHITACRE, FEI SONG, RICHARD M. WARDROP III,
 KIM CAMPBELL, MELANIE MCCLAIN, JACQUELINE BENSON, ZHEN GUAN,
 AND INGRID GIENAPP.. 172

Natural and Induced Regulatory T Cells. *By* EMMA J. O'NEILL, ANETTE SUNDSTEDT, GRAZIELLA MAZZA, KIRSTY S. NICOLSON, MARY PONSFORD, LESLIE SAURER, HEATHER STREETER, STEVE ANDERTON, AND DAVID C. WRAITH 180

ADP-Ribosylating Bacterial Enzymes for the Targeted Control of Mucosal Tolerance and Immunity. *By* NILS LYCKE. 193

In Vivo Effectors: Summary of Part IV. *By* MITCHELL KRONENBERG 209

Part V. Oral Tolerance: Animal Disease Models and Human Trials

Current Issues in the Treatment of Human Diseases by Mucosal Tolerance. *By* HOWARD L. WEINER 211

Failure to Induce Oral Tolerance in Crohn's and Ulcerative Colitis Patients: Possible Genetic Risk. *By* THOMAS A. KRAUS, LISA TOY, LISA CHAN, JOSEPH CHILDS, ADAM CHEIFETZ, AND LLOYD MAYER 225

Oral Glatiramer Acetate in Experimental Autoimmune Encephalomyelitis: Clinical and Immunological Studies. *By* DVORA TEITELBAUM, RINA AHARONI, ETY KLINGER, RIVKA KREITMAN, EMANUEL RAYMOND, ARTHUR MALLEY, RONA SHOFTI, MICHAEL SELA, AND RUTH ARNON 239

Constraints on the Efficacy of Mucosal Tolerance in Treatment of Human and Animal Arthritic Diseases. *By* NORMAN A. STAINES, CATHERINE J. DERRY, LILIA MARINOVA-MUTAFCHIEVA, NADIRA ALI, D. HUW DAVIES, AND JOHN J. MURPHY. 250

Oral Insulin Therapy to Prevent Progression of Immune-Mediated (Type 1) Diabetes. *By* BERRIN ERGUN-LONGMIRE, JOHN MARKER, ADINA ZEIDLER, ROBERT RAPAPORT, PHILIP RASKIN, BRUCE BODE, DESMOND SCHATZ, ALFONSO VARGAS, DOUGLAS ROGERS, SHERWYN SCHWARTZ, JOHN MALONE, JEFFREY KRISCHER, AND NOEL K. MACLAREN 260

Orally and Nasally Induced Tolerance Studies in Ocular Inflammatory Disease: Guidance for Future Interventions. *By* ROBERT NUSSENBLATT .. 278

Oral Immune Regulation toward Disease-Associated Antigens: Results of Phase I Clinical Trials in Crohn's Disease and Chronic Hepatitis. *By* YARON ILAN 286

Oral Tolerance in Humans: Failure to Suppress an Existing Immune Response by Oral Antigen Administration. *By* ZINA MOLDOVEANU, FRED OLIVER, JIRI MESTECKY, AND CHARLES O. ELSON 299

Oral Tolerance: Animal Disease Models and Human Trials—Summary of Part V. *By* WARREN STROBER 310

Part VI. Short Papers

Class II MHC–Expressing Myofibroblasts Play a Role in the Immunopathogenesis Associated with Staphylococcal Enterotoxins. *By* C.A. BARRERA, I.V. PINCHUK, J.I. SAADA, G. SUAREZ, D.A. BLAND, E. BESWICK, P.A. ADEGBOYEGA, R.C. MIFFLIN, D.W. POWELL, AND V.E. REYES 313

Early Upregulation of T Cell IL-10 Production Plays an Important Role in Oral Tolerance Induction. *By* Y. CONG, C. LIU, C.T. WEAVER, AND C.O. ELSON 319

Study of Oral Tolerance and Its Indirect Effects in Adoptive Cell Transfer Experiments. *By* ANDRÉ PIRES DA CUNHA, NELSON MONTEIRO VAZ, AND CLÁUDIA ROCHA CARVALHO 321

Differential Immune Induction with Subcutaneous versus Oral Administration of a Diabetogenic Insulin Peptide in the NOD Mouse. *By* DEVASENAN DEVENDRA, JOHANNA PARONEN, EDWIN LIU, HIROAKI MORIYAMA, DONGMEI MIAO, LIPING YU, AND GEORGE S. EISENBARTH 328

Comparative Study of Oral versus Subcutaneous B:9–23 Insulin Peptide in Balb/c Mice as an Experimental Model for Autoimmune Diabetes. *By* DEVASENAN DEVENDRA, JOHANNA PARONEN, EDWIN LIU, HIROAKI MORIYAMA, ROBERT TAYLOR, DONGMEI MIAO, LIPING YU, AND GEORGE EISENBARTH 331

CCL25 Enhances CD103-Mediated Lymphocyte Adhesion to E-Cadherin. *By* ANNA ERICSSON, ANU ARYA, AND WILLIAM AGACE 334

Bacterial Translocation in the Normal Human Appendix Parallels the Development of the Local Immune System. *By* JAN-OLAF GEBBERS AND JEAN-ALBERT LAISSUE 337

Hyporesponsiveness of CD4 T Cells Induced in Oral Tolerance Is Maintained by Selective Impairment in the TCR-Induced Calcium/NFAT Signaling Pathway Resulting from Caspase Activation. *By* SATOSHI HACHIMURA, TOMOHIRO KAJI, KAZUMI ASAI, WATARU ISE, TOSHINORI NAKAYAMA, AND SHUICHI KAMINOGAWA 344

The Presentation of Haptenated Proteins and Activation of T Cells in the Mesenteric Lymph Nodes by Dendritic Cells in the TNBS Colitis Rat. *By* YOH ISHIGURO, HIROTAKE SAKURABA, KAZUFUMI YAMAGATA, AND AKIHIRO MUNAKATA 346

Macrophage Migration Inhibitory Factor and Activator Protein-1 in Ulcerative Colitis. *By* YOH ISHIGURO, KAZUFUMI YAMAGATA, HIROTAKE SAKURABA, AKIHIRO MUNAKATA, AKIO NAKANE, TAKAYUKI MORITA, AND JUN NISHIHIRA 348

Genetic Selection for Resistance or Susceptibility to Oral Tolerance to Ovalbumin Affects General Mechanisms of Tolerance Induction in Mice. *By* ALICE O. KAMPHORST, MARIA F.S. DA SILVA, ANTÔNIO C. DA SILVA, CLAUDIA R. CARVALHO, AND ANA MARIA C. FARIA 350

CD45 Knockout Mice, Diet, and Colitis: In the Absence of CD45, Colitis Follows Dietary Changes. *By* MARÍA C. LÓPEZ AND NICK HOLMES 355

Noise and Microflora Behavior. *By* MÁXIMO LORENZO, PABLO SÁNCHEZ, AND ENRIQUE REWALD 358

Decreased Nasal Tolerance to Allergic Asthma in Mice Fed an Amino Acid–Based Protein-Free Diet. *By* DANIEL SOUSA MUCIDA, DUNIA RODRÍGUEZ, ALEXANDRE CASTRO KELLER, ELIANE GOMES, JUSCILENE SILVA MENEZES, ANA MARIA CAETANO DE FARIA, AND MOMCHILO RUSSO 361

Peyer's Patch Dendritic Cells Capturing Oral Antigen Interact with Antigen-Specific T Cells and Induce Gut-Homing $CD4^+CD25^+$ Regulatory T Cells in Peyer's Patches. *By* KATSUYA NAGATANI, KAYO SAGAWA, YOSHINORI KOMAGATA, AND KAZUHIKO YAMAMOTO 366

The Role of Transforming Growth Factor–β in a Model of Oral Tolerance to the Diet Antigen Dextrin. *By* SOFÍA OLMOS, MARIA GABRIELA MARQUEZ, MARÍA C. LÓPEZ, AND MARIA ESTELA ROUX 371

Commonly Used Drugs Impair Oral Tolerance in Mice. *By* SOPHIE PECQUET, GUÉNOLÉE PRIOULT, JOHN CAMPBELL, BRUCE GERMAN, AND MARCO TURINI 374

Intestinal Myofibroblasts and Immune Tolerance. *By* J.I. SAADA, C.A. BARRERA, V.E. REYES, P.A. ADEGBOYEGA, G. SUAREZ, R.A. TAMERISA, K.F. PANG, D.A. BLAND, R.C. MIFFLIN, J.F. DI MARI, AND D.W. POWELL 379

Transforming Growth Factor–β Regulates Susceptibility of Epithelial Apoptosis in Murine Model of Colitis. *By* HIROTAKE SAKURABA, YOH ISHIGURO, KAZUFUMI YAMAGATA, YOH-ICHI TAGAWA, YOICHIRO IWAKURA, KENJI SEKIKAWA, AKIHIRO MUNAKATA, AND AKIO NAKANE. 382

Early Events in Antigen-Specific Regulatory T Cell Induction via Nasal and Oral Mucosa. *By* JANNEKE N. SAMSOM, FEMKE HAUET-BROERE, WENDY W.J. UNGER, LISETTE A. VAN BERKEL, AND GEORG KRAAL 385

Stochastic Resonance-Like Phenomena in the Context of the Alimentary Tract. *By* PABLO SÁNCHEZ, MÁXIMO LORENZO, AND ENRIQUE REWALD . . . 390

Is Oral Tolerance Correlated with IgE Levels and Mast Cell Numbers? *By* ANTONIO CARLOS DA SILVA, MARIA F.S. SILVA, CRISTINA BIANCHI, RICARDO C. RIBEIRO, ALBERTO NÓBREGA, AND OSVALDO SANT'ANNA . . . 394

Genetic Selection for Susceptibility to Oral Tolerance Leads to a Profound Reduction of the Acute Inflammatory Response. *By* MARIA DE FÁTIMA SARRO DA SILVA, ALBERTO DA NÓBREGA, TEREZA CRISTINA BARJA-FIDALGO, ALINE C. BRANDO-LIMA, FERNANDO CUNHA, AND ANTONIO CARLOS DA SILVA 398

The Thymus Plays a Role in Oral Tolerance Induction in Experimental Autoimmune Encephalomyelitis. *By* FEI SONG, INGRID E. GIENAPP, TODD SHAWLER, ZHEN GUAN, AND CAROLINE C. WHITACRE 402

Selective Generation of Gut-Tropic T Cells in Gut-Associated Lymphoid Tissues: Requirement for GALT Dendritic Cells and Adjuvant. *By* MARCUS SVENSSON, BENGT JOHANSSON-LINDBOM, MARC-ANDRÉ WURBEL, BERNARD MALISSEN, GABRIEL MÁRQUEZ, AND WILLIAM AGACE 405

Long-Term Follow-Up of Oral Tolerance Induction with HLA-Peptide B27PD in Patients with Uveitis. *By* STEPHAN R. THURAU, HARALD FRICKE, CHRISTIAN BURCHARDI, MARIA DIEDRICHS-MÖHRING, AND GERHILD WILDNER. 408

IL-18 and Antigen-Specific $CD4^+$ Regulatory T Cells in Peyer's Patches. *By* NORIKO M. TSUJI AND BERNADETA NOWAK. 413

Gamma-Delta T Cells as Orally Induced Suppressor Cells in Rats: *In Vitro* Characterization. *By* GERHILD WILDNER, STEPHAN R. THURAU, AND MARIA DIEDRICHS-MÖHRING 416

Index of Contributors 423

Financial assistance was received from:

Major Funders
- AUTOIMMUNE INC.
- SERONO, INC.
- TEVA NEUROSCIENCE, INC.

Supporters
- BIOGEN, INC.
- CENTOCOR, INC.
- CROHN'S & COLITIS FOUNDATION OF AMERICA
- NATIONAL INSTITUTE OF ALLERGY AND INFECTIOUS DISEASES/NIH

Contributors
- AMGEN INC.
- FOUNDATION FOR NEUROLOGIC DISEASES
- NATIONAL MULTIPLE SCLEROSIS SOCIETY
- PEPGEN CORPORATION

The New York Academy of Sciences believes it has a responsibility to provide an open forum for discussion of scientific questions. The positions taken by the participants in the reported conferences are their own and not necessarily those of the Academy. The Academy has no intent to influence legislation by providing such forums.

Preface

Less than ten years ago we came together to build a bridge from animal models of oral tolerance to their clinical application in humans. The goal was to use oral tolerance to treat a variety of autoimmune/inflammatory disorders. On the basis of the initial findings there was enormous enthusiasm for the potential of this approach in treating human disease. Over the past decade we have seen significant progress in our understanding of mechanisms involved in tolerance induction in mice. We have also seen studies defining tolerance induction in people. What has not yet lived up to its promise has been the translation of the approach of oral tolerance in mice to treating inflammatory diseases in humans. Although positive results were observed in phase II trials, large-scale phase III trials in rheumatoid arthritis, multiple sclerosis, and diabetes yielded limited or no positive outcomes. The reason for these failures is poorly understood, but it occurs in the face of expanding murine models in which mucosal tolerance prevents or treats a variety of diseases, for example, stroke, graft rejection, atherosclerosis, and autoimmune thyroid disease.

So the primary questions remain: Is it possible to translate oral tolerance as a therapy for autoimmune and inflammatory conditions to humans? And if so, what is required? The answer is likely to be multifold, starting from the dose of antigen, the background genes, the nature of the antigen, the requirement for an effective mucosal adjuvant, and the timing. Even in murine models, oral ingestion of antigen is more effective in preventing disease than in ameliorating established disease or modifying an ongoing immune response. This suggests that oral tolerance may be most effective as a preventative therapy or following a course of global immunotherapy or immunosuppression.

The goal of this second conference on oral tolerance was to synthesize the large number of advances that have been made in understanding mechanisms of oral tolerance in animal models over the past decade and to help determine what is required to successfully bring oral tolerance to the treatment of human disease.

—LLOYD MAYER

Immunobiology Center
The Mount Sinai Medical Center
New York, New York

Oral Tolerance: Overview and Historical Perspectives

ALLAN McI. MOWAT, LUCY A. PARKER, HELEN BEACOCK-SHARP, OWAIN R. MILLINGTON, AND FERNANDO CHIRDO

Department of Immunology and Bacteriology, University of Glasgow, Western Infirmary, Glasgow, Scotland

ABSTRACT: Oral tolerance was first detailed almost 100 years ago, and since then, it has been shown repeatedly that feeding a wide variety of nonpathogenic antigens can inhibit subsequent systemic immune responses. All systemic immune responses are susceptible, but the degree and scope of the suppression depends on the nature and dose of the fed antigen. Oral tolerance has been described in most mammals, including humans, and it may be the homeostatic mechanism that prevents hypersensitivity to food antigens, as is found in celiac disease. A similar process may prevent the aberrant immune responses to commensal bacteria that occur in inflammatory bowel disease. The ability of oral tolerance to modulate experimental models of autoimmune and inflammatory disease has led to clinical trials in such diseases as rheumatoid arthritis, multiple sclerosis, and type I diabetes, with only variable success. Despite intense research, the exact mechanisms responsible for the systemic tolerance and the reasons why tolerance is the default response to many fed antigens remain controversial. Early studies suggested that CD8+ "suppressor" T cells were important, but it is now accepted that it may involve either anergy/deletion of CD4+ T cells, or the induction of regulatory CD4+ T cells that produce IL-10 and/or TGFβ. There may also be a role for CD4+ CD25+ T_{reg}, but how and when all these different mechanisms operate is still unclear. The ability of fed antigens to induce tolerance probably reflects their uptake by "quiescent" antigen-presenting cells in the intestine, with presentation to specific CD4+ T cells in the absence of costimulation, or with the involvement of inhibitory costimulatory molecules. Dendritic cells in the Peyer's patches or mucosal lamina propria are the most likely APCs involved, but it remains to be determined exactly where these interactions occur and what the precise nature of the relevant dendritic cells is.

KEYWORDS: systemic immune response; celiac disease; Crohn's disease; experimental autoimmune encephalomyelitis; antigen-presenting cells; intestine

Oral tolerance is the oldest recognized model of peripheral tolerance, having been first referred to in a study of anaphylactic sensitization to milk proteins by Besredka in 1909[1] and then studied extensively by Wells and Osborne in 1911.[2] It also has the

Address for correspondence: Allan McI. Mowat, Department of Immunology and Bacteriology, University of Glasgow, Western Infirmary, Glasgow, Scotland. Voice: +44-141-2112728; fax: +44-141-3373217.
a.m.mowat@clinmed.gla.ac.uk

distinction of being one of the few experimental systems of this kind with genuine physiological relevance, as it is clear that the normal intestinal immune system maintains a state of unresponsiveness to dietary proteins throughout adult life. A breakdown in this process is believed to underlie such diseases as celiac disease, in which aberrant $CD4^+$ T lymphocyte responses to gliadin peptides in wheat produce small intestinal damage in genetically susceptible individuals.[3] Although never proven formally, it is commonly believed that similar regulatory mechanisms exist toward the commensal bacterial flora of the large intestine, preventing the hypersensitivity reactions that can cause inflammatory bowel diseases such as Crohn's disease.[4] Although it was interest in these crucial physiological processes that provoked early studies in the field, much recent work has been driven by the possibility that oral tolerance could be exploited for administering therapy against inflammatory and autoimmune diseases.[5] Initially tried in experimental models of experimental autoimmune encephalomyelitis (EAE) and experimental arthritides, oral tolerance has been applied to a wide variety of experimental diseases, including type I diabetes, thyroiditis, uveitis, and, most recently, atherosclerosis and cerebrovascular stroke. There have also been clinical trials in rheumatoid arthritis, diabetes, and multiple sclerosis, and other papers in this volume will discuss the clinical applications of oral tolerance in more depth. Finally, the fact that orally administered antigens induce immunological tolerance so readily is an important theoretical and practical obstacle to the development of new generation mucosal vaccines containing recombinant proteins.

Oral tolerance has been described in most monogastric mammals, including humans (for review see Ref. 4). However only limited studies have been conducted in humans, and the relative lack of success in the clinical trials has led to continuing debate as to the potency of the phenomenon in humans. Given the rarity of clinical food hypersensitivities and the substantial evidence that food antigens are recognized by the human immune system, it seems most likely that oral tolerance does indeed occur in humans, and more work should be performed to study its basis and effects in human subjects. A vast range of antigens has been shown to induce tolerance when given by the oral route, although most of these share the property of being inert and/or soluble thymus-dependent antigens, such as proteins. Conversely, particulate materials, invasive pathogens, and inflammatory agents, such as toxins prime the local and systemic immune system to generate productive immunity. Virtually all aspects of systemic immune responses can be suppressed by feeding antigen, although there are differences in susceptibility between different effector components. In general, T cell–mediated responses such as delayed-type hypersensitivity and tissue immunopathology are exquisitely sensitive to even low doses of antigen, while antibody production is less easily inhibitible.[4] Although this has sometimes been used to support the idea that there is a Th1 versus Th2 dichotomy in oral tolerance, it is important to point out that IgE production is usually extremely easy to suppress by feeding antigen, indicating that the regulatory processes in tolerance are distinct from simple crosstalk between the two major subsets of $CD4^+$ T cell. Together with the fact that it is also possible to tolerize $CD8^+$ T cell–mediated cytotoxic T cell (CTL) responses, it is tempting to conclude that these findings support the idea that oral tolerance has evolved mainly to prevent immune effector responses that are potentially harmful to the intestine. An area of continuing controversy has been the status of local IgA responses in oral tolerance, and it is still not clear whether these are also suppressed, or if feeding antigen actually primes the production of local antibody production.

Despite its profound effects on systemic immunity and its practical importance, several decades of research have left the mechanisms responsible for oral tolerance unclear. During the first phase of intense immunological interest in the 1970s and 1980s, oral tolerance was held to be an example of the action of $CD8^+$ suppressor T cells.[6] As these T cells went out of favor, evidence began to accumulate that the "regulatory" T cell involved was a subset of the $CD4^+$ T cell, and a number of candidates have been proposed. These include Th3 cells, which produce transforming growth factor β (TGF-β) and/or interleukin 10 (IL-10);[7] and Trl cells, which produce mainly IL-10[8] and $CD4^+CD25^+$ T cells, whose mode of action is obscure, but could involve cytokine secretion, surface expression of cytokines, or other cell contact–dependent mechanisms such as CTLA-4.[9–12] No clear consensus has been reached about the overall contribution of each of these, and it is important to point out that they have generally been identified using very different *in vivo* or *in vitro* approaches. It is possible that there is indeed a wide range of different regulatory mechanisms that may either be important under different circumstances, or that together are needed to ensure the lack of systemic response. However, more information on the nature of the regulatory T cells and the conditions under which they are induced is needed.

Work during the 1980s and 1990s led to the idea that the mechanism responsible for oral tolerance depended on the feeding regime used to induce tolerance.[13,14] Single high doses of antigen were considered to cause clonal anergy (or deletion) of antigen-specific T cells, whereas repeated feeds of low doses of antigen appeared to induce regulatory T cell activity. This idea provided a useful theoretical basis for exploring the phenomenon and was also of potential practical use in designing clinical therapies, as most of these rely on the activity of regulatory T cells, which can suppress T cells of other specificities in a "bystander" manner.[14] However, the reasons underlying the apparently distinctive effects of the different feeding regimes have never been established, and it is now clear from other systems that there may be no clear distinction between anergy and regulatory activity in T lymphocytes. In particular, the earlier work on oral tolerance needs to be interpreted in the light of the evidence that T cells previously considered "anergic" are capable of secreting inhibitory cytokines and suppressing other lymphocytes.[15]

A further major question that remains unanswered is how the intestinal immune system can discriminate between harmless and invasive antigens. In common with other parts of the immune system, the status of antigen-presenting cells (APCs) seems to determine whether an antigen induces tolerance or productive immunity. APCs could play several roles in the regulation of mucosal immunity and tolerance. First, the activation status or lineage of the APCs may be important, by virtue of the fact that the levels of expression of costimulatory molecules and immunomodulatory cytokines are controlled by the presence of "danger signals," such as pathogen-associated molecules and proinflammatory cytokines.[16] CD28-mediated recognition of the upregulated levels of B7.I (CD80) and B7.2 (CD86) on activated APCs favors productive priming of T cells, whereas CTLA 4–mediated recognition of lower levels of B7.I/B7.2 on resting APCs appears to induce tolerance selectively. The recently discovered receptor-ligand pairs PD-1 and PDL-l/2 seem to play similar inhibitory roles in T cell activation.[17] Second, APCs are central to the induction and expression of regulatory T cell activity, as the balance between the production of IL-

12 and IL-10 production by APCs determines the differentiation of naive T cells after the initial contact with antigen.[18] Several pieces of evidence also indicate that APCs may be the principal target of regulatory T cell activity, transducing their effects to naive T cells.[19] Finally, the anatomical source of the APCs also controls the subsequent anatomical redistribution of the T cell, with dendritic cells (DCs) derived from Peyer's patches (PPs) and mesenteric lymph nodes (MLN) having a selective ability to induce the expression of the $\alpha_4\beta_7$ integrin and CCR9 chemokine receptor required for the localization of activated T cells into the small intestinal mucosa.[20–22]

In older work, we found that agents that produce generalized activation of APCs *in vivo* prevented the induction of tolerance by feeding ovalbumin (OVA) to mice,[6,23] but the cellular basis of these effects were not determined. More recently, evidence has accumulated that local DCs are the key players in these decision-making processes in the intestinal immune system. The intestine and its lymphoid organs contain large numbers of DCs, including a number of unique subsets,[24,25] and expansion of DC numbers in mice using the cytokine flt3 ligand (flt3L) markedly increases their susceptibility to the induction of oral tolerance.[26,27]

The location of the DCs involved in taking up soluble antigens from the intestine and inducing tolerance is currently a matter of debate. Conventional opinion is that M cells in the follicle-associated epithelium (FAE) of PPs are the principal route for the uptake of antigens from the intestine,[28] and there are large numbers of DCs in the PPs, including in the region immediately under the FAE. Accumulating evidence also suggests that PP DCs comprise several distinct subsets, including some that produce IL-10 rather than IL-12 and polarize naive T cells to a Th2 or regulatory phenotype.[25,29,30] DCs in PPs are therefore attractive candidates as tolerogenic APCs in determining the outcome of oral administration of antigens. However, work on mice lacking PPs due to genetic knockouts or treatment with a blocking form of the lymphotoxin β receptor (LTβR) has produced conflicting findings on whether PPs are essential for the induction of oral tolerance.[31] Therefore it is possible that the critical site of antigen handling is in other tissues, such as the villus LP, MLN, or peripheral lymphoid organs.

In recent experiments, we have attempted to follow up our findings that the lamina propria (LP) appeared to show one of the largest proportional expansions in DC numbers after treatment with flt3L and have explored the contribution of LP DCs to the uptake of protein antigens in the intestine. After feeding mice OVA, antigen-loaded APCs can be isolated from the LP within 15 minutes of feeding, with high levels of APC activity being detectable in this tissue at 1 hour, before declining and being almost completely absent by 20 hours. A similar time course of antigen loading was found in PPs and MLN, but the levels of APC activity in these tissues are of a much lower magnitude than in LP, even when the numbers of DCs in the different tissues are corrected for. This uptake into LP was much larger in flt3L-treated mice than in normal animals, suggesting that DCs were responsible. Subsequent studies confirmed this idea, as DCs purified from the LP of antigen-fed mice could present the antigen to $CD4^+$ T cells *in vitro* and *in vivo*. A number of distinct subsets of DCs are present in the LP. Although the majority are CDIIb$^+$ CD8α^-, similar to those found in other peripheral tissues, there are also small numbers of CDIIb$^-$ CD8α^+ DCs and a population of CDIIb$^-$ CD8α^+ similar to that found in the subepithelial compartment of PP DCs.[25] In addition, we consistently found significant numbers of $CD11c^{lo}$ class II MHC^{lo} DCs, some of which are $B220^+$ $Ly6C/G^+$, and which together are reminiscent of the recently described populations of regulatory DCs that may be tolerogenic in other murine models.[32–34] Consistent with this evidence that LP DCs may be important in oral tolerance, *in vivo* loaded LP DCs appear to induce antigen-specific tolerance when transferred into naive recipients. In parallel, LP DCs constitutively produce immunoregulatory cytokines, such as IL-10 and type 1 IFN, rather than proinflammatory mediators, such as IL-12. DCs from other tissues do not share these properties, and for these reasons, we believe LP DCs may be the principal APCs involved in ensuring that tolerance is the default response to orally administered protein antigens.

Together with other recent findings of regulatory DCs in mucosal tissues, such as the lung, MLN, and PPs,[35–38] these data suggest that the local microenvironment of the intestine has a specialized conditioning effect that polarizes DC maturation toward a "quiescent" or tolerogenic phenotype. This may reflect the physiological presence of immunomodulatory mediators, such as IL-10, TGF–β, or PGE_2, or the effects of products of intestinal bacteria that interact with toll-like receptors or other surface receptors, as has been described for certain pathogen-associated molecules, such as filamentous hemagglutinin from *Bordetella pertussis*.[40] Importantly, the phenotype of intestinal DCs is not fixed, as agents such as adjuvants or inflammatory cytokines, which can activate DCs *in vivo* can prevent the induction of oral tolerance, even when DC numbers have been expanded with flt3L.[27]

Despite the fact that LP DCs may play the central role in the induction of oral tolerance, it seems unlikely that the initial interaction between these APCs and $CD4^+$ T cells occurs in the mucosa itself. Naive $CD4^+$ T cells are rare in the LP, and T cells that encounter antigen here would not be able to mediate the systemic effects of tolerance. Therefore, it is more likely that antigen-loaded DCs migrate from the intestinal mucosa to meet naive $CD4^+$ T cells in the MLN. This would not only be consistent with disappearance of antigen-loaded APCs from the mucosa of antigen-fed mice, but also with the absolute requirement for intact MLN in the induction of oral tolerance and with other evidence for regulatory DCs in the MLN.[31] In addition, all studies using the adoptive transfer of antigen-specific TcR transgenic T cells have shown recognition of antigen in the MLN within a few hours of feeding tolerogenic doses of antigen.[31] Of course it also remains feasible that antigen itself may gain access to the MLN in the draining lymph.

One further route that should not be forgotten in considering the ways in which fed antigen can induce systemic tolerance is by the dissemination of antigen from the intestine to peripheral lymphoid organs via the bloodstream. We showed many years ago that antigenic protein was present in the blood one to two hours after feeding OVA to mice, and dietary proteins can be detected in the circulation of normal humans.[4,41] More recent work has shown the presence of antigen-loaded APCs in the spleen of protein-fed mice, presumably resulting from blood-borne spread,[42] and in mice, the material in serum induces specific tolerance when transferred into naive recipients.[43] Uptake of this material by quiescent DCs in peripheral lymphoid tissues could account for at least part of the systemic consequences of oral tolerance, particularly when high doses of antigen are administered.

Currently, there is no unifying hypothesis that can explain the apparent association between feeding regime and the induction of distinctive regulatory mechanisms in oral tolerance. If the preferential activation of regulatory T cells by low doses of antigen can be confirmed at the cellular level, it is tempting to speculate that this may reflect presentation of antigen that has been taken up only by DCs that have been conditioned by the specialized microenvironment of the mucosa to drive T cell differentiation toward a regulatory phenotype. According to this idea, low doses of soluble antigens will be taken up across the epithelium of PPs or the villus, before gaining access to quiescent, IL-10–producing DCs in the immediate vicinity. As we have discussed, in the LP this will result in emigration of the DCs to meet naive $CD4^+$ T cells in the MLN. In the PPs, the lack of danger signals will mean that the DCs are not stimulated to enter the thymus-dependent area (TDA), and any presentation to $CD4^+$ T cells will occur outside the TDA of the PPs, or after migration of the quiescent APCs to the MLN. One might predict that these conditions may also allow the induction of local IgA antibody production. On the other hand, high doses of soluble antigen may induce tolerance associated with widespread "anergy" of T cells, because they gain access not only to the DCs in the subepithelial compartments of the mucosa and PPs, but also to resting APCs in the TDA of the PPs, MLN, and peripheral lymphoid tissues. Presentation in these more distal sites may be relatively protected from the unique conditioning effects of the mucosa and so may occur under more "neutral" conditions, resulting in inactivation of antigen-specific T cells without acquisition of regulatory properties. It would be anticipated that local IgA production might also be inhibited as part of this global suppression. These ideas can be tested by exploring the sites of antigen uptake in the gut, the nature of the APCs involved, and the anatomical basis of the resulting interactions with T cells. It will also be important to clarify the costimulatory molecules involved in determining the induction of mucosal immunity and tolerance, as the existing work in the field does not give a clear idea of whether these processes require distinct events, or if these can be manipulated to tailor the response resulting from different regimes of feeding antigens.

REFERENCES

1. BESREDKA, A.M. 1909. De L'Anaphylaxie. Sixieme memoire de l'anaphylaxie lactique. Ann. Institute Pasteur **23:** 166.
2. WELLS, H.G. & T.B. OSBORNE. 1911. The biological reactions of the vegetable proteins. I. Anaphylaxis. J. Infect Dis. **8:** 66.
3. SOLLID, L.M. 2002. Coeliac disease: dissecting a complex inflammatory disorder. Nat. Rev. Immunol. **2:** 647.
4. MOWAT, A.M. & H.L. WEINER. 1999. Oral tolerance: basic mechanisms and clinical implications. *In* Mucosal Immunology, 2nd edit. P.L. Ogra, J. Mestecky, M.E. Lamm, W. Strober, J.R. McGhee & J. Bienenstock, Eds.: p. 587. Academic Press. San Diego.
5. FARIA, A.M.C. & H.L. WEINER. 1999. Oral tolerance: mechanisms and therapeutic applications. Adv. Immunol. **73:** 153.
6. MOWAT, A.M. 1987. The regulation of immune responses to dietary protein antigens. Immunol. Today **8:** 93.
7. WEINER, H.L. 2001. Induction and mechanism of action of transforming growth factor-β-secreting Th3 regulatory cells. Immunol. Rev. **182:** 207.
8. GROUX, H., A. O'GARRA, M. BIGLER, *et al.* 1997. A $CD4^+$ T-cell subset inhibits antigen-specific T-cell responses and prevents colitis. Nature **389:** 737.
9. THORSTENSON, K.M. & A. KHORUTS. 2001. Generation of anergic and potentially immunoregulatory $CD25^+CD4^+$ T cells *in vivo* after induction of peripheral tolerance with intravenous or oral antigen. J. Immunol. **167:** 188.
10. NAKAMURA, K., A. KITANI & W. STROBER. 2001. Cell contact-dependent immunosuppression by CD4(+)CD25(+) regulatory T cells is mediated by cell surface bound transforming growth factor β. J. Exp. Med. **194:** 629.

11. ZHANG, X., L. LZIKSON, L. UU & H.L. WEINER. 2001. Activation of CD25+CD4+ regulatory T cells by oral antigen administration. J. Immunol. **167:** 4245.
12. FOWLER, S. & F. POWRIE. 2002. CTLA-4 expression on antigen-specific cells but not IL-10 secretion is required for oral tolerance. Eur. J. Immunol. **32:** 2997.
13. WHITACRE, C.C., I.E. GIENAPP, C.G. OROSZ & D.M. BITAR. 1991. Oral tolerance in experimental autoimmune encephalitis. lII. Evidence for clonal anergy. J. Immunol. **147:** 2155.
14. WEINER, H.L., A. FRIEDMAN, A. MILLER, et al. 1994. Oral tolerance: immunologic mechanisms and treatment of animal and human organ-specific autoimmune diseases by oral administration of autoantigens. Annu. Rev. Immunol. **12:** 809.
15. SCHWARTZ, R.H. 2003. T cell anergy. Annu. Rev. Immunol. **21:** 305.
16. MEDZHITOV, R. & C. JANEWAY. 2000. Innate immune recognition: mechanisms and pathways. Immunol. Rev. **173:** 89.
17. SHARPE, A.H. & G.J. FREEMAN. 2002. The B7-CD28 superfamily. Nat. Rev. Immunol. **2:** 116.
18. GUERMONPREZ, P., J. VALLADEAU, L. ZITVOGEL, et al. 2002. Antigen presentation and T cell stimulation by dendritic cells. Annu. Rev. Immunol. **20:** 621.
19. VENDETTI, S., J.G. CHAI, J. DYSON, et al. 2000. Anergic T cells inhibit the antigen-presenting function of dendritic cells. J. Immunol. **165:** 1175.
20. STAGG, A.J., M.A. KAMM & S.C. KNIGHT. 2002. Intestinal dendritic cells increase T cell expression of $\alpha 4\beta 7$ integrin. Eur. J. Immunol. **32:** 1445.
21. JOHANSSON-LINDBOM, B., M. SVENSSON, M.A. WURBEL, et al. 2003. Selective generation of gut tropic T cells in gut-associated lymphoid tissue (GALT): requirement for GALT dendritic cells and adjuvant. J. Exp. Med. **198:** 963.
22. MORA, J.R., M.R. BONO, N. MANJUNATH, et al. 2003. Selective imprinting of gut-homing T cells by Peyer's patch dendritic cells. Nature **424:** 88.
23. STROBEL, C., A.M. MOWAT & A. FERGUSON. 1985. Prevention of oral tolerance induction to ovalbumin and enhanced antigen presentation during a graft-versus-host reaction in mice. Immunology **56:** 57.
24. MOWAT, A.M. & J.L. VINEY. 1997. The anatomical basis of mucosal immune responses. Immunol. Rev. **156:** 145.
25. IWASAKI, A. & B.L. KELSALL. 2001. Unique functions of CDllb+, CD8α+ and double negative Peyer's patch dendritic cells. J. Immunol. **166:** 4884.
26. VINEY, I.L., A.M. MOWAT, I.M. O'MALLEY, et al. 1998. Expanding dendritic cells *in vivo* enhances the induction of oral tolerance. J. Immunol. **160:** 5815.
27. WILLIAMSON, E., G.M. WESTRICH & I.L. VINEY. 1999. Modulating dendritic cells to optimize mucosal immunization protocols. J. Immunol. **163:** 3668.
28. NEUTRA, M.R., A. FREY & I.-P. KRAEHENBUHL. 1996. Epithelial M cells: gateways for mucosal infection and immunisation. Cell **86:** 345.
29. IWASAKI, A. & B.L. KELSALL. 1999. Freshly isolated Peyer's patch, but not spleen, dendritic cells produce interleukin 10 and induce the differentiation of T helper type 2 cells. J. Exp. Med. **190:** 229.
30. IWASAKI, A. & B.L. KELSALL. 2000. Localization of distinct Peyer's patch dendritic cell subsets and their recruitment by chemokines macrophage inflammatory protein (MIP)-3a, MIP-3β, and secondary lymphoid organ chemokine. J. Exp. Med. **191:** 1381.
31. MOWAT, A.M. 2003. Anatomical basis of tolerance and immunity to intestinal antigens. Nat. Rev. Immunol. **3:** 331.
32. MARTIN, P., G.M. DEL HOYO, F. ANJUERE, et al. 2002. Characterization of a new subpopulation of mouse CD8α+ B220+ dendritic cells endowed with type 1 interferon production capacity and tolerogenic potential. Blood **100:** 383.
33. STEINMAN, R.M., D. HAWIGER & M.C. NUSSENZWEIG. 2003. Tolerogenic dendritic cells. Annu. Rev. Immunol. **21:** 685.
34. WAKKACH, A., N. FOURNIER, V. BRUN, et al. 2003. Characterization of dendritic cells that induce tolerance and T regulatory 1 cell differentiation in vivo. Immunity **18:** 605.
35. STUMBLES, P.A., I.A. THOMAS, C.L. PIMM, et al. 1998. Resting respiratory tract dendritic cells preferentially stimulate helper cell type 2 (Th2) responses and require obligatory cytokine signals for induction of Th 1 immunity. J Exp. Med. **188:** 2019.
36. ALPAN, O., G. RUDOMEN & P. MATZINGER. 2001. The role of dendritic cells, B cells and M cells in gut-oriented immune responses. J. Immunol. **166:** 4843.

37. AKBARI, O., R.H. DEKRUYFF & D.T. UMETSU. 2001. Pulmonary dendritic cells producing IL-10 mediate tolerance induced by respiratory exposure to antigen. Nat. Immunol. **2:** 725.
38. BILSBOROUGH, J., T.C. GEORGE, A. NORMENT & J.L. VINEY. 2003. Mucosal CD8α+ DC, with a plasmacytoid phenotype, induce differentiation and support function of T cells with regulatory properties. Immunology **108:** 481.
39. KALINSKI, P., C.M.U. HILKENS, E.A. WIERENGA & M.L. KAPSENBERG. 1999. T-cell priming by type-1 and type-2 polarized dendritic cells: the concept of a third signal. Immunol. Today **20:** 561–567.
40. MCGUIRK, P., C. MCCANN & K.H. MILLS. 2002. Pathogen-specific T regulatory 1 cells induced in the respiratory tract by a bacterial molecule that stimulates interleukin 10 production by dendritic cells: a novel strategy for evasion of protective T helper type 1 responses by *Bordetella pertussis*. J. Exp. Med. **195:** 221.
41. STROBEL, S., A.M. MOWAT, H.E. DRUMMOND, *et al.* 1983. Immunological responses to fed protein antigens in mice. 2. Oral tolerance for CMI is due to activation of cyclophosphamide sensitive cells by gut processed antigen. Immunology **49:** 451.
42. GÜTGEMANN, I., A.M. FAHRER, M.M. DAVIS & Y-H. CHIEN. 1998. Induction of rapid T cell activation and tolerance by systemic presentation of an orally administered antigen. Immunity **8:** 667.
43. STROBEL, S. & A.M. MOWAT. 1998. Immune responses to dietary antigens: oral tolerance. Immunol. Today **19:** 173.

The Anatomy of Mucosal Immune Responses

PAUL GARSIDE, OWAIN MILLINGTON, AND KAREN M. SMITH

Division of Immunology, Infection, and Inflammation,
University of Glasgow, Glasgow, G11 6NT, United Kingdom

ABSTRACT: It remains unclear how and where unresponsiveness to fed antigens is induced. This "oral tolerance" is probably necessary to prevent the array of immune effector mechanisms required to counteract pathogens of the mucosae from being misdirected against food antigens or commensal flora. It will obviously be important to dissect where, when, and how such immunological homeostasis is maintained in the gut, but it will also be necessary to determine whether similar inductive and effector mechanisms are required for the therapeutic applications of oral tolerance systemically. This may be influenced by anatomical and microenvironmental effects on the phenotype and/or activation state of the antigen-presenting cell (APC), which presents orally delivered antigen. Fed antigen passes from the intestinal lumen either via the villus epithelium and M cells in the Peyer's patches (PP) or the mucosal lamina propria to the organized lymphoid tissues of the PP and mesenteric lymph nodes (MLN). In addition, there is evidence that mucosally administered antigen also gains access directly to peripheral lymphoid organs. Each of these sites contains distinctive populations of APCs and has unique local microenvironments that may influence the immune response in different ways. We propose that feeding antigen in high doses may induce clonal anergy, deletion, or altered differentiation because it gains direct access to resting APCs in the T cell areas of both the gut-associated lymphoid tissues (GALT) and peripheral lymphoid organs, with presentation occurring in the absence of productive costimulation. By contrast, low doses of tolerizing antigen may be taken up and presented preferentially by APCs in the GALT, where the local environment may favor the induction of regulatory T cells. This is consistent with our own and others findings, using adoptive transfer of TcR tg T cells. These studies have shown that antigen-specific CD4[+] T cells are activated simultaneously in all peripheral and gut-associated lymphoid organs after feeding high doses of proteins, but that this may be more restricted to local tissues when lower doses are used. Another level of anatomical control is imposed within lymphoid organs, where migration of T cells through distinct anatomical compartments can affect their differentiation. We find that, in contrast to orally primed T cells, orally tolerized T cells are unable to migrate into B cell follicles during their initial exposure to antigen. This affects their differentiation as upon subsequent challenge with antigen in adjuvant, tolerized T cells can be found in follicles but are unable to provide the B cell help that primed T cells can deliver. We hypothesize that the initial defective migration of tolerized T cells prevents them from receiving signals from antigen-specific B cells in follicles and results in abortive

Address for correspondence: Paul Garside, Division of Immunology, Infection and Inflammation, University of Glasgow, Glasgow, G11 6NT, United Kingdom. Voice: +44-141-211-2153; fax: +44-141-337-3217.
 p.garside@clinmed.gla.ac.uk

differentiation. Thus, both gross and fine anatomical location of fed antigen presentation may be important in mucosal immunoregulation.

KEYWORDS: anatomy; mucosa; tolerance; T cells; B cells; migration

GROSS ANATOMICAL LOCATION OF ANTIGEN PRESENTATION

The sites of oral priming and tolerance induction and the antigen-presenting cell (APC) involved remain unclear, but their identification will have important implications for the design of oral vaccines and if oral tolerance is to be used therapeutically. It has been proposed that fed antigen stimulates T cells in the gut-associated lymphoid tissues (GALT), which subsequently disseminate to the periphery.[1-4] However, T cells activated in the GALT preferentially home back to mucosal sites,[5-7] and it is therefore difficult to envisage how this could lead to systemic priming or tolerance. Fed antigen may also reach the periphery directly, and antigen can be detected in the blood very soon after feeding.[8] Antigen-laden APCs could also migrate from the GALT to the periphery, and dendritic cells (DC) carrying ovalbumin (OVA) have been detected in lymph after feeding.[9] To address some of these issues a number of groups have studied the activation of adoptively transferred TcR tg T cells[10] as a readout of where antigen is presented.

It is well established that feeding OVA alone induces systemic tolerance in adoptively transferred mice, as demonstrated by a reduction in a range of immune responses upon challenge, whereas feeding OVA with a mucosal adjuvant such as cholera toxin (CT) results in systemic priming.[11] Examination of the phenotypic and functional consequences of these contrasting immunological states at the single cell level by FACS analysis of TcR tg T cells has revealed increased numbers of primed and tolerized T cells both locally and systemically after feeding antigen.[12] Further studies with CFSE-labeled tg T cells showed that they divided locally and systemically as early as two days after feeding antigen, with or without adjuvant.[12] As no lag in division was seen between local and systemic tissues, this suggested that T cells recognize antigen and are induced to divide in both sites simultaneously. Interestingly, in some situations tolerized T cells divided significantly less than primed cells.[12]

To more definitively characterize where a T cell first encounters fed antigen, a number of groups have analyzed the expression of the early activation marker CD69 on tg T cells.[1-4,12,13] Though there are some contrasts in the published work, we found that T cells were activated, both systemically and locally, within six hours of feeding OVA or OVA/CT. CD69 has previously been shown to be upregulated on T cells three to six hours after feeding OVA.[3] Given that the time required for T cells to express CD69 is two to three hours,[14] the possibility that T cells and/or APCs migrate from the gut to peripheral sites is unlikely. Thus, it seems probable that fed antigen can be distributed throughout the body and cause T cell activation locally and systemically. More recently, we have confirmed these findings with anti-peptide-MHC antibodies, which showed orally administered antigen being presented in peripheral lymphoid organs within hours of feeding.[15]

Similar findings to those described above were obtained with a range of doses of antigen.[12] Interestingly, acquisition of a CD45RB^{lo} phenotype appeared to be dose dependent, with fewer tg cells in the peripheral lymph nodes (PLNs) downregulating CD45RB as the dose of antigen fed was decreased.[12] This suggests that after feeding higher doses, more antigen is presented in the PLN, which causes T cells to acquire different phenotypic characteristics. Whether the tolerizing antigen dose affects the functional characteristics of T cells differently in the GALT versus the periphery remains to be determined.

Thus, we have shown that after oral exposure to immunogenic or tolerogenic antigen, T cell activation, division, and expansion occurs simultaneously locally and systemically, suggesting that fed antigen is presented throughout the animal during priming and tolerance induction. Though these studies have indicated the location and kinetics of antigen presentation, they do not provide any direct evidence of the phenotype or activation state of the APCs involved. Progress in this area has been made with immunohistochemical analysis[16] and purification of APC populations.[17] However, these approaches have their limitations and definitive identification and characterization of the APCs involved in oral tolerance and priming will require *in situ* analysis of MHC-peptide expressing APCs using techniques such as laser scanning cytometry[18] and multiphoton microscopy.[19]

DEFECTIVE MIGRATION OF TOLERIZED T CELLS

These studies of the location of antigen presentation in oral tolerance and priming highlighted the requirement to assess the functional consequences of this directly *in vivo*. The mechanisms of oral tolerance of T and B cells are unknown. However, it is widely believed that the B cell unresponsiveness induced occurs because of a lack of T cell help and that the B cell remains potentially active. We therefore cotransferred TcR tg T cells and BcR tg B cells.

Our studies[11] showed that orally primed and tolerized T cells displayed similar abilities to clonally expand in response to challenge. Despite this similar clonal expansion, orally tolerized T cells were unable to support B cell responses adequately. Initially, by contrast, naive T cells, or those previously primed with antigen and adjuvant, showed no impairment in their ability to support B cell clonal expansion and antibody production. The B cell response was also directly visualized *in vivo*. Again, it was noted that tg B cell numbers increase in PLNs after challenge of both naive and primed groups. However, there was very little increase in tg B cells in tolerized groups following challenge. Thus, previously naive and primed T cells are capable of providing help for B cell clonal expansion and antibody production, but tolerized T cells are unable to provide such help, supporting the hypothesis that the B cell unresponsiveness observed after feeding results from a defect in tolerized tg T cells to provide cognate help for B cells.

A possible explanation for the defective capacity of orally tolerized T cells to provide B cell help may lie in their relative ability to migrate to B cell follicles. Previous studies have shown that during primary immune responses T cells proliferate in T cell areas, then move toward B cell follicles to help B cells.[10,20–22] Antigen-specfic T and B cells then meet at the border between the T and B cell areas.[20,23,24] The antigen-specific T cells are then well placed to provide cognate help for B cells that subsequently clonally expand and produce antibody.[20] However, previous studies have indicated that TcR tg T cells tolerized by intravenous (i.v.) administration of antigen are unable to undergo follicular migration.[10] Following oral or systemic priming we observed significant numbers of TcR tg T cells in follicular regions of local and PLNs, but such localization was not apparent following the induction of oral tolerance.[11] However, following systemic challenge with antigen in adjuvant tolerized as well as primed, T cells were apparent in B cell follicles.[11] This suggests that tolerized T cells display an initial defect in migration that is overcome by subsequent challenge, and that the effects of orally administered antigen are apparent systemically in both situations.

The migration of T cells is controlled by chemokines. Naive T cells are held in the paracortex, as they express the chemokine receptor CCR7, the ligands of which, SLC and ELC, are produced by stromal cells in the T cell area.[25] The CXCR5 chemokine receptor is expressed by antigen-specific T cells after exposure to antigen plus adjuvant but not antigen alone.[26] The ligand for CXCR5, BLC, is produced by follicular stromal cells[25] and may be responsible for recruiting antigen-stimulated T cells to B cell areas. Interestingly, signals through CD28 and OX40 are required for CXCR5 induction on T cells and subsequent migration to follicles. Furthermore, the ligands for CD28 and OX40 (B7 and OX40L) are induced on DC by inflammation.[27] These findings may explain why tolerized T cells do not migrate into B cell follicles during primary immune responses (as no inflammation is present), whereas following challenge, tolerized T cells acquire the ability to enter B cell follicles, as a consequence of acquiring CXCR5 expression after interaction with adjuvant activated DC. However, despite being able to migrate into B cell follicles, tolerized T cells remain unable to support fulminant B cell clonal expansion and antibody production. The defect in tolerized T cells remains unclear but may lie in defective and/or differential chemokine and/or chemokine receptor expression or disruption of chemokine responsiveness. In the latter case it is possible that nonsignaling or secreted chemokine receptors could modify lymphocyte migration.[28] Alternatively, tolerized T cells could preferentially express molecules that cleave chemokines, as has been described for anergic human T cells.[29]

POTENTIAL CONSEQUENCES OF DEFECTIVE MIGRATION OF TOLERIZED T CELLS

The consequences of the failed migration of tolerized T cells for B cell responses is clear, but there may also be a price to pay for the T cells themselves. A number of studies have demonstrated that normal secondary lymphoid architecture and migration within it are essential for the development of immune responses.[10–12,20,30–37] However, exactly how these responses are influenced by anatomy and migration remains unclear. This is particularly true in the case of T cells, where, for example, whether follicular homing is a cause or effect of immunological priming has not been determined. As the activation status of T cells (e.g., tolerized versus primed) may influence their follicular homing[10,11] and their functional capacity[11] and that this may be related to their division history,[38] the location of T cells could regulate the interactions they undergo, which could, in turn, determine the number of divisions they make and hence their differentiation and functional status.

As noted above the activated T and B lymphocytes migrate toward each other, facilitating a cognate interaction, which ultimately leads to the formation of a germinal center.[39,40] Throughout this process, antigen-specific T cells provide important signals for the survival and differentiation of the hypermutating B cells. The importance of these interactions for the B cell and germinal center response is clear, but it is less apparent if there is any benefit for the T cell. Several of the costimulatory molecules expressed by activated antigen-specific B cells (see below) could influence T cell survival and differentiation, and we propose that T cells require passage through a B cell follicle to undergo maximal clonal expansion, terminal differentiation, and acquire effector and memory function. Without this, they may default to a tolerant phenotype. Thus by somehow modulating follicular migration of T cells, antigen fed in a tolerogenic form promotes an alternative differentiation down an anergic or regulatory pathway.

A similar conclusion was reached from the earliest studies using adoptive transfer of TcR tg T cells, which showed that immunological priming was associated with clonal expansion of T cells in the paracortex and subsequent migration into B cell follicles.[10] By contrast, the induction of T cell tolerance by i.v. administration of antigen resulted in a failure of this migration.[10] As discussed above, our recent studies of oral tolerance using the same adoptive transfer system have revealed a similar pattern, with a failure or orally tolerized T cells to migrate into B cell follicles after the initial antigen feed.[11] Although these orally tolerized T cells can migrate into B cell follicles upon subsequent challenge with antigen in adjuvant, they are unable to provide B cell help.[11] We propose that this may be because of their failure to enter B cell follicles after their first exposure to antigen. Importantly, whether the lack of memory T cell responses found in B cell depleted mice is also associated with the induction of antigen-specific tolerance remains unclear.

We therefore hypothesize that because the fate and differentiation of T cells are dependent upon the number of divisions they make and that this also correlates with whether the T cells migrate into a B cell follicle, these two functions may be causally related. We propose that T cells require passage through a B cell follicle and that the cellular interactions they undergo there are necessary for maximal clonal expansion, terminal differentiation, and acquisition of effector and memory function. According to this idea, an encounter with the tolerogenic or immunogenic form of antigen will stimulate T cells to undergo up to four to six divisions in the paracortex of the lymph node. However, the presence of adjuvant is needed to allow these T cells to migrate into the B cell follicle via upregulated expression of costimulatory molecules (e.g., CD40, OX40L, CD80, and CD86). In turn these endow the T cells with the ability to home into follicles by downregulating CCR7 and upregulating CXCR5. Once in the follicle, the T cells can interact with antigen-specific B cells that provide the signals (e.g., costimulation, such as B7RP-1, CD40, and OX40L) that are essential to permit full clonal expansion and terminal differentiation. During the first exposure to antigen, T cells may have a limited window of opportunity to migrate into follicles and undergo terminal differentiation. If this does not occur the T cells may default to anergy/deletion or differentiation into some form of regulatory/suppressive T cell. A potential role for antigen-specific B cells in this scenario is supported by their accumulation, antigen-induced migration, and high-affinity receptors that may all aid to give them primacy over APCs, such as DC by this stage of a response.

These models and predictions might have more than academic value. For example, promoting migration of T cells into follicles would enhance clonal expansion and differentiation and could therefore promote immunity in the context of vaccination. Conversely, blocking such migration may not only prevent responses in the presence of, for example, fed antigen, it may actually enhance or promote the development of antigen-specific T cell tolerance with obvious therapeutic implications.

ACKNOWLEDGMENTS

P.G. would like to acknowledge the continued financial support of the MRC, BBSRC, and the Wellcome Trust.

REFERENCES

1. BILSBOROUGH, J. & J.L. VINEY. 2002. Getting to the guts of immune regulation. Immunology **106:** 139–143.
2. WILLIAMSON, E., J.M. O'MALLEY & J.L. VINEY. 1999. Visualizing the T-cell response elicited by oral administration of soluble protein antigen. Immunology **97:** 565–572.
3. SUN, J. *et al.* 1999. Antigen-specific T cell activation and proliferation during oral tolerance induction. J. Immunol. **162:** 5868–5875.
4. BLANAS, E. *et al.* 2000. A bone marrow-derived APC in the gut-associated lymphoid tissue captures oral antigens and presents them to both CD4+ and CD8+ T cells. J. Immunol. **164:** 2890–2896.
5. PARROTT, D.M. & M. DE SOUSA. 1971. Thymus-dependent and thymus-independent populations: origin, migratory patterns and lifespan. Clin. Exp. Immunol. **8:** 663–684.
6. PARROTT, D.M. & A. FERGUSON. 1974. Selective migration of lymphocytes within the mouse small intestine. Immunology **26:** 571–588.
7. SALMI, M. & S. JALKANEN. 1999. Molecules controlling lymphocyte migration to the gut. Gut **45:** 148–153.
8. PENG, H.J., M.W. TURNER & S. STROBEL. 1990. The generation of a 'tolerogen' after the ingestion of ovalbumin is time-dependent and unrelated to serum levels of immunoreactive antigen. Clin. Exp. Immunol. **81:** 510–515.
9. LIU, L.M. & G.G. MACPHERSON. 1993. Antigen acquisition by dendritic cells: intestinal dendritic cells acquire antigen administered orally and can prime naive T cells in vivo. J. Exp. Med. **177:** 1299–1307.
10. KEARNEY, E.R. *et al.* 1994. Visualization of peptide-specific T cell immunity and peripheral tolerance induction in vivo. Immunity **1:** 327–339.
11. SMITH, K.M., F. MCASKILL & P. GARSIDE. 2002. Orally tolerized T cells are only able to enter B cell follicles following challenge with antigen in adjuvant, but they remain unable to provide B cell help. J. Immunol. **168:** 4318–4325.
12. SMITH, K.M., J.M. DAVIDSON & P. GARSIDE. 2002. T-cell activation occurs simultaneously in local and peripheral lymphoid tissue following oral administration of a range of doses of immunogenic or tolerogenic antigen although tolerized T cells display a defect in cell division. Immunology **106:** 144–158.
13. GUTGEMANN, I. *et al.* 1998. Induction of rapid T cell activation and tolerance by systemic presentation of an orally administered antigen. Immunity **8:** 667–673.
14. TESTI, R. *et al.* 1994. The CD69 receptor: a multipurpose cell-surface trigger for hematopoietic cells. Immunol. Today **15:** 479–483.
15. KOBETS, N., K. KENNEDY & P. GARSIDE. 2003. An investigation of the distribution of antigen fed in tolerogenic or immunogenic forms. Immunol. Lett. **88:** 147–155.
16. IWASAKI, A. & B.L. KELSALL. 2000. Localization of distinct Peyer's patch dendritic cell subsets and their recruitment by chemokines macrophage inflammatory protein (MIP)-3alpha, MIP-3beta, and secondary lymphoid organ chemokine. J. Exp. Med. **191:** 1381–1394.
17. IWASAKI, A. & B.L. KELSALL. 2001. Unique functions of CD11b+, CD8 alpha+, and double-negative Peyer's patch dendritic cells. J. Immunol. **166:** 4884–4890.

18. DARZYNKIEWICZ, Z. *et al.* 1999. Laser-scanning cytometry: A new instrumentation with many applications. Exp. Cell Res. **249:** 1–12.
19. CAHALAN, M.D. *et al.* 2003. Real-time imaging of lymphocytes in vivo. Curr. Opin. Immunol. **15:** 372–377.
20. GARSIDE, P. *et al.* 1998. Visualization of specific B and T lymphocyte interactions in the lymph node. Science **281:** 96–99.
21. GULBRANSON-JUDGE, A. & I. MACLENNAN. 1996. Sequential antigen-specific growth of T cells in the T zones and follicles in response to pigeon cytochrome c. Eur. J. Immunol. **26:** 1830–1837.
22. ZHENG, B., S. HAN & G. KELSOE. 1996. T helper cells in murine germinal centers are antigen-specific emigrants that downregulate Thy-1. J. Exp. Med. **184:** 1083–1091.
23. FULCHER, D.A. *et al.* 1996. The fate of self-reactive B cells depends primarily on the degree of antigen receptor engagement and availability of T cell help. J. Exp. Med. **183:** 2313–2328.
24. CYSTER, J.G. & C.C. GOODNOW. 1995. Antigen-induced exclusion from follicles and anergy are separate and complementary processes that influence peripheral B cell fate. Immunity **3:** 691–701.
25. CYSTER, J.G. 1999. Chemokines and cell migration in secondary lymphoid organs. Science **286:** 2098–2102.
26. ANSEL, K.M. *et al.* 1999. In vivo-activated CD4 T cells upregulate CXC chemokine receptor 5 and reprogram their response to lymphoid chemokines. J. Exp. Med. **190:** 1123–1134.
27. BROCKER, T. *et al.* 1999. CD4 T cell traffic control: in vivo evidence that ligation of OX40 on CD4 T cells by OX40-ligand expressed on dendritic cells leads to the accumulation of CD4 T cells in B follicles. Eur. J. Immunol. **29:** 1610–1616.
28. GORTZ, A. *et al.* 2002. The chemokine ESkine/CCL27 displays novel modes of intracrine and paracrine function. J. Immunol. **169:** 1387–1394.
29. JAMES, M.J. *et al.* 2003. Anergic T cells exert antigen-independent inhibition of cell-cell interactions via chemokine metabolism. Blood **102:** 2173–2179.
30. RON, Y. & J. SPRENT. 1987. T cell priming in vivo: a major role for B cells in presenting antigen to T cells in lymph nodes. J. Immunol. **138:** 2848–2856.
31. KURT-JONES, E.A. *et al.* 1988. The role of antigen-presenting B cells in T cell priming in vivo. Studies of B cell-deficient mice. J. Immunol. **140:** 3773–3778.
32. LUTHER, S.A. & J.G. CYSTER. 2001. Chemokines as regulators of T cell differentiation. Nat. Immunol. **2:** 102–107.
33. PAPE, K.A. *et al.* 2003. Visualization of the genesis and fate of isotype-switched B cells during a primary immune response. J. Exp. Med. **197:** 1677–1687.
34. SHARPE, A.H. & G.J. FREEMAN. 2002. The B7-CD28 superfamily. Nat. Rev. Immunol. **2:** 116–126.
35. FILLATREAU, S. & D. GRAY. 2003. T cell accumulation in B cell follicles is regulated by dendritic cells and is independent of B cell activation. J. Exp. Med. **197:** 195–206.
36. CYSTER, J.G. 2003. Lymphoid organ development and cell migration. Immunol. Rev. **195:** 5–14.
37. SMITH, K.M. *et al.* 2003. Inducible costimulatory molecule-B7-related protein 1 interactions are important for the clonal expansion and B cell helper functions of naive, Th1, and Th2 T cells. J. Immunol. **170:** 2310–2315.
38. BIRD, J.J. *et al.* 1998. Helper T cell differentiation is controlled by the cell cycle. Immunity **9:** 229–237.
39. MACLENNAN, I.C. *et al.* 1997. The changing preference of T and B cells for partners as T-dependent antibody responses develop. Immunol. Rev. **156:** 53–66.
40. CLARK, E.A. & J.A. LEDBETTER. 1994. How B and T cells talk to each other. Nature **367:** 425–428.

How the Gut Links Innate and Adaptive Immunity

MARTIN RUMBO,[a] PASCALE ANDERLE,[a] ARNAUD DIDIERLAURENT,[a] FRÉDÉRIC SIERRO,[a] NATHALIE DEBARD,[a] JEAN-CLAUDE SIRARD,[b] DANIELA FINKE,[c] AND JEAN-PIERRE KRAEHENBUHL[a]

[a]*Swiss Institute for Experimental Cancer Research and the Institute of Biochemistry, University of Lausanne, CH-1066 Epalinges, Switzerland*

[b]*Equipe AVENIR-INSERM d'Immunité Anti-Microbienne des Muqueuses, Institut de Biologie de Lille, 1 rue du Professeur Calmette-BP 447-59021 Lille, France*

[c]*Pharmacenter-DKBW, University of Basel, Klingelbergstrasse 50-70, CH-4056 Basel, Switzerland*

ABSTRACT: Mucosal surfaces represent the main sites in which environmental microorganisms and antigens interact with the host. Sentinel cells, including epithelial cells, lumenal macrophages, and intraepithelial dendritic cells, continuously sense the environment and coordinate defenses for the protection of mucosal tissues. The mucosal epithelial cells are crucial actors in coordinating defenses. They sense the outside world and respond to environmental signals by releasing chemokines and cytokines that recruit inflammatory and immune cells to control potential infectious agents and to attract cells able to trigger immune responses. Among immune cells, dendritic cells (DC) play a key role in controlling adaptive immune responses, due to their capacity to internalize foreign materials and to present antigens to naive T and B lymphocytes, locally or in draining organized lymphoid tissues. Immune cells recruited in epithelial tissues can, in turn, act upon the epithelial cells and change their phenotype in a process referred to as epithelial metaplasia.

KEYWORDS: dendritic cell; lipopolysaccharide; pathogen-associated molecular pattern; Peyer's patch; pathogen recognition receptors; T helper; Toll-like receptor; T regulatory

INTRODUCTION

Mucosal epithelial tissues form efficient barriers that prevent environmental pathogens and antigens from gaining access to the host internal milieu. Because of their large surface area, mucosal tissues represent major sites of infection by pathogenic microbes.[1] Mammals have evolved defense mechanisms, including innate and adaptive immunity, to prevent and contain infection by highly diverse microbes.

Address for correspondence: Jean-Pierre Kraehenbuhl, Swiss Institute for Experimental Cancer Research, CH-1066 Epalinges, Switzerland. Voice: +41-21-692-5856; fax: +41-21-652-6933.

jean-pierre.kraehenbuhl@isrec.unil.ch

Commensal bacteria are harmless as long as they remain in the outside world. If they invade the host, they elicit strong inflammatory responses. Therefore, innate mechanisms have evolved that contribute to preventing invasion by commensals and eliminating potential intruders. When constitutive innate defenses are overwhelmed by pathogens, inducible immune responses are switched on. Innate and adaptive mechanisms are thus concomitantly and coordinately stimulated by mucosal sentinel cells responding to danger signals.[2]

CROSSTALK BETWEEN THE ENVIRONMENT AND EPITHELIAL CELLS

In mucosal tissues, microorganisms act on epithelial cells that, in turn, release signals that attract inflammatory and immune cells (FIG. 1). Intestinal epithelial cells express various pathogen-recognition receptors (PRR), including Toll-like receptors (TRL) that recognize the microbial molecular pattern (referred to as pathogen-associated molecular pattern or PAMP). TLR2, TLR3, TLR4, and TLR5, as well as Nod1, are associated with both human and mouse intestinal epithelium.[3] Signaling by epithelial TLRs provokes secretion of various mediators, including proinflammatory chemokines and cytokines, antimicrobial defensins, and tissue remodeling enzymes.[4,5] Activation of microbe-induced pathways in epithelia mediates the

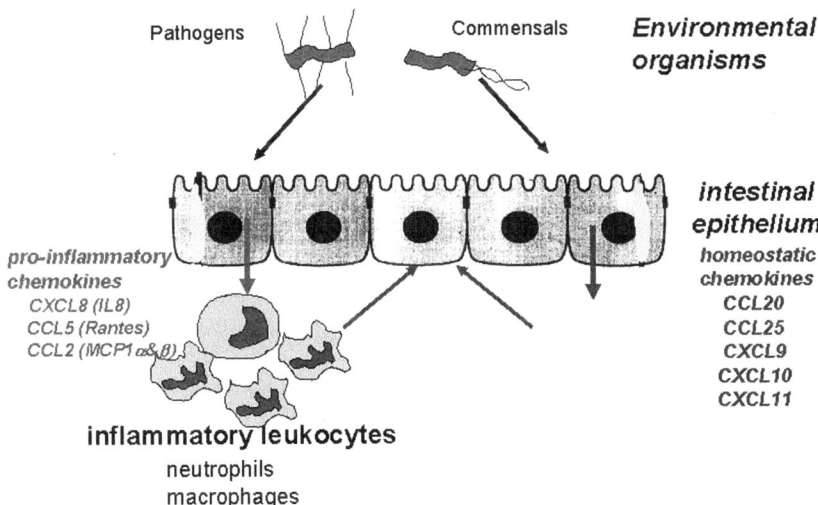

FIGURE 1. Microbial–epithelial cell crosstalk. The intestinal epithelium is in contact with a large number of commensals that are tolerated as long as they remain outside the host. Pathogens elicit strong proinflammatory epithelial responses that result in the recruitment of inflammatory cells (neutrophils and macrophages) that participate in the elimination of the pathogens. Flagellated microorganisms, including commensals, trigger epithelial homeostatic chemokine responses that recruit antigen-presenting cells to the epithelium, thus linking innate and adaptive immune responses.

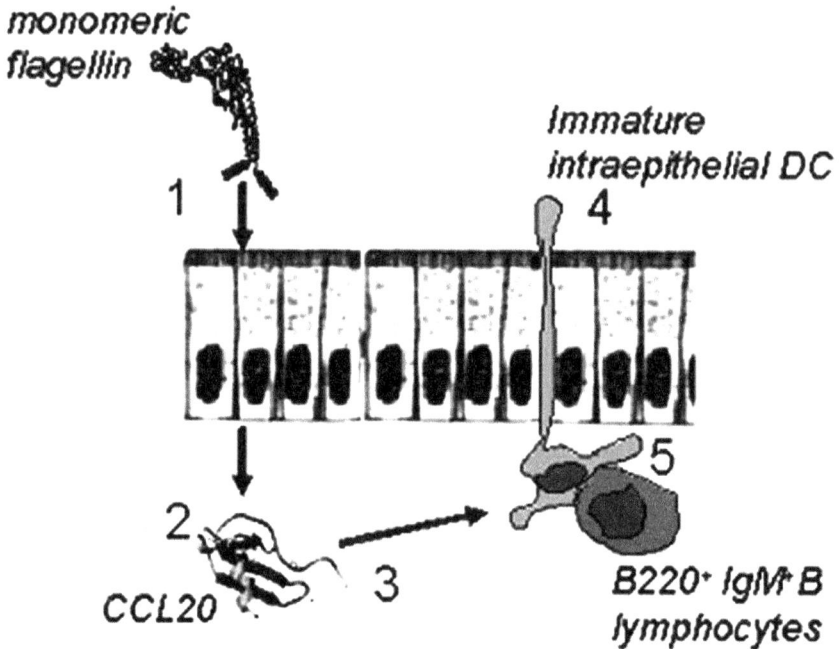

FIGURE 2. Potential role of intraepithelial dendritic cells. (**1**) Flagellin interacts with TLR5 expressed on the lumenal surface of gut epithelial cells; (**2**) engagement of TLR5 triggers NKκB-mediated release of the homeostatic chemokine CCL20; (**3**) CCL20 recruits immature myeloid DC into the epithelium; (**4**) DC open up the epithelial tight junctions and sample microorganisms, including commensals; (**5**) DC present the microbial antigens to local B220 IgM B lymphocytes, which may undergo T cell–independent IgA isotype switch to produce IgA antibodies that participate in barrier function by keeping the bacteria in the lumen or by eliminating IgA-opsonized microbes by phagocytosis.

recruitment of proinflammatory cells (neutrophils and macrophages), as well as immature dendritic cells (DC). Flagellin from flagellated bacteria triggers the production and release of CCL20, a homeostatic chemokine that selectively recruits immature myeloid dendritic cells that express the chemokine receptor CCR6 into the gut epithelium.[6] The induction is mediated by the canonical NFkB pathway. Intraepithelial DC may play a major role in the barrier function of the gut. DC in the intestinal epithelium are able to open up junctional complexes and send dendrites into the lumen that internalize lumenal microorganisms, in particular commensals.[7] It has recently been proposed that DC may present the internalized microorganisms to B cells in the gut lamina propria that undergo the T cell–independent IgA isotype switch.[8] Secreted IgAs contribute to the elimination of bacteria that have crossed the epithelial layer by opsonin-mediated degradation in Fcα/μ receptor-bearing phagocytes[9] (FIG. 2). This probably represents an innate mechanism that evolved as commensal microorganisms began to colonize vertebrates. Mucosal DC are also able to migrate to draining mesenteric lymph nodes and initiate adaptive immune responses.

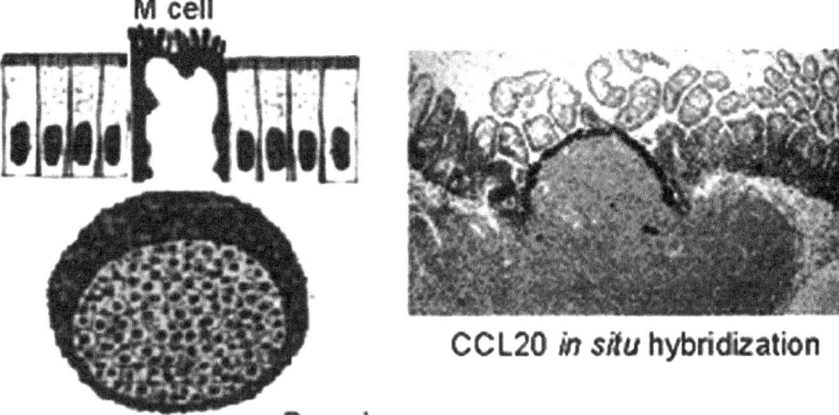

FIGURE 3. The follicle-associated epithelium constitutively expresses CCL20. The FAE contains M cells and enterocytes with downregulated digestive functions. The FAE constitutively expresses CCL20 (*in situ* hybridization with CCL20-specific probes).

CROSSTALK BETWEEN EPITHELIA AND IMMUNE CELLS

The follicle-associated epithelium (FAE) that overlies Peyer's patches (PPs) expresses distinct features, when compared to the adjacent villus epithelium. Besides the presence of antigen-sampling M cells and enterocytes with downregulated digestive functions, the FAE constitutively expresses the chemokine CCL20[10] (FIG. 3). CCL20 is responsible for the recruitment of DC in the subepithelial region of PPs.[11,12] The mechanisms that induce FAE differentiation and CCL20 expression are poorly understood. It has been suggested that the phenotypic changes seen in the FAE are the result of interactions with immune cells. Because LTβ receptor signaling plays a major role in Peyer's patch ontogeny,[13,14] and because intestinal epithelial cells express LTβ receptors, we tested whether LTß receptor signaling mediates the phenotypic changes typical of the FAE. LTβR and LT$\alpha_1\beta_2$, as well as CCL20 expression, were monitored during embryonic development by *in situ* hybridization of mouse intestine.[15] CCL20 was expressed in the FAE before birth at the time the first hematopoietic $CD4^+CD3^-LT\beta^+$ cells home to sites corresponding to PP anlage.

GLOBAL ASSESSMENT OF GENE PROFILE REGULATION UPON CCL20, TNFα, AND FLAGELLIN TREATMENT

We tested whether LT$\alpha_1\beta_2$ stimulation induced expression of CCL20 using T84 human intestinal epithelial cells. CCL20 was induced in T84 cells upon LTβR signaling using an agonistic ligand or anti-LTβ receptor agonistic antibodies. We compared the influence of the various treatments in T84 cells with untreated cells on the expression levels of genes using a self-organization map (SOM) approach. T84 cells were dynamically regulated upon the various treatments. The order of dynamic changes on the genomic profiles in T84 cells was as follows: TNFα < flagellin < LTα$_1$β$_2$. TNFα treatment induces the broadest spectrum of chemokines in T84 cells, eliciting CCL20, IL-8 and CXCL2 (neutrophils), and CXCL10 (T cells). LTα$_1$β$_2$ upregulated CCL20 expression and IL-8, whereas flagellin induced only CCL20 expression. TNFα and LTα$_1$β$_2$ induced NFkB family members, such as p100, Rel B, c Rel, IκBα, and IκBε. Flagellin upregulated only IκBα and IκBε.

Gene expression following agonistic anti-LTβR antibody treatment *in vivo* was studied by laser microdissection and quantitative RT-PCR. Genes showing high correlation with CCL20 across the different conditions tested were detected by clustering analysis. Quantitative PCR was optimized for the TNIP, TNAIP3, BIRC3, BTG3, ezrin, and syndecan-4 genes, and differential expression on microdissected tissue was measured. In addition, the expression of some selected chemokines upregulated in T84 upon TNFα treatment was also assessed. For the set of genes we tested, only CCL20 was significantly upregulated in the FAE compared to the crypts or the villus epithelium. None of the genes whose gene expression profile highly correlated with CCL20 in the microarray experiments was specific for the FAE.

Our results show that LTβR signaling induces CCL20 expression in intestinal epithelial cells, suggesting that this pathway triggers constitutive production of Ccl20 in the mouse FAE. More analysis and *in vivo* validation will be required to identify additional LTα$_1$β$_2$ -induced FAE-specific genes.

In conclusion, the gut epithelium, as probably most mucosal epithelia, integrates signals from the outside and inside world (FIG. 4). Flagellin induces a selective homeostatic CCL20 chemokine response recruiting immature DC to the epithelium.

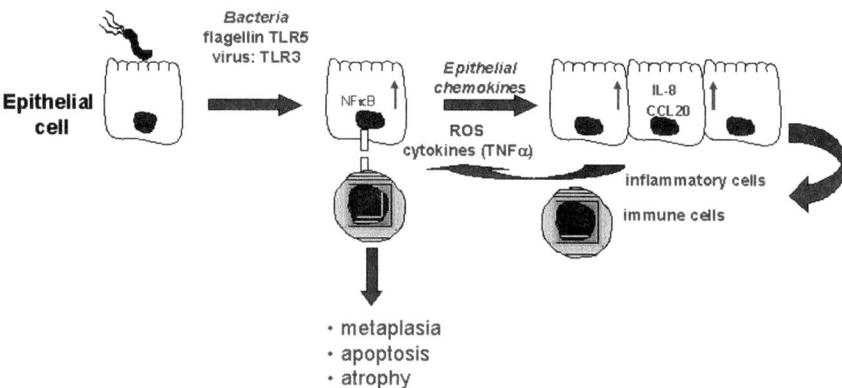

FIGURE 4. The gut epithelium intergrates signals from the outside and inside world. Microbial (bacteria and viruses) known as PAMPs interact with Toll-like receptors (TLR3 and TLR5) expressed on the lumenal surface of the enterocytes. Engagement of the receptors induces through the NFκB pathway the production of epithelial cytokines and chemokines that recruit immune and inflammatory cells. The recruited cells, in turn, act directly or via cytokines on epithelial cells changing their gene expression patterns and inducing phenotypic changes known as epithelial metaplasia.

Whether such recruited cells are able to pick up commensals and present them to lamina propria B cells remains to be established. A large number of genes, including CCL20, are also induced in the gut epithelium by recombinant $LT\alpha_1\beta_2$- or $LT\alpha_1\beta_2$-bearing immune cells recruited to the mucosal environment, indicating that immune cell/epithelial cell crosstalk dramatically affects the gut epithelium.

ACKNOWLEDGMENTS

We wish to thank Corinne Tallichet-Blanc, Monique Reinhardt, Isabelle Surbek, and Catherine Roger for their skillful technical assistance. M.R. was partially supported by scholarships from the Roche Research Foundation, the Consejo Nacional de Investigaciones Cientificas y Tecnicas (CONICET), and the Antorchas Foundation. This work was supported by grants from the Swiss National Science Foundation to JPK (3100-067926.02) and to DF (PPOOA—68855), and from an OncoSwiss grant to DF.

REFERENCES

1. NEUTRA, M.R., N.J. MANTIS & J.P. KRAEHENBUHL. 2001. Collaboration of epithelial cells with organized mucosal lymphoid tissues. Nature Immunol. **2:** 1004–1009.
2. JANEWAY, C.A. & R. MEDZHITOV. 2002. Innate immune recognition. Annu. Rev. Immunol. **20:** 197–216.
3. CARIO, E. & D.K. PODOLSKY. 2000. Differential alteration in intestinal epithelial cell expression of toll-like receptor 3 (TLR3) and TLR4 in inflammatory bowel disease. Infect. Immun. **68:** 7010– 7017.
4. LOPEZ-BOADO, Y.S., C.L. WILSON & W.C. PARKS. 2001. Regulation of matrilysin expression in airway epithelial cells by Pseudomonas aeruginosa flagellin. J. Biol. Chem. **276:** 41417– 41423.
5. OGUSHI, K. et al. 2001. Salmonella enteritidis FliC (flagella filament protein) induces human beta-defensin-2 mRNA production by Caco-2 cells. J. Biol. Chem. **276:** 30521–30526.
6. SIERRO, F. et al. 2001. Flagellin stimulation of intestinal epithelial cells triggers CCL20-mediated migration of dendritic cells. Proc. Natl. Acad. Sci. USA **98:** 13722–13727.
7. RESCIGNO, M. et al. 2001. Dendritic cells express tight junction proteins and penetrate gut epithelial monolayers to sample bacteria. Nature Immunol. **2:** 361–367.
8. FAGARASAN, S. et al. 2001. In situ class switching and differentiation to IgA-producing cells in the gut lamina propria. Nature **413:** 639–643.
9. SHIBUYA, A. et al. 2000. Fc alpha/mu receptor mediates endocytosis of IgM-coated microbes. Nature Immunol. **1:** 441–446.
10. TANAKA, Y. et al. 1999. Selective expression of liver and activation-regulated chemokine (LARC) in intestinal epithelium in mice and humans. Eur. J. Immunol. **29:** 633– 642.
11. COOK, D.N. et al. 2000. CCR6 mediates dendritic cell localization, lymphocyte homeostasis, and immune responses in mucosal tissue. Immunity **12:** 495–503.
12. IWASAKI, A. & B.L. KELSALL. 2000. Localization of distinct Peyer's patch dendritic cell subsets and their recruitment by chemokines macrophage inflammatory protein (MIP)-3 alpha, MIP-3 beta, and secondary lymphoid organ chemokine. J. Exp. Med. **191:** 1381–1393.
13. FINKE, D. & J.P. KRAEHENBUHL. 2001. Formation of Peyer's patches. Curr. Opin. Genet. Devel. **11:** 562–569.
14. FINKE, D. et al. 2002. CD4[+] CD3[−] cells induce Peyer's patch development: role of alpha4beta1-integrin-activation by CXCR5. Immunity **17:** 363–373.
15. RUMBO, M. et al. 2004. Lymphotoxin β receptor signaling induces the chemokine CCL20 in intestinal epithelium. Gastroenterology **129:** 213–223.

Activation of a Unique Population of CD8$^+$ T Cells by Intestinal Epithelial Cells

MATTHIEU ALLEZ, JENS BRIMNES, LING SHAO, IRIS DOTAN, ATSUSHI NAKAZAWA, AND LLOYD MAYER

Immunobiology Center, Mount Sinai School of Medicine, New York, New York 10029, USA

ABSTRACT: Intestinal epithelial cells may play a role in the regulation of immune responses toward luminal antigens. We show that a subset of CD8$^+$ T cells undergoes oligoclonal expansion in the intestinal mucosa, probably through interaction with a unique complex expressed on epithelial cells, formed by a CEA subfamily member (gp180) and CD1d. This subset, which is regulatory *in vitro*, may play a role in the control of intestinal immune responses toward luminal antigens. A lack of expansion of these CD8$^+$ regulatory T cells, probably related to the defective expression of the gp180/CD1d complex, is observed in inflammatory bowel disease.

KEYWORDS: intestinal epithelial cell; T regulatory cell; CD8; CD1D; gp180

INTRODUCTION

The regulation of T lymphocyte activation in the gut requires a complex network of stimulatory and inhibitory signals. Classical mechanisms described for the regulation of adaptive immune responses in the peripheral lymph nodes or spleen appear to be nonfunctional in the gut-associated lymphoid tissue (GALT), and there is a chronic state of lymphocyte activation (controlled or physiologic inflammation). This control may exist at many levels. There is emerging evidence that novel nonclassical MHC class I–like (nonclassical class I) molecules play important roles in the local environment of the gut epithelium. The intestinal epithelial cell (IEC) is capable of expressing many nonclassical class I molecules. It is tempting to hypothesize that the presence of this diverse repertoire of molecules, associated with innate immunity, is important for the activation of a variety of regulatory T (Tr) cells that are involved in controlled/physiologic inflammation. A number of novel Tr cells have been defined, many of which were identified first in the intestine. Defects in Tr cells can result in the development of mucosal inflammation (e.g., CD45Rb^{hi}→SCID transfer model of colitis). Regulatory T cells may contribute by helping to control inflammation and maintain the mucosal barrier. The presence or absence of the various Tr cells has not been assessed in human disease.

Address for correspondence: Lloyd Mayer, Immunobiology Center, Mount Sinai School of Medicine, 1425 Madison Avenue, New York, NY. 10029. Voice: 212-659-9266; fax: 212-987-5593.
  lloyd.mayer@mssm.edu

Ann. N.Y. Acad. Sci. 1029: 22–35 (2004). © 2004 New York Academy of Sciences.
doi: 10.1196/annals.1309.004

Over the past 10 years, the field of regulatory T cells (formerly called suppressor cells) has been resurrected. Interestingly, this rebirth has come largely from the study of mucosal immune responses and, interestingly, predominantly in CD4+ T cells. Th3 cells (secreting TGF-β) were first described in oral tolerance models.[1–3] Tr1 cells (secreting IL-10) were identified in intestinal graft versus host disease and in the CD45Rb^{hi}→SCID transfer model of colitis.[4–6] In this and a number of other animal models of inflammatory bowel disease (IBD), transfer of regulatory T cells prevents the onset of disease. In other models, neonatal depletion of regulatory T cells (CD4+CD25+ Tr cells by neonatal thymectomy) provides the substrate for the development of mucosal inflammation (autoimmune gastritis).[7] The list of such cells is growing but includes both CD4+ and CD8+ T cells (as well as non–T cells: B cells, macrophages, dendritic cells, and NKT cells).[8,9] Where each of these populations exerts its effects is unknown, and the requirement for such redundancy is not understood. Furthermore, the nature of the interactions between these populations is controversial (i.e., is one a precursor population for another?). The antigen specificity and MHC restriction of these cells has also been questioned. Cecal bacteria-specific Tr1 cells have been defined in mouse models of IBD,[10] and soluble antigen-specific Th3 cells (to the oral tolerogen) have been isolated. CD4+CD25+ Tr cells are anergic but are postulated to be self-reactive.[11,12] Regardless of their initial antigen reactivity, most investigators agree that their effector function is antigen nonspecific (mediated by cytokines or cell contact). CD8+ Tr cells were the "suppressor cells" originally described in the 1980s. Their validity (and existence) was questioned when specific T cell receptor (TcR) rearrangements were not noted and attempts to grow these cells in long-term culture were unsuccessful. However, more recently a number of regulatory CD8+ T cells have been reported as well. These include CD8αα+ T cells in the IEL population[13] and CD8+28− cells in alloantigen restimulation studies.[14] Our group has defined the CD1d/gp180-restricted TrE cells that are the result of T cell interactions with normal intestinal epithelial cells. All CD8+ T regs described exert their effects, like their CD4+ counterparts, in an antigen-nonspecific fashion. Although the restriction element for TrE cells is known, those regulating CD8αα+ T cells are not and, as alluded to above, IELs may be restricted by a number of nonclassical restriction elements.

In concert with the unique lymphoid populations present in the mucosa-associated lymphoid tissue (MALT), there appear to be a number of distinct antigen presenting cells (APCs) as well. Mucosal macrophages express an activated phenotype but respond poorly to lipopolysaccharide (LPS), and are weak stimulators of T cell proliferation.[15,16] Dendritic cells (DCs) of several subtypes exist within the lamina propria and Peyer's patches, however these, too, have been poorly characterized functionally. In the rat and mouse, the submucosal DCs extend their dendrites into the epithelial layer, expressing tight junction proteins, but this does not appear to be the case in humans.[17] Difficulty in isolating and growing these cells from the mucosa has hampered more careful studies.

In 1986, Bland and colleagues described a novel function for rat IECs, that of APCs.[18,19] Early studies had documented that normal IECs could express MHC class II molecules constitutively. These were the only non-DC, non-monocyte, or non–B cell specialized APCs shown to constitutively express these critical immunoregulatory molecules. Interestingly, in the initial studies in rats and humans, IECs were found to selectively activate CD8+ T cells. These cells were suppressive functionally and in humans did not express the cytolytic proteins perforin and granzyme. Several studies have documented the capacity of normal IECs to take up soluble antigens *in vitro* and *in vivo*.[20–25] Thus, there is evidence to support the contention that IECs might function as unique APCs in mucosal immune responses. Hershberg's group constructed a novel system, transfecting the class II regulator CIITA and HLA-DR4 into a malignant human IEC line, T84.[26–28] Stimulation of these cells with IFNγ results in the expression of class II MHC molecules and confers the capacity to present antigen to a human TcR-transfected murine T cell hybridoma or T cell lines. These studies suggest that not only can IECs take up antigen but they can process antigen appropriately and present it to class II–restricted T cells. However, several caveats exist here. First, most studies have failed to demonstrate the expression of critical costimulatory molecules (e.g., B7-1, B7-2, CD40[29,30]), so that activation of primary cells via IECs would more likely result in the induction of anergy. Second, in studies using primary cells (normal), stimulation of $CD4^+$ T cells by IECs has been weak (even alloreactive T cells). This might relate to the lower expression of MHC class II on IECs than conventional APCs. $CD8^+$ T cells can be activated by antigen presented by IECs.[31] The predominant T cell population activated in IEC:T cell cocultures appears to be $CD8^+ CD28^-$ T cells.[31] More recent studies suggest that the activation of these cells is regulated by a series of novel interacting molecules. We have identified a novel CD8 ligand, a glycoprotein within the CEA family, termed gp180.[32] This molecule engages CD8 at sites distinct from classical class I, and results in the activation of the CD8-associated kinase, p56lck. It also forms an association with the nonclassical class I molecule CD1d.[33,34] The complex of CD1d and gp180 appears to be recognized by a subpopulation of regulatory $CD8^+$ T cells in peripheral blood and perhaps in the lamina propria. The characterization of these novel Tr cells is the focus of this manuscript.

METHODS

Isolation of Human Intestinal Epithelial Cells

Surgical specimens from patients undergoing bowel resection for cancer (at least 10 cm away from the tumor) at the Mount Sinai Medical Center were used as a source of intestinal epithelial cells (IECs). IECs were isolated by a method described previously. Resected surgical specimens were washed extensively with PBS. The mucosa was stripped off from the submucosa, minced into small pieces, and placed in 1 mM dithiothreitol (DTT, Sigma Chemical Co) for 10 min at room temperature to remove mucus. The pieces were washed in PBS and incubated twice in medium (RPMI) containing 3 mg/mL Dispase II (Roche Diagnostics, Mannheim, Germany) for 30 min at 37°C, and vortexed every 5 minutes. The cell suspension was collected and centrifuged on a Percoll (Amersham Biosciences, Piscataway, NJ) density gradient and IECs were collected from the 0–30% interface. Cells were washed with PBS and resuspended in serum free medium (Aim V, 50 u/mL penicillin, 50 mg/mL streptomycin, 2 mM glutamine, all from GIBCO BRL). The purified IECs were greater than 95% viable and contained less than 2% IELs. Preparations of IECs were irradiated (3000 rads) prior to culture with T cells.

Lymphocyte Isolation from Lamina Propria, Intraepithelium, and Peripheral Blood

Lamina propria mononuclear cells (LPMCs) were isolated from the tissue remaining after the dispase treatment. The tissue was incubated for 1 h at 37°C in medium containing 1 mg/mL collagenase (clostridiopeptidase A). The cell suspension was collected and centrifuged on a Percoll density gradient and the LPMCs were harvested from the 40–60% interface. Viability was greater than 90%. In functional studies, LP $CD4^+$ and $CD8^+$ T cells were sorted after staining (FITC-conjugated anti-CD8, PE-conjugated anti-CD4, and APC-conjugated anti-CD3) using a MoFlo sorter (Cytomation, Ft. Collins, CO). IELs were isolated in some experiments: briefly, resected surgical specimens were incubated for 30 min at 37°C in RPMI 1640 containing 1.5 mmol/L $MgCl_2$ and 1 mmol/L EDTA. The supernatant containing the IELs was passed through a nylon filter (Falcon 2360; Becton Dickinson), and IELs were washed twice in PBS. Peripheral blood mononuclear cells (PBMCs) were isolated on a Ficoll-Hypaque density gradient according to standard procedures. Cells were resuspended in RPMI and the cell density adjusted to 5×10^6 cells/mL. T cells were separated by a rosetting technique using neuraminidase-treated sheep red blood cells and Ficoll-Hypaque density gradient centrifugation. Rosetted T cells were treated with 0.75% ammonium chloride on ice for 5–10 minutes to lyse sheep red blood cells. The T cell suspension was then washed with PBS and resuspended in Aim V culture medium.

Membrane Labeling of T Cells with CFSE

T cells were resuspended in PBS at 5×10^6/mL for staining with CFSE. CFSE (Molecular Probes, Eugene, OR), in the form of a 5 mM stock solution in DMSO, was added at the final concentration of 1 mM for 10 min at 37°C. T cells were then washed twice in RPMI, and resuspended in culture medium (Aim V, 50 u/mL penicillin, 50 mg/mL streptomycin, and 2 mM glutamine).

Cocultures of Peripheral T Cells and IECs

Mixed cell culture was performed as previously described using irradiated IECs (3000 rad) as stimulator cells and allogeneic T cells as responder cells. CFSE-labeled T cells and IECs were cocultured at 1×10^6/mL and 0.5×10^6/mL, respectively, in culture medium at 37°C in a 5% CO_2 humidified incubator for 5 to 10 days. These cells are referred to as IEC-activated T cells. At the same time, T cells were cultured alone (referred to as nonactivated T cells—negative control) or with allogeneic non–T cells (MLR-positive control).

Experiments with Blocking Antibodies

In some experiments, IECs were preincubated for 1 h at 4°C with an anti-gp180 monoclonal antibody (B9), anti-CD1d (mAb D5), anti–class I (W6/32), or an IgG1 control (626.1, anti-CD40 antibody, was used as an isotype control; CD40 is not expressed on IECs). The suspension of IECs was washed and irradiated before addition to the culture with T cells. Blocking experiments with the same monoclonal antibodies (mAbs) were also performed in MLR (control) cultures; allogeneic non–

T cells were preincubated with mAbs (B9, D5, W6/32) or isotype controls as described for IECs.

Flow Cytometric Analysis

CFSE-labeled T cells from cocultures, freshly isolated mucosal lymphocytes (IELs, MLN cells, and LPL), and T cell lines were resuspended in PBS and incubated for 30 min with antibodies. The following antibodies, conjugated with FITC, PE, PerCP, or APC, were used: anti-CD3, anti-CD8, anti-CD4, anti-VB antibodies specific for 17 VB subfamilies, anti-CD28, anti-CD94, anti-CD56, anti-CD25 (all from Becton-Dickinson), anti-CD152 (CTLA4) (Pharmingen), and relevant isotype controls. Anti-CD101 (18F7) and anti-CD103 (28C12) were a gift from Drs. Michael Brenner and Gary Russell (Brigham and Womens Hospital, Boston). A Becton Dickinson FACScalibur was used for the flow cytometric analysis. A MoFlo Cytomation cell sorter was used for sorting. Four-color analyses were performed using Cell Quest software (Becton Dickinson).

Lines of IEC-Activated $CD8^+$ T Cells

Different populations of T cells were sorted from cocultures (using a Cytomation Moflo) in order to generate lines. $CD3^+CD8^+$ T cells were cultured with IECs for 8 d (proliferating-CFSE low– versus nonproliferating-CFSE high–), allogeneic non–T cells (MLR), or in medium alone. Sorted populations were stimulated just after sorting, and every 3 weeks, using PHA (1 μg/mL), IL-2 (100 U/mL), IL-7 (10 ng/mL), IL-15 (20 ng/mL), and feeder cells (irradiated allogeneic PBMCs) in Aim V medium. Preliminary studies using various cytokine combinations had shown that IL-7 and IL-15 were critically important for the development of long-term lines in these cocultures. Lines of lamina propria lymphocytes (LPL) were grown under the same conditions.

Suppressor Assays

We studied the effect of $CD8^+$ T cells (cell lines or freshly isolated LPL) on pokeweed-stimulated PBMC (10^5 per 100 μL in Aim V). PBMCs were either unstimulated or stimulated with pokeweed mitogen (PWM, 1 mg/mL). The $CD8^+$ T cells were added to PBMCs, before PWM stimulation, at a ratio of 1:1 and 1:5 (1 $CD8^+$ T cell to 5 PBMC). Supernatants were harvested at day 7, and IgG secretion was measured by ELISA. In some experiments, these populations of $CD8^+$ T cells were added to an unrelated mixed lymphocyte reaction (MLR), with CFSE-labeled T cells, at a ratio of 1:5 and 1:10, and the proliferation of $CD4^+$ T cells was analyzed by flow cytometry.

CDR3 Length Analysis and Sequencing

mRNA was extracted from the different T cell populations to generate cDNA. Primers specific for each VB subfamily and a fluorescent CBR primer were used for DNA amplification. The CDR3 coding region length distributions of the VB transcripts were analyzed on an ABI377DNA sequencer. For sequencing, the appropriate PCR products were subcloned using a TOPO TA cloning kit (Invitrogen,

Carlsbad, CA), and approximately 20 clones were processed. Sequencing and analyses were performed as previously described.

RESULTS

Normal IECs activate a subpopulation of $CD8^+$ $CD28^-$ $CD101^+$ $CD103^+$ regulatory T cells restricted by the CD1d/gp180 complex. We initiated experiments to define the nature of the $CD8^+$ regulatory T cell(s) activated by the gp180/CD1d complex. We used a CFSE system to identify T cells proliferating in response to coculture with normal IECs. Using this system, we were able to reconfirm our original observation that normal IECs preferentially activate $CD8^+$ T cells.[35] However, given the sensitivity of this system and the potential for other phenotypic and functional characterization of cells proliferating in these cocultures, we were able to identify additional proliferating T cell populations and test the role that gp180/CD1d played in the activation of each of these subpopulations. We identified a population of $CD8^+CD28-CD101^+CD103^+$, $CD8^+CD28^+$, $CD4^+CD28^+CD25^{+/-}$ T cells proliferating in these cocultures. The precursor frequency of responder $CD8^+CD28^-$ T cells was surprisingly high (0.3 to 0.9% of PB T cells).[35] Only the population of $CD8^+CD28^-$ T cells was blocked (no proliferation) in the presence of either anti-gp180 or anti-CD1d mAbs (but not anti–class I mAbs). We were able to sort the proliferating $CD8^+CD28^-$ T cells and show that, as we initially described, they exhibited antigen-nonspecific suppressor activity and required cell:cell contact to mediate the suppression. Using cytokines shown to be relevant to the expansion of mucosal T cells (IL-7) and $CD8^+$ T cells (IL-15) we were able to generate lines from these sorted cells. These lines retained the phenotypic and functional characteristics of the initially sorted cells (FIG. 1).

Because CD1d is nonpolymorphic and may have a limited set of antigens that it can present, we next assessed the TcR repertoire of both the proliferating $CD8^+$ cells and cell lines. In eight experiments (IEC:T cell cocultures) we noted an increase in $CD8^+V\beta5.1^+$ T cells, as well as $V\beta16$, $V\beta23$, and $V\beta7^+$ T cells (staining with specific anti-$V\beta$ mAbs). Importantly, previous studies have shown that $V\beta5.1$ is rarely used by $CD8^+$ T cells. We therefore asked whether the expansion of any of the $V\beta$-expressing T cells could be inhibited by anti-gp180 or CD1d mAbs. In all experiments, only proliferation of the $V\beta5.1^+CD8^+$ T cells was inhibited by these mAbs (FIG. 2).

Expansion of a specific $V\beta$-expressing T cell population can reflect either conventional antigen or superantigen stimulation. To assess this directly, we performed CDR3 length analysis of proliferating versus nonproliferating $CD8^+$ T cells in these cocultures. As seen in TABLE 1, there was a clonal expansion of $V\beta5.1^+$ T cells (CDR3 = 8–9 AAs) and $V\beta16$ in 6 of 8 and 7 of 8 experiments respectively. The CDR3 sequence was then determined. As seen in TABLE 1, there was a common motif seen in the more N-terminal sequence of the CDR3 region and there was a biased usage of $J\beta2.1$ and 2.7.

We then went back to the IEC-activated T cell lines that had been expanded over a three-week period with IL-7, IL-15, IL-2, PHA, and irradiated allogeneic PBMCs (every three weeks). One line generated by this approach expressed $V\beta5.1^+CD8^+$ T cells only. This line had a surface phenotype consistent with what we had previously

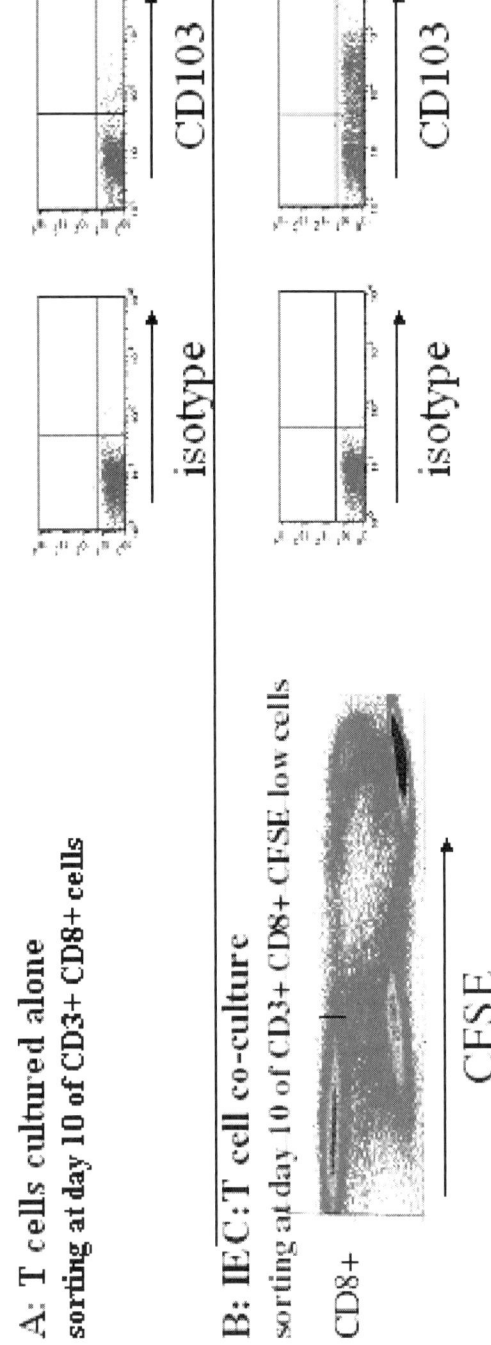

FIGURE 1. IEC:T cell (CFSE-labeled) cocultures were established on day 0. Proliferation was assessed by flow on day 10, and CD8+CSFE[lo] (proliferating) and CD8+CSFE[hi] (nonproliferating) cells were sorted and grown for 3 months in the presence of IL-7/IL-15/PHA/IL-2 and allogeneic-irradiated PBMC (every 3 weeks). After 3 months in culture, the cells were analyzed for cell surface markers, including CD28, CD101, CD103 (shown here), IL-2R, and Vβ repertoire (see below). Cells maintained their phenotype in these long-term cultures.

TABLE 1.

	Common Motif in the CDR3β?					Sequence in the CDR3α			
016 IEC act CD8+ T Vβ5.1						**016 IEC act CD8+T Vα18**			
LINE	CAS	SLVWGEKLF	**FGSG**	9αα	Jβ1.4	LINE	CAP	WHGGAATNKLI	FGTG	10αα	Jα23
017 IEC act CD8+ T Vβ5.1						**036 IEC act CD8+T Vα18**			
1,2,5,6,9	CAS	SLVWGELF	**FGEG**	8αα	Jβ2.2	LINE	CAF	VPGNTGKLI	FGQG	9αα	Jα37
011 IEC act CD8+ T Vβ5.1						**044 IEC act CD8+T Vα18**			
7,9	CAS	SLGGLEQF	**FGPG**	8αα	Jβ2.1	3	CAP	LGGATNKLI	FGTG	9αα	Jα23
010 IEC act CD8+ T Vβ5.1									
4	CAS	SFGGANEQF	**FGPG**	9αα	Jβ2.1	4	CAP	VFYNQGGKLI	FGQG	10αα	Jα37

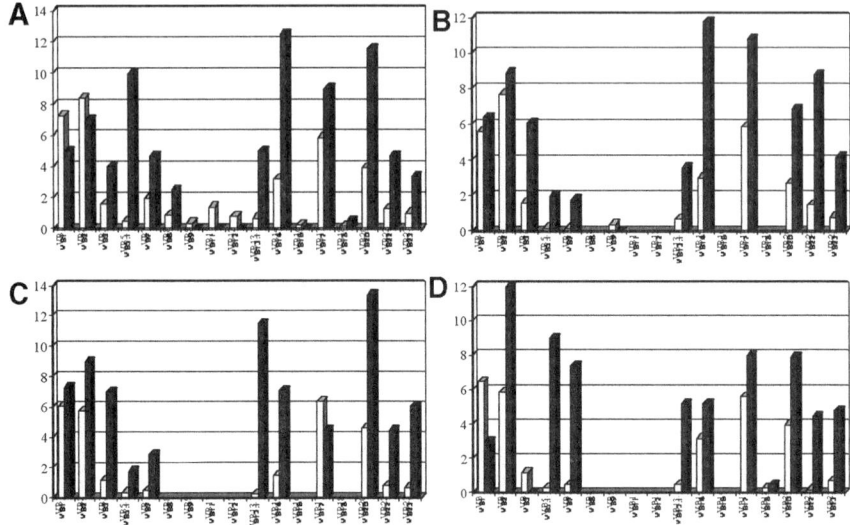

FIGURE 2. CSFE-labeled T cells cocultured with normal irradiated IECs in the presence of monoclonal antibodies to (**a**) an isotype control, (**b**) gp180, (**c**) CD1d, or (**d**) class I. Proliferating (*black*) and nonproliferating (*gray*) CD8$^+$ T cells (gated on CD3$^+$CD8$^+$ T cells) were analyzed for BV expression using a panel of anti-BV mAbs (BD).

described for IEC-activated T cells and was capable of suppressing immunoglobulin secretion by PWM-stimulated PBMCs. This line was then analyzed for Vα usage. We determined that these cells used Vα18, an uncommon Vα in CD8$^+$ T cells. The other lines (nonclonal) were analyzed as well for the presence of Vα18. In 4 of 5 lines from IEC-activated proliferating CD8$^+$ T cells Vα18 mRNA was detectable (FIG. 3). This TcR was not detected in nonproliferating cells expanded with IL-7, IL-15, PHA, and IL-2 (data not shown), or in CD8$^+$ T cells proliferating in MLRs. Sequence of the CDR3 region of Vα18 from these cells did not reveal an invariant sequence (TABLE 1), although the more C-terminal sequence was hydrophobic in nature in all of the sequences obtained. Furthermore, there was a biased usage of Jα23 and 37, evolutionarily related Jαs. Taken together, these data suggest that there are Vα18/Vβ5.1 expressing CD8$^+$ T cells expanded after interaction with normal IECs. These cells appear to be gp180/CD1d-restricted, but are not clonal in nature, and may reflect activation following presentation of a limited set of antigens by IECs. We have defined these cells as TrE cells.

We next looked to see whether these cells were present in normal mucosa. This was a critically important set of experiments required to validate the results of our *in vitro* model. Isolated normal IELs, LPL, and MLN cells were subjected to enrichment of CD8$^+$ T cells. Vβ5.1$^+$CD8$^+$ T cells were detected in LPL at much higher frequency than in PB (4 to 10% versus 0.1 to 0.5% PB) and to a lesser extent in IELs (1 to 2%). No enrichment was seen in MLN cells (same percentage as PB). Interestingly, the percentage of these cells was decreased in the lamina propria of patients with inflammatory bowel disease, even in areas where there was no active

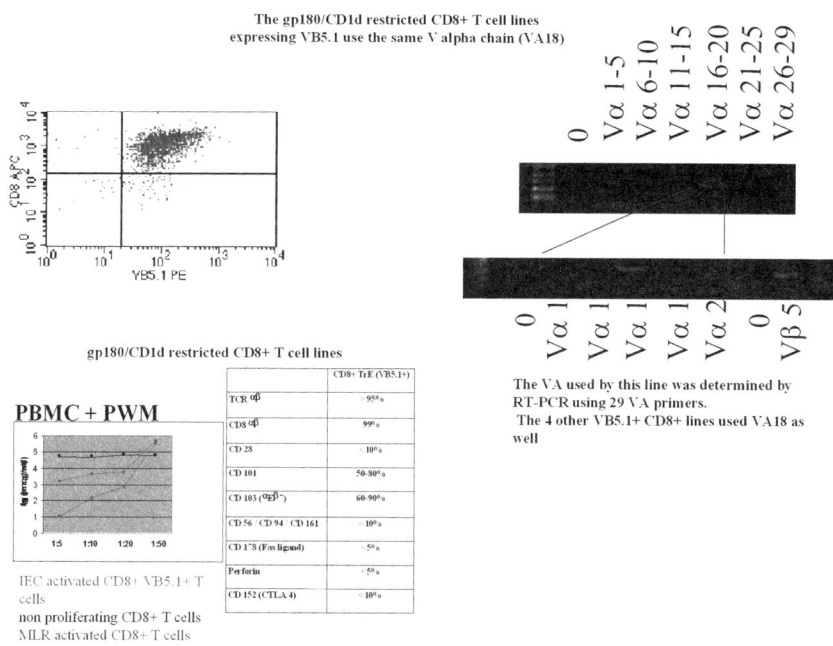

FIGURE 3. Cocultures were established as described above and grown in the presence of IL-7 and IL-15. Cell lines were then stained with anti-Vβ monoclonal antibodies. *Top left panel* shows a line that is 100% Vβ5.1+. This line was analyzed for Vα usage and was found to express Vα18. *Bottom panel* represents the phenotype of this line (TcRα/β+, CD8α/β+ CD28−, CD101 and 103+, CTLA4−, perforin−, FasL−). Functionally, these cells suppressed nonspecifically (seen here as suppression of PWM-induced immunoglobulin secretion by human B cells). Four other lines expressing Vβ5.1 coexpressed Vα18.

inflammation (TABLE 2). These findings are consistent with the lack of expression of gp180 by IBD IECs previously reported.[36]

DISCUSSION

The nature of the immune response in the gastrointestinal tract is quite distinct from its counterpart in the systemic immune system. The large and chronic antigenic exposure dictates the necessity for tight regulation. Over the past decade, there has been renewed interest in cells that mediate such regulation, Tr cells. Interestingly, all of the Tr cells identified to date have been either described in the GI tract or in association with some GI pathology (e.g., CD4+CD25+ Tr cells and autoimmune gastritis; Th3 cells in oral tolerance; Tr1 cells in colitis, etc.).[2–4,6,7,10,13] In addition to these CD4+ Tr cells, a number of regulatory CD8+ T cells have been identified as well.[13,14,19,31]

As alluded to above, the immunological tone of the GALT is one of suppression or dampened inflammatory responses. Given the chronic exposure of the various

TABLE 2. Lack of activation/expansion of CD8$^+$ Vβ5.1$^+$ T lymphocytes in cocultures with IECs isolated in IBD patients: decreased frequency of Vβ5.1$^+$ CD8$^+$ LPL

	IBD ($n = 5$)	Normal ($n = 8$)
In vitro (IEC:PB T coculture) % Vβ5.1/IEC activated CD8$^+$ T cells (CFSE^{lo})	1.52 ± 1.33%*	4.36 ± 2.42%
In vivo (LPL) % Vβ5.1/CD8$^+$ LPL	2.23 ± 1.04%**	4.72 ± 1.41%

$P = .02$
$P = .0018$

components of the GALT to luminal bacteria, it is likely that diverse regulatory mechanisms exist to allow for peaceful coexistence. While many factors account for the immunologic nonresponsiveness of the GI tract, the nature of the antigens and the antigen presenting cells are key to this process. In addition to tolerogenic DCs and poorly responsive macrophages (i.e., not responding to LPS), nonprofessional APCs have been described as well. The intestinal epithelium has long been viewed as a physical (nonimmune) barrier to infection and to access by antigen to the GALT. More recently, several groups have described novel activities for these cells that relate to both innate and adaptive immune responses (i.e., chemokine synthesis in response to bacterial invasion, antigen presentation by classical and nonclassical MHC molecules). In terms of adaptive immune responses, IECs have been shown to selectively activate antigen-nonspecific CD8$^+$ suppressor T cells when presenting soluble antigens to local T cell populations.[8,31] This event appears to be regulated by a series of novel cell surface interactions: a ligand for CD8 (gp180) and the nonclassical class I molecule CD1d. This complex appears to be recognized by a subpopulation of CD8$^+$CD28$^-$ T cells causing their activation and effector function, suppression, which potentially downregulates inflammatory and immune responses locally. The IEC can regulate inflammation via the innate system as well. Activated IECs have been shown to secrete TGF-β, IL-10, and PGE$_2$, all inhibitory factors for immune activation.[37] Thus, the IEC may be a critical control point for regulating intestinal inflammatory responses. The key is the identity of cells capable of interacting with the IEC. Given their location, a prime target for the IEC is the intraepithelial lymphocyte, which has been demonstrated to be difficult to activate *in vitro* and may require a unique set of activating stimuli. Lamina propria lymphocytes also have the capacity to interact with IECs, but they are similarly resistant to signals mediated via their antigen receptors.[38–40] Several groups have speculated that the IEC might be the appropriate APC for these cell populations.

The intestinal epithelial cell expresses MHC class I and class II molecules but, possibly more important, expresses a wide array of nonclassical class I molecules as well. In this paper, we document that normal IECs activate a selected subpopulation of CD8$^+$ Tr cells that are restricted by the complex of CD1d and gp180. CD1d, by its nonpolymorphic nature and large hydrophobic groove, likely presents a limited set of antigens (lipids, glycolipids, lipoproteins) to a restricted population of T cells. The cells described here, expressing Vβ5.1/Vα18, may recognize antigens of bacterial origin and may be involved in the phenomenon of controlled/physiologic inflammation in the normal lamina propria. In any given coculture of freshly isolated

IECs and PB T cells there are a number of expanded clones. Only the Vβ5.1/Vα18+ T cells are consistently inhibited by antibodies to either CD1d or gp180 (but not classical class I). The absence of an invariant Vα, as seen in CD1d-restricted NKT cells,[41–43] may reflect differences in the antigens carried within the groove of the CD1d molecule by the IECs isolated from different individuals. Interestingly the same epithelial cell preparation expands similar clones from peripheral T cells derived from two different controls. These data suggest that the IEC, and the antigens presented by these cells, dictate the T cell clone that is activated.

The real question is whether such cells exist *in vivo*. Preliminary studies suggest that Vβ5.1/Vα18 CD8+ T cells are present in the normal lamina propria, and that these cells suppress by a contact-dependent antigen-nonspecific manner, as reported for TrE cells. Interestingly, the number of TrE cells are reduced in the lamina propria of IBD patients. This may reflect the reported defects in both gp180 and CD1d expression.

Different Tr cells may exhibit different functions. Some may be more important in the stomach versus the small bowel or colon, whereas others may be involved in systemic tolerance versus local controlled inflammation. The relationship between these different Tr cells, and whether these cells work alone or in combination, has not yet been clarified. As we define the antigen specificity and immunologic signatures, we should be able to ascertain the answers to these questions.

ACKNOWLEDGMENTS

This work was supported by NIH Grants AI 23504, AI 24671, AI 44236, and AI 07605. M.A. and I.D. were supported by the CCFA (fellowship award) and M.A. additionally by the Société Nationale Française de Gastroentérologie. J.B. was supported by the Danish Medical Research Agency. I.D. was supported by CCFA (fellowship award). L.S. was supported by Training Grant AI 07605.

REFERENCES

1. MILLER, A., A. AL-SABBAGH, L.M. SANTOS, *et al.* 1993. Epitopes of myelin basic protein that trigger TGF-beta release after oral tolerization are distinct from encephalitogenic epitopes and mediate epitope-driven bystander suppression. J. Immunol. **151:** 7307–7315.
2. KHOURY, S.J., HANCOCK, W.W. & H.L. WEINER. 1992. Oral tolerance to myelin basic protein and natural recovery from experimental autoimmune encephalomyelitis are associated with downregulation of inflammatory cytokines and differential upregulation of transforming growth factor beta, interleukin 4, and prostaglandin E expression in the brain. J. Exp. Med. **176:** 1355–1364.
3. SANTOS, L.M., A. AL-SABBAGH, A. LONDONO & H.L. WEINER. 1994. Oral tolerance to myelin basic protein induces regulatory TGF-beta-secreting T cells in Peyer's patches of SJL mice. Cell. Immunol. **157:** 439–447.
4. GROUX, H., A. O'GARRA, M. BIGLER, *et al.* 1997. A CD4+ T-cell subset inhibits antigen-specific T-cell responses and prevents colitis. Nature **389:** 737–742.
5. GROUX, H., M. BIGLER, J.E. DE VRIES & M.G. RONCAROLO. 1996. Interleukin-10 induces a long-term antigen-specific anergic state in human CD4+ T cells. J. Exp. Med. **184:** 19–29.
6. ASSEMAN, C., S. MAUZE, M.W. LEACH, *et al.* 1999. An essential role for interleukin 10 in the function of regulatory T cells that inhibit intestinal inflammation. J. Exp. Med. **190:** 995–1004.

7. SAKAGUCHI, S. & N. SAKAGUCHI. 1990. Thymus and autoimmunity: capacity of the normal thymus to produce pathogenic self-reactive T cells and conditions required for their induction of autoimmune disease. J. Exp. Med. **172:** 537–545.
8. MIZOGUCHI, E., A. MIZOGUCHI, F.I. PREFFER & A.K. BHAN. 2000. Regulatory role of mature B cells in a murine model of inflammatory bowel disease. Int. Immunol. **12:** 597–605.
9. HUANG, F.P. & G.G. MACPHERSON. 2001. Continuing education of the immune system—dendritic cells, immune regulation and tolerance. Curr. Mol. Med. **1:** 457–468.
10. CONG, Y., C.T. WEAVER, A. LAZENBY & C.O. ELSON. 2002. Bacterial-reactive T regulatory cells inhibit pathogenic immune responses to the enteric flora. J. Immunol. **169:** 6112–6119.
11. KITANI, A., K. CHUA, K. NAKAMURA & W. STROBER. 2000. Activated self-MHC-reactive T cells have the cytokine phenotype of Th3/T regulatory cell 1 T cells. J. Immunol. **165:** 691–702.
12. SHEVACH, E.M., C.A. PICCIRILLO, A.M. THORNTON & R.S. MCHUGH. 2003. Control of T cell activation by CD4+CD25+ suppressor T cells. Novartis Found. Symp. **252:** 24–36; discussion 36–44, 106–14.
13. POUSSIER, P., T. NING, D. BANERJEE & M. JULIUS. 2002. A unique subset of self-specific intraintestinal T cells maintains gut integrity. J. Exp. Med. **195:** 1491–1497.
14. LIU, Z., B. YU, J. FAN, et al. 2001. CD8(+)CD28(-) T cells suppress alloresponse of CD4(+) T cells both in primates and rodents. Transplant. Proc. **33:** 82–83.
15. SMITH, P.D., E.N. JANOFF, M. MOSTELLER-BARNUM, et al. 1997. Isolation and purification of CD14-negative mucosal macrophages from normal human small intestine. J. Immunol. Methods **202:** 1–11.
16. SMITH, P.D., L.E. SMYTHIES, M. MOSTELLER-BARNUM, et al. 2001. Intestinal macrophages lack CD14 and CD89 and consequently are down-regulated for LPS- and IgA-mediated activities. J. Immunol. **167:** 2651–2656.
17. RESCIGNO, M., G. ROTTA, B. VALZASINA & P. RICCIARDI-CASTAGNOLI. 2001. Dendritic cells shuttle microbes across gut epithelial monolayers. Immunobiology **204:** 572–581.
18. BLAND, P.W. & L.G. WARREN. 1986. Antigen presentation by epithelial cells of the rat small intestine. II. Selective induction of suppressor T cells. Immunology **58:** 9–14.
19. BLAND, P.W. & L.G. WARREN. 1986. Antigen presentation by epithelial cells of the rat small intestine. I. Kinetics, antigen specificity and blocking by anti-Ia antisera. Immunology **58:** 1–7.
20. LAIPING SO, A., K. PELTON-HENRION, G. SMALL, et al. 2000. Antigen uptake and trafficking in human intestinal epithelial cells. Dig. Dis. Sci. **45:** 1451–1461.
21. SIMINOSKI, K., P. GONNELLA, J. BERNANKE, et al. 1986. Uptake and transepithelial transport of nerve growth factor in suckling rat ileum. J. Cell Biol. **103:** 1979–1990.
22. GONNELLA, P.A., K. SIMINOSKI, R.A. MURPHY & M.R. NEUTRA. 1987. Transepithelial transport of epidermal growth factor by absorptive cells of suckling rat ileum. J. Clin. Invest. **80:** 22–32.
23. BRANDEIS, J.M., M.H. SAYEGH, L. GALLON, et al. 1994. Rat intestinal epithelial cells present major histocompatibility complex allopeptides to primed T cells. Gastroenterology **107:** 1537–1542.
24. HUGHSON, E.J. & C.R. HOPKINS. 1990. Endocytic pathways in polarized Caco-2 cells: identification of an endosomal compartment accessible from both apical and basolateral surfaces. J. Cell Biol. **110:** 337–348.
25. SO, A.L., G. SMALL, K. SPERBER, et al. 2000. Factors affecting antigen uptake by human intestinal epithelial cell lines. Dig. Dis. Sci. **45:** 1130–1137.
26. HERSHBERG, R.M. & L.F. MAYER. 2000. Antigen processing and presentation by intestinal epithelial cells—polarity and complexity. Immunol. Today **21:** 123–128.
27. HERSHBERG, R.M. 2002. The epithelial cell cytoskeleton and intracellular trafficking. V. Polarized compartmentalization of antigen processing and Toll-like receptor signaling in intestinal epithelial cells. Am. J. Physiol. Gastrointest. Liver Physiol. **283:** G833–839.
28. HERSHBERG, R.M., D.H. CHO, A. YOUAKIM, et al. 1998. Highly polarized HLA class II antigen processing and presentation by human intestinal epithelial cells. J. Clin. Invest. **102:** 792–803.

29. NAKAZAWA, A., I. DOTAN, J. BRIMNES, et al. 2004. The expression and function of costimulatory molecules B7H and B7-H1 on colonic epithelial cells. Gastroenterology **126:** 1347–1357.
30. NAKAZAWA, A., M. WATANABE, T. KANAI, et al. 1999. Functional expression of costimulatory molecule CD86 on epithelial cells in the inflamed colonic mucosa. Gastroenterology **117:** 536–545.
31. MAYER, L. & R. SHLIEN. 1987. Evidence for function of Ia molecules on gut epithelial cells in man. J. Exp. Med. **166:** 1471–1483.
32. YIO, X.Y. & L. MAYER. 1997. Characterization of a 180-kDa intestinal epithelial cell membrane glycoprotein, gp180. A candidate molecule mediating t cell-epithelial cell interactions. J. Biol. Chem. **272:** 12786–12792.
33. CAMPBELL, N.A., H.S. KIM, R.S. BLUMBERG & L. MAYER. 1999. The nonclassical class I molecule CD1d associates with the novel CD8 ligand gp180 on intestinal epithelial cells. J. Biol. Chem. **274:** 26259–26265.
34. CAMPBELL, N.A., M.S. PARK, L.S. TOY, et al. 2002. A non-class I MHC intestinal epithelial surface glycoprotein, gp180, binds to CD8. Clin. Immunol. **102:** 267–274.
35. ALLEZ, M., J. BRIMNES, I. DOTAN & L. MAYER. 2002. Expansion of CD8+ T cells with regulatory function after interaction with intestinal epithelial cells. Gastroenterology **123:** 1516–1526.
36. TOY, L.S., X.Y. YIO, A. LIN, et al. 1997. Defective expression of gp180, a novel CD8 ligand on intestinal epithelial cells, in inflammatory bowel disease. J. Clin. Invest. **100:** 2062–2071.
37. SANTOS, L.M., O. LIDER, J. AUDETTE, et al. 1990. Characterization of immunomodulatory properties and accessory cell function of small intestinal epithelial cells. Cell. Immunol. **127:** 26–34.
38. TARGAN, S.R., R.L. DEEM, M. LIU, et al. 1995. Definition of a lamina propria T cell responsive state. Enhanced cytokine responsiveness of T cells stimulated through the CD2 pathway. J. Immunol. **154:** 664–675.
39. QIAO, L., G. SCHURMANN, M. BETZLER & S.C. MEUER. 1991. Activation and signaling status of human lamina propria T lymphocytes. Gastroenterology **101:** 1529–1536.
40. BOIRIVANT, M., I. FUSS, C. FIOCCHI, et al. 1996. Hypoproliferative human lamina propria T cells retain the capacity to secrete lymphokines when stimulated via CD2/CD28 pathways. Proc. Assoc. Am. Physicians **108:** 55–67.
41. TANIGUCHI, M., H. KOSEKI, T. TOKUHISA, et al. 1996. Essential requirement of an invariant V alpha 14 T cell antigen receptor expression in the development of natural killer T cells. Proc. Natl. Acad. Sci. USA **93:** 11025–11028.
42. TANIGUCHI, M., Y. MAKINO, J. CUI, et al. 1996. V alpha 14+ NK T cells: a novel lymphoid cell lineage with regulatory function. J. Allergy Clin. Immunol. **98:** S263–269.
43. EXLEY, M., J. GARCIA, S.P. BALK & S. PORCELLI. 1997. Requirements for CD1d recognition by human invariant Valpha24+ CD4-CD8- T cells. J. Exp. Med. **186:** 109–120.

Compartmentalization of the Mucosal Immune Responses to Commensal Intestinal Bacteria

ANDREW J. MACPHERSON AND THERESE UHR

Institut für Experimentelle Immunologie, Universitätsspital Zürich, Zürich, Switzerland

ABSTRACT: Mammals coexist with a luxuriant load of bacteria in the lower intestine (up to 10^{12} organisms/g of intestinal contents). Although these bacteria do not cause disease if they remain within the intestinal lumen, they contain abundant immunostimulatory molecules that trigger immunopathology if the bacteria penetrate the body in large numbers. The physical barrier consists only of a single epithelial cell layer with overlying mucus, but comparisons between animals kept in germ-free conditions and those colonized with bacteria show that bacteria induce both mucosal B cells and some T cell subsets; these adaptations are assumed to function as an immune barrier against bacterial penetration, but the mechanisms are poorly understood. In mice with normal intestinal flora, but no pathogens, there is a secretory IgA response against bacterial membrane proteins and other cell wall components. Whereas induction of IgA against cholera toxin is highly T help dependent, secretory IgA against commensal bacteria is induced by both T independent and T dependent pathways. When animals are kept in clean conditions and free of pathogens, there is still a profound intestinal secretory IgA response against the commensal intestinal flora. However, T dependent serum IgG responses against commensal bacteria do not occur in immunocompetent animals unless they are deliberately injected intravenously with 10^4 to 10^6 organisms. In other words, unmanipulated pathogen-free mice are systemically ignorant but not tolerant of their commensal flora despite the mucosal immune response to these organisms. In mice that are challenged with intestinal doses of commensal bacteria, small numbers of commensals penetrate the epithelial cell layer and survive within dendritic cells (DC). These commensal-loaded DC induce IgA, but because they are confined within the mucosal immune system by the mesenteric lymph nodes, they do not induce systemic immune responses. In this way the mucosal immune responses to commensals are geographically and functionally separated from systemic immunity.

KEYWORDS: IgA; commensal bacteria; dendritic cells; compartmentalization; gnotobiotic animal; recolonization

INTRODUCTION

There is an abundant flora of nonpathogenic commensal intestinal bacteria in the lower intestine of mammals, with densities rising to 10^{12} organisms/g intestinal

Address for correspondence: Andrew J. Macpherson, Institut für Experimentelle Immunologie, Universitätsspital Zürich, Schmelzbergstrasse, 12, CH8091 Zürich, Switzerland. Voice: +41-1-255-3788; fax: +41-1-255-4420.
amacpher@pathol.unizh.ch

contents.[1] This means that the number of bacterial cells exceeds the number of eukaryotic cells in the host. Moreover, the total gene load from commensal bacteria is several orders of magnitude greater than the number of genes in the host chromosomes. This remarkable mutualism is the more striking because commensal bacteria share molecular patterns recognized by the Toll-like receptor family of the innate immune system to detect and respond to dangerous pathogens, yet the mucosal immune system of the healthy intestine has evolved to contain these bacteria within the intestinal lumen and avoid intestinal inflammation or sepsis.

It is clear that the host does not ignore its load of commensal intestinal bacteria. Animals can be bred and maintained in entirely sterile conditions in positive pressure isolators, in which case they lack intestinal commensal organisms. Compared with specific pathogen-free animals of the same genetic strain, germ-free animals have an undeveloped mucosal immune system: the Peyer's patches and isolated lymphoid follicles are small with few germinal centers; there are very few IgA-secreting plasma cells in the lamina propria;[2] and the numbers of lamina propria $CD4^+$ and intraepithelial $CD8\alpha\beta^+$ cells are markedly reduced.[3–6] More generally, the intestinal epithelial differentiation program is altered[7,8] and gnotobiotes are relatively hypogammaglobulinemic with poorly formed systemic secondary lymphoid structures.[9–13]

A gnotobiotic animal is an excellent culture medium: if it is exposed to microorganisms merely by placing an animal with normal intestinal flora in the same cage, commensal bacteria will start to colonize the germ-free intestine within 24 hours. Germ-free recolonizations have been used experimentally to study the sequential alterations of the mucosal immune system and their functional importance in preventing penetration of commensals to the underlying systemic tissues. The induction of B and T cell responses by the mucosal immune system takes two to three weeks, and live commensal organisms penetrate the mucosa to deeper tissues in the period before intestinal defenses have fully adapted.[14] After adaptation, the deeper tissues once again become sterile. T cell–deficient animals have also been found to show increased spontaneous penetration of commensals through the intestinal mucosa.[15,16] Yet although commensal bacteria are certainly sensed by the mucosa and its immune system, the detailed mechanisms of the diverse immunological and epithelial changes in containing these organisms are poorly understood.

PRODUCTION AND FUNCTION OF IgA IN THE INTESTINAL MUCOSA

IgA is the most abundantly produced immunoglobulin in the body; it is mainly secreted as a dimer across the epithelial cell layer through a specialized transport system.[17] Classical experiments showed that IgA^+ B cells are induced in the Peyer's patches[18] and circulate through the mesenteric lymphatics to enter the blood stream via the thoracic duct and home back to the intestinal mucosa.[19,20] Similar recirculation also occurs with many intestinal T cells.[21]

Studies on the functional importance of secreted IgA show that it can neutralize viruses[22,23] or toxins[24,25] intraluminally or during transport via the polymeric immunoglobulin receptor (pIgR).[26] This presumably accounts for only a tiny proportion of the IgA, as the comparisons between germ-free and specific pathogen-free (SPF) mice show that the abundance of intestinal IgA-secreting plasma cells depends on the presence of commensal bacteria. Despite this, there is only scant evidence that IgA has a role in preventing commensal bacterial penetration or limiting the growth of bacteria and their densities in the lumen of the intestine.[27]

Initial studies of the mechanisms of IgA induction and the cytokine requirements were carried out using cell culture systems. These showed that TGF-β and IL-4 promoted the switch from surface IgM to IgA expression,[28,29] and that IL-2, IL-6, and IL-10 worked in a synergistic fashion.[30–32] Experiments in which cellular components (B and T lymphocytes and dendritic cells) were purified from different secondary lymphoid structures and reconstituted *in vitro* showed that the IgA switch was much more efficient when leukocytes—especially dendritic cells—were derived from Peyer's patches than from other cellular sources.[33,34]

IgA induction mechanisms have also been studied *in vivo* by measuring antigen-specific and total IgA levels in strains of mice with selective immune deficiencies as a result of gene targeting. To induce antigen-specific IgA, soluble proteins have been administered into the stomach together with cholera toxin, an oral adjuvant: in these circumstances IgA is induced both in the mucosa and the serum.[35,36] However, this oral immunization regime is not confined to the mucosal immune system (and, therefore, may not be entirely representative of normal mucosal B cell induction), as it also induces serum IgG and IgE.[37] Nude mice with very limited T cell numbers have reduced IgA levels,[38] and cholera toxin-dependent IgA induction is abrogated in mice selectively deficient in CD4,[39] IL-4,[40] MHC class II,[41] or CTLA4-Hγ1 transgenic animals in which CD28-CD80/86 signaling is blocked.[42] Although these studies show the importance of CD4 T cells, costimulation, and cytokine mechanisms for IgA induction, paradoxically the CD4$^{-/-}$, IL-4$^{-/-}$ MHC II$^{-/-}$, and CTLA4-Hγ1Tg animals had relatively preserved total IgA levels, supporting the notion that T help-dependent IgA induction with cholera toxin may not reveal all IgA induction pathways.

Using Western blots of proteins prepared from the cell walls of *Enterobacter cloacae* (the main aerobic commensal in the Zürich colony of SPF mice), we found that intestinal IgA was induced to a wide range of bacterial proteins.[43,44] Although the total levels of secreted IgA were reduced to about a quarter of wild-type levels in animals deficient for the β and δ chains of the T cell receptor (TCR-β$^{-/-}$ δ$^{-/-}$, lacking both αβ and γδ T cells), the same anticommensal specificities were generated. T independent IgA induction against commensal bacteria was also seen against crystallographically pure OmpF outer membrane protein and chimeric proteins expressed in live bacteria in the intestine under the control of the nirB *in vivo* inducible promoter. In addition, IgA induction to commensals does not need conventional organization of secondary lymphoid structures in the mucosal immune system—it is extremely efficient in the tumor necrosis factor I–deficient strain that lacks follicular dendritic cells and has a very limited number of highly disorganized Peyer's patches. However, lymphotoxin α-deficient or alymphoplastic (aly/aly) mice that have no B cell structures whatsoever in the intestine lack intestinal IgA. This suggests that IgA$^+$ B cell induction takes place locally within the mucosa, although the system is primitive in terms of T independence and the superfluity of compartmentalized B, T, and follicular zones within the intestinal lymphoid follicles.

The earliest site of B cell production is the fetal liver, but after birth B cells are produced in both the bone marrow and pleuropericardial cavities of mice.[45–49] The progeny of these different sites can be distinguished according to their surface markers: B1 cells from the pleuropericardium stain strongly for IgM, Mac-1, and CD5

(B1a), but weakly for B220 and IgD. The situation is reversed for B2 cells from the bone marrow, in which strong B1 markers stain weakly and vice versa. B1 cells are a major source for IgM antibodies specific for bacterial cell wall components. The surface markers that characterize B1 and B2 cells are downregulated as plasma cells differentiate, but the relative contribution of each has been assessed indirectly by reconstituting radiation chimeras with allotypically marked bone marrow and peritoneal leukocytes. In most cases, this has shown that B1 cells are the source of up to half the secretory intestinal IgA,[50–52] although much lower proportions ($\leq 10-15\%$) have also been found after recolonization of gnotobiotic chimeras in which neonatal antibody depletion preceded reconstitution.[53] Our reconstitution experiments in TCR$\beta^{-/-}$ $\delta^{-/-}$ mice showed that peritoneal B1 cells reconstituted most of the T independent IgA.[43] The interpretation of these reconstitution experiments relies on the independence of the adult B1 and B2 lineages; this is in itself controversial, as in immunoglobulin transgenic and "knock-in" mice B cells can be generally distributed with B1 or B2 phenotypes predominating depending on their B cell receptor specificity and surface density rather than site of origin.[54] However, in an independent approach a substantial contribution of B1 cells to intestinal IgA production was also detected in MHC class II$^{-/-}$ mice, where antigen-specific intestinal IgA was abrogated when the strain was made deficient of Bruton kinase (*xid*), which causes deficiency of B1a cells.[41]

MUCOSAL AND SYSTEMIC RESPONSES AGAINST COMMENSALS ARE INDEPENDENT

The same Western blots that detect secretory IgA that binds to commensal bacterial cell wall proteins are negative when used to detect serum IgG binding in unmanipulated SPF animals. This is ignorance rather than tolerance, because deliberate injection of 10^4 to 10^6 c.f.u. bacteria into the tail vein induces a specific IgG response within 14 days.[43] In other words, the mucosal immune system has an excellent IgA response to the presence of commensal intestinal bacteria, but this is separate from the systemic immune response. Immune responses to commensals are, therefore, a function of exposure to the organisms, and immune responses are very efficiently induced if the organisms succeed in penetrating. Penetration presumably represents only the tip of the iceberg, as systemic tissues are normally sterile.

When mice are challenged with experimental doses of commensal bacteria, small numbers of these commensals penetrate the epithelial layer to be taken up by, and survive in, dendritic cells of the Peyer's patches.[55] These commensal-loaded DC effectively induce IgA$^+$ B cells in *ex vivo* assays, in the presence or absence of added T cells.[55] Commensal bacteria can survive within mucosal DC for up to 60 h, whereas they are rapidly killed by intestinal macrophages; this contrasts with intestinal pathogens, which are generally able to subvert phagocytic biocidal mechanisms.[56] Although the bacteria-loaded mucosal DC can migrate to the mesenteric lymph nodes, they do not penetrate further to reach systemic secondary lymphoid structures, except in mice where the mesenteric lymph nodes have been surgically removed four to six weeks previously.[55] The geographical compartmentalization of commensal-loaded DC explains how induction of IgA responses to commensals is achieved within the mucosal immune system, yet at the same time preserving systemic ignorance, given that extraintestinal responses are avoided.

Mice that are deficient in B and/or T cell arms of the adaptive immune system are stable in a pathogen-free animal house despite dense bacterial flora (Zürich cecal culturable bacterial densities: $RAG^{-/-}$, $7.1\pm3.5\times10^7$ aerobes, $7.2\pm2.1\times10^{10}$ anaerobes; $J_H^{-/-}$, $3.7\pm2.3\times10^7$ aerobes, $8.1\pm1.5\times10^{10}$ anaerobes; C57BL/6, $6.9\pm6.5\times10^7$ aerobes, $1.7\pm1.3\times10^{10}$ anaerobes; $\bar{x}\pm SD$, $n = 9$ to 14; all animals 6 to 10 weeks old). By contrast, mice in which the oxygen-free radical and inducible nitric oxide biocidal mechanisms of phagocytes are severely deficient die soon after weaning as a result of sepsis from the commensals.[57] In other words, systemic adaptive responses against commensals are not essential, as the innate immune system is very efficient at clearing the few commensals that do penetrate.

Does the secretion of IgA across the intestinal mucosa limit the penetration of commensals into the body, resulting in tolerance to these organisms, either by directly blocking penetration or by limiting luminal bacterial densities? Selectively deficient $IgA^{-/-}$ mice have a relatively mild phenotype,[58] and selective deficiency of IgA in humans is often without clinical consequences, probably because IgM can substitute for IgA. However, deficiency of the pIgR transporter that conveys IgA (or IgM) across the epithelial cell layer to the intestinal lumen results in an intestinal enteropathy,[59] suggesting that without protective secretion of antibody into the intestinal lumen, bacteria or bacterial products trigger intestinal inflammation. One way of detecting the presence of low levels of penetrating commensal intestinal bacteria is to look at the priming of serum IgG responses against commensal proteins, which, as described above, do not occur in C57BL/6 wild-type mice unless the commensal is deliberately injected intravenously. We found that $IgA^{-/-}$ mice, and other strains such as aly/aly deficient in IgA expression, show spontaneous systemic priming even in unmanipulated animals, indicating (indirectly) that IgA plays a role in limiting the exposure of central body tissues to penetration by the luxuriant load of commensals in the intestinal lumen. This is supported by experiments in which germ-free C57BL/6 wild-type mice and germ-free antibody-deficient $J_H^{-/-}$ mice are recolonized with commensal bacteria in parallel by adding a sentinel animal containing an SPF flora.[55] Both wild-type and antibody-deficient animals acquire the commensal bacteria within days of exposure to the SPF animal, and penetration of commensal bacteria through the intestinal epithelial layer can be measured before the mucosa has had chance to adapt to the presence of the intestinal flora. Antibody-deficient animals show increased penetration of commensals for the first 30 d, measured by culturable organisms in the mesenteric lymph nodes, although their cecal bacterial densities are similar. After 40 d, the mesenteric lymph nodes of even the antibody-deficient animals become sterile, showing that the IgA response is only one component of intestinal adaptation to the commensal flora.

CONCLUSIONS

In this article we have argued that the concept of oral tolerance does not apply to commensal intestinal bacteria. Clean animals are ignorant, but not tolerant, of their commensals despite an excellent mucosal immune response to these organisms, and the systemic immune system is perfectly capable of mounting a rapid response to penetrating commensals. Penetration is the exception rather than the rule, because the intestinal epithelium and the mucosal immune system are highly adapted to the presence of the commensals; even when penetration occurs, commensals do not subvert the biocidal mechanisms of phagocytes,[60] and they are rapidly cleared by the innate immune system. Commensal bacteria can survive within intestinal DC for extended periods, and these bacteria-loaded DC do induce mucosal responses to the commensals. However, the commensal-loaded DC are confined by the mesenteric lymph nodes to the mucosal immune system, which results in geographical and functional compartmentalization of adaptive anticommensal immune responses.

ACKNOWLEDGMENTS

We would like to acknowledge the constant support and encouragement of Rolf Zinkernagel and Hans Hengartner. Joanna Massacand helped with the experiments cited in the mucosal and systemic responses section. Work in our laboratory is supported by the Swiss National Science Foundation and the Kanton of Zürich.

REFERENCES

1. MACKIE, R., A. SGHIR & H.R. GASKINS. 1999. Developmental microbial ecology of the neonatal gastrointestinal tract. Am. J. Clin. Nutr. **69:** 1035S–1045S.
2. BENVENISTE, J. *et al.* 1971. Immunoglobulins in intact, immunized, and contaminated axenic mice: study of serum IgA. J. Immunol. **107:** 1647–1655.
3. GUY-GRAND, D. *et al.* 1991. Two gut intraepithelial CD8+ lymphocyte populations with different T cell receptors: a role for the gut epithelium in T cell differentiation. J. Exp. Med. **173:** 471–481.
4. UMESAKI, Y. *et al.* 1993. Expansion of alpha beta T-cell receptor-bearing intestinal intraepithelial lymphocytes after microbial colonization in germ-free mice and its independence from thymus. Immunology **79:** 32–37.
5. HELGELAND, L. *et al.* 1997. Regional phenotypic specialization of intraepithelial lymphocytes in the rat intestine does not depend on microbial colonization. Scand. J. Immunol. **46:** 349–357.
6. HELGELAND, L. *et al.* 1996. Microbial colonization influences composition and T-cell receptor V beta repertoire of intraepithelial lymphocytes in rat intestine. Immunology **89:** 494–501.
7. HOOPER, L.V. & J.I. GORDON. 2001. Commensal host-bacterial relationships in the gut. Science **292:** 1115–1118.
8. HOOPER, L.V. *et al.* 2001. Molecular analysis of commensal host-microbial relationships in the intestine. Science **291:** 881–884.
9. CRABBE, P.A. *et al.* 1970. Immunohistochemical observations on lymphoid tissues from conventional and germ-free mice. Lab. Invest. **22:** 448–457.
10. MANOLIOS, N., C.L. GECZY & L. SCHRIEBER. 1988. High endothelial venule morphology and function are inducible in germ-free mice: a possible role for interferon-gamma. Cell Immunol. **117:** 136–151.
11. WOSTMANN, B.S. & J.R. PLEASANTS. 1991. The germ-free animal fed chemically defined diet: a unique tool. Proc. Soc. Exp. Biol. Med. **198:** 539–546.
12. WOSTMANN, B.S., J.R. PLEASANTS & P. BEALMEAR. 1971. Dietary stimulation of immune mechanisms. Fed. Proc. **30:** 1779–1784.
13. BAKKER, R., E. LASONDER & N.A. BOS. 1995. Measurement of affinity in serum samples of antigen-free, germ-free and conventional mice after hyperimmunization with 2,4-dinitrophenyl keyhole limpet hemocyanin, using surface plasmon resonance. Eur. J. Immunol. **25:** 1680–1686.

14. SHROFF, K.E., K. MESLIN & J.J. CEBRA. 1995. Commensal enteric bacteria engender a self-limiting humoral mucosal immune response while permanently colonizing the gut. Infection & Immunity **63:** 3904–3913.
15. OWENS, W.E. & R.D. BERG. 1980. Bacterial translocation from the gastrointestinal tract of athymic (nu/nu) mice. Infect. Immun. **27:** 461–467.
16. BERG, R.D. 1996. The indigenous gastrointestinal microflora. Trends Microbiol. **4:** 430–435.
17. BRANDTZAEG, P. & H. PRYDZ. 1984. Direct evidence for an integrated function of J chain and secretory component in epithelial transport of immunoglobulins. Nature **311:** 71–73.
18. CRAIG, S.W. & J.J. CEBRA. 1971. Peyer's patches: an enriched source of precursors for IgA-producing immunocytes in the rabbit. J. Exp. Med. **134:** 188–200.
19. HUSBAND, A.J. & J.L. GOWANS. 1978. The origin and antigen-dependent distribution of IgA-containing cells in the intestine. J. Exp. Med. **148:** 1146–1160.
20. PIERCE, N.F. & J.L. GOWANS. 1975. Cellular kinetics of the intestinal immune response to cholera toxoid in rats. J. Exp. Med. **142:** 1550–1563.
21. GUY-GRAND, D., C. GRISCELLI & P. VASSALLI. 1978. The mouse gut T lymphocyte, a novel type of T cell. Nature, origin, and traffic in mice in normal and graft-versus-host conditions. J. Exp. Med. **148:** 1661–1677.
22. RENEGAR, K.B. & P.A. SMALL. 1991. Passive transfer of local immunity to influenza-virus infection by IgA antibody. J. Immunol. **146:** 1972–1978.
23. RENEGAR, K.B. & P.A. SMALL, JR. 1991. Immunoglobulin A mediation of murine nasal anti-influenza virus immunity. J. Virol. **65:** 2146–2148.
24. LYCKE, N., L. ERIKSEN & J. HOLMGREN. 1987. Protection against cholera toxin after oral immunisation is thymus dependent and associated with intestinal production of neutralising IgA antitoxin. Scand. J. Immunol. **25:** 413–419.
25. LYCKE, N. *et al.* 1999. Lack of J chain inhibits the transport of gut IgA and abrogates the development of intestinal antitoxic protection. J. Immunol. **163:** 913–919.
26. BURNS, J.W. *et al.* 1996. Protective effect of rotavirus VP6-specific IgA monoclonal antibodies that lack neutralizing activity [see comments]. Science **272:** 104–107.
27. FAGARASAN, S. *et al.* 2002. Critical roles of activation-induced cytidine deaminase in the homeostasis of gut flora. Science **298:** 1424–1427.
28. COFFMAN, R.L., D.A. LEBMAN & B. SHRADER. 1989. Transforming growth factor β specifically enhances IgA production by lipopolysaccharide stimulated murine B lymphocytes. J. Exp. Med. **170:** 1039–1044.
29. KUNIMOTO, D.Y., G.R. HARRIMAN & W. STROBER. 1988. Regulation of IgA differentiation in CH12LX B cells by lymphokines: IL-4 induces membrane IgM-positive CH12LX cells to express membrane IgA and IL-5 induces membrane IgA-positive CH12LX cells to secrete IgA. J. Immunol. **141:** 713–720.
30. BEAGLEY, K.W. *et al.* 1988. Recombinant murine IL-5 induces high rate IgA synthesis in cycling IgA-positive Peyer's patch B cells. J. Immunol. **141:** 2035–2042.
31. KUNIMOTO, D.Y., R.P. NORDAN & W. STROBER. 1989. IL-6 is a potent cofactor of IL-1 in IgM synthesis and of IL-5 in IgA synthesis. J. Immunol. **143:** 2230–2235.
32. DEFRANCE, T. *et al.* 1992. Interleukin 10 and transforming growth factor beta cooperate to induce anti-CD40-activated naive human B cells to secrete immunoglobulin. J. Exp. Med. **175:** 671–682.
33. WEINSTEIN, P.D. & J.J. CEBRA. 1991. The preference for switching to IgA expression by Peyer's patch germinal centre B cells is likely due to the influence of their microenvironment. J. Immunol. **147:** 4126–4135.
34. SCHRADER, C.E. & J.J. CEBRA. 1993. Dendritic cell dependent expression of IgA by clones in T/B microcultures. Adv. Exp. Med. Biol. **329:** 59–64.
35. ELSON, C.O. & W. EALDING. 1984. Cholera toxin feeding did not induce oral tolerance in mice and abrogated oral tolerance to an unrelated protein antigen. J. Immunol. **133:** 2892–2897.
36. ELSON, C.O. & W. EALDING. 1984. Generalized systemic and mucosal immunity in mice after mucosal stimulation with cholera toxin. J. Immunol. **132:** 2736–2741.
37. SNIDER, D.P. *et al.* 1994. Production of IgE antibody and allergic sensitization of intestinal and peripheral tissues after oral immunization with protein Ag and cholera toxin. J. Immunol. **153:** 647–657.

38. GUY-GRAND, D., C. GRISCELLI & P. VASSALLI. 1975. Peyer's patches, gut IgA plasma cells and thymic function: study in nude mice bearing thymic grafts. J. Immunol. **115:** 361–364.
39. HÖRNQUIST, C.E. *et al.* 1995. Paradoxical IgA immunity in CD4-deficient mice. J. Immunol. **155:** 2877–2887.
40. VAJDY, M. *et al.* 1995. Impaired mucosal immune responses in interleukin 4-targeted mice. J. Exp. Med. **181:** 41–53.
41. SNIDER, D.P. *et al.* 1999. IgA production in MHC class II-deficient mice is primarily a function of B-1a cells. Int. Immunol. **11:** 191–198.
42. GARDBY, E., P. LANE & N.Y. LYCKE. 1998. Requirements for B7-CD28 costimulation in mucosal IgA responses: paradoxes observed in CTLA4-H gamma 1 transgenic mice. J. Immunol. **161:** 49–59.
43. MACPHERSON, A.J. *et al.* 2000. A primitive T cell-independent mechanism of intestinal mucosal IgA responses to commensal bacteria. Science **288:** 2222–2226.
44. MACPHERSON, A.J. *et al.* 2001. IgA B cell and IgA antibody production in the absence of mu and delta heavy chain expression early in B cell ontogeny. Nat. Immunol. **2:** 625–631.
45. HAYAKAWA, K. *et al.* 1983. The "Ly-1 B" cell subpopulation in normal immunodefective, and autoimmune mice. J. Exp. Med. **157:** 202–218.
46. HAYAKAWA, K. *et al.* 1984. Ly-1 B cells: functionally distinct lymphocytes that secrete IgM autoantibodies. Proc. Natl. Acad. Sci. USA **81:** 2494–2498.
47. HAYAKAWA, K., R.R. HARDY & L.A. HERZENBERG. 1985. Progenitors for Ly-1 B cells are distinct from progenitors for other B cells. J. Exp. Med. **161:** 1554–1568.
48. HAYAKAWA, K. *et al.* 1986. Immunoglobulin-bearing B cells reconstitute and maintain the murine Ly-1 B cell lineage. Eur. J. Immunol. **16:** 1313–1316.
49. HAYAKAWA, K. & R.R. HARDY. 1988. Normal, autoimmune, and malignant CD5+ B cells: the Ly-1 B lineage? Annu. Rev. Immunol. **6:** 197–218.
50. KROESE, F.G.M. *et al.* 1988. Many of the IgA producing plasma cells in the murine gut are derived from self-replenishing precursors in the peritoneal cavity. Int. Immunol. **1:** 75–84.
51. KROESE, F.G., W.A. AMMERLAAN & A.B. KANTOR. 1993. Evidence that intestinal IgA plasma cells in mu, kappa transgenic mice are derived from B-1 (Ly-1 B) cells. Int. Immunol. **5:** 1317–1327.
52. BOS, N.A. *et al.* 1996. Monoclonal immunoglobulin A derived from peritoneal B cells is encoded by both germ line and somatically mutated VH genes and is reactive with commensal bacteria. Infect. Immun. **64:** 616–623.
53. THURNHEER, M.C. *et al.* 2003. B1 cells contribute to serum IgM but not to intestinal IgA production in gnotobiotic Ig allotype chimeric mice. J. Immunol. **170:** 4564–4571.
54. MACPHERSON, A.J. & T. UHR. 2004. Induction of protective IgA by intestinal dendritic cells carrying commensal bacteria. Science **303:** 1662–1665.
55. SANSONETTI, P. 2001. Phagocytosis of bacterial pathogens: implications in the host response. Semin. Immunol. **13:** 381–390.
56. SHILOH, M.U. *et al.* 1999. Phenotype of mice and macrophages deficient in both phagocyte oxidase and inducible nitric oxide synthase. Immunity **10:** 29–38.
57. HARRIMAN, G.R., *et al.* 1999. Targeted deletion of the IgA constant region in mice leads to IgA deficiency with alterations in expression of other immunoglobulin isotypes. J. Immunol. **162:** 2521–2529.
58. JOHANSEN, F.E. *et al.* 1999. Absence of epithelial immunoglobulin A transport, with increased mucosal leakiness, in polymeric immunoglobulin receptor/secretory component-deficient mice. J. Exp. Med. **190:** 915–922.
59. MACPHERSON, A.J., M.M. MARTINIC & N. HARRIS. 2003. The functions of mucosal T cells in containing the indigenous flora of the intestine. Cell. Mol. Life Sci. **59:** 2088–2096.

Isolated Lymphoid Follicles Can Function as Sites for Induction of Mucosal Immune Responses

ROBIN G. LORENZ[a] AND RODNEY D. NEWBERRY[b]

[a]*Department of Pathology, University of Alabama at Birmingham, Birmingham, Alabama 35294-2170, USA*

[b]*Department of Internal Medicine, Division of Gastroenterology, Washington University School of Medicine, St. Louis, Missouri 63110, USA*

ABSTRACT: Isolated lymphoid follicles (ILFs) are organized lymphoid structures in the small intestine. ILFs were recently identified in the murine small intestine; however, the function of ILFs is unknown. To better understand ILFs and the role they play in the intestinal immune response, we have examined the composition of ILFs, the factors that are involved in the genesis of ILFs, and the ability of ILFs to support antigen-specific immunoglobulin production. We found that ILFs contain predominantly B-2 B lymphocytes, and CD4$^+$ TCRβ$^+$ T lymphocytes. Similar to the formation of Peyer's patches (PPs), lymphotoxin β receptor (LTβR)–dependent events are required for ILF formation; however, the timing of these events and the cellular source of LT differ. ILF formation can occur *de novo* in response to luminal stimuli and requires LT-sufficient B lymphocytes and TNF receptor I function for full maturation. The epithelium over ILFs resembles the PP follicle-associated epithelium, as M cells are present and pathogens such as *Yersinia* can be bound and taken up into the underlying follicle. Total fecal IgA production is not augmented in animals possessing ILFs; however, the production of antigen-specific IgA is increased in animals possessing ILFs orally challenged with *Salmonella typhimurium*. Similar to PPs, ILFs can support antigen-specific IgA production following oral immunization. These findings support the concept that ILFs are formed in response to mucosal challenges, and may play a physiological role in the production of antigen-specific intestinal IgA.

KEYWORDS: gastrointestinal tract; Peyer's patches; murine; follicles; IgA

INTRODUCTION

Traditionally, the gastrointestinal-associated lymphoid tissue (GALT) has been divided into loosely organized effector sites, including the lamina propria (LP) and intraepithelial lymphocytes (IEL), and more structured tissues, such as the Peyer's

Address for correspondence: Robin G. Lorenz, Department of Pathology, University of Alabama at Birmingham, 845 19th Street South BBRB 730, Birmingham, AL 35294-2170. Voice: 205-934-0676; fax: 205-975-8310.
 rlorenz@uab.edu

patches (PPs), which have been assigned an induction function.[1] The loosely organized LP is mainly composed of CD4$^+$ T cells and IgA-producing plasma cells, while the IEL compartment is primarily CD8$^+$ T cells. The exact functions of either of these compartments are still under investigation; however, they do contain T cells with a "memory" surface phenotype, and the cells have recently been reported to have a regulatory phenotype.[2] Trafficking of cells into these effector sites is directed by the adhesion molecule pair α4β7:MAD-CAM1 and the chemokine-receptor pair CCL25(TECK):CCR9. A third effector site is the lymphocyte-filled villi (LFV), which has been only characterized in humans and is primarily composed of memory T cells, with a limited B cell contribution (TABLE 1).[3] It has been suggested that these structures function in antigen presentation to memory T cells; however, there has been no direct investigation of either their function or their developmental requirements. The small intestine can also function as a primary lymphoid organ supporting the extrathymic development of T lymphocytes. This primary lymphoid organ function is attributed to a structure found at the base of intestinal crypts, known as a cryptopatch (CP) (TABLE 1).[4–6] These structures are the developmental site of progenitor T cells for extrathymic IEL descendants and require the interaction of CD25(TECK) and CCR9 for their formation.[7]

The most widely studied lymphoid structure found in the small intestine is the PPs. PPs are secondary lymphoid structures, and their development has been extensively investigated. PP development shares with other secondary lymphoid structures the requirements for lymphotoxin (LT)α$_1$β$_2$, LTβR, and CXCR5.[8–10] PP development is also dependent upon interleukin (IL)-7 and IL-7R, and recent evidence suggests that this requirement may extend to other secondary lymphoid structural development as well.[11–13] The LT/LTβR and IL-7/IL-7R interactions necessary for PP formation occur prior to birth, but complete PP development also requires subsequent exposure to bacterial flora.[8,14,15] The requirements for the development of PPs, and other secondary lymphoid structures, form the basis for identifying and categorizing PP and ILFs.

PPs can be seen without the aid of a microscope in the submucosa of the small intestine. Depending on the strain of mouse analyzed, the average number of PPs per small intestine ranges from six to ten.[16] A PP is a collection of multiple large B cell follicles with intervening T cell areas. This organization of lymphocytes is covered by a layer of intestinal epithelial cells known as the follicle-associated epithelium (FAE). This FAE is noted for the presence of microfold (M) cells, which are specialized transport cells that are known to bind pathogens such as reovirus, HIV, *Salmonella*, and *Yersinia*.[17,18] It is still controversial whether M cells and PPs are essential for mucosal immune responses and tolerance to luminal antigens. Early work with soluble antigens implied that PPs were not essential for local intestinal antibody responses to KLH; however, recent work with the bacteria *Salmonella* demonstrated a need for entry via FAE and M cells for the stimulation of specific mucosal IgA.[19,20] Oral tolerance to protein antigens such as ovalbumin has been reported to either require PPs or to occur in the absence of PPs, depending on the study.[21–23] For these experiments, mice lacking PPs were generated by *in utero* treatment with LTβR-Ig or anti-IL-7Rα. As recent publications show, these treatments do not block the development of isolated lymphoid follicles (ILFs), only the development of PPs.[24,25] Therefore, part of the confusion over the role of M cells and PPs in mucosal immune responses may be due to the unappreciated presence of ILFs.

TABLE 1. Lymphocyte-containing structures in the intestine

Structure	Cellular Composition	Type of Lymphoid Structure	Location	Appearance	Developmental Requirements
Loosely Organized Gastrointestinal Lymphoid Tissue					
Lamina propria	Plasma cells T cells (60% CD4$^+$; 40% CD8$^+$)	Tertiary	Stroma between intestinal villi	Loosely structured	$\alpha_4\beta_7$/MAD-CAM1 CCL25 (TECK) / CCR9
Intraepithelial compartment	T cells (40% CD8$\alpha\beta^+$; 60% CD8$\alpha\alpha^+$)	Tertiary	Above the epithelial basement membrane throughout the small intestine	Scattered isolated cells	IL-7 CD103
Lymphocyte-filled villus (human)	Memory T cells	Tertiary	Stroma between intestinal villi in the jejunum	Fat villus	ND^a
Structured Gastrointestinal Lymphoid Tissue					
Peyer's patch	B cells (60%) T cells (35%)	Secondary	Antimesenteric border, distal>proximal	Multiple domes (3 or more)	$LT\alpha_1\beta_2$ (CD3$^-$CD4$^+$ cell) IL-7 CXCR5 $LT\beta R$
Cryptopatches	T cells and T cell precursors (few/no B cells)	Primary	Base of villi throughout the small intestine	Collection of cells at the base of a crypt	CCL25 (TECK) / CCR9
Isolated lymphoid follicle	B cells (B220$^+$), few T cells	Tertiary	Distal>proximal	1–2 domes	$LT\beta R$ TNFRI $LT\alpha_1\beta_2$ (B cell)

^{a}ND, not determined

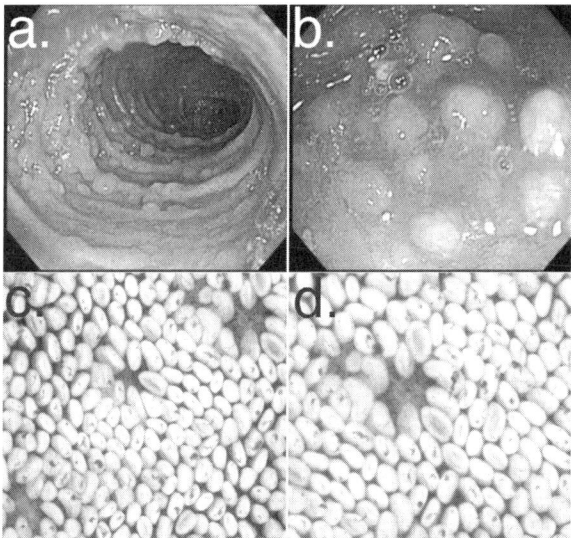

FIGURE 1. Isolated lymphoid aggregates are present in humans and mice. Isolated lymphoid aggregates are present in the terminal ileum of normal individuals undergoing endoscopy (panels **a** and **b**). Analogous structures can be seen on whole mounts of the distal small intestine of unmanipulated Balb/c mice (panels **c** and **d**). Original magnification 25×.

Lymphoid aggregates resembling a single dome of a PP have been described in humans and can be seen on endoscopic examination of the small intestine (FIG. 1a and b). These aggregates have been assumed to represent a solitary follicular unit similar to that found in PPs.[26] These lymphoid aggregates are hypertrophied in patients with increased colonization of the small intestine, and this hyperplasia can be replicated in mouse models with expansion of anaerobic flora.[26] Isolated lymphoid aggregates resembling a single dome of a PP have also been described in normal murine small intestines (FIG. 1c and d).[25] These structures have both germinal centers and an overlying FAE, suggesting that they can function as inductive sites for the mucosal immune response (FIG. 2).[24]

Whether isolated lymphoid aggregates represented single-domed PPs or distinct structures was unclear until recently. To better understand the differences between these isolated lymphoid aggregates and PPs, we have studied the nature and factors required for isolated lymphoid aggregate formation.[24] We have found distinct differences between the formation of PPs and some isolated lymphoid aggregates, which we will term ILFs. We recognize that in humans, and in some mouse strains, not all isolated lymphoid aggregates may be formed in the same manner as ILFs, and may in fact represent single-domed PPs. For this reason, we have limited our investigations involving the formation and function of ILFs to the C57BL/6 mouse strain, which does not spontaneously form isolated lymphoid aggregates. Therefore, isolated lymphoid aggregates formed in this animal strain represent inducible lymphoid aggregates, as opposed to single-domed PPs.

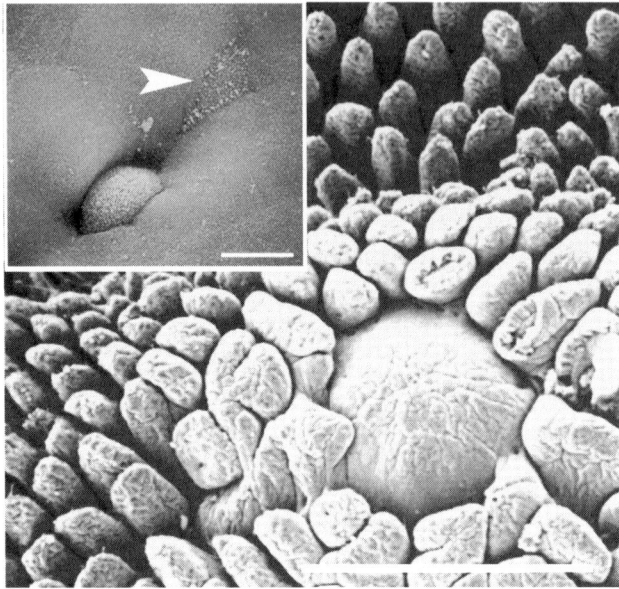

FIGURE 2. Follicular-associated epithelium and M cells overlie isolated lymphoid follicles. Intestines from C57BL/6 mice receiving LTβR-Ig *in utero* to block PP formation were examined by scanning electron microscopy as previously described.[24] The epithelium overlying mILFs contain a FAE with cells fitting the morphologic criteria of M cells. Scale bars: 500 μm; inset, 5 μm.

We have observed a range of structures that fit the published descriptions of ILFs, including immature ILFs (iILFs), which are clusters of $B220^+$ cells, as well as completely organized lymphoid nodules, or mature ILFs (mILFs) that are similar to nodules found in Peyer's patches. In the C57BL/6 mouse strain we have designated PPs as consisting of three or more similar-sized lymphoid nodules grouped together, and mILF as consisting of a single nodule or two nodules of differing size. We have found that these designations can accurately differentiate between PPs and mILF in this mouse strain, as all lymphoid aggregates induced by the ablation of PPs or by the adoptive transfer of wild type bone marrow to $LT\alpha^{-/-}$ mice fit the above description of mILF, and mILF are rare or absent in untreated C57BL/6 mice. The requirements for formation of ILFs are similar in some ways to PP formation, in that LT and LTβR are essential. However, in contrast to PP formation, these events can occur in adulthood and require LT-sufficient B lymphocytes and tumor necrosis factor (TNF)-RI function. Given our findings, we feel ILFs are tertiary lymphoid structures that can be formed in response to lumenal stimuli, including normal flora.

In considering these results, there are several questions left unanswered. First, it is still unclear whether these ILFs are pathologic structures or whether they perform physiologic functions. The formation of tertiary lymphoid structures occurs in many chronic inflammatory and autoimmune conditions, including rheumatoid arthritis,

Sjogren's syndrome, primary sclerosing cholangitis, chronic hepatitis C infection, myasthenia gravis, multiple sclerosis, Hashimoto's thyroiditis, and *Helicobacter pylori* gastritis.[27,28] The function of these tertiary lymphoid structures is unclear, but they have been suggested to provide local sites for interactions between lymphocytes, antigens, and antigen-presenting cells. It has also been suggested that these tertiary lymphoid structures contribute to the formation of autoreactive and neoplastic lymphocytes, as the regulatory mechanisms normally present in lymph nodes are absent.[27] This may explain the association of *de novo* formation of tertiary lymphoid structures with conditions having autoimmune features and increased neoplastic potential. Another observation is that the number of ILFs varies widely between different inbred murine strains, even when raised in identical SPF animal facilities. This variation raises further questions: What is controlling the number of ILFs? and What triggers the increase in ILF formation in the absence of PPs? This manuscript addresses these questions.

MATERIALS AND METHODS

Mice

All mice used for this study were housed in a specific pathogen-free facility and fed routine chow diet. Animal procedures and protocols were carried out in accordance with the institutional review board at Washington University School of Medicine. Balb/c, SJL, C3H/SnJ, C57BL/6, and JH deficient mice on the C57BL/6 background were purchased from The Jackson Laboratory, Bar Harbor, Maine.[29] LTα-deficient mice, a gift from Dr. D. Chaplin, were bred onto the C57BL/6 background for greater than 10 generations prior to use in experiments.[30] Treatment of C57BL/6 mice with LTβR-Ig *in utero* to ablate PP formation was performed as previously described.[24,31]

Infection with Salmonella and Assessment of Antigen-Specific Fecal IgA Production

Wild-type *Salmonella typhimurium* strain 14028 carrying the puc18 vector to confer antibiotic resistance (gift from Dr. J. Pfeiffer, Washington University School of Medicine, St. Louis, MO) were cultured overnight at 37°C in Luria-Bertani broth containing ampicillin. A dose of 5×10^5 live organisms, as determined by counting using a Petroff-Hausser counter (Hausser Scientific, Horsham, PA), was administered orally to mice at four-week intervals. Mice were given ampicillin 0.06 mg/mL in drinking water for the duration of the experiment. Feces were collected from infected animals, and fecal supernatants were extracted as previously described.[31] Fecal supernatants diluted in PBS containing 0.05% Tween-20 (Sigma-Aldrich, St. Louis, MO) were incubated in 96-well Immulon 4 plates (Fisher Scientific, Pittsburgh, PA) previously coated with 10 μg/mL protein extract from sonicated *Salmonella typhimurium* strain 14028 and blocked with PBS containing 5% bovine serum albumin and 0.05% Tween-20 at room temperature for two hours. Plates were washed three times with PBS containing 0.05% Tween-20, then goat anti-mouse IgA alkaline phosphatase-conjugated antibody (Southern Biotechnology Associates,

Inc., Birmingham, AL) diluted in PBS containing 5% bovine serum albumin, and 0.05% Tween-20 was added to the plate and incubated for two hours at room temperature. Plates were washed three times with PBS containing 0.05% Tween-20, and *p*-nitrophenyl phosphate alkaline phosphatase substrate (Sigma-Aldrich) was added. Plates were read at 405 nm using Bio-Tek Instruments Microplate Reader (Winooski, VT). Each sample was measured in duplicate; data shown is the mean absolute OD at 405 nm.

Infection with Yersinia

Yersinia enterocolitica strain JB580v, a restriction-minus derivative of a virulent American strain 8081v, serogroup O:8 Nal^r,[32] (a kind gift from V. Miller, Washington University, St. Louis, MO), was grown at 26°C overnight with aeration in Luria-Bertani (LB) broth, or on LB agar plates supplemented with 20 µg/mL nalidixic acid (Sigma-Aldrich). Mice were orally infected with 0.1 mL bacteria (infectious dose = 5×10^8 as determined from serial dilutions of the starting culture) via a 21-gauge feeding tube attached to a 1.0 mL syringe. Tissues were collected 24 hours postinfection. Detection of *Y. enterocolitica* within the tissues of infected mice was performed using the avidin-biotin complex procedure as previously described.[33]

Oral Immunization with Sheep Red Blood Cells and Determination of Antigen-Specific IgA Production

C57BL/6 mice were used as a source for PP cellular populations. C57BL/6 mice receiving 100 µg of LTβR-Ig *in utero* to block PP formation were used as a source of mILF cellular populations as previously described.[24] Sheep red blood cells (Colorado Serum Company, Denver Colorado) were washed three times in PBS, and 4×10^9 sRBC or vehicle (PBS) was administered to mice by gavage following an overnight fast on two consecutive days. Two days later, mice were sacrificed and PPs or ILF cellular populations were isolated as previously described.[24] PP and ILF cellular populations were cultured in 96-well plates at a density of 2×10^6 cells/mL in RPMI 1640 media (BioWhittaker, Walkersville, MD) containing 10% fetal calf serum (Hyclone, Logan, UT), 2 mM Glutamax I (Gibco Life Technologies, Grand Island, NY), 10 mM HEPES (BioWhittaker), 1 mM sodium pyruvate (BioWhittaker), 50 U/mL penicillin–50 mg/mL streptomycin (Gibco Life Technologies), and 50 mM 2-mercaptoethanol (Fisher Scientific) at 37°C and 5% CO_2. Four days later, supernatants were removed and anti-sRBC antibody production was measured as previously described.[34]

All other methods were performed as previously described.[24,31]

RESULTS AND DISCUSSION

Composition of Peyer's Patches and Mature Isolated Lymphoid Follicles

Using flow cytometric analysis, we demonstrated that like PPs, mILFs contain predominantly IgA-negative B-2 ($CD19^+$, $CD11b^-$) B lymphocytes and a smaller population of $CD4^+TCR\beta^+$ T lymphocytes (TABLE 2).[24] The majority of antigen-pre-

TABLE 2. Cellular Composition of mILFs[a]

Cell Type	Cell Surface Markers[b]		
B cells	CD19$^+$	CD19$^+$, IgA$^+$	CD19$^+$, CD11b$^+$
	75%	1%	2%
T cells	TCRβ$^+$	TCRβ$^+$, CD4$^+$	TCRβ$^+$, CD8α$^+$
	15%	12%	3%
APCs	MHCII$^+$, CD19$^-$	MHCII$^+$, CD11c$^+$	MHCII$^+$, F480$^+$
	12%	10%	2%

[a]mILF cellular populations isolated from C57Bl/6 mice that received LTβR-Ig *in utero* to block PP formation.

[b]Flow cytometric analysis compiled from authors' observations and previously published data.[24] Data expressed as percentage of the viable cell population as determined by forward and side scatter. Gates for positive staining were set such that 1% of the examined population stained positive with isotype control antibodies.

senting cells found in mILFs appear to be conventional dendritic cells (CD11c$^+$), although a small population of macrophages (F4/80$^+$) is also present. It has recently been shown that the dendritic cells found in classical PPs are critical in the imprinting of small intestinal lamina propria–homing T cells.[35] These structures are also essential for initiating murine acute and lethal graft-versus-host reactions.[36] However, structures such as PP or mILFs are not necessary for the proper homing and composition of the IEL compartment, as demonstrated by the normal IEL cell populations in LTα$^{-/-}$ (data not shown) and aly/aly mice.[37]

The Presence of ILFs in Different Mouse Strains

The physiologic role of ILFs has been questioned due to the presence of few to no ILFs in normal C57BL/6 small intestines. In order to address this question, we investigated the number of mILFs in several inbred mouse strains. As shown in FIGURE 3b, mouse strains other than C57BL/6, such as SJL, C3H/HeSnJ, and Balb/c, have numerous mILFs without any experimental manipulation. The distribution of these ILFs in Balb/c mice is slightly altered from what we previously described for C57BL/6 mice. In C57BL/6 mice, the formation of mILFs can be induced and are predominantly located in the distal small intestine and randomly oriented with respect for the mesenteric border. However, in Balb/c mice, mILFs occur spontaneously, are larger, are found preferentially on the antimesenteric border, and are distributed more proximally. Intriguingly, there appears to be an inverse relationship between the number of mILFs and the number of B220$^+$ clusters (immature ILFs) present: the C57BL/6 strain has few mILFs and numerous B220$^+$ clusters, whereas the Balb/c strain has numerous ILFs and few B220$^+$ clusters (FIG. 3).

In interpreting the differences in the numbers of mILFs in various mouse strains, it is important to note that the designation used to identify mILFs was developed in C57BL/6 mice, and may not be applicable to all mouse strains; some single-domed lymphoid aggregates in other strains may be PPs. We have previously demonstrated

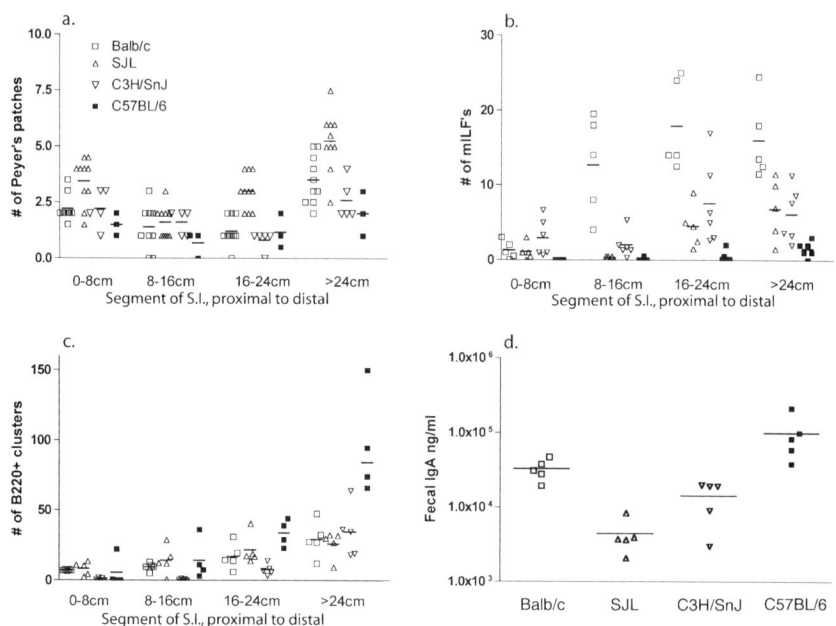

FIGURE 3. IgA levels and lymphoid nodules in inbred mouse strains. Intestines from untreated Balb/c (*open squares*), SJL (*open triangles*), C3H/HeSnJ (*open inverted triangles*), and C57BL/6 (*closed squares*) mice were examined as whole mounts (**a**, **b**), by a modified whole mount technique (**c**), or by analysis of fecal IgA levels (**d**), as previously described.[24,31] All mouse strains examined have a small range of numbers of PPs, but differ dramatically in the number of mILFs and immature ILFs ($B220^+$ clusters). There is an inverse ratio between the number of mILFs and immature ILFs, and between the number of mILFs and the total amount of fecal IgA.

that mILFs can be induced in response to luminal stimuli, and we have postulated that this may be an attempt to compensate for the absence of PPs and PP functions, such as fecal IgA production.[24] In support of this hypothesis, we observed that Balb/c mice have significantly lower total fecal IgA levels when compared with C57BL/6 mice ($P<.05$, FIG. 3d). These observations suggest that loss of the protective effects of fecal IgA may promote an inflammatory response to luminal stimuli, leading to the formation of mILFs and induction of the mucosal immune response. Consistent with this hypothesis is the recent description of a novel IgA receptor on murine PP M cells that mediates the transepithelial transport of secretory IgA from the intestinal lumen to the underlying lymphoid nodule.[38] Also supporting this hypothesis is the observation that some patients with common variable immunodeficiency syndrome have nodular lymphoid hyperplasia in their gastrointestinal tract.[39] However, it should be emphasized that based upon our previously published observations, ILFs (and PPs) are not essential for the production of total fecal IgA, but as we demonstrate below, mILFs may act as inductive sites for antigen-specific mucosal immune responses.[24] A potential explanation for these seemingly contradictory observations is that the fecal IgA may arise from two sources, B-1 and B-2 B lymphocytes. B-2 B lymphocytes are dependent upon interactions in organized lymphoid structures for their maturation, while B-1 B lymphocytes are not. It is possible that in the absence of organized lymphoid structures there is a compensatory increase in the fecal IgA production by the B-1 B lymphocyte pool, thus diminishing differences in total fecal IgA levels produced in the presence and absence of organized lymphoid structures. Consistent with this hypothesis, we observed diminished, but not significantly different, total fecal IgA levels in mice lacking PP, lymph nodes (LN), and ILFs when compared with mice lacking PPs and LN, but possessing ILFs.[31]

Function of Mature Isolated Lymphoid Follicles

PPs are believed to be the primary site for the induction of antigen-specific mucosal immune responses in the small intestine. *Salmonella typhimurium*, the causative agent of murine typhoid fever, and *Yersinia enterocolitica* selectively adhere to and use M cells in the FAE as portals of entry into the host.[40,41] Based upon the presence of germinal centers in ILFs and an overlying FAE containing M cells, it appears that ILFs have the potential to function as inductive sites for the mucosal immune response. In order to assess the potential of ILFs to act as inductive sites for mucosal immune responses, we infected $LT\alpha^{-/-}$ recipients of C57BL/6 bone marrow as well as $LT\alpha^{-/-}$ recipients of a combined $JH^{-/-}$ and $LT\alpha^{-/-}$ bone marrow. Both groups of

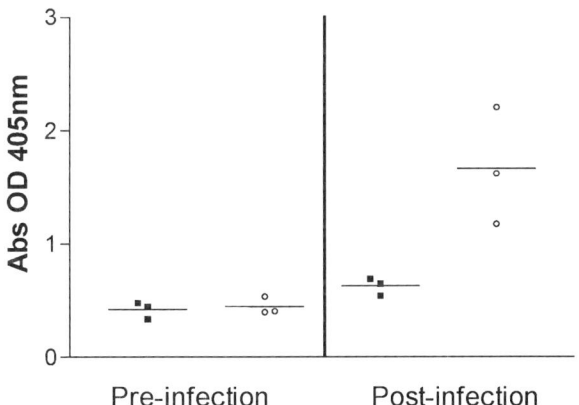

FIGURE 4. mILFs can act as inductive sites for antigen-specific mucosal immune responses. $LT\alpha^{-/-}$ mice reconstituted with a combination of $JH^{-/-}$ and $LT\alpha^{-/-}$ bone marrow (*filled squares*) and $LT\alpha^{-/-}$ mice reconstituted with C57BL/6 bone marrow (*open circles*) were infected with wild-type *Salmonella typhimurium* as described in MATERIALS AND METHODS. Feces were collected prior to infection and 8 weeks following the initial infection, and fecal IgA specific for *S. typhimurium* was detected as described in MATERIALS AND METHODS. Recipients of a combination of $JH^{-/-}$ and $LT\alpha^{-/-}$ bone marrow (lacking PPs, LN, and ILFs) did not produce *Salmonella*-specific fecal IgA, whereas recipients of C57BL/6 bone marrow (lacking PPs and LN, but possessing ILFs) produced *Salmonella*-specific fecal IgA. These findings document that ILFs, like PPs, can act as inductive sites for antigen-specific mucosal immune responses.

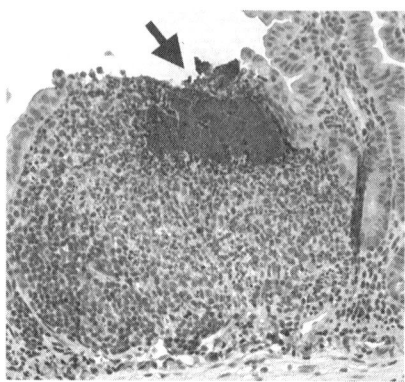

FIGURE 5. *Yersinia enterocolitica* invasion of mILFs. Intestines from C57BL/6 mice that received LTβR-Ig *in utero* to block PP formation were removed 24 hours after oral infection with 5×10^8 *Y. enterocolitica* strain JB580v. Intestine sections were prepared and stained for the presence of *Y. enterocolitica* as previously described.[24,33] The arrow indicates the site of *Y. enterocolitica* invasion of an ILF. Original magnification 200×.

mice lack PPs and LN and produce comparable levels of total fecal IgA.[31] Following the infection with wild-type *Salmonella* we observed the production of antigen-specific fecal IgA in $LT\alpha^{-/-}$ mice receiving C57BL/6 bone marrow (possessing mILFs but lacking PP and LN) (FIG. 4). $LT\alpha^{-/-}$ recipients of combined $JH^{-/-}$ and $LT\alpha^{-/-}$ bone marrow (lacking mILFs, PPs, and LN) did not produce detectable antigen-specific fecal IgA.

These observations suggest that mILFs, like PPs, can act as inductive sites for antigen-specific mucosal immune responses. Additional support for the involvement of mILFs in the mucosal immune response to luminal bacteria is shown in FIGURE 5. The initial site of *Y. enterocolitica* infection has been shown to be the PPs. To gain entry to the PPs, the bacteria must first bind to and then cross the specialized intestinal epithelial cell, the M cell, that overlies the PPs. The binding and translocation event is mediated by the bacterial invasin protein (Inv).[33] Therefore, we determined whether *Y. enterocolitic* invasion in C57BL/6 mice receiving LTβR-Ig *in utero* could occur via the FAE and M cells of mILFs. After a 24-hour oral infection, *Y. enterocolitica* specifically localizes to mILFs, indicating that similar to the FAE of PPs, the FAE of mILFs can function as a site for *Y. enterocolitica* invasion.

In addition to their role in the formation of ILFs, both LT and TNFR-I are required for the formation of clusters of follicular dendritic cells (FDC) within the primary and secondary follicles of the spleen white pulp.[34] FDC clusters are critical to the formation of germinal centers in the spleen and other secondary lymphoid structures, and are required for the mature isotype-switched Ig response after immunization with T cell–dependent antigens, such as sheep RBCs (sRBCs), when administered without adjuvants. Therefore, in order to determine whether mILFs contained functional FDC clusters and germinal centers, we immunized C57BL/6 mice (PP source) or C57BL/6 mice that had been treated with 100 μg of LTβR-Ig *in utero* (ILF source) with sRBC and measured the ability of cells isolated from the PPs or the

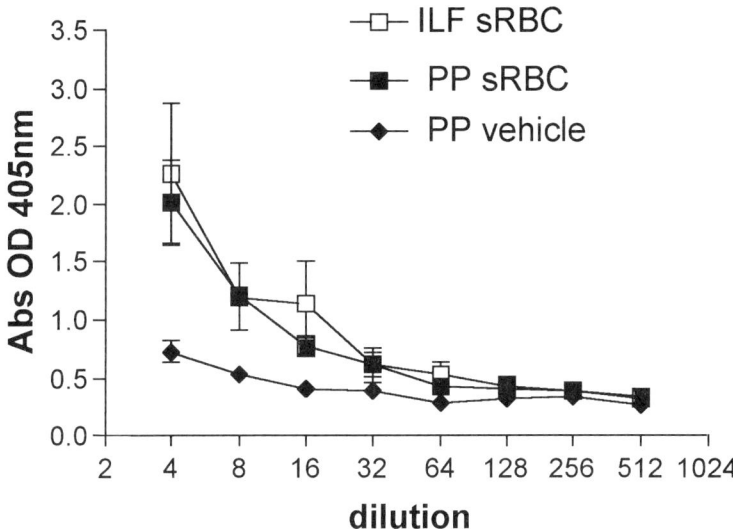

FIGURE 6. Antigen-specific IgA production by Peyer's patch and mILF cellular populations following oral immunization. C57BL/6 mice (source of Peyer's patch cells) and C57BL/6 mice that received 100 μg of LTβR-Ig *in utero* to block Peyer's patch formation (source of mILF cells) were administered sheep red blood cells (sRBC) or vehicle by gavage as described in MATERIALS AND METHODS. Peyer's patch and mILF cellular populations were isolated and cultured with sRBC and the supernatants assayed for IgA anti-sRBC antibody production. mILF and Peyer's patch cellular populations from mice given sRBC demonstrated antigen-specific IgA production when compared to mice given vehicle alone. Supernatants were measured in duplicate at each dilution, and results are displayed as the mean OD ± SEM.

mILF to produce sRBC-specific, isotype-switched IgA. As shown in FIGURE 6, both PP cells and mILF cells were able to produce a specific IgA response to sRBC. This result implies that not only can mILFs bind and respond to pathogenic bacteria, but they also can develop fully functional germinal centers and participate fully as inductive immune sites. Therefore, in conclusion, mILFs are organized tertiary lymphoid structures that are formed in response to mucosal challenges and can function as sites of induction of the mucosal immune response.

ACKNOWLEDGMENTS

This work was supported by NIH Grants DK59911, DK02608, and DK60648; by RPG-99-086 from the American Cancer Society; by IBD-0042 from the Broad Medical Research Program; by the University of Alabama at Birmingham Digestive Diseases Research Development Centers Grant DK064400; and by Washington University School of Medicine Digestive Disease Research Core Center Grant DK52574. We would like to thank Virginia Miller and Scott Handley at Washington University School of Medicine, St. Louis, MO for technical support and discussions regarding the *Y. enterocolitica* system, and Jacquie McDonough and Keely McDonald for expert technical assistance.

REFERENCES

1. MOWAT, A.M. 2003. Anatomical basis of tolerance and immunity to intestinal antigens. Nat. Rev. Immunol. **3:** 331–341.
2. CONG, Y. *et al.* 2002. Bacterial-reactive T regulatory cells inhibit pathogenic immune responses to the enteric flora. J. Immunol. **169:** 6112–6119.
3. MOGHADDAMI, M., A. CUMMINS & G. MAYRHOFER. 1998. Lymphocyte-filled villi: comparison with other lymphoid aggregations in the mucosa of the human small intestine. Gastroenterology **115:** 1414–1425.
4. OIDA, T. *et al.* 2000. Role of gut cryptopatches in early extrathymic maturation of intestinal intraepithelial T cells. J. Immunol. **164:** 3616–3626.
5. SAITO, H. *et al.* 1998. Generation of intestinal T cells from progenitors residing in gut cryptopatches. Science **280:** 275–278.
6. SUZUKI, K. *et al.* 2000. Gut cryptopatches. Direct evidence of extrathymic anatomical sites for intestinal T lymphopoiesis. Immunity **13:** 691–702.
7. ONAI, N. *et al.* 2002. Pivotal role of CCL25 (TECK)-CCR9 in the formation of gut cryptopatches and consequent appearance of intestinal intraepithelial T lymphocytes. Int. Immunol. **14:** 687–694.
8. RENNERT, P.D. *et al.* 1996. Surface lymphotoxin alpha/beta complex is required for the development of peripheral lymphoid organs. J. Exp. Med. **184:** 1999–2006.
9. ANSEL, K.M. *et al.* 2000. A chemokine-driven positive feedback loop organizes lymphoid follicles. Nature **406:** 309–314.
10. CUPEDO, T., G. KRAAL & R.E. MEBIUS. 2002. The role of $CD45^+CD4^+CD3^-$ cells in lymphoid organ development. Immunol. Rev. **189:** 41–50.
11. YOSHIDA, H. *et al.* 1999. IL-7 receptor alpha+ CD3(–) cells in the embryonic intestine induces the organizing center of Peyer's patches. Int. Immunol. **11:** 643–655.
12. FINKE, D. & J.P. KRAEHENBUHL. 2001. Formation of Peyer's patches. Curr. Opin. Genet. Dev. **11:** 561–567.
13. LUTHER, S.A., K.M. ANSEL & J.G. CYSTER. 2003. Overlapping roles of CXCL13, interleukin 7 receptor alpha, and CCR7 ligands in lymph node development. J. Exp. Med. **197:** 1191–1198.
14. WOSTMANN, B.S. 1996. Germfree and gnotobiotic animal models: background and applications. CRC Press. Boca Raton.
15. MCCRACKEN, V.J. & R.G. LORENZ. 2001. The gastrointestinal ecosystem: a precarious alliance among epithelium, immunity and microbiota. Cell. Microbiol. **3:** 1–11.
16. GOLOVKINA, T.V. *et al.* 1999. Organogenic role of B lymphocytes in mucosal immunity. Science **286:** 1965–1968.
17. NEUTRA, M.R., E. PRINGAULT & J.P. KRAEHENBUHL. 1996. Antigen sampling across epithelial barriers and induction of mucosal immune responses. Annu. Rev. Immunol. **14:** 275–300.
18. KRAEHENBUHL, J.P. & M.R. NEUTRA. 2000. Epithelial M cells: differentiation and function. Annu. Rev. Cell. Dev. Biol. **16:** 301–332.
19. VAZQUEZ-TORRES, A. *et al.* 1999. Extraintestinal dissemination of Salmonella by CD18-expressing phagocytes. Nature **401:** 804–808.
20. HAMILTON, S.R. *et al.* 1981. No impairment of local intestinal immune response to keyhole limpet haemocyanin in the absence of Peyer's patches. Immunology **42:** 431–435.
21. FUJIHASHI, K. *et al.* 2001. Peyer's patches are required for oral tolerance to proteins. Proc. Natl. Acad. Sci. USA **98:** 3310–3315.
22. SPAHN, T.W. *et al.* 2002. Mesenteric lymph nodes are critical for the induction of high-dose oral tolerance in the absence of Peyer's patches. Eur. J. Immunol. **32:** 1109–1113.
23. KUNKEL, D. *et al.* 2003. Visualization of peptide presentation following oral application of antigen in normal and Peyer's patches-deficient mice. Eur. J. Immunol. **33:** 1292–1301.

24. LORENZ, R.G. et al. 2003. Isolated lymphoid follicle formation is inducible and dependent upon lymphotoxin-sufficient B lymphocytes, lymphotoxin beta receptor, and TNF receptor I function. J. Immunol. **170:** 5475–5482.
25. HAMADA, H. et al. 2002. Identification of multiple isolated lymphoid follicles on the antimesenteric wall of the mouse small intestine. J. Immunol. **168:** 57–64.
26. FAGARASAN, S. et al. 2002. Critical roles of activation-induced cytidine deaminase in the homeostasis of gut flora. Science **298:** 1424–1427.
27. HJELMSTROM, P. 2001. Lymphoid neogenesis: de novo formation of lymphoid tissue in chronic inflammation through expression of homing chemokines. J. Leukoc. Biol. **69:** 331–339.
28. GRANT, A.J. et al. 2002. Hepatic expression of secondary lymphoid chemokine (CCL21) promotes the development of portal-associated lymphoid tissue in chronic inflammatory liver disease. Am. J. Pathol. **160:** 1445–1455.
29. GU, H., Y.R. ZOU & K. RAJEWSKY. 1993. Independent control of immunoglobulin switch recombination at individual switch regions evidenced through Cre-lox P-mediated gene targeting. Cell **73:** 1155–1164.
30. DE TOGNI, P. et al. 1994. Abnormal development of peripheral lymphoid organs in mice deficient in lymphotoxin. Science **264:** 703–707.
31. NEWBERRY, R.D. et al. 2002. Postgestational lymphotoxin/lymphotoxin beta receptor interactions are essential for the presence of intestinal B lymphocytes. J. Immunol. **168:** 4988–4997.
32. KINDER, S.A. et al. 1993. Cloning of the YenI restriction endonuclease and methyltransferase from Yersinia enterocolitica serotype O8 and construction of a transformable R-M+ mutant. Gene **136:** 271–275.
33. DUBE, P.H. et al. 2003. The rovA mutant of Yersinia enterocolitica displays differential degrees of virulence depending on the route of infection. Infect. Immun. **71:** 3512–3520.
34. FU, Y.X. et al. 1998. B lymphocytes induce the formation of follicular dendritic cell clusters in a lymphotoxin alpha-dependent fashion. J. Exp. Med. **187:** 1009–1018.
35. MORA, J.R. et al. 2003. Selective imprinting of gut-homing T cells by Peyer's patch dendritic cells. Nature **424:** 88–93.
36. MURAI, M. et al. 2003. Peyer's patch is the essential site in initiating murine acute and lethal graft-versus-host reaction. Nat. Immunol. **4:** 154–160.
37. NANNO, M. et al. 1994. Development of intestinal intraepithelial T lymphocytes is independent of Peyer's patches and lymph nodes in aly mutant mice. J. Immunol. **153:** 2014–2020.
38. MANTIS, N.J. et al. 2002. Selective adherence of IgA to murine Peyer's patch M cells: evidence for a novel IgA receptor. J. Immunol. **169:** 1844–1851.
39. BASTLEIN, C. et al. 1988. Common variable immunodeficiency syndrome and nodular lymphoid hyperplasia in the small intestine. Endoscopy **20:** 272–275.
40. DUBE, P.H., P.A. REVELL, D.D. CHAPLIN, et al. 2001. A role for IL-1 alpha in inducing pathologic inflammation during bacterial infection. Proc. Natl. Acad. Sci. USA **98:** 10880–10885.
41. NEUTRA, M.R., A. FREY & J.P. KRAEHENBUHL. 1996. Epithelial M cells: gateways for mucosal infection and immunization. Cell **86:** 345–348.

Anatomy and Physiology
Summary of Part I

JIRI MESTECKY

Departments of Microbiology and Medicine, University of Alabama at Birmingham, Birmingham, Alabama 35294-2170, USA

The type of response—mucosal and systemic immunity versus tolerance—induced as a consequence of the exposure of mucosa-associated lymphoepithelial structures to abundant food and microbial antigens depends on many factors. On the side of stimulation, the type of antigen, its form (soluble versus particulate), low versus high dose, commensal versus pathogenic bacterium, and longevity of the exposure profoundly influence the interactions with various populations of host mucosal cells and the ensuing type of immune responses.

Papers presented in this session by Drs. Garside, Kraehenbuhl, Mayer, Macpherson, Lorenz, and their coworkers addressed essential questions concerning these points. Specifically, the organization of lymphoepithelial structures of mucosal tissues, particularly in the intestinal tract, their cellular compositions, and intercellular ligand/receptor-mediated communications play a decisive role in the outcome of the response. In addition to the extensively studied Peyer's patches (PPs) with their characteristic localization, cellular composition, and function, isolated lymphoid follicles (ILFs) complement and extend or even substitute for the PP function as a mucosal inductive site, particularly with respect to the humoral, IgA-mediated responses induced by oral immunization with gram-negative intestinal bacteria. Thus, the absence of PPs in certain mouse strains does not seem to significantly compromise the quality and magnitude of humoral immune responses.

The potential participation of ILFs in the induction of mucosal tolerance has not been investigated. Furthermore, there may be important species and even mouse strain-dependent differences in the presence and function of PPs and ILFs that should be considered in the generalization and unbiased interpretation of results. Nevertheless, it is becoming quite clear that mucosal tissues with associated lymphoepithelial structures and unique cellular composition, such as PPs, ILFs, intestinal cryptopatches, as well as loosely organized structures in the lamina propria, intraepithelial compartment, and villi, independently or in concert fulfill their basic mission—induction of IgA-dominated humoral responses that restrict further antigen uptake, and at the same time induce a state of mucosal tolerance by various mechanisms (clonal anergy, deletion, or stimulation of various populations of immunoregulatory T cells).

Address for correspondence: Jiri Mestecky, Departments of Microbiology and Medicine, University of Alabama at Birmingham, 845 19th Street South, Birmingham, Alabama 35294-2170. Voice: 205-934-2225; fax: 205-934-3894.
  mestecky@uab.edu

Studies of the mechanisms involved in the induction (by commensal or pathogenic microbiota) and regulation (by T cells) of mucosal (IgA) and systemic (IgG) humoral responses have generated stimulating results. It appears that, at least in the murine model, secretory IgA responses against commensals are induced by both T cell–dependent or –independent pathways, while responses to pathogens and their products (such as cholera toxin) are strictly T cell dependent. Furthermore, commensal bacteria that remain localized in the intestinal lumen, or penetrate only in very small numbers and are captured by dendritic cells (DCs), stimulate secretory IgA but not concomitant systemic IgG responses, as is the case with pathogens. Implications of this principle may be of importance in the design of vaccines using bacterial vectors for delivery of antigens that stimulate responses involved in protective immunity or tolerance. Studies of the cell-mediated arm of the response to commensal versus pathogenic microbiota should also provide relevant data. It should be, however, recognized that researchers involved in studies of the T cell dependence of IgA production and antigen-specific responses are not united in their opinion and that the types of microorganisms and species (or strains) of experimental animals may contribute to the variances in the interpretation of data.

We are beginning to fully appreciate the crucial roles of specialized populations of epithelial cells separating the external and internal environment, in both antigen uptake and processing in antigen presentation to T cells, and in providing chemokine/cytokine and ligand/receptor-mediated signals for recruitment, homing, differentiation, and function of underlying cell populations. Thus, intestinal epithelial cells may play an important role in the regulation of T cell responses to luminal antigens, probably through unique interactions involving a member of the carcinoembryonic antigen subfamily (gp180) and CD1d expressed on epithelial cells. Interestingly, studies of interactions between epithelial and mucosal T cells from the intraepithelial and lamina propria compartments revealed several points pertinent to the preferential activation of T cells (mainly $CD8^+$) and expanded usage of selected V regions of the T cell receptor, which is probably influenced by the type and quantity of antigens encountered by epithelial cells in the intestinal lumen.

Therefore, in addition to the mechanical barrier function and the production of a large array of factors of innate immunity, the epithelial cells display novel functions essential for the induction of adaptive immune responses and tolerance through unique interactions with T cells that, in turn, regulate the quality and magnitude of the ensuing response. Alterations in these intercellular communications may contribute to the inflammatory reactions and/or exaggeration rather than physiological suppression of local immune responses as manifested in inflammatory bowel diseases. In addition to epithelial cells, mucosal DCs, found in abundance in the intraepithelial compartment of single or multilayered epithelial surfaces, continuously sample the external environment with their surface-reaching "arms" and send signals to other cells that play a key role in coordinated mucosal defenses.

Undoubtedly, further studies of the anatomic localization and distribution, cellular composition, intercellular communications (receptor/ligand), signaling pathways, and the ensuing production of regulatory substances, as related to the quality and magnitude of external stimuli, will generate information essential in the design of strategies for the induction of responses of the desired physiological impact—protective immunity or mucosal tolerance.

Involvement of Dendritic Cell Subsets in the Induction of Oral Tolerance and Immunity

MARINA FLEETON,[a] NIKHAT CONTRACTOR,[a] FRANCISCO LEON,[a] JIANPING HE,[a] DENISE WETZEL,[b] TERENCE DERMODY,[b] AKIKO IWASAKI,[a,c] AND BRIAN KELSALL[a]

[a]*Laboratory of Clinical Investigation, NIAID, NIH, Bethesda, Maryland 20892, USA*

[b]*Departments of Pediatrics, and Microbiology and Immunology, Vanderbilt University School of Medicine, Nashville, Tennessee 37232, USA*

ABSTRACT: Dendritic cells (DCs) play a central role in the generation of immune responses in the intestine. DCs induce differentiation and tolerance of T cells, and may have a direct role in B cell switching to IgA. Four distinct subsets of $CD11c^+$ DCs are present in murine Peyer's patches, which represent primary sites for the induction of mucosal T and B cell responses. Studies suggest that CD11b+ DCs or plasmacytoid DCs may be specialized for the induction of regulatory T cells, and $CD8\alpha^+$ DCs for the induction of clonal deletion in response to soluble oral antigen, while all DC subsets (including $CD8\alpha^-/CD11b^-$ DCs) may be involved in responses to pathogens. We are currently using reovirus type-1 Lang (T1L) to explore the role of DC populations in mucosal immunity *in vivo*, as oral administration of live T1L to mice induces strong mucosal and systemic antiviral immune responses, whereas oral administration of inactivated T1L results in tolerance to viral proteins. We found that primary infection with T1L occurs in epithelial cells of the PP follicle–associated epithelium, but that $CD8\alpha^-/CD11b^-$ DCs in the subepithelial dome region (SED) are loaded with T1L antigens in the absence of active DC infection. At least a portion of this antigen is associated with cell fragments from apoptotic epithelial cells, demonstrating that SED DCs cross-present antigens from apoptotic epithelial cells. *In vitro*, in contrast to exposure to several TLR-ligands or anti-CD40, exposure to T1L does not activate DCs to mature or to produce cytokines, despite clear loading of the DCs with viral antigens. These data suggest that T1L is taken up by a "silent" receptor on DCs, and that the induction of immunity to T1L is dependent on signals from non-DCs following active viral infection that induce DC maturation. Thus, the decision between tolerance and immunity to inactive and live virus, respectively, likely depends on whether there is active infection of epithelial cells by T1L, which results in the elaboration of molecules, such as cytokines, that induce DC maturation.

KEYWORDS: dendritic cell; tolerance; cytokines; reovirus

[c]Current address: Section of Immunobiology, Yale University School of Medicine, New Haven, CT 06520, USA.

Address for correspondence: Brian L. Kelsall, Senior Investigator, Mucosal Immunobiology Section, Laboratory of Molecular Immunology, 10/11N228, 10 Center Drive, Bethesda, MD 20892. Voice: 301-496-7473; fax: 301-480-6768.

Kelsall@nih.gov

INTRODUCTION

Exposure of mucosal tissues to antigens can result in antigen-specific T cell tolerance via the induction of anergy or deletion of antigen-specific cells, or the generation of regulatory T cells. In addition, responses against pathogens are required to protect the host. Exposures to commensal organisms normally results in a form of "tolerance" that includes the generation of specific antibodies that may help to exclude commensal organisms from mucosal tissues by preventing their uptake or enhancing their trapping within the mucus coat. Dysregulation of this tolerance to commensal organisms results in intestinal inflammation. The precise role of dendritic cells in the orchestration of these responses is not well understood; however, their overall importance is suggested by studies demonstrating that expansion of dendritic cells (DCs) with flt3-ligand[1] or enhancement of their survival with RANK-ligand[2] results in increased sensitivity to oral tolerance to soluble proteins, or to enhanced immune responses to immunizing regimens.

MUCOSAL DENDRITIC CELL POPULATIONS AND MODELS OF ORAL TOLERANCE AND IMMUNITY

The role of specific DC subsets in the induction of oral tolerance has been suggested by *in vitro* studies. In particular, at least five subpopulations of DCs have been identified in the intestine of the mouse. Three populations of $CD11c^{hi}$ "conventional" DCs have been identified in the murine Peyer's patch (PP) and mesenteric lymph node, which have also been described in the intestinal lamina propria (Ref. 3 and elsewhere in this volume). $CD11b^+/CD8\alpha^-$ DCs produce high levels of IL-10 and induce differentiation of IL-4– and IL-10–producing T helper (Th) 2 cells *in vitro*.[4] In contrast, $CD11b^{lo}/CD8\alpha^+$ and $CD11b^{lo}/CD8\alpha^-$ DCs produce low levels of IL-10, high levels of IL-12, and induce only IFNγ-producing Th1 cells.[4] Spatial as well as functional differences define these three DC subsets. The DC-rich region of the subepithelial dome underlying the follicle-associated epithelium (FAE) contains both $CD11b^+/CD8\alpha^-$ and $CD11b^{lo}/CD8\alpha^-$ DCs, the T cell-rich intrafollicular region contains both $CD11b^{lo}/CD8\alpha^+$ and $CD11b^{lo}/CD8\alpha^-$ DCs, and the B cell follicle contains only $CD11b^{lo}/CD8\alpha^-$ DCs.[5] In addition, two different subpopulations of $CD11c^{lo}/B220^+$ plasmacytoid DCs have been described in the intestine. One population expresses CD8 and has been shown to preferentially drive IL-10–producing T cells *in vitro* and also to be particularly capable of activating the suppressive function of $CD25^+$ regulatory T cells when these cells are cocultured with naive T cells (Ref. 6 and elsewhere in this volume).

These initial studies allow the formulation of models for the role of PP DC populations in the induction of oral tolerance and immunity to pathogens.[5,7] In one such model there is constitutive trafficking of DCs from sites of antigen uptake in the mucosa, such as the lamina propria or the PP subepithelial dome, to draining lymphoid tissues.[8] These DCs migrating in the steady-state (noninfected, noninflamed, nonvaccinated) are "quiescent" DCs that capture antigens in the mucosa and migrate to lymphoid sites, such as the MLNs or the PP T cell–rich intrafollicular region (IFR). These DCs, although having altered their chemokine receptor pattern (for example, to express CCR7), allow them to migrate to T cell–rich regions of the PPs or MLNs, and present antigen in the absence of costimulation and/or cytokines, such as IL-12, which results in tolerized or regulatory T cells. In contrast, exposure to pathogens drives DCs to both migrate and express high levels costimulatory molecules, resulting in effector T cell responses, the quality of which (e.g., Th1, Th2, CTL) will depend on the initial stimulus provided by the pathogen, as well as by constitutive or induced signals from the microenvironment. Because of their ability to drive IL-10–producing T cells *in vitro* in the absence of exogenous activating signals, it can be argued that the induction of regulatory cells in this model would most likely be the result of the $CD11c^{hi}CD8^-CD11b^+$ or the $CD11c^{lo}B220^+CD8^+$ DC subsets. Whereas any of the five DC subsets may be activated to induce effector T cell responses, depending on the organisms and the pattern-recognition receptors expressed by the particular DC subset.

In addition, $CD8\alpha^+$ DCs, which are primarily located in T cell zones of lymphoid tissues, are implicated in the induction of antigen-specific deletion of T cells because antigen targeting to these cells, at least in the spleen, results in peripheral T cell tolerance. Therefore, it is likely that tolerance to mucosal antigens occurs via a variety of mechanisms that act simultaneously, and that may be mediated by different DC subpopulations. What determines the extent to which the induction of regulatory T cells versus the induction of anergy and deletion occurs is not yet clear; however, one possibility is that regulatory cells are induced to oral antigens in the mucosal tissues, while anergy or deletion can occur at all lymphoid sites. In this scenario, very high antigen doses that result in early systemic antigen distribution would preferentially lead to anergy and deletion of a limited number of antigen-specific T cells, whereas low doses of antigens that are processed more proximally are likely to induce regulatory T cells. Finally, it is not at all clear how regulatory T cells induced with oral antigen are related to the naturally occurring $CD25^+$ regulatory T cells originally described by Sakaguchi, or to IL-10–producing TR1 cells,[9] which may require different DC subsets or differentiation states for their expansion and survival. Therefore, although models for how DCs are involved in the induction of oral tolerance or immunity can be developed based on *in vitro* findings,[5,7,10,11] the validity of these models has not yet been tested *in vivo*.

DENDRITIC CELL POPULATIONS IN IMMUNITY TO MURINE REOVIRUS INFECTION

To address the function of specific DC subsets *in vivo*, we studied mammalian reovirus infection of adult mice,[12] an important model of mucosal virus infection.[13] Studies of reovirus are of interest because oral adminstration of live reovirus type-1 lang results in infection of PPs and the induction of Th1 and cytotoxic T lymphocyte (CTL) responses, while oral administration of inactivated virus appears to cause reovirus-specific systemic tolerance.[14]

Following oral inoculation of mice with T1L, the outer capsid of the virus is processed by luminal proteases, resulting in generation of infectious subvirion particles that specifically enter PPs via M cells in the FAE.[15–17] Once inside the PPs, T1L productively infects columnar epithelial cells overlying both the PPs (in the FAE) and lamina propria via receptors on the epithelial cell basolateral membrane.[18,19] In addition, early in infection, viral antigen is detectable in a few poorly characterized mononuclear cells within the SED.[17,19] Later in infection, the virus spreads to systemic sites, including the central nervous system.[20] Infection of adult mice with T1L is short-lived, and virus is usually cleared by local and systemic immunity within two weeks of inoculation.[13] The immune response to reovirus is characterized by production of IgA in the mucosa and development of Th1 and CTL responses at both local and systemic sites.[21–23]

$CD11b^+$ and $CD11b^{lo}/CD8\alpha^-$ DCs in the SED are in close proximity to M cells in the FAE and are thus poised to capture both soluble antigens and pathogens, such as reovirus. In support of this possibility, *Listeria monocytogenes* and *Salmonella typhimurium* are detectable in PP DCs following oral inoculation.[24,25] In addition, oral administration of virus-sized fluorescent polystyrene microparticles to mice results in detection of fluorescent signal in $CD11b^{lo}/CD8\alpha^-$ DCs in the SED.[26] However, there is very little known about DC processing of enteric viral pathogens.

To explore the role of PP DC populations in the induction of immune responses to reovirus T1L, PP cryosections from T1L-infected mice were examined for expression of viral structural ($\sigma1$) and nonstructural (σNS) proteins by immunofluorescence and confocal microscopy. Cells located in the FAE were actively infected with reovirus, as these cells were positive for σNS. In contrast, $\sigma1$ could be detected both in the FAE and the SED in association with the $CD11b^{lo}/CD8\alpha^-$ subset of $CD11c^+$ DCs. In concordance with these data, purified PP DCs could not be productively infected by reovirus *in vitro*. We found that $\sigma1$ protein was associated with staining for fragmented DNA in the SED, suggesting that DCs within the SED capture reovirus antigen from infected apoptotic epithelial cells. Confocal microscopic analysis of FACS-purified PP DCs from infected mice demonstrated that a small proportion of DCs (<1%) contained $\sigma1$, while no cells contained detectable σNS. Furthermore, $\sigma1$ in some DCs was associated with activated caspase 3, an early marker of apoptosis, and the epithelial protein cytokeratin, suggesting that reovirus antigen originated in epithelial cells. Finally, purified DCs from PPs of infected mice induced reovirus-primed $CD4^+$ cells to proliferate and produce IFNγ. These studies thus suggested that $CD11b^{lo}/CD8\alpha^-$ DCs in the PP SED process reovirus antigen from infected apoptotic epithelial cells for presentation to $CD4^+$ T cells.[12]

In subsequent studies, we demonstrated that TIL cannot activate conventional $CD11c^{hi}$ DCs to make cytokines, such as IL-10 or IL-10, or plasmacytoid $CD11c^{lo}$ $B220^+$ DCs to make IL-12 or type I IFNs. In addition, maturation of bone marrow–derived DCs or the murine D1 DC cell line could not be detected following exposure to TIL *in vitro*. Therefore, TIL appears to be a virus that neither infects nor activates DCs directly, yet is still capable of inducing strong immune responses.

Our current working model is that following infection with TIL, epithelial cells produce factors, such as type I interferons, TNFα, or IL-1β, and then undergo apoptosis. Apoptotic bodies are processed by DCs, which are activated by either dsRNA that is present within apoptotic bodies via interactions with TLR 3 in phagocytic endosomes, or by epithelial cell–derived factors, such as those mentioned above. Therefore, the active infection of epithelial cells that results in the elaboration of DC-activating signals is responsible for driving effector T cell responses to TIL. In contrast, without active epithelial cell infection, inactivated TIL would be processed as an innocuous antigen that results in oral tolerance. This would place the decision of active immunity or tolerance on the ability of the antigen/pathogen to induce DC-activating factors by epithelial cells, and not by direct interactions with DCs.

REFERENCES

1. VINEY, J.L., A.M. MOWAT, J.M. O'MALLEY, et al. 1998. Expanding dendritic cells in vivo enhances the induction of oral tolerance. J. Immunol **160:** 5815–5825.
2. WILLIAMSON, E., J.M. BILSBOROUGH & J.L. VINEY. 2002. Regulation of mucosal dendritic cell function by receptor activator of NF-kappa B (RANK)/RANK ligand interactions: impact on tolerance induction. J. Immunol. **169:** 3606–3612.
3. MOWAT, A.M., A.M. DONACHIE, L.A. PARKER, et al. 2003. The role of dendritic cells in regulating mucosal immunity and tolerance. Novartis Found. Symp. **252:** 291–302.
4. IWASAKI, A. & B.L. KELSALL. 2001. Unique functions of $CD11b^+$, $CD8\alpha^+$, and double-negative Peyer's patch dendritic cells. J. Immunol. **166:** 4884–4890.
5. IWASAKI, A. & B.L. KELSALL. 2000. Localization of distinct Peyer's patch dendritic cell subsets and their recruitment by chemokines macrophage inflammatory protein (MIP)-3α, MIP-3β, and secondary lymphoid organ chemokine. J. Exp. Med. **191:** 1381–1393.
6. BILSBOROUGH, J., T.C. GEORGE, A. NORMENT, et al. 2003. Mucosal CD8alpha+ DC, with a plasmacytoid phenotype, induce differentiation and support function of T cells with regulatory properties. Immunology **108:** 481–492.
7. IWASAKI, A. & B.L. KELSALL. 1999. Mucosal immunity and inflammation. I. Mucosal dendritic cells: their specialized role in initiating T cell responses. Am. J. Physiol. **276:** G1074–1078.
8. LIU, L.M. & G.G. MACPHERSON. 1993. Antigen acquisition by dendritic cells: intestinal dendritic cells acquire antigen administered orally and can prime naive T cells in vivo. J. Exp. Med. **177:** 1299–1307.
9. ZHANG, X., L. IZIKSON, L. LIU, et al. 2001. Activation of CD25(+)CD4(+) regulatory T cells by oral antigen administration. J. Immunol. **167:** 4245–4253.
10. MOWAT, A.M. 2003. Anatomical basis of tolerance and immunity to intestinal antigens. Nat. Rev. Immunol. **3:** 331–341.
11. BILSBOROUGH, J. & J.L. VINEY. 2004. Gastrointestinal dendritic cells play a role in immunity, tolerance, and disease. Gastroenterology **127:** 300–309.
12. FLEETON, M.N., N. CONTRACTOR, F. LEON, et al. 2004. Peyer's patch dendritic cells process viral antigen from apoptotic epithelial cells in the intestine of reovirus-infected mice. J. Exp. Med. **200:** 235–245.
13. VIRGIN, H.W., T.S. DERMODY & K.L. TYLER. 1998. Reoviruses II. Cytopathogenicity and pathogenesis. In Current Topics in Microbiology and Immunology. K.L. Tyler & M.B.A. Oldstone, Eds.: 147-161. Springer Verlag. Berlin.
14. GREENE, M.I. & H.L. WEINER. 1980. Delayed hypersensitivity in mice infected with reovirus. II. Induction of tolerance and suppressor T cells to viral specific gene products. J. Immunol. **125:** 283–287.
15. BODKIN, D.K., M.L. NIBERT & B.N. FIELDS. 1989. Proteolytic digestion of reovirus in the intestinal lumens of neonatal mice. J. Virol. **63:** 4676–4681.
16. BASS, D.M., D. BODKIN, R. DAMBRAUSKAS, et al. 1990. Intraluminal proteolytic activation plays an important role in replication of type 1 reovirus in the intestines of neonatal mice. J. Virol. **64:** 1830–1833.
17. WOLF, J.L., D.H. RUBIN, R.S. FINBERG, et al. 1981. Intestinal M cells: a pathway for entry of reovirus into the host. Science **212:** 471–472.
18. RUBIN, D.H. 1987. Reovirus serotype 1 binds to the basolateral membrane of intestinal epithelial cells. Microb. Path. **3:** 215–219.
19. BASS, D.M., J.S. TRIER, R. DAMBRAUSKAS, et al. 1988. Reovirus type I infection of small intestinal epithelium in suckling mice and its effect on M cells. Lab. Investig. **55:** 226–235.
20. KAUFFMAN, R.S., J.L. WOLF, R. FINBERG, et al. 1983. The sigma 1 protein determines the extent of spread of reovirus from the gastrointestinal tract of mice. Virology **124:** 403–410.
21. FAN, J.-Y., C.S. BOYCE & C.F. CUFF. 1998. T-Helper 1 and T-Helper 2 cytokine responses in gut-associated lymphoid tissue following enteric reovirus infection. Cell. Immunol. **188:** 55–63.

22. MAJOR, A.S. & C.F. CUFF. 1997. Enhanced mucosal and systemic immune responses to intestinal reovirus infection in β2-microglobulin-deficient mice. J. Virol. **71:** 5782–5789.
23. LONDON, S.D., D.H. RUBIN & J.J. CEBRA. 1987. Gut mucosal immunization with reovirus serotype 1/L stimulates virus-specific cytotoxic T cell precursors as well as IgA memory cells in Peyer's patches. J. Exp. Med. **165:** 830–847.
24. HOPKINS, S.A., F. NIEDERGANG, I.E. CORTHESY-THEULAZ, et al. 2000. A recombinant *Salmonella typhimurium* vaccine strain is taken up and survives within murine Peyer's patch dendritic cells. Cell. Microbiol. **2:** 59–68.
25. PRON, B., C. BOUMALIA, F. JAUBERT, et al. 2001. Dendritic cells are early cellular targets of *Listeria monocytogenes* after intestinal delivery and are involved in bacterial spread in the host. Cell. Microbiol. **3:** 331–340.
26. SHREEDAR, V.K., B.L. KELSALL & M.R. NEUTRA. 2003. Cholera toxin induces migration of dendritic cells from the subepithelial dome region to T- and B-cell areas of Peyer's patches. Infect. Immun. **71:** 504–509.

Intestinal Epithelial Cells Control Dendritic Cell Function

MONICA RIMOLDI,[a] MARCELLO CHIEPPA,[b] MARISA VULCANO,[b] PAOLA ALLAVENA,[b] AND MARIA RESCIGNO[a]

[a]*Department of Experimental Oncology, European Institute of Oncology, 20141 Milano, Italy*

[b]*Department of Immunology, Istituto di Ricerche Farmacologiche "Mario Negri", 20157 Milan, Italy*

ABSTRACT: Dendritic cells (DCs) comprise a family of cells specializing in antigen capture and presentation to T cells. We have recently shown that DC play an active role in bacterial uptake across mucosal surfaces. Indeed, DC are able to open tight junctions and to sample antigens directly across epithelia, both *in vitro* and *in vivo*. Because DC express tight junction proteins, the integrity of the epithelial barrier is preserved. In this study we have analyzed the possible involvement of epithelial cells in controlling DC function. We developed an *in vitro* model in our laboratory consisting of a three-player system of dendritic cells, epithelial cell monolayers, and bacteria. The crosstalk between epithelial cells and dendritic cells was analyzed, and epithelial cells were tested for their capacity to release cytokines and chemokines that induce the migration and activation of DC. We show that the capacity of epithelial cells to produce cytokines and activate DC is dependent on the invasiveness of the bacteria tested. In particular, invasive bacteria stimulate epithelial cells to release proinflammatory cytokines and to induce the maturation state of DC. By contrast, noninvasive bacteria are unable to stimulate epithelial cells, but can activate DC directly when DC translocate to the apical side. In conclusion, epithelial cells are not simply a barrier to bacteria entering via the oral route, but actively influence the activating properties of bystander DC.

KEYWORDS: dendritic cells; epithelial cells; bacteria; intestine; mucosa; JAM; tight junctions

INTRODUCTION

Entry of pathogens across the intestinal mucosa occurs mainly through specialized epithelial cells, called M cells, that are located in Peyer's patches.[1] However, we have recently described a new mechanism for bacterial entry that is mediated by dendritic cells (DCs).[2] DCs are distributed as immature cells in nonlymphoid organs and in the blood where they perform a sentinel function for incoming pathogens.[3–8]

Address for correspondence: Maria Rescigno, Ph.D., European Institute of Oncology, Department of Experimental Oncology, Via Ripamonti, 435, 20141 Milano, Italy. Voice: +39-02-57489865; fax: +39-02-57489851.
 mrescigno@lar.ieo.it

Immature DCs are characterized by the capacity to take up antigens and to phagocytose macroparticles.[9,10] During infection or inflammation, DCs are mobilized in and out of peripheral tissues,[11,12] and activated DCs are targeted to secondary lymphoid organs.[13,14] Here, DCs have the unique ability, among antigen-presenting cells, to activate naive T cells. Thus, DCs play an important role in the induction of immune responses.

As often occurs, understanding the mechanisms underlying the physiology of the organism allows the unveiling of the uncontrolled steps that lead to some pathological condition, and vice versa. In this regard, the comparison of how microorganisms are handled by DCs in healthy or diseased environments can shed some light on the development of uncontrolled inflammatory responses to nondangerous commensal microorganisms. We have described how, during infection, lamina propria DCs are able to open tight junctions (TJ) between adjacent epithelial cells and to capture bacteria directly across the mucosal epithelium. The epithelial barrier remains preserved because DCs express TJ proteins, whose level is regulated by bacteria or bacterial products, and establish TJ-like structures with neighboring epithelial cells.[2] Interestingly, lamina propria DCs can discriminate between pathogenic and nonpathogenic bacteria. In fact, when the intestine is infected with nonpathogenic bacteria, DCs do not receive any migratory signal and stay *in situ,* whereas infection with pathogenic bacteria induces a large migration of DCs from the mucosa, presumably to the mesenteric nodes.[2] Thus, DCs play an active role in bacterial handling across mucosal surfaces.

But how can DCs "sense" the presence of bacteria on the apical side of the mucosal epithelium and discriminate between pathogenic and commensal bacteria? We know from previous studies that bacteria, regardless of their pathogenicity,[15] easily activate DCs from the spleen or from the bone marrow. This results in secretion of pro- and anti-inflammatory cytokines and in the upregulation of those molecules, which are necessary for their antigen-presenting function and for cell migration.[16,17] This suggests that DCs by themselves are unable to discriminate between pathogenic or nonpathogenic bacteria. Thus, what is the role of epithelial cells that are the first cells encountering bacteria in the intestinal lumen? Can they act to control DCs function according to the type of microorganism encountered?

In this study, we analyzed the role of epithelial cell–derived factors in mediating DC–epithelial cell crosstalk in terms of DC recruitment and activation. We used an *in vitro* co-culture model that we developed in our laboratory. Epithelial cells were tested for their capacity to release chemokines, such as IL-8 and MIP-3α, and to activate DCs after encountering *Salmonella typhimurium*. Epithelial cells or epithelial cell/DC co-cultures were incubated with several salmonella strains deficient in different pathways of pathogenicity and invasiveness.

MATERIALS AND METHODS

Cells and Reagents

DCs were derived from peripheral blood monocytes according to a slightly modified protocol.[18] Briefly, monocytes were purified by positive selection with anti-CD14 antibodies coupled to magnetic beads (Miltenyi). $CD14^+$ cells were incubated for six days in complete medium containing GM-CSF (50 ng/mL, Peprotech) and IL-4 (20 ng/mL, Endogen) in order to obtain immature DCs.

Bacterial Strains

Bacillus subtilis is an aerobe commonly found in soil or water sources, or associated with plants whose genome has been completely sequenced.[19] Lactic acid bacteria (LAB), including *Lactobacillus plantarum*, are present in the intestines of most animals. *Salmonella typhimurium* is a typical pathogen that enters the host across mucosal surfaces.[20] Listed below are the mutations carried by the attenuated salmonella strains that we used: msbB (lipid A), purE, AroA, surA, invA (SPI I deficient), ssaV (SPI II deficient), htrA, ompC-ompF, and ompR. These strains are impaired either in invasiveness (e.g., SPI I deficient), in their capacity to survive inside the phagosome (e.g., SPI II), in growth (e.g., purE), or in general toxicity (e.g., msbB).

Cells were incubated with live bacteria for one hour, and then bacteria were killed by the addition of antibiotics (gentamicin, 100 µg/mL; and tetracycline, 10 µg/mL).

Cytokine Assay and Cell Phenotype

The ability of DCs to produce pro- and anti-inflammatory cytokines (IL-10, IL-12, IL-8, IL-6) was tested by ELISA (R&D Systems) of culture supernatants 24 h after bacterial incubation. Cells were analyzed for acquisition of maturation markers (CD83, CD80, DC-LAMP, HLA-DR) by cytofluorimetry (FACScalibur, Becton Dickinson).

Dendritic Cell/Epithelial Cell Co-culture

Generation of an Epithelial Monolayer (Situations a and b)

In brief, Caco-2 cells were seeded in the upper chamber of a Transwell filter (3 µm pore diameter; Costar) for 5–7 d until a transepithelial resistance of 300 Ohm × cm^2 was achieved.

Situation a (Figure 1)

Epithelial cell monolayers were incubated with bacteria on the apical surface (upper chamber). After 1 h of incubation, bacteria were washed out and the medium changed to one containing antibiotics (gentamicin, 100 µg/mL; and tetracycline, 10 µg/mL). Culture supernatants were collected at different time points from the lower chamber (facing the basolateral membrane) and were tested for activation of DCs. DCs were incubated for 24 h in culture supernatant and then analyzed phenotypically for expression of surface activation markers (CD83, CD80, HLA-DR). Distinction between cytokines released by epithelial cells and dendritic cells was made by analyzing culture supernatants before and after DC incubation. Culture supernatants collected at different time points from the lower chamber were also analyzed for the presence of cytokines (IL-10, IL-12, IL-6, IL-8).

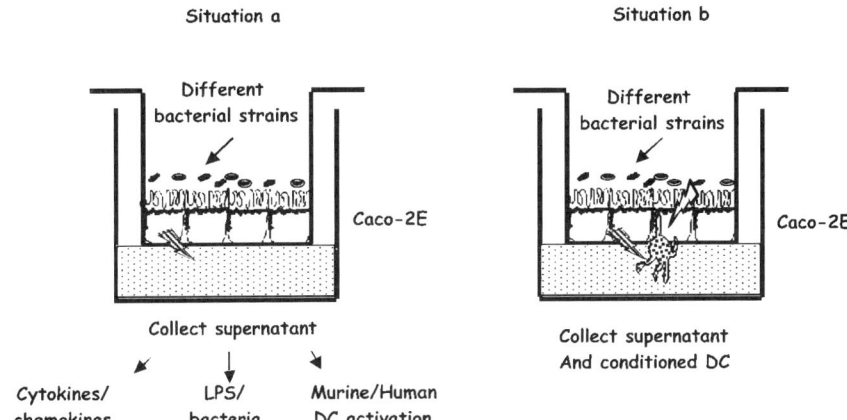

FIGURE 1. Schematic representation of experimental models. *Left*: Situation a; DCs are incubated with supernatants of epithelial cells previously treated with bacteria. *Right*: Situation b; the interaction of DCs with epithelial cells and bacteria is studied directly, across a monolayer of epithelial cells. (See text for details.)

Situation b (Figure 1)

Filters were turned upside down and DCs were seeded on the filter facing the basolateral membrane of epithelial cells for 4 h to let the cells attach to the filter. Filters were then turned upside down again into a 24-well plate. The Transwell filters were either left for 5 h before treatment with bacteria to allow the "conditioning" of DCs by epithelial cells or were treated directly with bacteria (bacteria/EC ratio = 10:1) from the apical surface (upper chamber). After 1 h of incubation, bacteria were washed out and the medium changed to one containing antibiotics (gentamicin, 100 µg/mL, and tetracycline, 10 µg/mL). DCs and culture supernatants were collected at different time points and analyzed as in situation a.

Analysis of the Ability of DCs to Creep between Epithelial Cells

The ability of DCs to intercalate between EC and to open tight junction proteins was analyzed by laser confocal microscopy after staining of filters for DCs (CD11c$^+$) or tight junction markers (occludin), as previously described.[2]

RESULTS AND DISCUSSION

DC–epithelial cell interactions were studied by using an *in vitro* system developed in our laboratory. This system is particularly suitable for dissecting out the contributions of epithelial cell–derived factors or bacterial products in the activation of DCs. It simplifies the mucosal barrier to just three players—DCs, epithelial cells, and bacteria—in a spatial arrangement similar to that found *in vivo*. Thus, it can help to identify possible interactions and factors responsible for the ability or inability of DCs to sense different bacterial strains. Two possible scenarios were considered

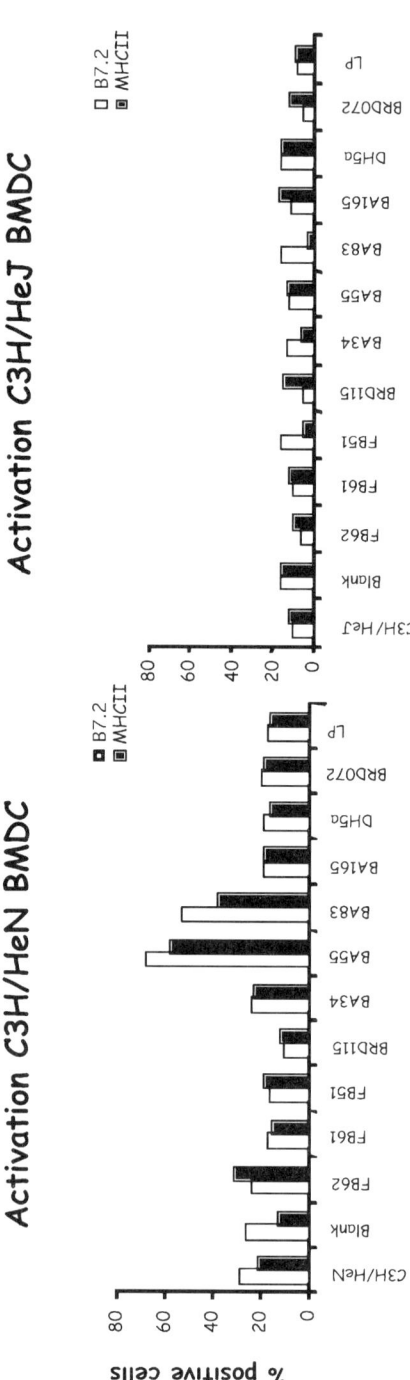

FIGURE 2. Bacterial LPS activation of murine BMDC incubated with supernatants from epithelial cell/bacteria co-cultures. Culture supernatants tested for activation of BMDC from wild-type C3H/HeN mice (*left*) or from TLR4-mutated C3H/HeJ mice (*right*). Expression of activation markers MHC II and B7.2 is shown. In cells from wild-type mice, DCs are partially activated only by supernatants from epithelial cells treated with competent invasive bacteria; mutation in TLR4 abrogates this effect. Bacterial strains: invasive salmonellae (FB62: WT; BA55: htrA; BA 83: SPI-II (ssaV); BA 165: ompC-ompF; FB51: purE); noninvasive salmonellae (FB61: msbB; BRD115: SurA; BA34: SPI-I (InvA⁻); noninvasive *E. coli* (DH5a); commensal *Lacobacillus plantarum* (LP). See text for details.

TABLE 1. Analysis of cell culture supernatants of epithelial cells activated with different bacterial strains in terms of IL-8 production and dendritic cells activating properties. The percent of CD83 high and DC-LAMP high cells is shown as an indicator of activated DCs

Bacterial Strains[a]	IL-8 (ng/mL)	%CD83^{hi} cells	%DC-LAMP^{hi} cells	MIP-3α (ng/mL)	Invasive
C5 WT	2.27	61.6	70.9	1.02	Yes
SL1344 WT	1.55	82.5	50.6	0.96	Yes
htrA	1.13	70.8	77	1.08	Yes
ssaV (SPI-II)	1.31	91.8	96	1.13	Yes
ompC-ompF	0.72	89.5	73.5	0.658	Yes
msbB	0.07	33.9	29.4	0.46	No
SurA	0.56	30.6	30.3	1.03	No
InvA (SPI-I)	0.16	47.6	52	0.88	No
DH5α	0	32	33.4	0.08	No
B. subtilis	0	N.D.	N.D.	1.2	No
untreated	0	27.2	28	0.04	—
LPS	—	85.8	98.8	—	—
iDCs	—	10.8	12.2	—	—

[a]Bacterial strains: Invasive: (a) Salmonella: C5 WT; SL1344 WT; htrA; SPI-II (ssaV); omp-CompF. Noninvasive: (a) Salmonella: msbB (lipid A mutant); SurA; SPI-I (InvA); (b) E. coli: DH5α; (c) B. subtilis.

(FIG. 1). In situation a, DCs were incubated with supernatants of epithelial cells previously treated with bacteria; in situation b, the interaction of DCs with epithelial cells and bacteria was studied directly, across a monolayer of epithelial cells.

We observed that incubation of invasive salmonellae, but not of noninvasive bacteria, on the apical side of epithelial cell monolayers in the absence of DCs (situation a) induced the release of proinflammatory cytokines, such as IL-8 (TABLE 1). As we could not detect any bacteria in the lower chamber of the epithelial monolayer, this suggests that the observed effect is the result either of bacteria remaining intracellularly or of translocation of bacterial products across the monolayer to basolateral membrane receptors. Interestingly, incubation of DCs with culture supernatant from epithelial cells treated with invasive bacteria, but not with noninvasive bacteria, induced DC activation, as attested by an increased number of cells expressing high levels of the activation markers, CD83 and DC-LAMP (TABLE 1). Activation of DCs could be due simply to bacterial products that have crossed the epithelial cell monolayer. However, when we incubated murine bone marrow–derived DCs (BMDC), which can respond to bacteria or bacterial products, together with the same epithelial cell supernatants, some cell activation was observed (FIG. 2, left graph). This correlated with the detection of traces of bacterial lipopolysaccharide (LPS). Indeed, when we incubated murine BMDC derived from C3H/HeJ mice that are mutated in the Toll-like receptor 4 gene and cannot respond to LPS, DC activation was abrogated (FIG. 2, right graph). This suggests that human DC activation that occurs only

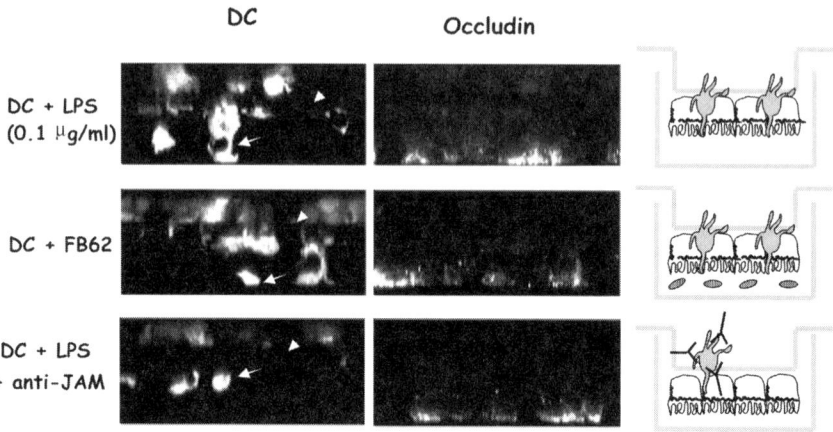

FIGURE 3. Anti-JAM antibodies block LPS-induced DC translocation. Invasive salmonella (FB62: WT) or LPS (0.1 μg/mL) induce DC migration across a monolayer of epithelial cells all the way to the apical face. Preincubation of DCs with anti-JAM 1 antibody (10 μg/mL) for 30 min before addition to the epithelial monolayer from the basolateral membrane blocks DC migration. Transwell filters were fixed 2 h after addition of bacteria and were processed for laser confocal microscopy. *Left*: CD11c staining of DCs. *White arrowheads* show the location of the filter (black); *white arrows* indicate the position of DCs that have migrated across the filters. *Center*: Occludin staining of epithelial tight junctions. *Right*: Schematic. Note that preincubation of DCs with anti-JAM 1 antibody does not block DC migration across the filter, but inhibits their ability to open tight junctions and reach the apical surface.

after incubation with supernatants of epithelial cells infected with invasive bacteria is the result of a combination of factors, including bacterial products and epithelial cell–derived molecules.

LPS was detected in the lower chamber of epithelial cell/bacteria co-cultures only when invasive bacteria were seeded from the apical side. LPS is the major bacterial component able to induce DC translocation across a monolayer of epithelial cells (FIG. 3), probably by upregulating the expression of tight junction proteins (not shown). In fact, LPS alone can induce the translocation of DCs (FIG. 3), and commensal bacteria, such as *Lactobacillus plantarum*, lacking LPS are unable to recruit DCs to the apical side (not shown). Tight junction proteins expressed by DCs are necessary to allow DC translocation. In fact, preincubation of DCs with antibodies to the extracellular portion of the tight junction protein, junctional adhesion molecule 1 (JAM1), inhibits the ability of DCs to open adjacent epithelial cell junctions (FIG. 3).

Interestingly, both invasive and noninvasive salmonellae, as long as they express flagellin, induce the release of MIP-3α, a chemokine responsible for the recruitment of immature DCs (TABLE 1). This is consistent with a recent report showing that flagellated salmonellae can induce the release of MIP-3α by epithelial cells.[21] This indicates that the presence of flagellated bacteria induces the recruitment of immature DCs, regardless of their invasiveness or pathogenicity. In fact, *Bacillus subtilis*, a flagellated soil bacterium, is also able to induce MIP-3α release by epithelial cells (TABLE 1). By contrast, only invasive bacteria induce DC activation. If, however, we switch to situation b in which DCs are coincubated with epithelial cells and can sense the bacteria directly across the monolayer, they are activated both by invasive and noninvasive bacteria (not shown), even by commensal bacteria, such as *Lactobacillus plantarum*, due to their capacity to cross the monolayer (not shown). This suggests that during infection two situations are generated. In the first one, invasive bacteria transduce activation signals to epithelial cells that release inflammatory chemokines, such as IL-8, and activating factors for DCs. As a consequence, DCs that have not encountered the bacteria will also be activated. By contrast, in the second situation, noninvasive bacteria that have not been sensed by epithelial cells will not induce bystander DC activation. In both cases, because invasive and noninvasive salmonellae both express flagellin, they will recruit immature DCs. Thus in the second situation, noninvasive bacteria induce the activation only of those DCs that have crept between epithelial cells and can contact them directly from the luminal side. Whether this activation then results in a different capability to polarize T cells remains to be established. The signals that induce DC migration across the monolayer after infection with noninvasive salmonellae also remain to be elucidated.

In conclusion, we have demonstrated that during a bacterial infection, DCs respond differently if they receive signals from invasive or noninvasive bacteria. In particular, invasive bacteria induce a broad DC activation due to a combination of epithelial cell–derived and bacteria-derived factors, whereas noninvasive bacteria induce activation only of those DCs that they have contacted directly. Whether noninvasive or commensal bacteria also modulate DC function by inducing an immunosuppressive effect on epithelial cells, as has been recently suggested,[22] remains to be established. Hence, epithelial cells are not simply a barrier to bacteria entering via the oral route, but are also actively influencing the activating properties of bystander dendritic cells.

ACKNOWLEDGMENTS

This work was supported by grants from the Italian Association for Cancer Research (AIRC), from the Crohn's and Colitis Foundation of America (CCFA), and from the Ministero della Salute (Ricerca finalizzata). We thank Drs. Gordon Dougan and Liljana Petrovska for providing *Salmonella typhimurium* mutant strains.

REFERENCES

1. NEUTRA, M.R. 1999. M cells in antigen sampling in mucosal tissues. Curr. Top. Microbiol. Immunol. **236:** 17–32.
2. RESCIGNO, M., M. URBANO, B. VALZASINA, *et al.* 2001. Dendritic cells express tight junction proteins and penetrate gut epithelial monolayers to sample bacteria. Nat. Immunol. **2:** 361–367.
3. PALUCKA, K. & J. BANCHEREAU. 2002. How dendritic cells and microbes interact to elicit or subvert protective immune responses. Curr. Opin. Immunol. **14:** 420–431.
4. BANCHEREAU, J., F. BRIERE, C. CAUX, *et al.* 2000. Immunobiology of dendritic cells. Annu. Rev. Immunol. **18:** 767–811.
5. RESCIGNO, M. 2002. Dendritic cells and the complexity of microbial infection. Trends Microbiol. **10:** 425.

6. PULENDRAN, B., K. PALUCKA & J. BANCHEREAU. 2001. Sensing pathogens and tuning immune responses. Science **293**: 253–256.
7. REIS E SOUSA, C. 2001. Dendritic cells as sensors of infection. Immunity **14**: 495–498.
8. WICK, M.J. 2003. The role of dendritic cells in the immune response to Salmonella. Immunol. Lett. **85**: 99–102.
9. INABA, K., M. INABA, M. NAITO, et al. 1993. Dendritic cell progenitors phagocytose particulates, including bacillus Calmette-Guerin organisms, and sensitize mice to mycobacterial antigens in vivo. J. Exp. Med. **178**: 479–488.
10. REIS E SOUSA, C. & J.M. AUSTYN. 1993. Phagocytosis of antigens by Langerhans cells. Adv. Exp. Med. Biol. **329**: 199–204.
11. DE SMEDT, T., B. PAJAK, E. MURAILLE, et al. 1996. Regulation of dendritic cell numbers and maturation by lipopolysaccharide in vivo. J. Exp. Med. **184**: 1413–1424.
12. ROBERT, C., R.C. FUHLBRIGGE, J.D. KIEFFER, et al. 1999. Interaction of dendritic cells with skin endothelium: a new perspective on immunosurveillance. J. Exp. Med. **189**: 627–636.
13. SAEKI, H., A.M. MOORE, M.J. BROWN, et al. 1999. Cutting edge: secondary lymphoid-tissue chemokine (SLC) and CC chemokine receptor 7 (CCR7) participate in the emigration pathway of mature dendritic cells from the skin to regional lymph nodes. J. Immunol. **162**: 2472–2475.
14. SOZZANI, S., P. ALLAVENA, G. D'AMICO, et al. 1998. Differential regulation of chemokine receptors during dendritic cell maturation: a model for their trafficking properties. J. Immunol. **161**: 1083–1086.
15. RESCIGNO, M., M. URBANO, M. RITTIG, et al. 2001. Interaction of dendritic cells with bacteria. *In* Dendritic Cell: Biology and Clinical Applications. M. Lotze & A. Thomson, Eds.: 473-486. Academic Press. San Diego, CA.
16. RESCIGNO, M., S. CITTERIO, C. THÉRY, et al. 1998. Bacteria-induced neo-biosynthesis, stabilization, and surface expression of functional class I molecules in mouse dendritic cells. Proc. Natl. Acad. Sci. USA **95**: 5229–5234.
17. RESCIGNO, M., F. GRANUCCI & P. RICCIARDI-CASTAGNOLI. 2000. Molecular events of bacterial-induced maturation of dendritic cells. J. Clin. Immunol. **20**: 161–166.
18. SALLUSTO, F. & A. LANZAVECCHIA. 1994. Efficient presentation of soluble antigen by cultured human dendritic cells is maintained by granulocyte/macrophage colony-stimulating factor plus interleukin 4 and downregulated by tumor necrosis factor alpha. J. Exp. Med. **179**: 1109–1118.
19. KUNST, F., N. OGASAWARA, I. MOSZER, et al. 1997. The complete genome sequence of the gram-positive bacterium Bacillus subtilis. Nature **390**: 249–256.
20. MASTROENI, P. & N. MENAGER. 2003. Development of acquired immunity to Salmonella. J. Med. Microbiol. **52**: 453–459.
21. SIERRO, F., B. DUBOIS, A. COSTE, et al. 2001. Flagellin stimulation of intestinal epithelial cells triggers CCL20-mediated migration of dendritic cells. Proc. Natl. Acad. Sci. USA **98**: 13722–13727.
22. NEISH, A.S., A.T. GEWIRTZ, H. ZENG, et al. 2000. Prokaryotic regulation of epithelial responses by inhibition of IkappaB-alpha ubiquitination. Science **289**: 1560–1563.

Uptake of Antigens from the Intestine by Dendritic Cells

GORDON MacPHERSON,[a] SIMON MILLING,[a] ULF YRLID,[a] LESLEY COUSINS,[a] EMMA TURNBULL,[b] AND FANG-PING HUANG[c]

[a]*Sir William Dunn School of Pathology, University of Oxford, Oxford, United Kingdom*

[b]*Edward Jenner Institute for Vaccine Research, Berkshire, United Kingdom*

[c]*Department of Pathology, University of Hong Kong, Hong Kong*

ABSTRACT: The intestinal immune system responds to ingested antigens in a variety of ways, ranging from tolerance to full immunity. How T cells are instructed to make these differential responses is still unclear. Dendritic cells (DCs) sample enteric antigens in the lamina propria and Peyer's patches, and transport them within the patch or to mesenteric nodes where they are presented to lymphocytes. It is probable that DCs also transmit information that influences the outcome of T cell activation, but the nature of this information and the factors in the intestine that regulate DC behavior and properties are far from clear. We have developed a model in the rat that permits analysis of DCs actually in the process of migration from the intestine to mesenteric nodes. In this paper we will review those aspects of our research that relate to antigen uptake and discuss these in the context of other experimental systems.

KEYWORDS: dendritic cell; antigen uptake; rat; lymph; lymph node; intestine; Peyer's patch; scrapie; prions; TSE; migration

INTRODUCTION

Naive $CD4^+$ T cells represent an immunological example of middle management. They have been educated and selected (thymus), but they move around randomly until told what to do (secondary lymphoid tissues). They can react in a variety of ways to instruction (tolerance, regulation, Th1, Th2), but in general they cannot do very much on their own (effector function); they have to tell others what to do. Understanding the regulation of $CD4^+$ T cell activation and differentiation is, however, crucial to understanding how to harness and modulate intestinal immune responses for therapeutic purposes. It is increasingly clear that dendritic cells (DCs) play central roles in these processes and, thus, understanding the biology of intestinal DCs is of major importance in these areas.

The intestine encounters a huge variety of antigens, mostly harmless under normal circumstances. Some, however, are inherently pathogenic, whereas others can

Address for correspondence: Dr. G. Gordon MacPherson, Sir William Dunn School of Pathology, University of Oxford, UK. Voice: +44-1865-275584; fax: +44-1865-275501.
gordon.macpherson@path.ox.ac.uk

become pathogenic if an inappropriate immune response is initiated, for example, to gluten in celiac disease or commensal bacteria in models of inflammatory bowel disease (IBD). It is likely that small proportions of all ingested proteins are absorbed intact and will thus interact with the adaptive immune system, either in Peyer's patches (PPs) or mesenteric nodes (MLN), and, thus, mechanisms must exist that determine how lymphocytes exposed to antigens subsequently differentiate: whether they induce active immunity, become unresponsive (tolerance), or become able to downregulate the activation of other naive, antigen-specific cells (regulation).

Sites of lymphocyte activation, apart from PPs, are anatomically distant from the sites of antigen entry, and even in PP, T cells are activated in areas to which antigen may not have direct entry. T cells, however, respond differentially to nonpathogenic and pathogenic antigens, and the types of active response that are initiated can show distinct polarization. For example, intestinal *Trichinella* induces a strong, protective Th2 immune response in rodents, whereas *Eimeria* induces a strong, protective Th1 response. These two parasites illustrate very clearly one of the central problems in intestinal immunity. Thus, in the early stages, at least, both are confined to the intestine, but the response to them is initiated in the MLN.[1] Not only must antigen be transported from the intestine to MLN, in addition, information must reach naive T cells that informs their differentiation pathways. We are still far from having a complete understanding of either of these processes; yet such an understanding is crucial if we are to develop effective intestinal vaccines and strategies for the immunotherapy of IBD and food hypersensitivities.

Increasing evidence suggests that DCs play a central and crucial role in both antigen uptake and delivery, and in regulating the outcomes of T cell activation. This paper will review the roles of intestinal DCs in the uptake, transport, and delivery of foreign antigens introduced into the intestinal lumen and of self-antigens in the form of apoptotic cells and will be based largely on our studies in the rat.[2–11]

DENDRITIC CELLS

DCs include several distinct subpopulations that differ in life history and functions.[12] The complexity of these cells is apparent, but unraveling the significance of this complexity is beset with difficulties: DCs are rare cells, difficult to isolate; they can exist at different stages of maturation and activation; and their isolation itself can induce changes in gene expression, phenotype, and function. In addition, it is proving difficult to relate DC subpopulations in rodents to their human counterparts.

DCs in the adult are mostly bone marrow derived, although murine Langerhans cells are self-renewing in the steady state.[13] However, the points at which DC lineages branch from other hemopoietic lineages are ill defined. Thus, murine DCs may have a CD11c blood precursor,[14] but under inflammatory conditions can derive from monocytes.[15]

INTESTINAL DENDRITIC CELLS

Intestinal DCs have been isolated from intestinal lamina propria of mice,[16] humans,[17–19] and rats.[7] They have also been isolated from PPs of the same and other species.[7,20–38] The isolation of DCs from the lamina propria is, however, inefficient (the proportion of DCs present that is actually isolated is unknown, but probably very small), may select for particular subsets, and can induce at least partial activation. In addition, such DCs represent cells at different stages of maturation. To compensate for these difficulties, we have developed a model that permits collection of DCs that are in the process of migration from the intestine to the MLN.

PSEUDOAFFERENT LYMPH DENDRITIC CELLS

DCs migrating in lymph from the intestine are normally extracted efficiently in the mesenteric nodes (>95%) and do not appear in significant numbers in efferent lymph.[39] If the MLN are removed in young rats, afferent and efferent lymphatics heal, permitting passage of DCs into the thoracic duct, from which they can be collected by insertion of a cannula. These cells can be collected over at least 48 h, placed on ice to "freeze" them metabolically, and purified by different combinations of density gradient centrifugation, magnetic bead sorting, and flow cytometric sorting (FACS). These DCs have only just left the intestine, are the ones involved in antigen transport and delivery, and are probably the ones that regulate T cell differentiation. They represent DCs "in action." We have characterized these DCs in detail.[2–6,8,9,40] Important findings from our lab include the following:

DCs are migrating continually from the intestine in the absence of any overt stimulation, as is in fact true for all peripheral tissues studied. In rats, DC output is maintained at a relatively constant rate for at least five days after cannulation.[2] Intestine-derived DCs can be found in T cell areas of MLN from germ-free rats,[10] showing that their migration is not dependent on commensal flora.

At least two distinct populations of DCs migrate from the intestine.[41] $CD4^+$/SIRPα^+ DCs resemble "classical" DCs and are strong antigen-presenting cells (APCs). In contrast, $CD4^-$/SIRPα^- DCs are weaker APCs, survive very poorly in culture, but carry remnants of apoptotic enterocytes to T cell areas of MLN,[10] and, thus, may be involved in constitutive presentation of self antigens to induce tolerance (see below). It is of interest that similar DC subpopulations are present in bovine skin lymph.[42]

DENDRITIC CELLS AND SELF-TOLERANCE

Several reports suggest that DCs play a crucial role in tolerance to peripheral self-antigens and, by analogy, to nonpathogenic intestinal antigens. Thus, IgG or a hen egg lysozyme peptide targeted to DCs in mice induces tolerance,[43,44] and a truncated, nonsecreted form of ovalbumin (OVA), expressed solely in enterocytes, induces tolerance in TCR transgenic $CD8^+$ T cells.[45] More direct evidence that DCs are the cell type involved in self-tolerance comes from studies of tolerance to pancreatic islet-expressed OVA, where $CD8\alpha^+$ DCs from pancreatic nodes were shown to be able to present OVA to T cells.[46]

UPTAKE OF ANTIGENS BY INTESTINAL DENDRITIC CELLS

Soluble Antigens

Soluble antigens introduced into the intestine can induce specific hyporesponsiveness in T lymphocytes (oral tolerance). We have shown that after giving antigen by gavage or direct injection into the intestine at laparotomy, DCs collected from pseudoafferent lymph between 6 and 18 to 24 h can present the antigen specifically to sensitized T cells *in vitro*.[5] More recently, we have found that following the injection of FITC-labeled OVA intraintestinally, FITC can be detected in 4 to 6% of lymph DCs between 6 and 18 h after injection. Both $CD4^+/SIRP\alpha^+$ and $CD4^-/SIRP\alpha^-$ DCs expressed fluorescence in approximately similar proportions, but in the former, the fluorescence had a fine granular appearance, whereas in the latter it was concentrated in large inclusions. We do not know whether DCs in which fluorescence could not be detected were devoid of antigen.

Particulate Antigens

The major portals of entry for particulate antigens are PPs, via M cells. Virus-sized latex particles given by gavage to mice are taken up by subepithelial dome DCs and remain in these cells for at least 14 days.[47] We have done similar experiments in rats using a variety of latex particles and were surprised to find virtually no translocation into PPs. Possibly this relates to the specific pathogen-free (SPF) status of our rats, as it has been shown that moving mice from SPF to conventional conditions stimulates a three-fold increase in M cell numbers.[48] An alternative mechanism for particulate transport has been suggested by Rescigno *et al*. They found that intralumenal bacteria could induce lamina propria DCs to extend processes between epithelial cells, and suggest that these processes can capture and translocate bacteria.[49]

Some pathogens, such as *Eimeria* and *Trichinella*, are confined to the intestine, at least in the early stages of infection, yet both induce strong immunity which, for *Trichinella* at least, commences in MLN.[50] Essentially, nothing is known about how antigens from these parasites are transported to the nodes.

UPTAKE OF PRION PROTEINS FROM THE INTESTINE

The protease-resistant form of prion-related protein (PrP), PrP^{Sc}, is thought to be the agent responsible for transmissible spongiform encephalopathies (TSEs). PrP^{Sc} accumulates in the central nervous system of infected individuals and is thought to be transmitted largely by consumption of infected material. PrP^{Sc} contains a large proportion of β-pleated sheets and aggregates spontaneously. The form that is absorbed from the intestine is not known, but it may well be handled as a particle rather than a soluble protein. Scrapie is a form of TSE that has been adapted to murine models. Following peripheral administration, PrP^{Sc} in the form of scrapie-associated fibrils (SAF), accumulates/replicates in secondary lymphoid tissues in or on follicular dendritic cells (FDC).[51] FDC are resident, long-lived cells in B cell follicles and are unrelated to the migratory DCs so far discussed. We suggested that DCs might acquire PrP^{Sc} from the intestine and transport it to mesenteric nodes. To test this, we injected mesenteric-lymphadenectomized cannulated rats with SAF and examined lymph at intervals afterwards.[11] PrP could be detected by immunolabeling in 4 to 6% of DCs between 6 and 24 h after injection. Immunoblotting showed that at least a proportion was protease resistant. PrP could not be detected in any other lymph cells, in lymph plasma, or in DCs from noninjected rats. Scrapie infectivity is tested by intracerebral injection into mice. Injection of lysates from DCs collected from intestinally injected rats did not, however, reveal significant infectivity. This probably relates to the very small amounts of PrP^{Sc} acquired by DCs (about 1 in 10,000 of the molecules injected).

PrP^{Sc} is rapidly degraded in macrophages.[52] We, however, had evidence that DCs could retain native protein antigens for long periods. Thus, following brief incubation of splenic DCs with horse radish peroxidase, active enzyme could be detected for over 24 hours.[53] In addition, when splenic DCs were isolated from rats up to 24 h after giving protein intravenously, injection of these DCs into naive rats stimulated an antibody response, showing that the transferred DCs contained intact antigen.[53,54] Recently, we have found that PrP^{Sc} accumulates similarly in DCs and macrophages during *in vitro* coincubation, but that the agent is rapidly degraded in macrophages, whereas immunodetectable PrP^{Sc} is retained for at least 72 h in DCs (Huang *et al*, in preparation).

DELIVERY OF ANTIGEN TO LYMPH NODES

How the antigens that are inducing tolerance or immunity are actually delivered to T cells is unclear. Molecules such as chemokines injected subcutaneously or into the intestinal wall rapidly enter lymph, but the great bulk of such molecules are excluded from the T cell areas of the draining nodes.[55–58] The lymph node cortex contains numerous channels that run from the subcapsular sinus to high-endothelial venules, and these serve as conduits for such molecules. Recent studies have shown that following subcutaneous injection of antigen, two waves of antigen appear in the node. The first appears rapidly in the conduits and labels T cell area DCs weakly. The second wave is delayed by several hours, and the antigen appears in strongly labeled DCs. This second wave and, crucially, sensitization for delayed-type hypersensitivity, is abolished by extirpating the antigen depot, suggesting that the labeled DCs had acquired antigen in the periphery and then migrated to the node.[59,60] It is not known whether the first wave of antigen can induce tolerance.

CONCLUSIONS

The mechanisms by which adaptive immune responses to intestinal antigens are regulated are as yet poorly understood. In the steady state, DCs are continually migrating from the intestine to MLN, carrying self- and food antigens, and during infection, they presumably carry antigens from intestinal pathogens. DCs represent the main mechanism by which antigen is transported and delivered to T cells, but DCs represent complex cell populations with different functions. DCs are recruited rapidly to inflamed tissues, and their properties may be modulated by cytokines released in these tissues. This modulation of DC properties may be central to inducing differential activation pathways in T cells, but, as yet, little is known about what is really going on under these circumstances in the periphery and in the node. Understanding these processes is, however, crucial to devising rational vaccination and immunotherapeutic strategies in the future.

REFERENCES

1. ROSE, M.E., D. WAKELIN & P. HESKETH. 1991. Interferon-gamma-mediated effects upon immunity to coccidial infections in the mouse. Parasite Immunol. **13:** 63–74.
2. PUGH, C.W., G.G. MACPHERSON & H. W. STEER. 1983. Characterization of nonlymphoid cells derived from rat peripheral lymph. J. Exp. Med. **157:** 1758–1779.
3. MACPHERSON, G.G., S. FOSSUM & B. HARRISON. 1989. Properties of lymph-borne (veiled) dendritic cells in culture. II. Expression of the IL-2 receptor: role of GM-CSF. Immunology **68:** 108–113.
4. MACPHERSON, G.G. 1989. Properties of lymph-borne (veiled) dendritic cells in culture. I. Modulation of phenotype, survival and function: partial dependence on GM-CSF. Immunology **68:** 102–107.
5. LIU, L.M. & G.G. MACPHERSON. 1993. Antigen acquisition by dendritic cells: intestinal dendritic cells acquire antigen administered orally and can prime naive T cells in vivo. J. Exp. Med. **177:** 1299–1307.
6. LIU, L.M. & G.G. MACPHERSON. 1995. Antigen processing: cultured lymph-borne dendritic cells can process and present native protein antigens. Immunology **84:** 241–246.
7. LIU, L.M. & G.G. MACPHERSON. 1995. Rat intestinal dendritic cells: immunostimulatory potency and phenotypic characterization. Immunology **85:** 88–93.
8. MACPHERSON, G.G. et al. 1995. Endotoxin-mediated dendritic cell release from the intestine. Characterization of released dendritic cells and TNF dependence. J. Immunol. **154:** 1317–1322.
9. LIU, L.M. et al. 1998. Dendritic cell heterogeneity in vivo: two functionally different dendritic cell populations in rat intestinal lymph can be distinguished by CD4 expression. J. Immunol. **161:** 1146–1155.
10. HUANG, F.P. et al. 2000. A discrete subpopulation of dendritic cells transports apoptotic intestinal epithelial cells to T cell areas of mesenteric lymph nodes. J. Exp. Med. **191:** 435–444.
11. HUANG, F.P. et al. 2002. Migrating intestinal dendritic cells transport PrP(Sc) from the gut. J. Gen. Virol. **83:** 267–271.
12. SHORTMAN, K. & Y.J. LIU. 2002. Mouse and human dendritic cell subtypes. Nat. Rev. Immunol. **2:** 151–161.
13. MERAD, M. et al. 2002. Langerhans cells renew in the skin throughout life under steady-state conditions. Nat. Immunol. **3:** 1135–1141.
14. DEL HOYO, G.M. et al. 2002. Characterization of a common precursor population for dendritic cells. Nature **415:** 1043–1047.
15. RANDOLPH, G.J. et al. 1998. Differentiation of monocytes into dendritic cells in a model of transendothelial trafficking [see comments]. Science **282:** 480–483.
16. PAVLI, P. et al. 1990. Isolation and characterization of antigen-presenting dendritic cells from the mouse intestinal lamina propria. Immunology **70:** 40–47.
17. PAVLI, P. et al. 1996. Distribution of human colonic dendritic cells and macrophages. Clin. Exp. Immunol. **104:** 124–132.
18. BELL, S.J. et al. 2001. Migration and maturation of human colonic dendritic cells. J. Immunol. **166:** 4958–4967.
19. STAGG, A.J., M.A. KAMM & S.C. KNIGHT. 2002. Intestinal dendritic cells increase T cell expression of alpha4beta7 integrin. Eur. J. Immunol. **32:** 1445–1454.
20. SPALDING, D.M. et al. 1983. Accessory cells in murine Peyers patch. I. Identification and enrichment of a functional dendritic cell. J. Exp. Med. **157:** 1646–1659.
21. WILDERS, M.M. et al. 1983. Large mononuclear Ia-positive veiled cells in Peyer's patches. II. Localization in rat Peyer's patches. Immunology **48:** 461–467.

22. SPALDING, D.M. et al. 1984. Peyer's patch dendritic cells: Isolation and functional comparison with murine spleen dendritic cells. Immunobiology **168**: 380–390.
23. SPALDING, D.M. et al. 1984. Preferential induction of polyclonal IgA secretion by murine Peyer's patch dendritic cell-T cell mixtures. J. Exp. Med. **160**: 941–946.
24. BARR, W.G. et al. 1985. The accessory cell function of murine Peyer's patches. Cell Immunol. **92**: 41–52.
25. EVERSON, M.P., W.J. KOOPMAN & K.W. BEAGLEY. 1993. Divergent T-cell cytokine profiles induced by dendritic cells from different tissues. Adv. Exp. Med. Biol. **329**: 47–52.
26. RAO, A.S. et al. 1993. Isolation of dendritic leukocytes from non-lymphoid organs. Adv. Exp. Med. Biol. **329**: 507–512.
27. EVERSON, M.P. et al. 1996. Dendritic cells from different tissues induce production of different T cell cytokine profiles. J. Leukoc. Biol. **59**: 494–498.
28. KELSALL, B.L. & W. STROBER. 1996. Distinct populations of dendritic cells are present in the subepithelial dome and T cell regions of the murine Peyer's patch. J. Exp. Med. **183**: 237–247.
29. KELSALL, B.L. & W. STROBER. 1996. The role of dendritic cells in antigen processing in the Peyer's patch. Ann. N.Y. Acad. Sci. **778**: 47–54.
30. RUEDL, C. et al. 1996. Phenotypic and functional characterization of CD11c+ dendritic cell population in mouse Peyer's patches. Eur. J. Immunol. **26**: 1801–1806.
31. EVERSON, M.P. et al. 1997. FACS-sorted spleen and Peyer's patch dendritic cells induce different responses in Th0 clones. Adv. Exp. Med. Biol. **417**: 357–362.
32. RUEDL, C. & S. HUBELE. 1997. Maturation of Peyer's patch dendritic cells in vitro upon stimulation via cytokines or CD40 triggering. Eur. J. Immunol. **27**: 1325–1330.
33. RUEDL, C. et al. 1997. The role of CD11c+ cells as possible candidates for immature dendritic cells in the murine Peyer's patches. Adv. Exp. Med. Biol. **417**: 111–114.
34. EVERSON, M.P. et al. 1998. Dendritic cells from Peyer's patch and spleen induce different T helper cell responses. J. Interferon Cytokine Res. **18**: 103–115.
35. MAKALA, L.H. et al. 1998. Isolation and characterisation of pig Peyer's patch dendritic cells. Vet. Immunol. Immunopathol. **61**: 67–81.
36. ANJUERE, F. et al. 1999. Definition of dendritic cell subpopulations present in the spleen, Peyer's patches, lymph nodes, and skin of the mouse. Blood **93**: 590–598.
37. IWASAKI, A. & B.L. KELSALL. 1999. Freshly isolated Peyer's patch, but not spleen, dendritic cells produce interleukin 10 and induce the differentiation of T helper type 2 cells. J. Exp. Med. **190**: 229–239.
38. DE BAEY, A. et al. 2003. A subset of human dendritic cells in the T cell area of mucosa-associated lymphoid tissue with a high potential to produce TNF-alpha. J. Immunol. **170**: 89–94.
39. MATSUNO, K. & T. EZAKI. 2000. Dendritic cell dynamics in the liver and hepatic lymph. Int. Rev. Cytol. **197**: 83–136.
40. TURNBULL, E. & G. MACPHERSON. 2001. Immunobiology of dendritic cells in the rat. Immunol. Rev. **184**: 58–68.
41. LIU, L. et al. 1998. Dendritic cell heterogeneity in vivo: two functionally different dendritic cell populations in rat intestinal lymph can be distinguished by CD4 expression. J. Immunol. **161**: 1146–1155.
42. HOWARD, C.J. et al. 1997. Identification of two distinct populations of dendritic cells in afferent lymph that vary in their ability to stimulate T cells. J. Immunol. **159**: 5372–5382.
43. FINKELMAN, F.D. et al. 1996. Dendritic cells can present antigen in vivo in a tolerogenic or immunogenic fashion. J. Immunol. **157**: 1406–1414.
44. HAWIGER, D. et al. 2001. Dendritic cells induce peripheral T cell unresponsiveness under steady state conditions in vivo. J. Exp. Med. **194**: 769–779.
45. VEZYS, V., S. OLSON & L. LEFRANCOIS. 2000. Expression of intestine-specific antigen reveals novel pathways of CD8 T cell tolerance induction. Immunity **12**: 505–514.
46. BELZ, G.T. et al. 2002. The CD8alpha(+) dendritic cell is responsible for inducing peripheral self-tolerance to tissue-associated antigens. J. Exp. Med. **196**: 1099–1104.
47. SHREEDHAR, V.K., B.L. KELSALL & M.R. NEUTRA. 2003. Cholera toxin induces migration of dendritic cells from the subepithelial dome region to T- and B-cell areas of Peyer's patches. Infect. Immun. **71**: 504–509.

48. SMITH, M.W., P.S. JAMES & D.R. TIVEY. 1987. M cell numbers increase after transfer of SPF mice to a normal animal house environment. Am. J. Pathol. **128:** 385–389.
49. RESCIGNO, M. *et al.* 2001. Dendritic cells express tight junction proteins and penetrate gut epithelial monolayers to sample bacteria. Nat. Immunol. **2:** 361–367.
50. LEVIN, D.M. *et al.* 1976. Cellular immunity in Peyer's patches of rats infected with *Trichinella spiralis*. Infect. Immun. **13:** 27–30.
51. BRUCE, M.E. *et al.* 2000. Follicular dendritic cells in TSE pathogenesis. Immunol. Today **21:** 442–446.
52. CARP, R.I. & S.M. CALLAHAN. 1982. Effect of mouse peritoneal macrophages on scrapie infectivity during extended in vitro incubation. Intervirology **17:** 201–207.
53. WYKES, M. *et al.* 1998. Dendritic cells interact directly with naive B lymphocytes to transfer antigen and initiate class switching in a primary T-dependent response. J. Immunol. **161:** 1313–1319.
54. MACPHERSON, G.G., N. KUSHNIR & M. WYKES. 1999. Dendritic cells, B cells and the regulation of antibody synthesis. Immunol. Rev. **172:** 325–334.
55. GRETZ, J.E. *et al.* 1996. Sophisticated strategies for information encounter in the lymph node: the reticular network as a conduit of soluble information and a highway for cell traffic. J. Immunol. **157:** 495–499.
56. GRETZ, J.E., A.O. ANDERSON & S. SHAW. 1997. Cords, channels, corridors and conduits: critical architectural elements facilitating cell interactions in the lymph node cortex. Immunol. Rev. **156:** 11–24.
57. GRETZ, J.E. *et al.* 2000. Lymph-borne chemokines and other low molecular weight molecules reach high endothelial venules via specialized conduits while a functional barrier limits access to the lymphocyte microenvironments in lymph node cortex. J. Exp. Med. **192:** 1425–1440.
58. KALDJIAN, E.P. *et al.* 2001. Spatial and molecular organization of lymph node T cell cortex: a labyrinthine cavity bounded by an epithelium-like monolayer of fibroblastic reticular cells anchored to basement membrane-like extracellular matrix. Int. Immunol. **13:** 1243–1253.
59. ITANO, A.A. *et al.* 2003. Distinct dendritic cell populations sequentially present antigen to CD4 T cells and stimulate different aspects of cell-mediated immunity. Immunity **19:** 47–57.
60. ITANO, A.A. & M.K. JENKINS. 2003. Antigen presentation to naive CD4 T cells in the lymph node. Nat. Immunol. **4:** 733–739.

In Vivo Enhancement of Dendritic Cell Function

JANINE BILSBOROUGH AND JOANNE L. VINEY

Department of Autoimmunity and Vascular Biology, Amgen, Seattle, Washington 98119, USA

ABSTRACT: Despite the apparent positive recognition of antigen by mucosal T cells after ingesting food, the default functional response in the gut is tolerance. Although dendritic cells (DCs) are classically defined as potent stimulatory antigen-presenting cells, we have previously shown that tolerance is enhanced *in vivo* in the presence of elevated numbers of DCs. In order to more closely investigate the mechanistic basis of tolerance induction, we have focused our subsequent studies on identifying features peculiar to mucosal dendritic cells and the functional involvement of mucosal DCs in driving the early T cell response to fed antigen. These studies have revealed a population of DCs in the mucosae that exhibit the plasmacytoid phenotype and secrete IFN-α following stimulation with CpG, and can drive differentiation of naive T cells into cells that exhibit regulatory properties. The activity of these DCs also failed to sustain robust T cell proliferation and, rather, functioned to enhance the suppressive efficacy of $CD4^+CD25^+$ T regulatory cells. Given their significant presence in mucosal tissue, these DCs likely provide a mechanistic basis for the homeostatic regulation prominent in the gut, presumably by eliciting regulatory cell suppressor function and poorly supporting T helper cell proliferation. These studies further underscore the critical role for intestinal DCs in promoting tolerogenic antigen presentation at a site of high antigenic stimulation.

KEYWORDS: plasmacytoid DC; regulatory T cells; oral tolerance; intestinal homeostasis; Tr1 cells

The cells of the gastrointestinal immune system are exposed to a plethora of antigens, including food proteins and microbial antigens from both commensal microorganisms and potentially harmful pathogens. In order to maintain homeostasis in the gut, the immune system must tightly regulate cellular responsiveness and maintain a balance between active immunity and tolerance. Loss of tolerance to food antigens can result in food allergy or celiac disease, whereas loss of tolerance to the normal gut flora can be the underlying cause of inflammatory bowel disease (IBD). In normal individuals, despite the apparent positive recognition of antigen by mucosal T cells after ingesting food, the default functional response in the gut is tolerance.[1,2]

Address for correspondence: Joanne L. Viney, Amgen, 1201 Amgen Court West, Seattle, WA 98119. Voice: 206-265-7178; fax: 206-217-0494.
vineyj@amgen.com

Dendritic cells are central to the generation of adaptive immunity, and, although DCs are classically defined as potent stimulatory antigen-presenting cells, tolerance is enhanced in the presence of elevated numbers of DCs *in vivo*.[3] How intestinal DCs function to promote tolerogenic immune responses has been the focus of our laboratory's research in recent years. Accumulating evidence suggests that different DC populations may differ in their capacity to activate T cells. For example, when stimulated with the TNFR family member RANKL, mucosal DCs upregulate the transcript for IL-10, while splenic DCs upregulate IL-12.[4] Furthermore, different DC populations in the Peyer's patch can produce different cytokine profiles following exposure to the same stimuli.[5] This differential responsiveness in the context of cytokine production may be key to the control of the subsequent immune response, because cytokines such as IL-10, interferon-alpha (IFN-α), and transforming growth factor-β (TGF-β) can all be produced by DCs and have each been used to generate T cells that can regulate T cell proliferation *in vitro*.[6,7] Apart from cytokines, DCs can exhibit other mechanisms by which to regulate T cell proliferation. Stimulation of T cells with DCs that overexpress the ligand for Notch 1 or stimulation with immature DCs can induce T cells that exhibit regulatory properties,[8,9] and DCs expressing enzymes such as prostaglandin E_2 (PGE_2) or indoleamine 2,3 dioxygenase (IDO) can suppress T cell proliferation.[10–12] Like PGE_2, IDO is expressed in the intestine, and early studies on IDO suggested that peripheral $CD8\alpha^+$ DC expressed IDO and could inhibit the immunogenic properties of $CD8\alpha^-$ DC.[13] More recent data suggests that a number of other mouse DC populations in the periphery express IDO.[14]

We assessed mucosal lymphoid tissue for the presence of both $CD8\alpha^+$ DCs and DCs that express IDO. Flow cytometry (FACS) analysis of DC populations in the mucosal lymphoid departments highlighted two populations of DCs that expressed $CD8\alpha$: one $CD8\alpha^+$ population expressed low levels of CD11c, whereas the other $CD8\alpha^+$ population expressed high levels of CD11c. In the mesenteric lymph nodes (MLNs), spleen, and the peripheral lymph nodes (PLNs), $CD8\alpha^+$ DCs exhibited both low and high levels of CD11c (CD11c lo and CD11c hi, respectively), whereas in the Peyer's patch, the majority of $CD8\alpha^+$ DC were CD11c lo.[15] Analysis of IDO mRNA in these different $CD11c^+$ DC subsets showed that the CD11c lo subset of DCs expressed significantly higher levels of IDO than the CD11c hi subset (TABLE 1). The increase in IDO expression correlated with the decreased ability of these DCs to induce antigen-specific T cell proliferation (TABLE 1). Furthermore, phenotypic analysis of these DCs suggested they displayed a plasmacytoid DC phenoytpe, as they were positive for B220 and Gr-1, but negative for CD19, showed low levels of Class II, CD40, CD80, and CD86, and secreted IFNα following stimulation with CpG.

Because IFN-α and IL-10 have been shown to support the differentiation of Tr1 cells *in vitro*,[6] we tested whether CD11c lo DC from mucosal tissues could support the *de novo* differentiation of mouse Tr1 cells. To this end, we generated ovalbumin (OVA)-specific T cell lines (depleted of $CD25^+$ T cells) with freshly isolated DC populations in the presence of OVA peptide and IL-2. After three weeks, the resulting cells lines were assayed for regulatory activity by measuring their ability to inhibit antigen-specific T cell proliferation by naive OVA T cell receptor (TCR) Tg T cells. T cell lines generated with mucosal CD11c lo DCs could significantly suppress the proliferation of naive T cells to antigen (TABLE 2), whereas those T cell lines

TABLE 1. Levels of IDO mRNA expressed by DC populations correlate with inefficient induction of antigen-specific T cell proliferation

Tissue of Origin	CD8α+ DC Subset	Relative Expression of IDO mRNA^a ($\times 10^{-3}$)	T cell proliferation^b (cpm)
Spleen	CD11c hi	1.01 + 0.3	140,180 ± 60,529
	CD11c lo	1.5 + 0.3	112,330 ± 7,696
MLN	CD11c hi	0.73 + 0.2	255,775 ± 74,902*
	CD11c lo	3.1 + 1.4*	109,679 ± 12,542
PLN	CD11c hi	0.82 + 0.3	249,723 ± 27,408
	CD11c lo	3.5 + 0.6*	150,371 ± 57,293
PP^c	CD8α-	0.97 + 0.4	233,125 ± 59,859*
	CD11c lo	3.6 + 0.78*	86,030 ± 33,265

^{a}IDO mRNA expression was measured relative to HPRT using real-time quantitative PCR.
^{b}T cell proliferation by naive OVA TCR Tg T cells was assessed at 375 nM of OVA peptide.
^{c}PP do not have sufficiently significant numbers of CD11c hi CD8α$^+$ DC to allow for comparisons between CD11c hi and CD11c lo DC for this tissue.
*Indicates statistical significance ($P < .05$, Student's t test) between levels of CD11c lo and CD11c hi DCs from the same tissue.

TABLE 2. Inhibition of proliferation of naive OVA TCR Tg T cells in the presence of T cell lines generated with CD8α$^+$ plasmacytoid DCs

OVA Peptide Concentration (nM)	T Cell Line Alone (cpm)	Naive OVA TCR Tg T Cells Alone (cpm)	Naive TCR Tg T cells + T Cell Line (cpm)
5	173 ± 68	806 ± 574	220 ± 112
50	155 ± 40	29,395 ± 12,483	587 ± 474
500	224 ± 93	93,958 ± 19.368	2,996 ± 1,431^a

^{a}Levels of proliferation of naive OVA TCR Tg alone and combined with the T cell line generated by CD8α$^+$ CD11c lo DCs are statistically significant at $P < .05$ (Welch's t test).

generated by CD8α$^+$ nonplasmacytoid DCs could not (data not shown). The suppressive T cell lines were found to produce IL-4, IL-10, and IFN-γ following stimulation with plate-bound anti-CD3, suggesting a Tr1-like phenotype, with the difference that these cell lines appear to produce IL-4. In addition to their ability to induce *de novo* differentiation of Tr1-like cells, T cell suppression induced by classical CD4$^+$CD25$^+$ T regulatory cells was enhanced in the presence of CD11c lo DCs, probably owing to the fact that CD11c lo DCs are poor stimulators of T cell proliferation (TABLE 3). Thus, CD8α$^+$ CD11c lo DCs from the gut exhibiting a plasmacytoid DC phenotype express higher levels of IDO mRNA than the nonplasmacytoid CD8α$^+$ DCs present in these tissues. They are inefficient at inducing T cell proliferation and, as a result, are supportive of CD4$^+$CD25$^+$ T regulatory–mediated suppression of proliferation. Furthermore, they induce the differentiation of T cells that exhibit a suppressive phenotype. The latter point is of particular

TABLE 3. Enhanced suppression of T cell proliferation of naive OVA TCR Tg T cells by CD4+CD25+ T regulatory cells in the presence of CD8α+ CD11c lo plasmacytoid DCs

Tissue of Origin	DC Subset	Proliferation (cpm)		Percent Inhibition of Proliferation
		Naive OVA TCR Tg T Cells Alone	Naive OVA TCR Tg T cells + CD4+CD25+ T Regulatory Cells	
Spleen	CD11c hi	149,756 ± 14,906	51,367 ± 8,524	66
	CD11c lo	104,309 ± 7,914	14,685 ± 4,470	86
MLN	CD11c hi	170,181 ± 3 602	55,865 ± 4,065	67
	CD11c lo	72,072 ± 13,576	5,853 ± 343	88
PLN	CD11c hi	183,040 ± 18,188	64,359 ± 7,376	65
	CD11c lo	88,654 ± 14,174	5,822 ± 2,332	94
PP	CD8α-	161,262 ± 1,219	75,669 ± 787	53
	CD11c lo	42,054 ± 3,315	2,541 ± 6,122	94

significance in the light of recent data demonstrating that gut-derived DCs can selectively imprint gut-homing characteristics on T cells, thus maintaining local tissue immunosuppressiveness.[16]

Our studies in the past have demonstrated that mucosal dendritic cells appear to preferentially promote tolerogenic responses.[3] Our present studies suggest that a single DC subset within the gut may not only play a pivotal role in the downregulation of new immune responses in the gut, but may also be involved in the differentiation and maintenance of the resident regulatory population.[15]

REFERENCES

1. SMITH, K.M., J.M. DAVIDSON & P. GARSIDE. 2002. T-cell activation occurs simultaneously in local and peripheral lymphoid tissue following oral administration of a range of doses of immunogenic or tolerogenic antigen although tolerized T cells display a defect in cell division. Immunology **106:** 144–158.
2. WILLIAMSON, E., J.M. O'MALLEY & J. L. VINEY. 1999. Visualizing the T-cell response elicited by oral administration of soluble protein antigen. Immunology **97:** 565–572.
3. VINEY, J.L., A.M. MOWAT, J.M. O'MALLEY, et al. 1998. Expanding dendritic cells in vivo enhances the induction of oral tolerance. J. Immunol. **160:** 5815–5825.
4. WILLIAMSON, E., J.M. BILSBOROUGH & J.L. VINEY. 2002. Regulation of mucosal dendritic cell function by receptor activator of NF-kappa B (RANK)/RANK ligand interactions: impact on tolerance induction. J. Immunol. **169:** 3606–3612.
5. IWASAKI, A. & B.L. KELSALL. 2001. Unique functions of CD11b+, CD8 alpha+, and double-negative Peyer's patch dendritic cells. J. Immunol. **166:** 4884–4890.
6. LEVINGS, M.K., R. SANGREGORIO, F. GALBIATI, et al. 2001. IFN-alpha and IL-10 induce the differentiation of human type 1 T regulatory cells. J. Immunol. **166:** 5530–5539.
7. YAMAGIWA, S., J.D. GRAY, S. HASHIMOTO & D.A. HORWITZ. 2001. A role for TGF-beta in the generation and expansion of CD4+CD25+ regulatory T cells from human peripheral blood. J. Immunol. **166:** 7282–7289.
8. HOYNE, G.F., I. LE ROUX, M. CORSIN-JIMENEZ, et al. 2000. Serrate1-induced notch signalling regulates the decision between immunity and tolerance made by peripheral CD4(+) T cells. Int. Immunol. **12:** 177–185.

9. JONULEIT, H., E. SCHMITT, G. SCHULER, et al. 2000. Induction of interleukin 10-producing, nonproliferating CD4(+) T cells with regulatory properties by repetitive stimulation with allogeneic immature human dendritic cells. J. Exp. Med. **192:** 1213–1222.
10. NEWBERRY, R.D., W.F. STENSON & R.G. LORENZ. 1999. Cyclooxygenase-2-dependent arachidonic acid metabolites are essential modulators of the intestinal immune response to dietary antigen. Nat. Med. **5:** 900–906.
11. NEWBERRY, R.D., J.S. MCDONOUGH, W.F. STENSON & R.G. LORENZ. 2001. Spontaneous and continuous cyclooxygenase-2-dependent prostaglandin E2 production by stromal cells in the murine small intestine lamina propria: directing the tone of the intestinal immune response. J. Immunol. **166:** 4465–4472.
12. MUNN, D.H., E. SHAFIZADEH, J.T. ATTWOOD, et al. 1999. Inhibition of T cell proliferation by macrophage tryptophan catabolism. J. Exp. Med. **189:** 1363–1372.
13. GROHMANN, U., R. BIANCHI, M.L. BELLADONNA, et al. 2000. IFN-gamma inhibits presentation of a tumor/self peptide by CD8 alpha-dendritic cells via potentiation of the CD8 alpha+ subset. J. Immunol. **165:** 1357–1363.
14. MELLOR, A.L., B. BABAN, P. CHANDLER, et al. 2003. Cutting edge: induced indoleamine 2,3 dioxygenase expression in dendritic cell subsets suppresses T cell clonal expansion. J. Immunol. **171:** 1652–1655.
15. BILSBOROUGH, J., T.C. GEORGE, A. NORMENT & J.L. VINEY. 2003. Mucosal CD8alpha+ DC, with a plasmacytoid phenotype, induce differentiation and support function of T cells with regulatory properties. Immunology **108:** 481–492.
16. MORA, J.R., M.R. BONO, N. MANJUNATH, et al. 2003. Selective imprinting of gut-homing T cells by Peyer's patch dendritic cells. Nature **424:** 88–93.

Regulation of Tolerance in the Respiratory Tract

TIM-1, Hygiene, and the Environment

DALE T. UMETSU AND ROSEMARIE H. DeKRUYFF

Division of Immunology and Allergy, Stanford University, Stanford, California 94305-5208, USA

ABSTRACT: In this chapter we will discuss the regulation of immune responses in the respiratory mucosal system, rather than in the gastrointestinal mucosal system. However, because the lung and gastrointestinal tracts derive developb-mentally from a common endoderm, immune mechanisms in the respiratory and gastrointestinal tracts are likely to be very similar. Therefore, concepts that are learned about the respiratory tract are likely to benefit the understanding of tolerance in the gastrointestinal tract. We will discuss the regulation of immune responses in asthma, the role of respiratory tolerance, mediated by dendritic cells and regulatory T cells in the lung. In addition, we will discuss a genetic approach to better understand respiratory tolerance and the discovery of the TIM gene family, which regulates the development of Th2 responses, asthma, and tolerance. Finally, we will discuss the association in humans of TIM-1 and atopy, and the relationship between TIM1, hygiene, and the environment.

KEYWORDS: asthma; atopy; dendritic celll; regulatory T cell

ASTHMA, ATOPY, AND TOLERANCE

Asthma is an immunological disease caused by Th2-driven inflammation that is characterized by increased mucus production in the bronchioles, and by an inflammatory process in the peribronchiolar space that consists of eosinophils, basophils, mast cells, and Th2 lymphocytes. Respiratory exposure to allergen can induce the development of tolerance that protects against the development of airway hyperreactivity (AHR), a cardinal feature of asthma. This tolerance process is mediated by dendritic cells (DC) within the respiratory tract that take up allergen and migrate to the draining lymph nodes, where they mature, express high levels of costimulatory molecules (including B7-1, B7-2, and ICOS-L), and transiently produce IL-10 (as detected by RT-PCR or by intracellular staining).[1] These IL-10–producing DC induce the production of IL-10 in antigen-specific T cells (as detected by intracellular cytokine staining), but not IFN-γ, and induce transient production of IL-4. When these IL-10–producing regulatory T cells (Tr) are adoptively transferred, they prevent the development of AHR.[2] The tolerance induction phase and the inhibitory function of the Tr are both dependent on the ICOS-ICOS-ligand pathway. In contrast, control mice sensitized and challenged with allergen develop severe AHR, as expected. The inhibitory effect is due in part to IL-10, as treatment of these mice with an anti-IL-10 monoclonal antibody abolishes this effect. Thus, respiratory tolerance is mediated by DC and Tr cells, which produce IL-10 and protect against the development of asthma.

GENETIC APPROACH TO BETTER UNDERSTAND TOLERANCE

To better understand how respiratory tolerance mechanisms protect against asthma, we took a genetic approach to evaluating this system that also took into account the epidemiological factors involved in the pathogenesis of asthma. Like inflammatory bowel diseases, the prevalence of asthma has increased dramatically over the past two decades. Since 1980, the prevalence of asthma, and all atopic diseases, has essentially doubled in industrialized countries, while at the same time the incidence of a number of infectious diseases has decreased dramatically.[3] These infectious diseases include measles, mumps, tuberculosis, and hepatitis A virus, to which we will return later. This inverse relationship between infection and atopy is the basis for the "hygiene hypothesis," but the specific infectious agents responsible for this relationship are not fully known.

Asthma and atopy are complex genetic traits, the expression of which is triggered by environmental factors, including infections.[4] Together, these effects result in a Th2 response and asthma in some individuals, and a protective response with no asthma in others, presumably related to tolerance to allergens. Asthma susceptibility has been linked in human genome-wide scans to at least a dozen chromosomal regions, including regions on chromosomes 5, 6, 7, 11, 12, 14, and 20. However, identification of specific genes within these chromosomal regions has been extremely difficult because each of the dozen or so asthma susceptibility gene exerts only a small effect in the overall pathogenesis of asthma, interacts with other genes on other chromosomes in nonadditive ways, interacts with the environment in nonadditive ways, and, finally, segregates independently. Because of these problems, only a few asthma susceptibility genes have been identified with any degree of certainty. However, we believed that identification of asthma susceptibility genes might provide very important insights into the regulation of Th2 responses, tolerance, and asthma, and, therefore, we set out to find an asthma susceptibility gene that might protect against asthma and allergy. It was clear that in order to be successful, the task had to be simplified by reducing the number of interacting genes. We accomplished this by developing a congenic mouse model of asthma.

We repeatedly backcrossed one mouse strain, DBA/2, with another strain, BALB/c, resulting in congenic strains that had discrete chromosomal segments from DBA/2 on the BALB/c background. On immunization with allergen, BALB/c mice develop Th2-dominated immune responses, with high IL-4 production and severe AHR, whereas DBA/2 mice develop low IL-4 responses and have normal airway reactivity when sensitized and challenged with allergen. The congenic HBA mice that we developed from these backcrosses contained a discrete segment from chromosome 11 of the DBA/2 mouse on the BALB/c background. This chromosomal segment is syntenic to the human chromosomal region 5q23-35, a region that has been linked repeatedly to asthma, as well as to inflammatory bowel disease. Most important, having this particular chromosomal segment converted the BALB/c mouse into one that produced low IL-4 levels and resisted the development of airway AHR. Our goal, therefore, was to identify the gene within this region, and the polymorphisms in that gene, that were responsible for these differences.

POSITIONAL CLONING OF THE TIM GENES

First, we analyzed the chromosome 11 region in HBA mice inherited from DBA/2 mice by the use of 25 simple sequence length polymorphism (SSLP) microsatellite markers and found that the HBA mice had, in fact, inherited two discrete segments of chromosome 11. We also confirmed that the rest of the genome in HBA mice was identical to that of BALB/c. The proximal chromosomal segment inherited from DBA/2 mice is about 20 centimorgans (cM). We used an additional 22 microsatellite markers to analyze this region in higher resolution. This region is homologous to human chromosome 5q23-35, and contains several potentially interesting genes, including those for IL-3, IL-5, IL-13, IL-4, and IL-12p40.

In the next step of the analysis, we generated N2 mice and linked IL-4 production and AHR with genotype. These N2 mice were generated by first breeding F1 mice, and then backcrossing these Fl mice to HBA mice. In about 80% of the N2 progeny, no recombination occurred within the proximal segment inherited from DBA/2 mice. However, about 20% of the N2 mice had recombination in this region, owing to crossover events in the F1 parent, which allowed us to map the allergic phenotype to specific genes in this region.

We genotyped about 3,000 N2 mice to find recombinant mice, which we then phenotyped. In these mice, IL-4 production and AHR segregated into high responders and low responders. The bimodal distribution indicated that IL-4 production and AHR segregated as if a single gene was responsible for both traits in these mice. This means that in our model we were able to simplify several very complex genetic traits into a single gene trait.

Using linkage analysis, we narrowed the region of interest to less than 0.5 cM, then sequenced all of the genes and ESTs in this region. By doing this, we discovered a new gene family. All members of this family are expressed in T cells, and their gene products contain an immunoglobulin domain and a mucin domain; for this reason, we refer to these genes as members of the TIM family of genes.[5] The predicted amino acid sequence of the first member of this family, TIM-1, has significant polymorphisms, including a 23–amino acid deletion in the HBA sequence. We believe that these differences in the sequence of this gene are responsible for the phenotypic differences observed between BALB/c and HBA mice.

The mucin domains of the TIM gene family products are heavily glycosylated at o-linked sites and at N-linked sites. In addition, each TIM protein has a transmembrane domain and an intracellular domain, and three of the four TIM proteins have a tyrosine phosphorylation motif, suggesting that these proteins are involved in transmembrane signaling. In mice, TIM-1 encodes a 305–amino acid protein, which regulates the development of asthma and allergy, possibly by inducing tolerance.

TIM-3 encodes a 281–amino acid protein that appears to regulate the development of autoimmune disease.[6,7] TIM-1 is preferentially expressed on Th2 cells, and TIM-3 is preferentially expressed on Th1 cells. These findings indicate that the TIMs are critically involved in the regulation of adaptive immunity and the function of CD4 T cells.[8]

HUMAN TIMS

We next determined whether the human TIM genes were polymorphic, as they are in mice, and whether they might be involved in regulating the development of atopy. The TIMs are located on human chromosome region 5q33.2, which is a chromosomal region that has been repeatedly linked to asthma in humans. We sequenced TIM-1 in 40 individuals and found significant polymorphisms, including a 6–amino acid insertion/deletion polymorphism.

HEPATITIS A VIRUS RECEPTOR

It has emerged that the human TIM-1 is the receptor for the hepatitis A virus (HAV).[9] This finding is important because in humans, infection with HAV has been associated with protection against asthma.[10,11] In one study, Matricardi *et al.* showed that the prevalence of asthma, and atopy in general, in individuals who are seropositive for HAV is about one half of that of individuals who are seronegative for HAV.[10] In another study of 30,000 individuals in the United States, the prevalence of asthma in HAV-seropositive individuals was shown to be about one-fourth that of individuals who were seronegative.[11] However, because HAV is not a respiratory pathogen, and because HAV is transmitted through fecal-oral routes, many people have assumed that infection with HAV is merely a marker of poor hygiene, and that it is poor hygiene and not HAV that protects against the development of asthma.

THE ASSOCIATION OF TIM-1, ATOPY, AND HAV

To examine the association of TIM-1 with atopy, we enrolled 375 subjects in a study that assessed these individuals for atopy by history, evaluation of allergy to 16 different aeroallergens, and total IgE level. We also obtained HAV titers and genotyped these individuals for the 6–amino acid insertion/deletion polymorphism in TIM-1. We used stratified Mantel-Haenszel chi-square tests to quantify the association between atopy and the 6–amino acid insertion/deletion in TIM-1. In our study population, about 15% had two copies of the insertion in TIM-1, whereas about 40% had one copy of the insertion, and about 40% had no copies of the insertion.[12] This indicated that this polymorphism is very common in the general population. Further, the frequency of the polymorphism varied slightly with racial background, with Asians having the lowest frequency, Caucasians an intermediate frequency, and African-Americans the highest frequency of the insertion polymorphism.

In the total population, we were initially very disappointed to find that there was no association of the TIM-1 insertion with atopy. Thus, if an individual had one or two copies of the insertion polymorphism in TIM-1, he or she was as likely to be atopic as those who had no copies of the insertion polymorphism. However, when we separated the subjects into those who were HAV seropositive and those who were HAV seronegative, we found that there was a significant inverse association of the insertion and atopy. Thus, in the HAV-seropositive subjects, those who had one or two copies of the insertion were much less likely to be atopic than those who had no copies of the insertion. This was highly significant, with a P value of .0005.[12] On the other hand, in the HAV seronegative population, the insertion was not associated with any protection against atopy.

These results indicate that TIM-1 is a very significant atopy susceptibility gene, but only in HAV-infected or HAV-exposed individuals. Further, these results suggest that HAV directly prevents the development of atopy, perhaps by binding to TIM-1, its receptor, and decreasing the development of Th2 cells and asthma. However, HAV protects against atopy only in individuals with the long form of TIM-1. We believe that HAV binds more efficiently to the longer form of TIM-1. We believe that this interaction between HAV and the longer form of TIM-1 results in more efficient infection in T cells by HAV, and decreased Th2 cell development or possible deletion of Th2 cells, resulting in decreased atopy and decreased asthma. Alternatively, it is possible that this interaction induces a form of tolerance that suppresses the development of Th2-driven inflammation. In contrast, we believe that HAV binds less efficiently to the short form of TIM-1, resulting in less efficient HAV infection, greater Th2 cell development, and more atopy. These studies, therefore, provide a molecular mechanism for the hygiene hypothesis. Moreover, because the incidence of HAV infection is greatly reduced in industrialized countries, this protective effect of HAV is much less common today compared with 20 years ago.

SUMMARY

Using a genetic approach, we identified the TIM gene family that regulates CD4 T cell differentiation, airway inflammation, AHR and EAE, and possibly IBD. Much more work is required to understand the function of the TIMs. Second, we found that the human TIM-1 gene lies in chromosome region 5q33.2 and is associated with protection against atopy in HAV-seropositive individuals. We suspect HAV may also protect against IBD, but this needs to be examined closely. Finally, we suggest that TIM-1 provides a molecular mechanism for the hygiene hypothesis.

REFERENCES

1. AKBARI, O., R.H. DEKRUYFF & D.T. UMETSU. 2001. Pulmonary dendritic cells secreting IL-10 mediate T cell tolerance induced by respiratory exposure to antigen. Nature Immunol. **2:** 725–731.
2. AKBARI, O., G.J. FREEMAN, E.H. MEYER, *et al.* 2002. Antigen-specific regulatory T cells develop via the ICOS-ICOS-Ligand pathway and inhibit allergen-induced airway hyperreactivity. Nat. Med. **8:** 1024–1032.
3. BACH, J.F. 2002. The effect of infections on susceptibility to autoimmune and allergic diseases. N. Engl. J. Med. **347:** 911–920.

4. UMETSU, D., J. MCINTIRE, C. MACAUBAS, *et al.* 2002. Asthma: an epidemic of dysregulated immunity. Nat. Immunol. **3:** 715–720.
5. McIntire, J.J., S.E. Umetsu, O. Akbari, *et al.* 2001. Identification of Tapr (an airway hyperreactivity regulatory locus) and the linked Tim gene family. Nat. Immunol. **2:** 1109–1116.
6. MONNEY, L., C.A. SABATOS, J.L. GAGLIA, *et al.* 2002. Th1-specific cell surface protein Tim-3 regulates macrophage activation and severity of an autoimmune disease. Nature **415:** 536–541.
7. SANCHEZ-FUEYO, A., J. TIAN, D. PICARELLA, *et al.* 2003. Tim-3 inhibits T helper type 1-mediated auto- and alloimmune responses and promotes immunological tolerance. Nat. Immunol. **4:** 1093–1101.
8. KUCHROO, V.K., M.P. DAS, J.A. BROWN, *et al.* 1995. B7-1 and B7-2 costimulatory molecules activate differentially the Th1/Th2 developmental pathways: application to autoimmune disease therapy. Cell **80:** 707–718.
9. KAPLAN, G., A. TOTSUKA, P. THOMPSON, *et al.* 1996. Identification of a surface glycoprotein on African green monkey kidney cells as a receptor for hepatitis A virus. EMBO J. **15:** 4282–4296.
10. MATRICARDI, P., F. ROSMINI, S. RIONDINO, *et al.* 2000. Exposure to foodborne and orofecal microbes versus airborne viruses in relation to atopy and allergic asthma: epidemiological study. BMJ **320:** 412–417.
11. MATRICARDI, P.M., F. ROSMINI, L. FERRIGNO, *et al.* 1997. Cross sectional retrospective study of prevalence of atopy among Italian military students with antibodies against hepatitis A virus. BMJ **314:** 999–1003.
12. MCINTIRE, J., S. UMETSU, C. MACAUBAS, *et al.* 2003. Immunology: hepatitis A virus link to atopic disease. Nature **425:** 576.

Mechanisms of Oral Tolerance: Dendritic Cells
Summary of Part II

TERRENCE A. BARRETT

Department of Medicine and Microbiology/Immunology,
Northwestern University Feinberg School of Medicine, Chicago, Ilinois 60611, USA

THE DICHOTOMY OF DENDRITIC CELL RESPONSES

In the opening remarks of the mucosal dendritic cell (DC) session, Brian Kelsall proposed a paradigm for immature DC development: Immature DCs arise in the bone marrow (BM) and enter the circulation, where they localize to such tissues as the intestine and peripheral lymph nodes. Activation of immature DCs upon phagocytosis of microbial antigens may be influenced by toll-like receptor (TLR), CD40, and/or interferon α (IFN-α) receptor[1] signaling. Antigen acquisition under activating conditions upregulates surface molecules important for T cell activation, such as CD80, CD86, and major histocompatibility complex (MHC) class II molecules. In contrast, DCs that acquire soluble antigen in tissues (generally lymphoid) under steady state conditions transition into mature, quiescent cells. Data suggest that recruitment of immature DCs to steady state lymphoid tissue alter function and expression of MHC. Thus, Dr. Kelsall presented a dichotomous model of DC maturation where the outcome is determined by the level of threat appreciated. If antigen is acquired under activating conditions, DCs upregulate cofactors needed to generate effector T cells efficiently. By comparison, less alarming forms of antigen (e.g., soluble or oral) are presented by DCs in steady state tissues to promote tolerance.

On the basis of accessory signals received, type of pathogen encountered, and signals received in local tissue environments (e.g., cytokine/chemokine receptor ligation), DCs develop into subsets that express distinct surface and functional phenotypes.[2] As recently described by Kelsall and colleagues,[3] there are three subsets of CD11c[+] Peyer's patch (PP) DCs.[4–6] CD8α[−]CD11β[hi] DCs produce high levels of IL-10 and induce differentiation of IL-4– and IL-10–producing Th2 cells *in vitro*.[5] In contrast, CD8α[+]CD11β[lo] and CD8α[−]CD11β[lo] DCs produce low levels of IL-10, high levels of IL-12, and induce only IFN-γ–producing Th1 cells.[5] Spatial as well as functional differences define the three DC subsets. The DC-rich region of the subepithelial dome (SED) underlying the follicle-associated epithelium (FAE) contains both CD8α[−]CD11β[hi] and CD8α[−]CD11β[lo] DCs, the T cell–rich intrafollicular region contains both CD8α[+]CD11β[lo] and CD8α[−]CD11β[lo] DCs, and the B cell follicle con-

---

Address for correspondence: Terrence Barrett, M.D., Associate Professor, Dept. of Medicine and Microbiology/Immunology, Division of Gastroenterology, Northwestern University Medical School, 303 E. Chicago, Searle 10-526, Chicago, IL 60611. Voice: 312-503-0293; fax: 312-908-6192.
  tabarrett@northwestern.edu

tains only $CD8\alpha^-CD11\beta^{lo}$ DCs.[6] Under the proposed paradigm, $CD11\beta^+$ or plasmacytoid DCs that encounter soluble food antigens under steady state conditions generate $CD25^+$ regulatory T (Tr) cells that produce IL-4 and IL-10. In contrast, activating forms of antigen acquired from pathogens induce IL-12 production by $CD8\alpha^+CD11\beta^{lo}$ and $CD8\alpha^-CD11\beta^{lo}$ DCs that drive Th1 differentiation.

To test the role of DC subpopulations in presenting viral antigen after enteric infection, Dr. Kelsall used a well-characterized model of intestinal reovirus infection.[7] Kelsall found that $CD8\alpha^-CD11b^{lo}$ DCs in the PP SED contained reovirus structural protein σ1 following infection. However, reovirus nonstructural protein σNS (associated with replication) was detected in follicle-associated epithelial cells. Further examination of DCs in the SED revealed that viral antigen colocalized with caspase-positive, keratin-positive material, suggesting that DCs acquired viral antigen from infected, apoptotic epithelial cells.[3] These findings were reminiscent of data from McPherson and colleagues in which keratin-positive material was detected in antigen-positive DCs isolated from mesenteric duct lymph.[8] Taken together, these data indicate that epithelial cells play an essential role in transferring antigen derived from enteric infections to mucosal DCs. For their part, mucosal DCs are capable of capturing and processing antigen used to activate and drive T cell proliferation.

EPITHELIAL GATEKEEPERS TO DENDRITIC CELL ACTIVATION

In the presentation that followed, Maria Rescigno summarized data showing the ability of subepithelial DCs to sample environmental microorganisms without compromising the epithelial barrier function. The groups used $CD11\beta^+CD8\alpha^-$ DCs to examine bacterial transport across colonic epithelial monolayers (CaCo-2) and followed $CD11c^+$ DC in ligated intestinal loops. Dr. Rescigno and coworkers used fluorescence-labeled bacteria to show that DCs sample bacteria by extending processes between epithelial cells. A major finding of these studies was the ability of DCs to send projections into the lumen without disrupting epithelial barrier function. The groups found that DCs upregulated tight junction (TJ) proteins and established TJ-like structures with epithelial cells. The formation of TJ complexes allowed DCs to take up antigen without changing transepithelial resistance (TER). Specifically, through binding to TJ proteins, such as occludin, claudin 1, and junctional adhesion molecule (JAM), DCs were able to maintain barrier function while sampling bacterial antigen at the mucosal surface.[9] Interestingly, $CD11c^+$ cells carrying bacteria were found deeper in the lamina propria (LP) at the base of the villi, which suggested that they migrated away from the epithelial layer after antigen acquisition. In summary, the data presented indicate that DCs are recruited to mucosal surfaces, likely via release of epithelial chemokine such as macrophage inflammatory protein 3α (MIP-3α), where they open tight junctions between epithelial cells, and send dendrites outside the epithelium to directly sample bacteria.[10]

A comparison presented by Dr. Rescigno of the effects of invasive and noninvasive bacteria on DC function resembled the "dichotomy of DC function" proposed by Dr. Kelsall. Dr. Rescigno's group found that epithelial exposure to invasive bacteria induced greater IL-8 production and recruited more DCs than noninvasive bacteria.[10] Similarly, exposure of DCs to culture supernatants from epithelia activated with invasive bacteria upregulated greater levels of activation markers CD83 and DC-LAMP. Findings that DC activation was reduced in cells with mutated toll-like receptor 4 suggest that direct exposure to endotoxin also contributed to DC activation. Importantly, invasive as well as noninvasive bacteria were capable of activating DCs via this direct pathway. Taken together, these findings indicate that direct (i.e., bacterial-mediated) and indirect (i.e., epithelial-mediated) pathways cooperate to activate mucosal DCs in the intestine. Exposure of the mucosal surface to invasive bacteria activates DCs via epithelial (indirect) as well as bacterial-derived (direct) factors, whereas DC activation by noninvasive bacteria relies on direct (bacterial) factors only. The system ensures that pathogens induce more robust (indirect and direct) host defense responses, whereas commensal organisms activate more specific responses, presumably more susceptible to regulation (up or down) by factors released in the mucosal microenvironment.

DENDRITIC CELLS AS INTESTINAL "TROJAN HORSES"

In opening remarks, Gordon MacPherson challenged previously held "dogma" that immature DCs reside in peripheral tissues until receiving a "danger sign." Drawing upon observations in cells collected from pseudoafferent lymph (i.e., from mesenteric-lymphadenectomized cannulated rats), he suggested that DCs migrate from peripheral tissue continuously. It was estimated that DCs spend 2 to 4 d in the intestine and up to 7 d in draining LNs. In rats, two types of DC were described: (1) the "classical" $CD4^+/SIRPa^+$ (strong APC), and (2) the weaker, tolerance-inducing $CD4^-/SIRP\alpha^-$ DCs that carry self-antigen. Previously, MacPherson's group found that $CD4^-/SIRP\alpha^-$ DCs leaving the intestine carried antigen derived from apoptotic epithelial cells.[8] Once in draining LNs, these cells induced tolerance in naive T cells. As similar behavior has been reported for DCs from other tissues, it was suggested that this pattern of migration was a common pathway for monitoring antigen expression throughout extralymphoid tissue. Thus, current data suggest that DCs are constantly "in action," migrating into the intestine as immature cells and carrying antigen from the intestine to naive T cells waiting within draining LNs.

To examine the role of migratory DCs in transferring infectious material to draining LNs, Dr. MacPherson's group used a rat model of scrapie injection (a transmissible spongiform encephalopathy). They noted that within 24 h of scrapie injection, scrapie antigen was detectable in 3 to 5% of lymph-borne DCs, but not in other APCs. Attempts to transfer infectious material were not productive using DCs infected *in vivo*. However, DCs (but not macrophages) given scrapie *in vitro* retained infectivity for up to 72 hours. Although data were preliminary, the findings suggest that DCs may participate in alarming the systemic immune system by carrying live organisms to inductive sites within draining LNs.

As a follow-up to questions regarding the mechanisms of how "danger" signals are interpreted, MacPherson's group examined the effects of intravenous lipopolysaccharide (LPS) on DC migration. In results presented at the meeting, Dr. MacPherson reported that increased numbers of migratory DCs were detected in draining lymph within 5 to 15 h of LPS injection. These findings suggested that "danger" signals induce mucosal DCs to leave peripheral sites and migrate to draining LNs. Whether changes in DC migration were due to direct effects of LPS within the LP microenvironment or secondary to indirect effects of LPS on LN chemoattractant release was unclear. Examination of distinct lymphoid tissue revealed that LPS produced little effect on CD80 and CD86 expression within LP DCs, yet enhanced expression of both markers in splenic DCs. It was not clear whether LPS differentially affected distribution of distinct DC subsets within LN tissue. In final remarks, Dr. MacPherson emphasized that comprehensive assessments of DC function required evaluations of migratory behavior as well as surface phenotype and cytokine production.

TOLERANCE INDUCTION BY DENDRITIC CELLS

In comments from Joanne Viney, it was pointed out that although historically DCs were considered to be the "most potent" APC, recent data suggest that the default pathway for most DC-induced responses is tolerance. Data from Dr. Viney's lab and others suggest that mucosal DCs promote tolerance through IL-10, IFN-α, and/or TGF-β release.[11] Furthermore, Dr. Viney's data suggested that tolerogenic properties of mucosal DCs relate to their expression of indoleamine 2,3 dioxygenase (IDO). The enzyme depletes tryptophan and reduces T cell proliferation. In the intestine (MLN and PP), IDO enzyme expression was greatest in $CD8\alpha^+$ DCs that express $CD11c^{lo}$ compared with $CD11c^{hi}$ surface phenotypes. These cells exhibited a plasmacytoid phenotype with expression of B220 and Gr-1, and low levels of class II, CD40, CD80, and CD86, and no CD19. In addition, Dr. Viney pointed out that $CD8\alpha^+CD11c^{lo}$ DCs expressed lower levels of toll-like receptor 3 (TLR3) and higher levels of TLR7 and TLR9 than $CD8\alpha^+CD11c^{hi}$ DCs. These cells, termed mucosal plasmacytoid DCs (pDCs), secreted IL-10 and IFN-α, cytokines previously shown to support the *de novo* differentiation of regulatory T cells. When used as APCs, mucosal $CD8\alpha^+CD11c^{lo}$ DCs induced 50% less T cell proliferation than $CD8\alpha^+CD11c^{hi}$ DCs. Thus, characterization of mucosal pDCs suggests that these cells are responsible for the tolerance-inducing responses to enteric antigen that lack key "danger signs" described earlier.

In studies to assess effects of pDCs on tolerance mediated by Tr cells, Dr. Viney's group cocultured $CD8\alpha^+CD11c^{lo}$ and $CD11^{hi}$ DCs with $CD25^+$ (Tr) DO11.10 cells. They found that tolerance in Tr cells could be broken with high levels of peptide antigen presented by $CD8\alpha^+CD11c^{hi}$ DCs. However, the "break" in tolerance was not observed when high peptide levels were presented by $CD8\alpha^+CD11c^{lo}$ DCs to Tr cells. Overall, the novel data presented by Dr. Viney supported the notion that mucosal pDCs preferentially supported the generation and activities of Tr cells. Thus, antigen presentation by mucosal pDCs appears to be an important tolerogenic mechanism in the intestine—arguably a pathway more commonly followed than induction of aggressive host defense responses.

TIM-1: A KEY TO UNLOCKING THE "HYGIENE HYPOTHESIS" QUANDARY?

As a matter of introduction, Dale Umetsu commented on the relationship between the respiratory tract and the gastrointestinal tract, and on the well-established relationship between Th2-driven responses and airway hyperreactivity (AHR), a cardinal feature of asthma. Previous data from his lab showed that tolerance induced by respiratory allergen exposure in mice was mediated by IL-10–producing regulatory Tr cells induced by IL-10–producing pulmonary DCs.[12] These Tr cells were very effective in inhibiting the development of allergen-induced airway hyperreactivity (AHR).

To examine the mechanisms of tolerance and their relationship to AHR, Dr. Umetsu and his team undertook a genetic approach using congenic mice. This congenic approach simplified the problem of asthma and tolerance, which are very complex genetic traits. Congenic BALB/c mice carrying discrete chromosomal segments inherited from DBA/2 mice were screened for IL-4 responsiveness and allergen-induced AHR. One strain, HBA, stood out as distinctly different from wild-type BALB/c mice, and carried a chromosome 11 segment from DBA/2, which is syntenic to human chromosome 5q23-35, a region that has been repeatedly linked with asthma in humans. Thus, the BALB/c:DBA-2 congenic HBA strain offered a unique opportunity to identify a specific gene that regulates the development of Th2 responses, asthma, and tolerance.

Using the HBA congenic mice, Dr. Umetsu and his team positionally cloned a new gene family, which he called TIMs. The first member of this family, Tim-1, regulates the development of asthma and tolerance in mice. Umetsu and his group then examined the possibility that human TIM-1 might be polymorphic as it is in mice, and that TIM-1 regulates the development of Th2 responses and asthma in humans. Analysis of human TIM-1 sequences revealed a six amino acid insertion/deletion polymorphism. However, their study failed to reveal an association between the TIM-1 insertion and asthma.

Serendipitously, it turns out that the human homologue of Tim-1 encodes the receptor for the hepatitis A virus. When the data collected were analyzed for individuals with the TIM-1 insertion and a history of hepatitis A infection, a remarkable association emerged. The findings indicated that those individuals expressing the six amino acid insertion were protected from atopy if they had previously been infected with hepatitis A. The association between protection from asthma and TIM-1 in this cohort compared with those with the TIM-1 insertion not exposed to hepatitis A was highly significant ($P = .0005$) (Ref. 13). Based on these findings, Dr. Umetsu suggested that TIM-1 is a very important gene in regulating asthma, but only in hepatitis A–infected individuals. Moreover, Dr. Umetsu's findings are consistent with previous studies showing that infection with hepatitis A virus (HAV) can reduce the likelihood of developing atopy. As TIM-1 is expressed by $CD4^+$ T cells, it was postulated that HAV transduces a signal that skews T cell functional differentiation away from disease-associated Th2 phenotypes, thereby reducing the risk for asthma and atopy. Dr. Umetsu discussed the idea that TIM-1 provides a molecular mechanism for the "hygiene hypothesis," which states that the increased prevalence of autoimmune/atopic illnesses in more sterile, Westernized societies compared with less sanitary third world environments derives from the loss of protection from various infectious diseases that are no longer common. Because the incidence of infection with HAV has been reduced dramatically over the past two decades as a result of improved hygiene, the protective effect of HAV infection on atopic disease induced through TIM-1 by HAV is much less common today than 20 years ago.

The session ended with active discussion between audience members and Dr. Umetsu regarding the potential mechanisms to explain these ground-breaking studies.

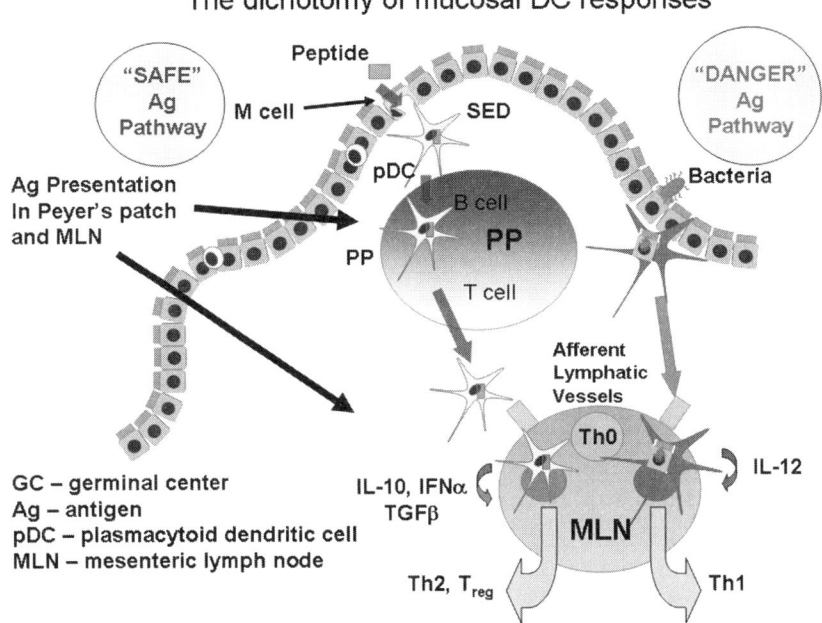

FIGURE 1. The dichotomy of mucosal DC responses. GC, germinal center; Ag, antigen; pDC, plasmacytoid dendritic cell; MLN, mesenteric lymph node.

SUMMARY

The session included talks and a discussion period in which novel paradigms for the role of DCs in generating tolerance as well as immunity at mucosal surfaces were proposed. Presentations raised questions on the dichotomy of DC responses to safe or pathogenic antigens (FIG. 1). Drs. Kelsall's and Rescigno's presentations helped attendees appreciate key roles played by DC subsets in monitoring mucosal surfaces for danger signs derived from enteric flora, local immune cells, and, especially, epithelial cells. A novel, yet fundamental view of DCs as migratory cells was presented by Dr. MacPherson, who elegantly delineated the role of DCs in shuttling antigen between mucosal tissue and inductive sites within draining LNs. Dr. Viney's presentation challenged the audience to consider how DCs affect responding T cells. Her examination of essential enzymes (e.g., IDO) expressed by DCs enhanced our understanding of the biochemical basis of tolerance versus immunity. Work by Dr. Umetsu and others suggested that innovative approaches to genetic research carry the potential to reveal novel relationships between genotype and phenotype in human disease. Taken together, the session allowed attendees to engage an international panel of speakers at the cutting edge of DC biology. Paradigms developed from newly generated model systems were discussed between researchers and participating audience members. Such interactions may potentially affect a range of clinically relevant areas, from enhanced host defense to mucosal pathogens, to improved mucosal vaccine development, to the development of new therapies for autoimmune disorders such as asthma and inflammatory bowel disease.

ACKNOWLEDGMENT

We thank Dr. Goo Lee, Northwestern University Medical School, for the generation of FIGURE 1.

REFERENCES

1. KELSALL, B.L. 2002. Dendritic cells at the host-pathogen interface. Nat. Immunol. **3:** 699–702.
2. IWASAKI, A. & B.L. KELSALL. 1999. Mucosal immunity and inflammation. I. Mucosal dendritic cells: their specialized role in initiating T cell responses. Am. J. Physiol. **276:** G1074–1078.
3. FLEETON, M.N., N. CONTRACTOR, F. LEON, et al. 2004. Peyer's patch dendritic cells process viral antigen from apoptotic epithelial cells in the intestine of reovirus-infected mice. J. Exp. Med. **200:** 235–245.
4. KELSALL, B.L. & W. STROBER. 1996. Distinct populations of dendritic cells are present in the subepithelial dome and T cell regions of the murine Peyer's patch. J. Exp. Med. **183:** 237–247.
5. IWASAKI, A. & B.L. KELSALL. 2001. Unique functions of CD11b$^+$, CD8α^+, and double-negative Peyer's patch dendritic cells. J. Immunol. **166:** 4884–4890.
6. IWASAKI, A. & B.L. KELSALL. 2000. Localization of distinct Peyer's patch dendritic cell subsets and their recruitment by chemokines macrophage inflammatory protein (MIP)-3α, MIP-3β, and secondary lymphoid organ chemokine. J. Exp. Med. **191:** 1381–1393.
7. FONTENEAU, J.F., M. LARSSON & N. BHARDWAJ. 2002. Interactions between dead cells and dendritic cells in the induction of antiviral CTL responses. Curr. Opin. Immunol. **14:** 471–477.
8. HUANG, F.P., N. PLATT, M. WYKES, et al. 2000. A discrete subpopulation of dendritic cells transports apoptotic intestinal epithelial cells to T cell areas of mesenteric lymph nodes. J. Exp. Med. **191:** 435–444.
9. RESCIGNO, M., G. ROTTA, B. VALZASINA & P. RICCIARDI-CASTAGNOLI. 2001. Immunobiology **204:** 572–581.
10. RESCIGNO, M., M. URBANO, B. VALZASINA, et al. 2001. Dendritic cells express tight junction proteins and penetrate gut epithelial monolayers to sample bacteria. Nat. Immunol. **2:** 361–367.
11. WILLIAMSON, E., J.M. BILSBOROUGH & J.L. VINEY. 2002. Regulation of mucosal dendritic cell function by receptor activator of NF-kappa B (RANK)/RANL ligand interactions: impact on tolerance induction. J. Immunol. **169:** 3606–3612.
12. AKBARI, O., G.J. FREEMAN, E.H. MEYER, et al. 2002. Antigen-specific regulatory T cells develop via the ICOS-ICOS-Ligand pathway and inhibit allergen-induced airway hyperreactivity. Nat. Med. **8:** 1024–1032.
13. MCINTIRE, J., S. UMETSU, C. MACAUBAS, et al. 2003. Immunology: hepatitis A virus link to atopic disease. Nature **425:** 576.

CD4$^+$ CD25$^+$ Regulatory T Cell Selection

ANDREW J. CATON, CRISTINA COZZO, JOSEPH LARKIN III,
MELISSA A. LERMAN, ALINA BOESTEANU, AND MARTHA S. JORDAN

The Wistar Institute, Philadelphia, Pennsylvania 10194, USA

ABSTRACT: Accumulating evidence indicates that regulatory T cells play a crucial role in preventing autoimmunity. To examine the processes by which regulatory CD4$^+$ T cells are produced during immune repertoire formation, we have developed transgenic mice that express the influenza virus hemagglutinin (HA) and coexpress major histocompatibility complex class II–restricted T cell receptors (TCRs) with varying affinities for the HA-derived CD4$^+$ T cell determinant S1. We show that interactions with a single self-peptide can induce thymocytes bearing an autoreactive TCR to undergo selection to become CD4$^+$ CD25$^+$ regulatory T cells, and that thymocytes bearing TCRs with low affinity for S1 do not undergo selection into this pathway. We show that CD4$^+$ thymocytes with identical specificity for the S1 self-peptide can undergo overt deletion versus abundant selection to become CD4$^+$ CD25$^+$ regulatory T cells in response to variations in expression of the S1 self-peptide in different lineages of HA transgenic mice. We also show that CD4$^+$ CD25$^+$ T cells proliferate in response to their selecting self-peptide in the periphery. Moreover, they do not proliferate in response to lymphopenia in the absence of the selecting self-peptide, reflecting a low level of expression of the high-affinity receptor for IL-7 (CD127) relative to conventional CD4$^+$ T cells. These studies are determining how specificity for self-peptides directs the thymic selection and peripheral expansion of CD4$^+$ CD25$^+$ regulatory T cells. Moreover, the differing responsiveness of CD4$^+$ CD25$^+$ regulatory T cells to cytokine- versus self-peptide–mediated signals may direct their accumulation to sites where the self-peptide is expressed.

KEYWORDS: regulatory T cells; self-tolerance; thymic selection; homeostasis; self-peptide

INTRODUCTION

The peripheral T cell repertoire is shaped by a series of selection events that are guided by the specificity and reactivity that T cell receptors (TCRs) exhibit toward complexes formed between major histocompatibility (MHC) molecules and self-peptides (reviewed in Ref. 1). T cell development begins in the thymus, where developing thymocytes rearrange their TCR genes. Positive selection rescues thymocytes from programmed cell death based on the ability of the TCR to react with host MHC molecules, which are mostly occupied by self-peptides. This ensures that

Address for correspondence: A.J. Caton, The Wistar Institute, 3601 Spruce St., Philadelphia, PA 19104. Voice: 215-898-3871; fax: 215-898-3868.
caton@wistar.upenn.edu

only those thymocytes whose TCRs have the capacity to recognize the host's MHC molecules when they are displaying foreign peptides will be exported to the periphery. However, additional processes have to occur to prevent these T cells from reacting toward the host's own cells and tissues, and these too must be guided by the reactivity of TCRs toward MHC molecules expressing self-peptides.[2] Ongoing interactions between the TCR and self-peptide:MHC molecules appear also to contribute to the maintenance of mature T cells in the periphery and can promote their expansion under lymphopenic conditions.[3,4] In healthy individuals, the immune system is able to maintain a repertoire of CD4$^+$ and CD8$^+$ T cells containing sufficient diversity and potential specificities to anticipate unknown and highly diverse pathogens. Yet, the healthy immune system must also occupy and remain unresponsive to a perhaps comparably diverse universe of self-antigens, and when it fails to do so autoimmune diseases can ensue.

Elegant studies performed by Le Douarin and her colleagues were among the first to show that the thymus generates regulatory T cells. In one series of experiments, allogeneic thymic epithelium from strain A mice was engrafted into athymic strain B mice; low numbers of CD4$^+$ cells from these engrafted animals would induce autoimmune disease when transferred into additional athymic strain A mice, but this did not occur when larger numbers of cells were transferred.[5,6] These results were interpreted to indicate that thymic epithelium normally generates mixed populations of autoreactive and regulatory T cells with overlapping specificities, and that insufficient regulatory T cells had been introduced to prevent autoimmunity when low doses of cells were transferred. Around this time, Sakaguchi and his colleagues showed that thymectomizing mice on their third day of life rendered these animals susceptible to autoimmune disease that could be prevented by adoptive transfer initially of CD4$^+$ T cells, and then of the CD4$^+$CD25$^+$ subset from normal mice.[7,8] These studies were quickly followed by the demonstration that CD4SP thymocytes contained a CD25$^+$ subset that could also confer regulatory function.[9] Mason and Powrie adopted a similar approach to demonstrate the existence of regulatory T cells, showing that splenocytes from normal mice could be fractionated into cells that would induce autoimmune disease in lymphopenic mice (CD45RBhi), and cells that were regulatory (CD45RBlow).[10] They went on to show that tissue-specific CD25$^+$ regulatory T cells (which largely but do not exclusively overlap with CD45RBlow regulatory T cells) arose in the thymus, but that if their target tissues were removed these regulatory cells were no longer detectable.[11] Collectively, these reports indicated that the thymus produces autoreactive CD4$^+$ T cells that exert regulatory function, and that interactions with target peptides in the periphery also contributed to the maintenance or functional development of regulatory T cells. However, the precise role that interactions with self-peptides play in the development of regulatory T cells, either in the thymus or the periphery, remained obscure.

We have developed a transgenic mouse system in which the development of self-peptide–specific regulatory T cells can be examined. We have generated lineages of transgenic mice that express the hemagglutinin (HA) molecule from influenza virus PR8 under the control of the SV40 early region promoter/enhancer.[12,13] These mice have been mated with additional transgenic mice (that we designate TS1 mice) expressing a TCR that recognizes the major I-Ed restricted determinant S1 from HA.[14] Studies analyzing CD4$^+$ T cell development in these TS1×HA Tg mice show that CD4$^+$CD25$^+$ regulatory T cell development is initiated by high specificity interactions with self-peptides in the thymus.[15,16] Moreover, $CD4^+$ thymocytes with identical specificity for a self-peptide can undergo overt deletion versus abundant selection to become $CD4^+CD25^+$ regulatory T cells in response to variations in expression of the self-peptide.[17] We have also shown that $CD4^+CD25^+$ regulatory T cells proliferate in response to their selecting self-peptide in the periphery, and that they do not proliferate in response to lymphopenia in mice that lack the selecting self-peptide.[18] These studies are more fully defining the mechanisms by which $CD4^+$ tolerance is established to self-peptides. They are also increasing our understanding of the development and activity of $CD4^+$ $CD25^+$ T regulatory cells, and may aid in their development as therapeutic agents.

RESULTS AND DISCUSSION

Thymic Selection of $CD4^+$ $CD25^+$ Regulatory T Cells and Deletion Are Alternative Mechanisms of $CD4^+$ T Cell Tolerance Induction

HA12 and HA28 mice express a polypeptide from the PR8 HA as a neo-self-antigen under the control of the SV40 early region promoter/enhancer.[12,13] These lineages were generated from different founder mice containing the same DNA construct; as a result, any differences in the expression of the HA transgene between these mice are a result of differences in the integration of these transgenes into the genomic DNA. Studies of transgene mRNA expression revealed diffuse, low-level expression of HA transgene mRNA in a wide variety of tissues, including the thymus.[12,13] To examine the effects of the HA transgene on $CD4^+$ T cell development, HA12 and HA28 mice were mated with TS1 mice, which express a transgene-encoded TCR that is specific for the major I-Ed determinant from HA (termed S1).[14] Initially, unfractionated lymph node (LN) cells from TS1, TS1×HA12, and TS1×HA28 mice were incubated *in vitro* with graded doses of the S1 peptide and their proliferative response was compared (FIG. 1a). The LN cells from TS1×HA12 and TS1×HA28 mice exhibited comparable reductions in their proliferative responses to S1 peptide relative to TS1 mice. This indicated that S1-specific $CD4^+$ T cells had been subjected to tolerance induction in both lineages, and it was noteworthy that these unfractionated LN cells from TS1×HA12 and TS1×HA28 mice yielded extremely similar responses to S1 peptide. However, addition of IL-2 to the cultures suggested that mechanistically distinct processes might be occurring in these different mice; the cultures from TS1×HA28 mice exhibited enhanced sensitivity to S1 peptide in the presence of exogenous IL-2, whereas the cultures obtained from TS1×HA12 mice were largely unaffected by its addition (FIG. 1a).

When the development of S1-specific $CD4^+$ T cells was examined using the anti-clonotypic monoclonal antibody 6.5 that detects the transgene-encoded TCR,[14] the mechanistic differences between TS1×HA12 and TS1×HA28 mice became much more evident. 6.5hi cells comprise approximately 20% of the CD4SP thymocytes and $CD4^+$ LN cells in TS1 mice (FIG. 1b). These cells are greatly reduced among both thymocytes and LN cells from TS1×HA12 mice, reflecting their deletion in response to the S1 peptide. By contrast, 6.5hi CD4 SP thymocytes and $CD4^+$ T cells were abundant in TS1×HA28 mice, although they exhibited modest (approximately twofold) reductions in the levels of TCR and CD4 relative to TS1 mice.[15,16] When

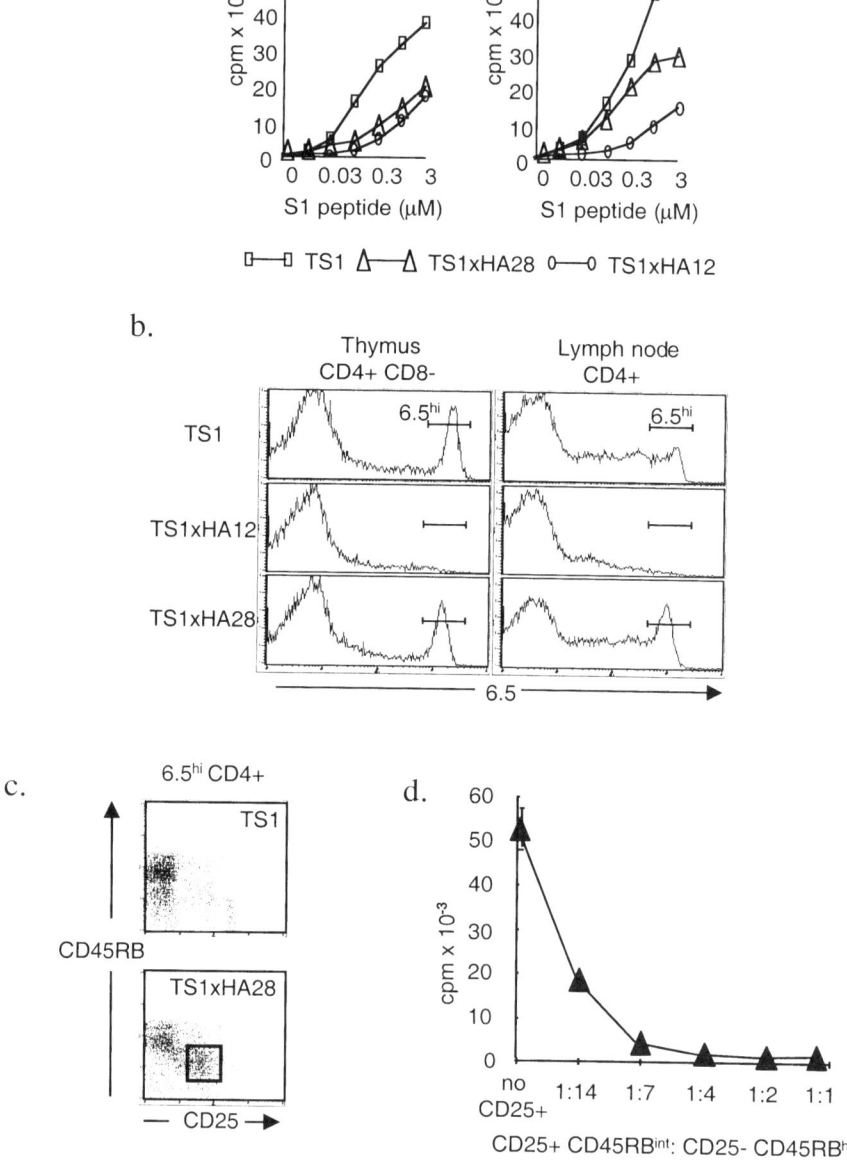

FIGURE 1. 6.5hi CD4+ T cells undergo overt deletion in TS1×HA12 mice, and abundant CD25+ regulatory T cell selection in TS1×HA28 mice. (**a**) Proliferative responses of unfractionated LN cells from TS1, TS1×HA12, and TS1×HA28 mice in response to *in vitro* stimulation with graded doses of S1 peptide in the presence or absence of exogenous IL-2. Values indicate [^{3}H]thymidine uptake after 56 to 72 h in culture. (**b**) Histograms show levels

the 6.5hi CD4$^+$ T cells from TS1×HA28 mice were examined in more detail, approximately half were found to be CD25$^+$CD45RBint (FIG. 1c). These cells were hyporesponsive to stimulation with S1 peptide when purified by flow cytometry. However, when they were purified away from CD25$^+$ CD45RBint cells, the CD25$^-$ CD45RBhi cells from TS1×HA28 mice proliferated comparably to CD25$^-$ CD45RBhi cells from TS1 mice.[15,16] Significantly, when purified CD25$^+$ CD45RBint cells from TS1×HA28 mice were mixed with purified CD25$^-$ CD45RBhi cells from either TS1 or TS1×HA28 mice, they inhibited proliferation even when added at low ratios relative to CD25$^-$ CD45RBhi cells (FIG. 1d). Thus, interactions with the S1 peptide in TS1×HA28 mice induced the selection of 6.5hi CD4$^+$ CD25$^+$ CD45RBint cells that share the same properties (impaired proliferative responses, and ability to suppress *in vitro* proliferation of effector CD4$^+$ T cells) as have been described for regulatory cells that can prevent the development of autoimmune disease *in vivo*.[19]

Thymic Selection of CD25$^+$ T Cells Occurs on Radioresistant Thymic Elements and Does Not Require Expression of Endogenous TCR α-Chains

To examine the thymic elements responsible for inducing the development of CD4$^+$ CD25$^+$ regulatory T cells, we generated radiation bone marrow (BM) chimeras. The 6.5hi CD4 SP thymocytes and 6.5hi CD4$^+$ LN cells from HA28 mice reconstituted with TS1 BM (TS1→HA28 chimeras) expressed decreased levels of 6.5, and roughly half of the 6.5hi CD4$^+$ LN cells from these chimeras expressed high levels of CD25 (FIG. 2). Conversely, the cell surface phenotypes of TS1×HA28→BALB/c and TS1→BALB/c chimeras were indistinguishable. These findings demonstrate that radioresistant thymic elements are both necessary and sufficient for the selection of CD4$^+$ CD25$^+$ T cells in TS1×HA28 mice.

Because radioresistant elements were responsible for the development of anergic/suppressor cells in TS1×HA28 mice, we repeated the TS1→HA28 BM chimera studies using BM cells from TS1 mice that were rendered incapable of allelic inclusion by mating onto a RAG-2–deficient background (TS1.RAG$^{-/-}$ mice). We performed these studies because allelic inclusion allows a large fraction of 6.5$^+$ T cells to express more than one TCR α-chain,[17] and the coexpression of endogenous α-chains could therefore be involved in the selection of CD4$^+$CD25$^+$ thymocytes in TS1×HA28 mice. In comparison with their TS1.RAG$^{-/-}$→BALB/c counterparts, CD4$^+$ T cells from TS1.RAG$^{-/-}$→HA28 chimeras expressed lower levels of 6.5, and approximately half of the 6.5hi T cells were CD25$^+$ (FIG. 2). The CD25$^+$ cells that arose in the TS1.RAG$^{-/-}$→HA28 chimeras also significantly inhibited the proliferation of the pu-

---

of 6.5 staining among CD4$^+$ SP thymocytes or CD4$^+$ LN T cells from TS1, TS1×HA12, and TS1×HA28 mice. Gates used to identify 6.5hi cells are shown. (**c**) Dot plots showing CD45RB versus CD25$^+$ staining of 6.5hi CD4$^+$ LN cells from TS1 and TS1×HA28 mice. Gates used to identify CD25$^+$ CD45RBint cells are shown. (**d**) Proliferative responses of purified CD4$^+$CD25$^-$ T cells from TS1 mice in response to *in vitro* stimulation with 0.3 μM S1 peptide (and irradiated splenocytes as antigen-presenting cells) in the presence of the indicated ratio of CD4$^+$CD25$^+$ cells purified from TS1×HA28 mice. Values indicate [^{3}H]thymidine uptake after 72 h in culture.

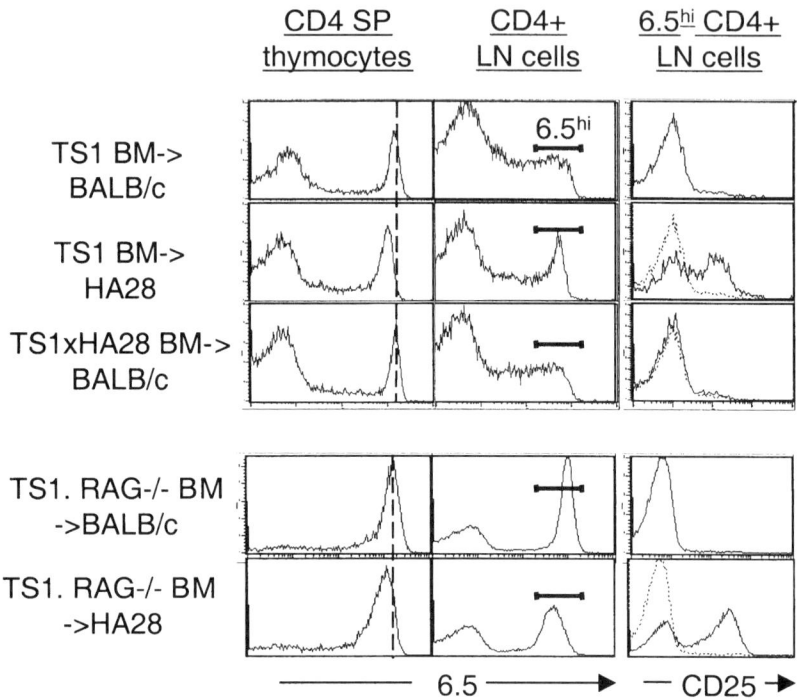

FIGURE 2. 6.5hi CD4+CD25+ regulatory T cells are selected by radioresistant thymic epithelial cells and are not dependent on allelic inclusion of endogenous TCR chains. Histograms show levels of 6.5 staining CD4+ CD8− thymocytes and CD4+ LN cells, and of CD25+ levels on 6.5hi cells, from radiation chimeras reconstituted with bone marrow cells as indicated. Gates used to identify 6.5hi cells are shown.

rified CD25− cells.[15] Together, these data indicate that thymocytes that can express only the 6.5 TCR undergo selection to become CD25+ T cells in TS1×HA28 mice.

Thymocytes Bearing a TCR with a Low Intrinsic Affinity for S1 Do Not Develop into CD4+ CD25+ T Cells

To examine the specificity with which thymocytes must react with self-peptides to undergo CD25+ regulatory T cell selection, we generated a second TCR transgenic mouse, TS1(SW). TS1(SW) T cells use a $V\alpha8/V\beta10$ TCR combination and are specific for an analogue of the S1 determinant, termed S1(SW), that contains two amino acid substitutions relative to the native S1 determinant (FIG. 3a). 6.5hi CD4+ LN cells from TS1 mice and Vα8hi CD4+ LN cells from TS1(SW) mice exhibited similar sensitivities for the S1 and SW(S1) determinants, respectively, differing ≤3-fold in the amount of peptide required for half-maximal stimulation. However, the TS1(SW) T cells were ~100-fold less sensitive to the S1 determinant than to S1(SW), indicating that the intrinsic affinity of the TS1(SW) TCR for the S1 determinant is ~100-fold lower than that of the 6.5 TCR (FIG. 3a). We mated TS1(SW)

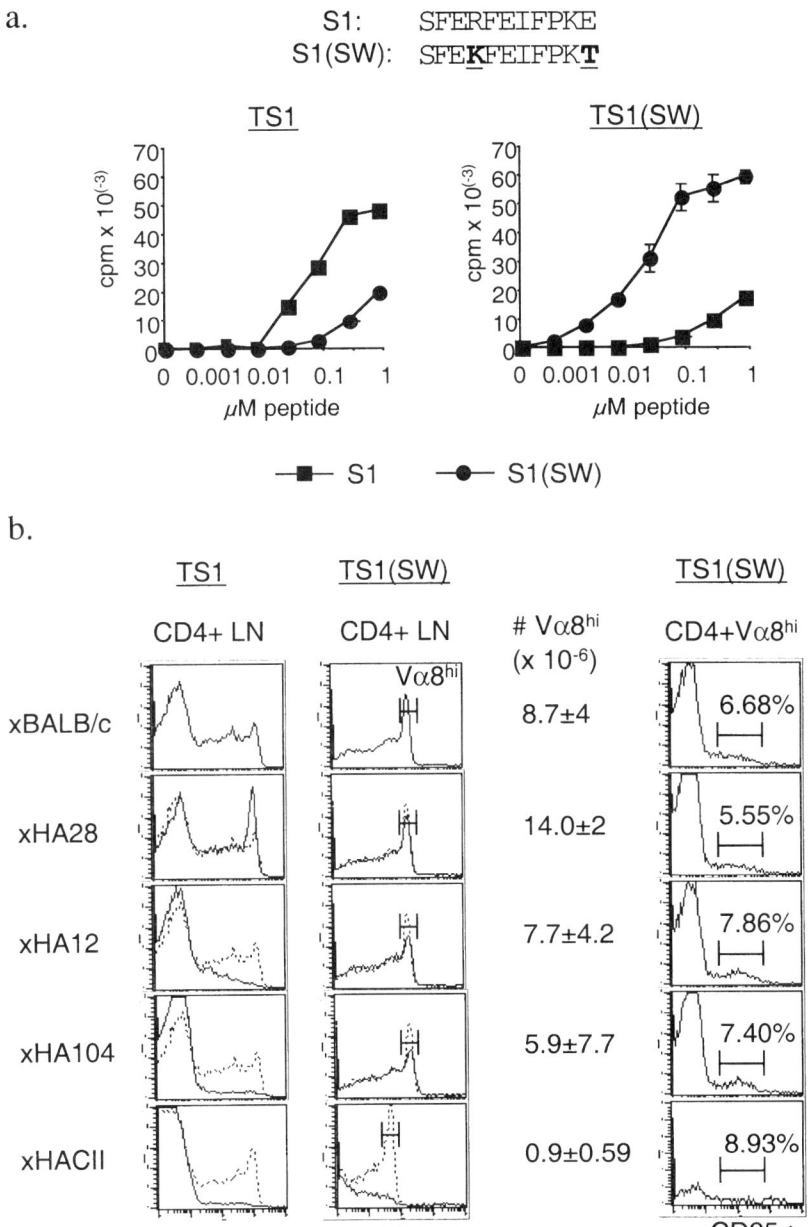

FIGURE 3. Thymocytes expressing a low-affinity TCR do not undergo selection to become CD25+ in response to S1 peptide. (**a**) Proliferative responses of purified 6.5hi CD4+ T cells from TS1 mice versus Vα 8hi CD4+ T cells from TS1(SW) mice in response to graded doses of S1 or S1(SW) peptides, whose sequences are shown. Values indicate [^{3}H]thymi-

mice with HA28 mice and compared LN cells from TS1(SW) and TS1(SW)×HA28 mice for their frequencies of $CD25^+$ cells. Both the absolute number and the percentage of $CD25^+$ cells among Vα8hi $CD4^+$ LN cells in TS1(SW)×HA28 mice were similar to those found in TS1(SW) mice (FIG. 3b). This is in contrast to TS1×HA28 mice, in which roughly half of the 6.5hi $CD4^+$ T cells were $CD25^+$ (FIG. 1c). Thus, thymocytes bearing a TCR with a low intrinsic affinity for the S1 peptide did not develop into $CD4^+CD25^+$ thymocytes in TS1(SW)×HA28 mice.

We next examined whether TS1(SW) T cells might develop into $CD4^+ CD25^+$ T cells in mice in which S1 mediates deletion of the 6.5 TCR. As described above, 6.5^+ thymocytes undergo substantial deletion in response to S1 peptide in HA12 mice, and we previously described another lineage of HA Tg mice (HA104) in which 6.5^+ thymocytes are deleted to a greater degree than in TS1×HA12 mice.[17] TS1(SW) mice were mated with HA12 and HA104 mice, and also with transgenic mice (HACII) that express the PR8 HA under the control of a MHC class II (I-Eα) promoter (FIG. 3b). Whereas 6.5^+ $CD4^+$ T cells were substantially deleted in TS1×HA12 mice, there was little or no reduction in the frequency of Vα8hi $CD4^+$ T cells in TS1(SW)×HA12 mice. There was a modest decrease in the number of Vα8hi $CD4^+$ T cells in TS1(SW)×HA104 mice that correlated with the increased deletion of 6.5^+ T cells in TS1×HA104 mice, and both TS1×HACII and TS1(SW)×HACII mice exhibited profound deletion of the respective clonotype-bearing T cells. Importantly, however, similar percentages of $CD4^+ CD25^+$ T cells were present in the LNs of TS1(SW) and TS1(SW)×HA transgenic mice. Thus, even when they develop in the presence of the S1 self-peptide under conditions that can to varying degrees induce deletion of the 6.5 TCR, thymocytes bearing the low affinity TS1(SW) TCR did not undergo selection into $CD25^+$ T cells. Under some circumstances they were deleted, but their low affinity for S1 appeared to preclude their development into $CD4^+ CD25^+$ T cells in response to S1 peptide.

S1 Peptide Drives the Peripheral Expansion of 6.5hi $CD4^+$ $CD25^+$ T Cells

Because signals received from cytokines and self-peptide:MHC complexes can each contribute to the maintenance of conventional $CD4^+$ T cells,[3,20] we were interested in determining how 6.5hi $CD4^+ CD25^+$ regulatory T cells respond to these signals in the periphery. We first examined whether 6.5hi $CD4^+ CD25^+$ and/or $CD4^+ CD25^-$ T cells would proliferate in response to lymphopenia in BALB/c mice, as is the case for conventional $CD4^+$ T cells. Accordingly, 6.5hi $CD4^+ CD25^+$ and $CD4^+ CD25^-$ T cells were purified from LNs of TS1×HA28 mice by cell sorting, labeled with the intracellular dye CFSE, and injected into normal or sublethally irradiated BALB/c mice. As a control population, we also coinjected CFSE-labeled LN cells from TS1(SW) mice. None of the transferred cell populations divided in nonirradiated BALB/c mice, but when transferred into lymphopenic BALB/c mice, both the

---

dine uptake after 72 h in culture. (**b**) Histograms show 6.5 or Vα 8 levels on $CD4^+$ LN cells from TS1 or TS1(SW) mice that have been crossed with the indicated HA Tg mice (*left panels*). The total numbers of Vα 8hi $CD4^+$ LN cells recovered from mice are shown. Histograms in the *right panels* show expression levels of CD25 on $CD4^+$ Vα 8hi cells from indicated TS1(SW)×HA Tg mice, and percentages that are $CD25^+$ are shown.

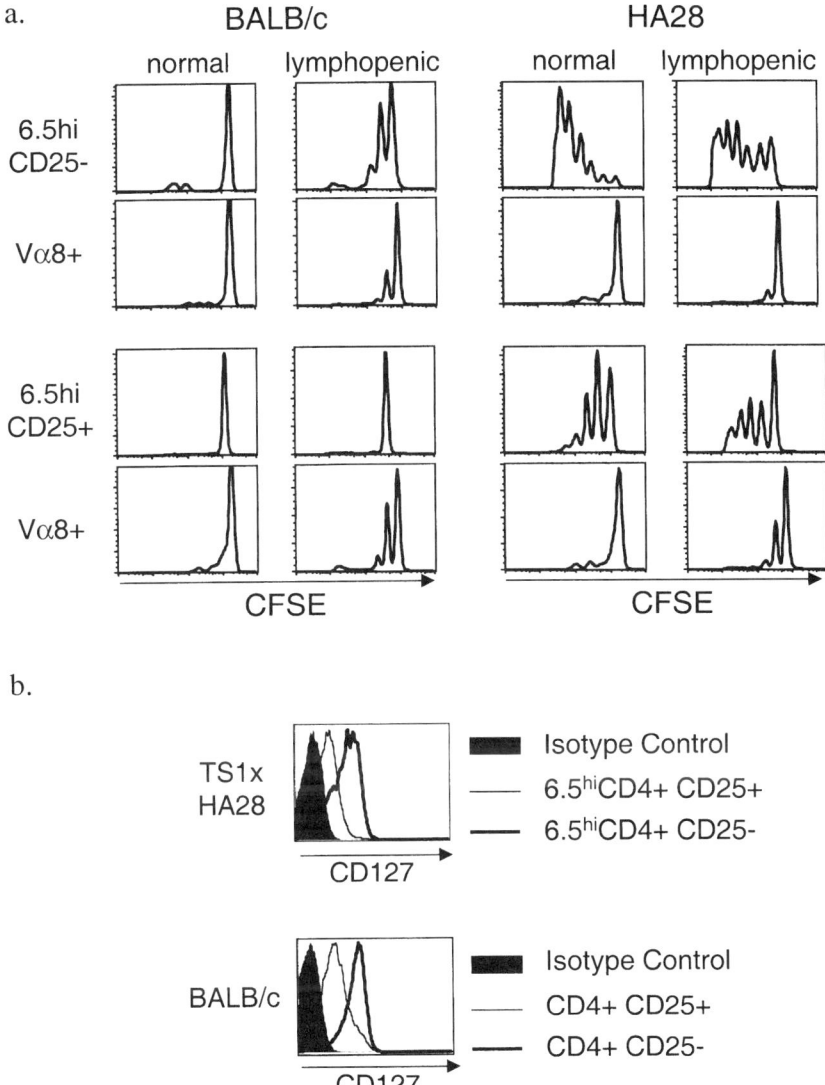

FIGURE 4. 6.5hi CD4+ CD25+ regulatory T cells proliferate in response to S1 peptide *in vivo*, but not in response to lymphopenia alone. (**a**) $1.5–2\times10^6$ CFSE-labeled CD4+ CD25+ or CD4+ CD25− cells from TS1×HA28 mice were mixed with $\sim 3\times 10^6$ CFSE-labeled LN cells from TS1(SW) mice and injected intravenously into normal or sublethally irradiated BALB/c (*left panels*) or HA28 (*right panels*) mice. Seven days later, LNs from recipient mice were harvested, stained, and analyzed by flow cytometry. Histograms are gated on CD4+ 6.5hi CFSE+ cells or CD4+ Vα8+ CFSE+ cells. (**b**) *Upper panel*: Histograms of CD127 expression on 6.5hi CD4+ CD25+ (*thin line*), 6.5hi CD4+ CD25− (*thick line*), or 6.5hi CD4+ LN cells stained with an isotype control antibody (*filled*) from TS1×HA28 mice. *Lower panel*: Histograms of CD127 expression on CD4+ CD25+ (*thin line*), CD4+ CD25− (*thick line*), or CD4+ LN cells stained with an isotype control antibody (*filled*) from BALB/c mice.

6.5hi $CD4^+CD25^-$ T cells from TS1×HA28 mice and the $CD4^+ V\alpha8^+$ T cells from TS1(SW) mice underwent one or two rounds of division (FIG. 4a). However, the 6.5hi $CD4^+CD25^+$ T cells from TS1×HA28 mice failed to proliferate in lymphopenic BALB/c mice. The recipient mice were indeed lymphopenic, because the $CD4^+ V\alpha8^+$ cells that were cotransferred went through one or two rounds of homeostatic division. Because IL-7 is critical for the homeostatic proliferation of conventional $CD4^+$ T cells,[21] we examined 6.5hi $CD4^+CD25^+$ and 6.5hi $CD4^+CD25^-$ T cells from TS1×HA28 mice for their levels of CD127, which is the high-affinity receptor for IL-7. CD127 levels were indeed markedly lower on 6.5hi $CD4^+CD25^+$ T cells, and $CD4^+CD25^+$ T cells from BALB/c mice showed similarly reduced levels of CD127 (FIG. 4b). These low levels of CD127 provide a basis by which $CD25^+$ T cells may fail to proliferate in response to lymphopenia.

In contrast to BALB/c mice, in which they failed to divide, the 6.5hi $CD4^+CD25^+$ cells from TS1×HA28 mice divided up to three times in nonirradiated HA28 mice (FIG. 4a). By contrast, $CD4^+ V\alpha8^+$ T cells from TS1(SW) mice did not divide in nonirradiated HA28 mice; this, and the failure of 6.5hi $CD4^+CD25^+$ T cells to divide in BALB/c mice, indicates that the proliferation of 6.5hi $CD4^+CD25^+$ T cells in HA28 mice is a specific response to S1 peptide. $CD4^+CD25^+$ cells that had undergone division in response to S1 peptide in HA28 mice were also as potent suppressors as freshly isolated $CD4^+CD25^+$ T cells from TS1×HA28 mice. This indicates that $CD4^+CD25^+$ T cells retain their regulatory properties following *in vivo* proliferation, and further shows that the regulatory $CD4^+CD25^+$ cells themselves (and not some other population of $CD4^+CD25^+$ cells) undergo division in response to S1 peptide in HA28 mice. 6.5hi $CD4^+CD25^+$ T cells also proliferated in lymphopenic HA28 mice. In this case, 6.5hi $CD4^+CD25^+$ T cells divided approximately four or five times, whereas $CD4^+ V\alpha8^+$ T cells went through one or two rounds of division (similar to their division in lymphopenic BALB/c mice). Together, these findings indicate that the peripheral expansion of 6.5hi $CD4^+CD25^+$ regulatory T cells in HA28 mice is both promoted by and dependent on interactions with the S1 peptide.

CONCLUSIONS

In TS1 mice, thymocytes bearing the 6.5 TCR are positively selected through interactions with MHC class II molecules expressing either a particular self-peptide, or a collection of self-peptides.[22] In TS1×HA28 mice, we introduced an additional self-peptide (S1) to the complex mixture of self-peptides that is expressed by the BALB/c thymus. S1 is an agonist peptide for the 6.5 TCR,[23] and its presence induced thymocytes bearing the 6.5 TCR to develop into $CD4^+CD25^+$ regulatory T cells. Accordingly, these studies in TS1×HA28 mice have shown that specificity for a single self-peptide can direct thymocytes bearing an autoreactive TCR to undergo selection into a distinct developmental pathway that results in the export of autoreactive regulatory T cells to the periphery. By contrast, interactions between the 6.5 TCR and S1 peptide induced substantial thymocyte deletion in TS1×HA12 mice, indicating that development into $CD4^+CD25^+$ regulatory T cells is also an alternative to deletion as a means to regulate thymocytes bearing a TCR with a high-intrinsic affinity for a self-peptide.

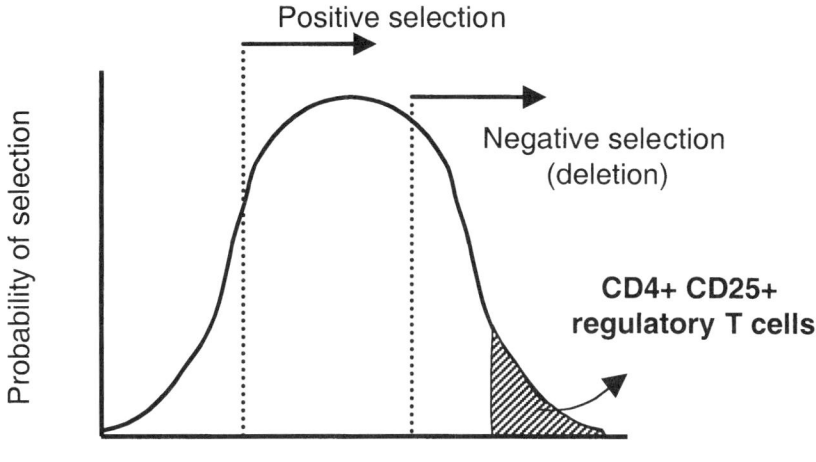

FIGURE 5. Role of TCR affinity in $CD4^+CD25^+$ T cell development. The graph shows a modified version of the avidity model of thymocyte development[1] in which thymocyte selection into the $CD4^+CD25^+$ regulatory T cell pathway requires a high intrinsic affinity of the TCR for the selecting self-peptide.

It is significant that differences in the expression of the S1 peptide between the HA28 and HA12 lineages play a decisive role in determining the fate of thymocytes expressing the 6.5 TCR. Previous studies aimed at characterizing how interactions with self-peptides direct thymocyte development have largely provided evidence that the avidity of the interaction between the thymocyte TCR and self-peptide MHC complexes play a crucial role in directing thymocyte development.[1] Low-avidity interactions appear to be required for positive selection, whereas high-avidity interactions have been found to induce thymocyte deletion. One prediction of this model was that $CD4^+CD25^+$ regulatory T cell development might occur when thymocytes bearing TCRs with low intrinsic affinities for self-peptides interacted with self-peptides that would induce deletion of thymocytes bearing high-affinity TCRs.[19,24] However, we found that thymocytes expressing the TS1(SW) TCR (whose affinity for the S1 peptide is ~100-fold lower than the 6.5 TCR) did not undergo $CD4^+CD25^+$ regulatory T cell selection in several lineages of HA Tg mice that induced varying degrees of deletion of the 6.5 TCR. This argues that $CD4^+CD25^+$ regulatory T cell selection requires a high intrinsic affinity of the TCR for the selecting peptide (FIG. 5), although some unknown differences between the 6.5 and TS1(SW) TCRs themselves (such as timing of expression) could contribute to the fate of developing thymocytes.

What is it, then, about the expression of S1 peptide in HA28 mice that differs from HA12 mice and induces thymocytes to undergo such abundant $CD4^+CD25^+$ selection? It remains possible that low doses of a peptide for which a thymocyte has a high intrinsic affinity provides a signal with an appropriate combination of high specificity and low overall avidity to direct or support selection into the $CD25^+$ pathway. Alternatively (although not exclusively), it may be that expression by different thymic cell types (e.g., cortical versus medullary epithelium) is important in determining the extent of deletion versus CD4$^+$ CD25$^+$ regulatory T cell selection. It is also not yet clear why 6.5$^+$ thymocytes are exported as mixtures of CD4$^+$ CD25$^+$ regulatory T cells and CD4$^+$ CD25$^-$ T cells in TS1×HA28 mice, although it is noteworthy that studies in non-transgenic systems have provided similar evidence that the thymus exports mixtures of regulatory and effector T cells with shared specificities.[6,11]

The studies described here also showed that the peptide that mediates the thymic selection of CD4$^+$ CD25$^+$ T cells induces their expansion in the periphery. Moreover, the peripheral expansion of 6.5hi CD4$^+$ CD25$^+$ T cells was shown to be dependent on interactions with S1 peptide, because unlike conventional CD4$^+$ T cells (and also 6.5hi CD4$^+$ CD25$^-$ T cells from TS1×HA28 mice), 6.5hi CD4$^+$ CD25$^+$ T cells did not proliferate in response to lymphopenia in BALB/c mice. The failure of CD4$^+$ CD25$^+$ T cells to proliferate in response to lymphopenia likely reflects the down-modulation of CD127, which is an important cytokine in directing division of conventional CD4$^+$ T cells under lymphopenic conditions.[21] In this respect, it is noteworthy that conventional CD4$^+$ T cells also downmodulate CD127 upon activation,[25] and that CD4$^+$ CD25$^+$ regulatory T cells exhibit other phenotypic characteristics, such as increased levels of CTLA-4 and glucocorticoid-induced thymocyte receptor (GITR), that they share with activated conventional CD4$^+$ T cells.[26–28] Whether CD4$^+$ CD25$^+$ regulatory T cells exhibit characteristics in common with activated CD4$^+$ T cells as a consequence of high-affinity interactions with self-peptides during their selection in the thymus and/or as a result of ongoing interactions with self-peptides in the periphery remains to be determined. Nevertheless, down-modulation of CD127 on CD4$^+$ CD25$^+$ regulatory T cells, coupled with the ability to proliferate in response to their selecting peptide, is likely to significantly affect how CD4$^+$CD25$^+$ regulatory T cells accumulate in the periphery.

6.5hi CD4$^+$ CD25$^+$ T cells accumulate in large numbers systemically in TS1×HA28 mice because S1 peptide is expressed in a wide variety of tissues,[12,13] and CD4$^+$ CD25$^+$ regulatory T cells directed toward ubiquitously expressed *bona fide* self-antigens are likely to be similarly represented in high numbers and to be systemically distributed. In the case of tissue-restricted antigens, however, their differing responsiveness to TCR- versus cytokine-mediated signals provides a mechanism by which CD4$^+$ CD25$^+$ regulatory T cells can accumulate selectively at sites of antigen expression. We have begun to examine CD25$^+$ T cell development in the thymus and periphery of additional lineages of HA Tg mice that express the S1 peptide under the control of tissue-specific promoters, in which CD4$^+$ CD25$^+$ T cells may undergo thymic selection via promiscuous expression in thymic epithelial cells.[29] Analyses of the development of CD4$^+$ CD25$^+$ T cells in different lineages of HA Tg mice provides an opportunity to explore how variations in the expression of self-peptides influence the selection and activity of CD4$^+$ CD25$^+$ regulatory T cells.

ACKNOWLEDGMENTS

We thank past and present members of the laboratory (particularly Heath Guay, Andrew Rankin, and Amy Reed) for discussion, and Andrea Holenbeck, Vicki

Scheinfeld, and Laura Panarey for support. This work was funded by grants from the National Institutes of Health.

REFERENCES

1. STARR, T.K., S.C. JAMESON & K.A. HOGQUIST. 2003. Positive and negative selection of T cells. Annu. Rev. Immunol. **21:** 139–176.
2. SPRENT, J. & H. KISHIMOTO. 2002. The thymus and negative selection. Immunol. Rev. **185:** 126–135.
3. ERNST, B., D.S. LEE, J.M. CHANG, et al. 1999. The peptide ligands mediating positive selection in the thymus control T cell survival and homeostatic proliferation in the periphery. Immunity **11:** 173–181.
4. BENDER, J., T. MITCHELL, J. KAPPLER & P. MARRACK. 1999. CD4+ T cell division in irraadiated mice requires peptides distinct from those reesponsible for thymic selection. J. Exp. Med. **190:** 367–374.
5. MODIGLIANI, Y., P. PEREIRA, V. THOMAS-VASLIN, et al. 1995. Regulatory T cells in thymic epithelium-induced tolerance. I. Suppression of mature peripheral non-tolerant T cells. Eur. J. Immunol. **25:** 2563–2571.
6. MODIGLIANI, Y., V. THOMAS-VASLIN, A. BANDEIRA, et al. 1995. Lymphocytes selected in allogeneic thymic epithelium mediate dominant tolerance toward tissue grafts of the thymic epithelium haplotype. Proc. Natl. Acad. Sci. USA **92:** 7555–7559.
7. ASANO, M., M. TODA, N. SAKAGUCHI & S. SAKAGUCHI. 1996. Autoimmune disease as a consequence of developmental abnormality of a T cell subpopulation. J. Exp. Med. **184:** 387–396.
8. SAKAGUCHI, S., N. SAKAGUCHI, M. ASANO, et al. 1995. Immunologic self-tolerance maintained by activated T cells expressing IL-2 receptor alpha-chains (CD25). Breakdown of a single mechanism of self-tolerance causes various autoimmune diseases. J. Immunol. **155:** 1151–1164.
9. PAPIERNIK, M., M.L. DE MORAES, C. PONTOUX, et al. 1998. Regulatory CD4 T cells: expression of IL-2R alpha chain, resistance to clonal deletion and IL-2 dependency. Int. Immunol. **10:** 371–378.
10. MASON, D. & F. POWRIE. 1998. Control of immune pathology by regulatory T cells. Curr. Opin. Immunol. **10:** 649–655.
11. SEDDON, B. & D. MASON. 1999. Peripheral autoantigen induces regulatory T cells that prevent autoimmunity. J. Exp. Med. **189:** 877–882.
12. CERASOLI, D.M., J. MCGRATH, S.R. CARDING, et al. 1995. Low avidity recognition of a class II-restricted neo-self peptide by virus-specific T cells. Int. Immunol. **7:** 935–945.
13. SHIH, F.F., D.M. CERASOLI & A.J. CATON. 1997. A major T cell determinant from the influenza virus hemagglutinin (HA) can be a cryptic self peptide in HA transgenic mice. Int. Immunol. **9:** 249–261.
14. KIRBERG, J., A. BARON, S. JAKOB, et al. 1994. Thymic selection of CD8+ single positive cells with a class II major histocompatibility complex-restricted receptor. J. Exp. Med. **180:** 2534.
15. JORDAN, M.S., A. BOESTEANU, A.J. REED, et al. 2001. Thymic selection of CD4+CD25+ regulatory T cells induced by an agonist self-peptide. Nat. Immunol. **2:** 301–306.
16. JORDAN, M.S., M.P. RILEY, H. VON BOEHMER & A.J. CATON. 2000. Anergy and suppression regulate CD4(+) T cell responses to a self peptide. Eur. J. Immunol. **30:** 136–144.
17. RILEY, M.P., D.M. CERASOLI, M.S. JORDAN, et al. 2000. Graded deletion and virus-induced activation of autoreactive CD4(+) T cells. J. Immunol. **165:** 4870–4876.
18. COZZO, C., J. LARKIN III & A.J. CATON. 2003. Cutting edge: self-peptides drive the peripheral expansion of CD4+ CD25+ regulatory T cells. J. Immunol. **11:** 5678-5682.
19. SHEVACH, E.M. 2000. Regulatory T cells in autoimmmunity. Annu. Rev. Immunol. **18:** 423–449.

20. JAMESON, S.C., K.A. HOGQUIST & M.J. BEVAN. 1994. Specificity and flexibility in thymic selection. Nature **369**: 750–752.
21. FRY, T.J. & C.L. MACKALL. 2001. Interleukin-7: master regulatort of peripheral T-cell homeostasis? Trends Immunol. **22**: 564–571.
22. BEVAN, M.J., K.A. HOGQUIST & S.C. JAMESON. 1994. Selecting the T cell repertoire. Science **264**: 796–797.
23. WEBER, S., A. TRAUNECKER, F. OLIVERI, *et al.* 1992. Specific low-affinity recognition of major histocompatibility complex plus peptide by soluble T-cell receptor. Nature **356**: 793–796.
24. ITOH, M., T. TAKAHASHI, N. SAKAGUCHI, *et al.* 1999. Thymus and autoimmunity: production of CD25+ CD4+ naturally anergic and suppressive t cells as a key function of the thymus in maintaining immunologic self-tolerance. J. Immunol. **162**: 5317–5326.
25. XUE, H.-H., P.E. KOVANEN, C.A. PISE-MASISON, *et al.* 2002. IL-2 negatively reulates IL-7 receptor a chain expression in activated T lymphocytes. Proc. Natl. Acad. Sci. USA **99**: 13759–13764.
26. READ, S., V. MALMSTROM & F. POWRIE. 2000. Cytotoxic T lymphocyte-associated antigen 4 plays an essential role in the function of CD25(+)CD4(+) regulatory cells that control intestinal inflammation. J. Exp. Med. **192**: 295–302.
27. TAKAHASHI, T., T. TAGAMI, S. YAMAZAKI, *et al.* 2000. Immunologic self-tolerance maintained by CD25(+)CD4(+) regulatory T cells constitutively expressing cytotoxic T lymphocyte-associated antigen 4. J. Exp. Med. **192**: 303–310.
28. SHIMIZU, J., S. YAMAZAKI, T. TAKAHASHI, *et al.* 2002. Stimulation of CD25(+)CD4(+) regulatory T cells through GITR breaks immunological self-tolerance. Nat. Immunol. **3**: 135–142.
29. DERBINSKI, J., A. SCHULTE, B. KYEWSKI & L. KLEIN. 2001. Promiscuous gene expression in medullary thymic epithelial cells mirrors the peripheral self. Nat. Immunol. **2**: 1032–1039.

Insights into the Mechanism of Oral Tolerance Derived from the Study of Models of Mucosal Inflammation

WARREN STROBER,[a] IVAN FUSS,[a] MONICA BOIRIVANT,[b] AND ATSUSHI KITANI[a]

[a]*The Mucosal Immunity Section, Laboratory of Host Defense, NIAID, National Institutes of Health, Bethesda, Maryland 20892, USA*

[b]*The Immune-Mediated Diseases Section, Department of Infectious, Parasitic and Immune-Mediated Diseases, Istituto Superiore di Sanita, Rome, Italy*

> ABSTRACT: Murine models of mucosal inflammation are frequently due to the inability of the mouse to mount a regulatory T cell response. To the extent that such responses arise from oral tolerance mechanisms, these models provide a unique way of studying oral tolerance. In this paper we focus on the regulatory cells generated in two of the most well-studied of such models, the cell-transfer model and the TNBS-colitis model. Our analysis leads to the view that regulatory cells generated by the oral tolerance seen in mucosal inflammation are, at least in part, cells that recognize self-antigens or antigens in the mucosal microflora whose effector function relies on the expression of TGF-β.
>
> KEYWORDS: regulatory T cells; cell-transfer colitis; TGF-β; TNBS-colitis; IL-10

INTRODUCTION

One rather unexpected consequence of the now decade-long study of models of mucosal inflammation is that such studies open a window on the mechanisms of oral tolerance. This relates to the fact that mucosal inflammation in most instances results from an imbalance between mucosal effector cell responses to ligands/antigens in the resident mucosal microflora and countervailing regulatory cell responses ultimately originating from oral tolerance. Because the effector cell response potentially resulting in mucosal inflammation is inevitably a robust phenomenon, it requires an equally robust regulatory cell response for its control. Thus, in studying mucosal inflammation, one has the opportunity to study oral tolerance under unusually telling conditions.

Address for correspondence: W. Strober, The Mucosal Immunity Section, Laboratory of Host Defense, NIAID, NIH, Bethesda, MD 20892. Voice: 301-496-6810; fax: 301-402-2240.
wstrober@niaid.nih.gov

REGULATION OF THE CELL-TRANSFER COLITIS MODEL

The role of regulatory cells in the control of mucosal inflammation has been very successfully studied in the "cell-transfer model" of colitis, wherein one induces a transmural, Th1 T cell-mediated (IL-12/IL-23–induced) colitis by adoptive transfer of antigen-naive (CD45RB^{hi}) CD4$^+$ T cells to severe combined immunodeficiency (SCID) or RAG2-deficient recipient mice, and prevents such colitis by cotransfer of antigen-experienced, mature (CD45RB^{lo}) CD4$^+$ T cells along with the naive cells.[1–3] This model of colitis lends itself to the study of regulatory cells because it allows one to elucidate the phenotype and function of the regulatory cells in the mature cell population that prevent the development of colitis. Among the facts concerning regulatory cells involved in mucosal inflammation that have been obtained with this model are that regulatory cells are CD25$^+$ T cells similar to "natural" regulatory cells identified previously in studies of thymectomized mice[4–6] and that such cells require TGF-β, IL-10, and interactions involving CTLA-4 costimulatory molecules to be functionally active.[7,8] In addition, studies of this model have disclosed that the regulatory cells act both in the lamina propria and in mesenteric lymph nodes by forming clusters containing both T cells and dendritic cells in these sites.[4,9]

Recent studies focusing on the role of TGF-β in the regulatory effect of CD45RB^{lo} cells in the cell-transfer model have shown that recipient mice that are adoptively transferred cells that lack the ability to respond to TGF-β because they bear a transgene gene encoding a dominant-negative protein suppressing the function of a TGF-β receptor component (TGF-βRII), cannot be suppressed by the transfer of CD45RB^{lo} cells;[10–12] thus, TGF-β is intrinsically a part of the regulatory mechanism operating in this model of mucosal inflammation. However, the origin of the TGF-β in this model is in some doubt. On the one hand, it has been shown that T cells that bear surface TGF-β (in the form of TGF-β1 bound to latency-associated protein) have been shown to mediate prevention of colitis, whereas cells that do not bear this surface molecule do not have this property; this implies that TGF-β–bearing cells are responsible for regulatory function and suggests that the TGF-β is produced by the regulatory cells.[13,14] On the other hand, it is still unclear whether cells from TGF-β knockout (KO) mice can exhibit regulatory function in the cell-transfer model: in one study such cells were capable of regulatory function in this model, whereas in other studies (using mice of other strains) they were not.[14,15] One resolution of this issue is that regulatory T cells in the cell transfer always operate via the expression of surface-bound TGF-β, but the latter does not necessarily have to arise from the T cell itself; it could arise from other cells that "arm" the regulatory cell. We will revisit this important question after we discuss the nature of regulatory T cells more generally.

A final point that needs to be made about the cell-transfer model in the present context is that the inflammation induced in the recipient mice is dependent on the presence of resident mucosal microflora, because no inflammation is induced in mice housed in a germ-free facility, and CD4$^+$ T cells from mice with cell-transfer colitis produce Th1 cytokines when stimulated by antigen-presenting cells pulsed with antigens in fecal extracts of normal, but not germ-free, mice.[16,17] The significance of this is that the effector cells in the CD45RB^{hi} cell population that cause the inflammation are being stimulated by antigens in the microflora or by self-antigens that cross-react with the latter. It is likely that the regulatory cells in the CD45RB^{lo}

cell population that can prevent the inflammation have a similar specificity, although in this case the antigens may also be "true" self-antigens that are released during the tissue destruction that accompanies inflammation. It should be noted, however, that the distinction between antigens associated with the intestinal microflora may be more apparent than real because microflora antigens are constantly present and have equal access to tolerogenic mechanisms in the thymus, as there is now good evidence that resident (commensal) organisms do penetrate the epithelial cell barrier.[18,19]

In any event, if the regulatory cells in the cell-transfer model are the same as the regulatory cells induced by oral tolerance, then one must draw the conclusion that oral tolerance functions in relation to antigens in the microflora or to self-antigens. Furthermore, it is likely that such regulatory cells are induced centrally in the thymus by the aforementioned microflora antigens that gain entry to the internal milieu and then traffic back to the mucosa where re-exposure to microflora antigens results in their expansion and control of effector cell responses induced by such antigens. Thus, in this case (and perhaps in all cases of oral tolerance) the apparent preferential development of regulatory cells in mucosal tissues is really due to the fact that these tissues are juxtaposed to a pool of antigens that can reinforce and expand the development of regulatory cells in the thymus.

This scenario of the origin of regulatory cells, including those that protect from the development of inflammation, would explain the fact that $CD45RB^{hi}$ cells do not contain a subpopulation of regulatory cells (and thus cause colitis when transferred alone) because regulatory cells that emerge from the thymus are cells that bear a mature $CD45RB^{lo}$ phenotype. An interesting implication of this conclusion bears on recent *in vitro* studies that suggest that regulatory cells can be induced in the periphery by TGF-β;[20–22] however, if this were the case in the cell-transfer model, one might expect that the naive $CD45RB^{hi}$ cell population would be induced to become regulatory cells and would not cause disease when transferred alone. It is therefore more likely that such induction of regulatory cells in the periphery in reality represents the expansion of pre-existing regulatory cells that have developed in the thymus. This, despite the fact that such induced regulatory cells can be $CD25^-$ cells that are otherwise indistinguishable for other $CD4^+$ cells, as it is likely that regulatory cells are not strictly defined by their expression of CD25.

REGULATION OF THE TNBS-COLITIS MODEL AND ITS RELATION TO ORAL TOLERANCE

Although the cell-transfer model has been an excellent vehicle for the study of regulatory cell *per se*, it is intrinsically incapable of linking the regulatory cell to oral tolerance. A better model in this respect is the hapten-induced colitis represented by TNBS-colitis in which colitis is induced by the intrarectal administration of trinitrobenzene sulfonic acid (TNBS) in ethanol solution.[23] This model is also a Th1-mediated (IL-12–induced) inflammation in the SJL/J and C57BL/10 mouse strains, both of which bear a disease susceptibility locus on chromosome 11 that encodes a gene or genes that leads to increased IL-12 responses to parenteral injection of lipopolysaccharide (LPS).[24] Thus, it is likely that the induction of inflammation in this model is initiated by an "innate" response to a bacterial component such as LPS or another ligand of one of the toll-like receptors (TLRs) that elicits a robust IL-12 response; this response is facilitated by the presentation of TNBS in ethanol because ethanol disrupts the epithelial barrier and leads to the introduction of bacterial components into the lamina propria proper. Having established an IL-12–rich environment, the TNBS/alcohol mixture then elicits an adaptive immune response to haptenated colonic proteins generated by chemical interaction between TNBS and protein components of the colon. In addition, as in the case of the cell-transfer model of colitis, inflammation in this model is furthered by response to antigens in the mucosal microflora, as mice with TNBS-colitis have been shown to contain cells that react with such antigens.[25,26] However, whether such antigens in the mucosal flora are limited to those that cross-react with TNP-haptenated colonic proteins or with a wider range of antigens in the flora is still unknown.

The property of TNBS-colitis that allows one to examine the influence of oral tolerance on inflammation is the fact that TNBS-haptenated protein can be administered orally at the time of colitis induction by intrarectal TNBS to determine whether such oral antigen influences the course of the inflammation. In fact, when this is done, induction of colitis is prevented and one sees the induction of a regulatory cell response in the lamina propria consisting of $CD4^+$ T cells that produce TGF-β.[26] One can prove that these cells are responsible for the prevention of colitis because

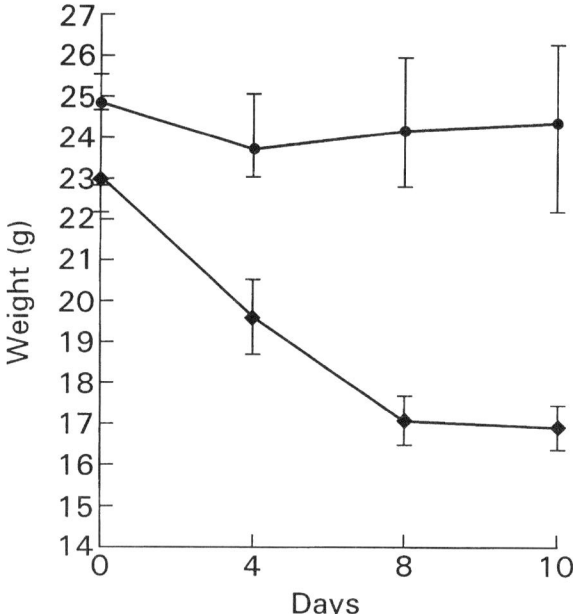

FIGURE 1. TNBS-induced colitis can be suppressed by the adoptive transfer of lamina propria (LP) $CD4^+$ T cells from HCP-fed mice. Weight changes of recipients of LP $CD4^+$ T cells obtained from mice fed HCP (HCP-fed $CD4^+$ T cells) (●) and mice with TNBS-colitis (TNBS $CD4^+$ T cells (♦). Recipient mice received TNBS per rectum 5 d after adoptive transfer of LP $CD4^+$ T cells. Data shown are from one representative experiment of three similar experiments. Each point represents the average weight of five mice; bars represent SD.

transfer of CD4$^+$ T cells from the lamina propria of mice fed haptenated-colonic protein confers protection from colitis on recipient mice undergoing TNBS-colitis induction[26,27] (FIG. 1). In addition, administration of anti–TGF-β to mice fed TNP-haptenated protein, or to mice transferred cells from such mice, abolishes the protective effect of feeding or feeding plus cell transfer on mice undergoing induction of TNBS-colitis.[26,27] Taken together, these data show that TNBS-colitis, no less than cell-transfer colitis, can be influenced by a regulatory response, but in this case the regulatory cells constituting the regulatory response are introduced into the system by feeding the colitis-inducing antigen(s) and inducing oral tolerance to these antigen(s).

One of the implications of this finding is that fed antigen has a markedly different effect on the mucosal immune response than intrarectal antigen accompanied by ethanol. The reason for this difference is fundamental to the understanding of the conditions that lead to oral tolerance on the one hand and mucosal effector cell responses on the other, at least within the context of TNBS-colitis. A general way of explaining this difference is that the response to the fed antigen is a "default" response that involves a noninflammatory presentation of antigen (TNP-haptenated colonic protein by dendritic cells that do not induce IL-12–mediated effector T cell responses). Such presentation may occur preferentially in mucosal inductive sites (Peyer's patches) or mesenteric lymph nodes or in both the latter sites as well as in mucosal effector sites (lamina propria) (reviewed in Ref. 28). In addition, it may involve dendritic cells with a propensity to produce IL-10 and IFN-α rather than IL-12, but this is by no means proven.[29] In contrast, the intrarectal antigen given with ethanol is associated with a break in the epithelial barrier that, as mentioned above, gives rise to a genetically determined hyper-responsiveness to some component of the mucosal microflora (e.g., LPS) in certain strains of mice.[24] This is associated with antigen presentation by dendritic cells producing increased amounts IL-12p70 that then generate a Th1-effector cell response capable of overriding the default response described above. Obviously, further work will be necessary to substantiate this scenario, particularly studies that focus on the types of presenting cells that predominate in the two kinds of antigen exposure.

THE RELATION OF IL-10 TO REGULATORY RESPONSES IN EXPERIMENTAL MUCOSAL INFLAMMATION

As discussed above in relation to the regulatory responses mediated by CD45RB^{lo} cells in the cell transfer model, IL-10 is a critical player because mice treated with anti–IL-10R or repleted by CD45RB^{lo} cells from IL-10$^{-/-}$ mice have little or no capacity to protect against the development of colitis.[30] However, the role of IL-10 in the cell transfer model has not yet been defined on a mechanistic level. One possibility is that T cells producing IL-10 (so-called Tr1 cells that do not express CD25 prior to activation) participate in the regulation of the colitis, as suggested by the fact that Tr1 cells induced *in vitro* and then transferred to SCID recipients along with CD45RB^{hi} cells prevent colitis induction by the latter cells.[31] However, the role of Tr1 cells in cell-transfer colitis is undermined by the fact that CD25$^-$ cells in the protective CD45RB^{lo} cell population do not account for the protection as one might predict if this cell subpopulation were to contain the precursors of IL-10–producing Tr1 cells.[30] In addition, RAG2 KO mice adaptively transferred with

CD45RB[hi] cells and then infected with *H. hepaticus* develop colitis when they are cotransferred CD25[−] cells, but not when the are cotransferred CD25[+] cells;[5] thus, again, cell populations containing putative Tr1 precursor cells are not protective, at least in the RAG2 host. It should be noted, however, that IL-10–producing T cells are induced during *H. hepaticus* infection of normal mice, and in this situation these cells, and not CD25[+] cells, are the protective regulatory cells, as defined in cell transfer studies.[32] Thus, IL-10–producing (Tr1) cells may be induced in the mucosa of normal mice in response to a pathogenic infection, but are not induced in RAG2 KO mice; furthermore, at least with respect to the cell-transfer model they do not play an effective regulatory role in inflammation induced by the mucosal microflora. On this basis, it seems more likely that the role of IL-10 in cell-transfer colitis is to support or facilitate the activity of CD25[+] regulatory cells that require TGF-β for their activity.

IL-10 also plays a role in the regulation of TNBS-colitis, and, in this case, some progress toward understanding this role on a mechanistic basis has been made. One fruitful approach to defining the latter has been to administer anti–TGF-β and anti–IL-10 to mice in whom regulatory cells are induced by feeding TNP-haptenated protein (TNP-HCP), or to mice transferred cells from the fed mice and then subjected to TNBS-colitis induction. In an initial series of studies of this kind, it was shown that mice fed TNP-HCP were not protected from the development of TNBS-colitis as described above when they were administered either anti–TGF-β or anti–IL-10.[27] However, the effect of these antibodies on cytokine production by CD4[+] T cells extracted from the lamina propria was very different. Whereas anti–TGF-β administration inhibited TGF-β secretion, it had no effect on IL-10 secretion; in contrast, anti–IL-10 administration inhibited both TGF-β and IL-10 secretion (FIG. 2). This result indicates quite clearly that TGF-β alone is necessary to mediate the protective effect of feeding and IL-10 is necessary to support TGF-β production, not to act as a suppressor cytokine by itself.

In additional studies in which the anti–TGF-β and anti–IL-10 were administered to either fed donor mice before cell transfer or to recipient mice, it was established that anti–IL-10 did not block the induction of regulatory cells, that is, anti–IL-10–treated fed mice still were a good source of regulatory cells that prevented colitis in most recipient mice.[27] However, anti–IL-10 did block the protective effect of transferred cells from fed mice when administered to the recipient mice. This indicates that IL-10 functions in a manner that facilitates the expansion and/or function of the regulatory cells after they are induced. However, it is still not clear how IL-10 provides this supportive function. One possibility is that IL-10 facilitates TGF-β signaling. This is suggested by the observation that IL-10 maintains TGF-βRII expression on activated cells that would otherwise downregulate this receptor.[33] In addition, because Smad7, a cytosolic intermediate that inhibits TGF-β signaling via Smad2 and Smad3, is upregulated by Th1 cytokines,[34] it is possible that IL-10 facilitates TGF-β signaling by overcoming this block. A third and perhaps most likely possibility is that IL-10 modulates the negative effect of Th1 cytokines on the expansion of regulatory cells producing TGF-β.[27] This view is supported by studies mentioned above showing that induction of TGF-β–producing cells by feeding TNP-HCP to donor mice in the absence of inflammation (i.e., in the absence of a Th1 cytokine milieu) is unhindered by anti–IL-10 administration, whereas expansion of TGF-β–producing cells in recipient mice in the presence of inflammation is blocked by anti–IL-10 administration. How can IL-10 have this effect on expansion of TGF-β–producing

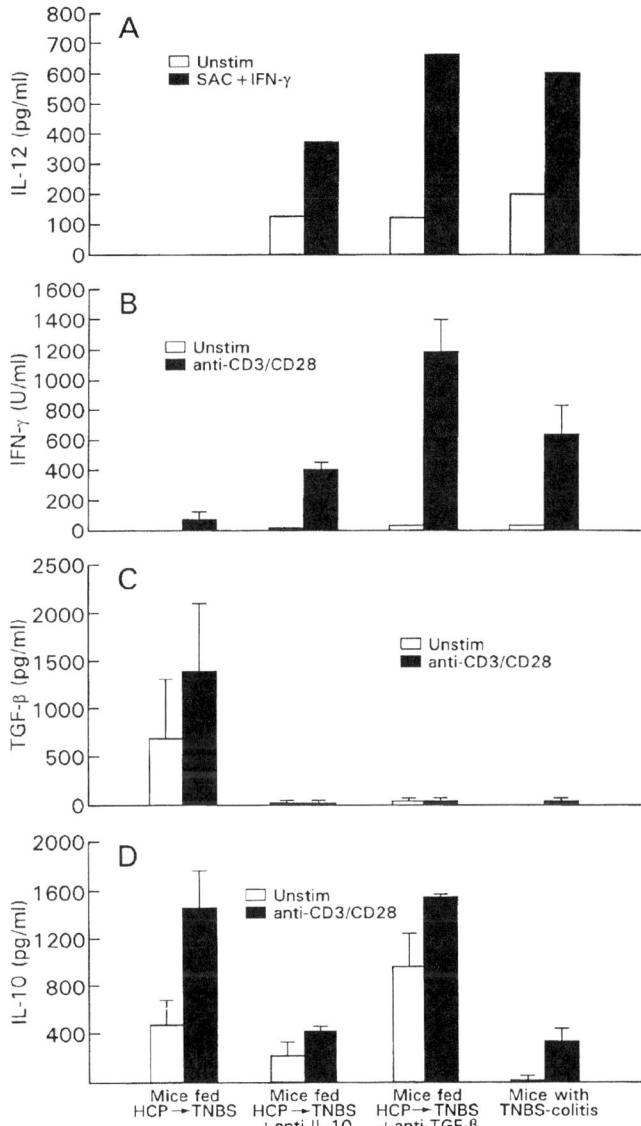

FIGURE 2. Cytokine secretion by lamina propria M cells isolated from colons of mice after HCP-feeding, either treated or untreated with anti–IL-10 or anti–TGF-β. Groups consisted of mice who were administered TNBS per rectum after HCP feeding, TNBS per rectum and anti–TGF-β IP after HCP feeding, TNBS per rectum and anti–IL-10 IP after HCP feeding, or TNBS per rectum without any previous treatment. Culture supernatants were assayed by specific ELISA for (**A**) IL-12 secretion, (**B**) IFN-γ secretion, (**C**) TGF-β secretion, (**D**) IL-10 secretion. Data of IFN-γ, TGF-β, and IL-10 represent mean values obtained from five independent experiments. In each experiment, culture supernatants from cultures of pooled cells extracted from five mice per group were analyzed. Bars represent SEM.

regulatory cells? One possibility is that it downmodulates Th1 cytokine production and its known negative effects on TGF-β production at a critical stage in the expansion cycle. In addition, because TGF-β may be necessary for the expansion of regulatory cells,[20–22] it is possible that IL-10 maintains TGF-β secretion in the face of Th1 cytokines that have been shown to inhibit such secretion.[35] In this context, it should be noted that we have found that TGF-β–producing T cells extracted from the lamina propria of fed mice when stimulated in the presence of certain Th1 cytokines do, in fact, exhibit reduced TGF-β production (unpublished data). A final possibility is that IL-10 inhibits TNF-α production by macrophages.

REGULATORY CELLS AND THE TREATMENT OF ESTABLISHED INFLAMMATION

So far in our discussion we have considered regulatory cells that prevent colitis in both the cell-transfer colitis model and in the TNBS-colitis model. An important question is whether these cells can also treat established inflammation. This has been answered in the affirmative in the cell-transfer model, where it has been very clearly shown that administration of regulatory CD25$^+$ cells to mice with severe colitis results in impressive amelioration/reversal of the colitis.[4] In this case, regulatory cells are found both in mesenteric lymph nodes and in the lamina propria of mice with inflammation and there is evidence that such cells interact with both T cells and dendritic cells in these sites to quell the inflammatory process. However, a different picture has been obtained with respect to TNBS-colitis, where recipients of simultaneously transferred effector cells (from mice administered intrarectal TNBS) and regulatory cells (from mice fed TNP-haptenated colonic protein) do not develop colitis, mice with established TNBS-colitis and then secondarily administered regulatory cells do not exhibit reversal of colitis (unpublished data). The reason for this discrepancy between the two models is not clear. As discussed above, the presence of a pre-existing Th1 cytokine milieu tends to suppress the function and/or the expansion of regulatory cells. The fact that it does not have this effect in the milieu of the cell-transfer colitis model but does in the TNBS-colitis model may indicate that the two models differ in some significant way that impacts on their susceptibility to regulation. One possible such difference is in the display of IL-10 in the two models, since we have seen that IL-10 is necessary for regulatory responses in both models. Another possibility is that the microenvironment of the SCID/RAG2 KO recipients used in the cell-transfer model may be more permissive of regulatory cell expansion than wild-type mice of the same strain used in the TNBS-model. This is suggested by the fact that whereas CD25$^+$ regulatory cells dependent on both TGF-β and IL-10 controlled inflammation induced by *H. hepaticus* in RAG2 KO mice, Tr1 regulatory cells dependent on IL-10 alone controlled inflammation in wild-type mice.[32] Obviously, further work will be necessary to resolve this important issue.

INDUCTION OF REGULATORY CELLS BY GENE TRANSFER

One way around the issue alluded to above regarding the problem of regulatory cell function/expansion in the face of an ongoing Th1 response is to induce regula-

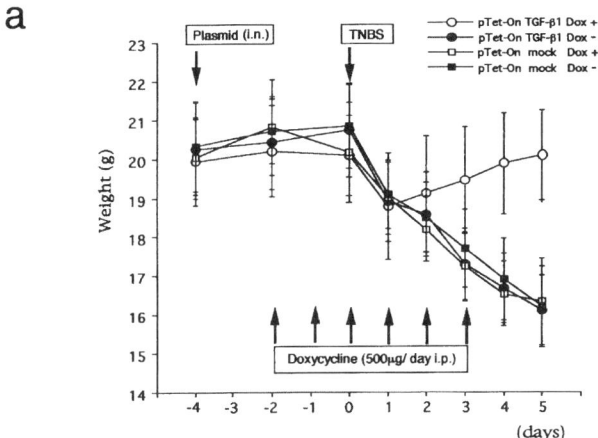

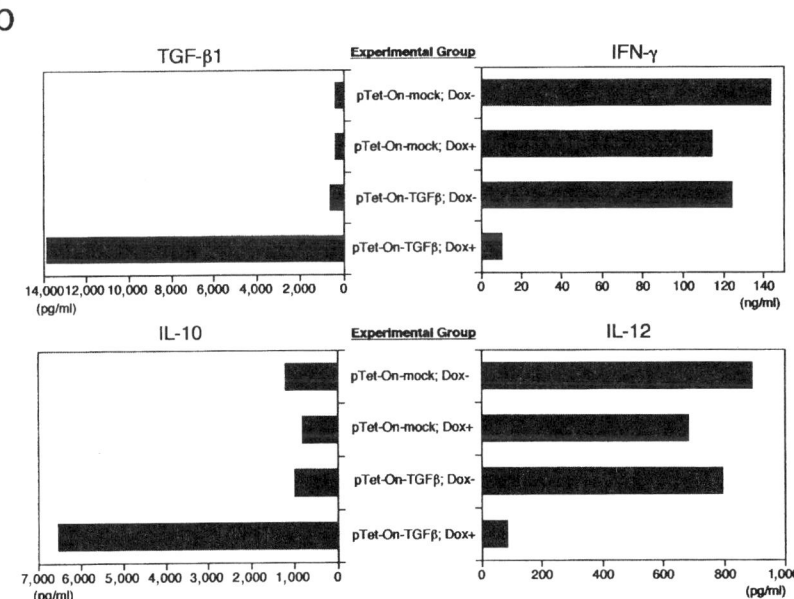

FIGURE 3. Effect of intranasal pTet-On–TGF-β1 administration on TNBS-induced colitis. (**a**) Weight changes of mouse groups administered intrarectal TNBS and intranasal pTet-On–TGF-β or pTet-On–mock (control plasmid) with or without doxycycline (Dox) i.p.; $n = 10$ for each group. (**b**) LP cells from mice 5 d after TNBS colitis induction were stimulated and cultured for ELISA assays of TGF-β1, IFN-γ, IL-10, and IL-12. As shown, LP cells from mice administered Dox plus pTet-On–TGF-β1 produced large amounts of TGF-β1 and IL-10 and exhibited suppressed IL-12 and IFN-γ production. Data shown are representative of three independent experiments.

tory cells by a method that would result in cells that would not be subject to normal requirements for expansion. This has, in fact, been accomplished by a form of "gene therapy" in which a plasmid vector encoding bioactive TGF-β under the control of a CMV promoter is administered to mice by intranasal inhalation.[36] It can be shown that such intranasal delivery of DNA results in the appearance of cells (both macrophages and T cells) in the spleen that express protein encoded by the delivered DNA. In addition, mice administered a plasmid encoding TGF-β and then subjected to TNBS-colitis exhibit T cells in the lamina propria that secrete TGF-β (FIG. 3). Using this technique to induce TGF-β–secreting regulatory cells, it could be shown that plasmid administered at the time of induction of TNBS-colitis very effectively prevented the development of TNBS-colitis in at least two ways: it suppressed the secretion of IL-12 and, by downregulating the IL-12Rβ2 signaling chain of the IL-12 receptor, it inhibited IL-12 signaling. In addition, it was shown that administration of the plasmid by the intranasal route also effectively abrogated established TNBS-colitis. Finally, in further studies it could be shown that a more sophisticated plasmid that was regulated by a Tet-on gene system and that required doxycycline for production of DNA encoding TGF-β could also both prevent and treat TNBS-colitis, but in this case, only when the mice were simultaneously administered doxycycline.[37] This latter experiment is important because it illustrates that TGF-β induced by plasmid administration can be tightly regulated so as not to expose the organism to the adverse effects of TGF-β itself.

INDUCTION OF IL-10 BY TGF-β

An important insight that emerged from the study of the effects of intranasal administration of a plasmid encoding TGF-β was that such administration was accompanied by the co-induction of IL-10, so that cells in treated mice not only secreted TGF-β, but also secreted IL-10 (Refs. 36 and 37; FIG. 4). This observation was explored in several ways. First, it was shown that both T cells and macrophage lines transfected with a TGF-β–expressing vector (either a plasmid or a retrovirus) produced substantial amounts of IL-10; in contrast, neither epithelial cells nor fibroblasts had this property.[36,37] Second, it was shown that Th1 cell lines infected with a retrovirus expressing both GFP and TGF-β and then analyzed by flow cytometry produced IL-10, whether or not they expressed the retrovirus (as indicated by their co-expression of GFP).[37] This means that TGF-β production induces IL-10 in both an autocrine and paracrine fashion. Parallel studies showed that IL-10 was also

---

FIGURE 4. TGF-β1 activates IL-10 promoter transcription through Smad4 in Th1 cells. (**a**) An electrophoretic mobility shift assay shows that TGF-β1–induced nuclear extracts exhibit binding activity to an SBE variant oligonucleotide as well as native SBE oligonucleotide. Anti-Smad4 antibody causes supershift of the complex with the SBE variant. (**b**) Schematic map of self-inactivating pBMN–IL-10 luciferase reporter genes. (**c**) Luciferase activity of IL-10 promoter was assayed by infection with self-inactivating retroviruses. Retrovirally expressed TGF-β1 induces IL-10 promoter activity in developing Th1 cells signaling through SBE variant sequence, but TGF-β1 is not required for activation of IL-10 promoter in developing Th2 cells.

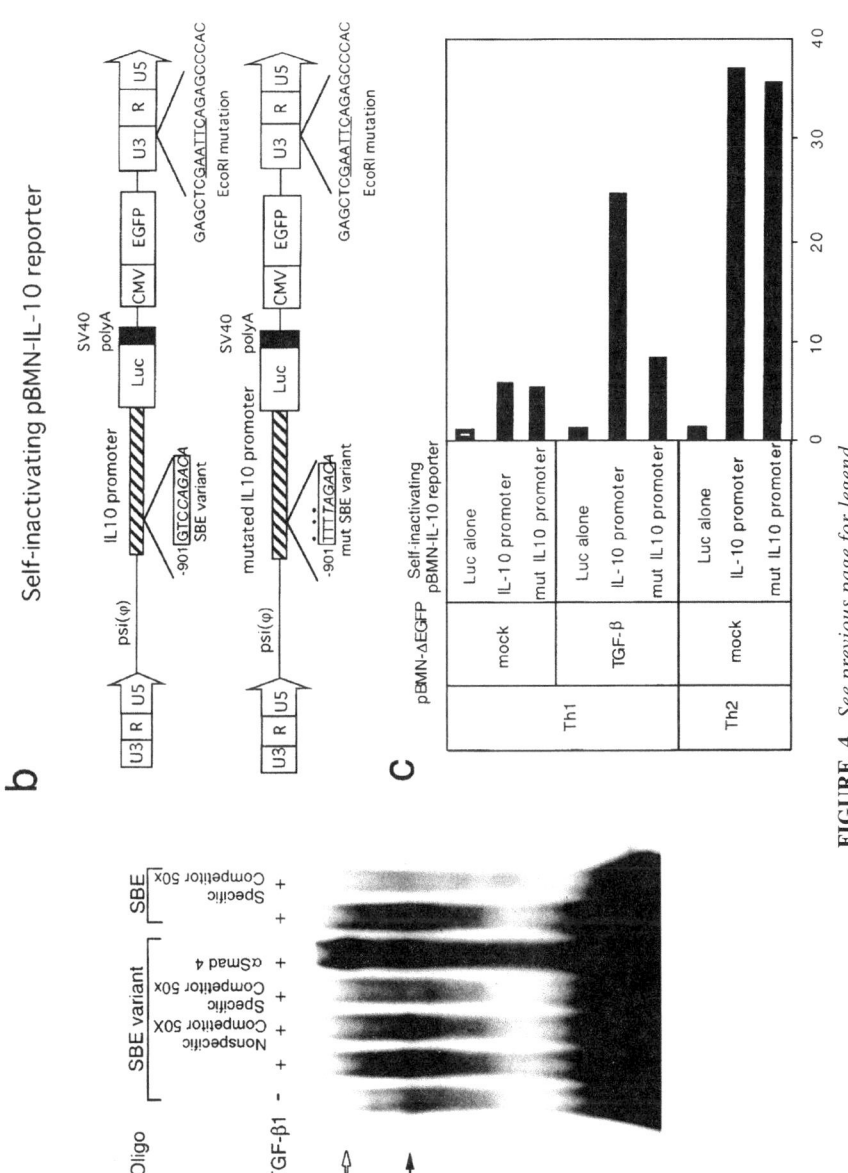

FIGURE 4. *See previous page for legend.*

secreted by Th1 cells lines after retroviral infection or, indeed, after exposure to soluble TGF-β[37] (FIG. 4). The reason for this induction of IL-10 secretion by TGF-β became apparent from subsequent studies showing that TGF-β–induced Smad4 binds to a Smad-binding consensus sequence in the IL-10 promoter and, more importantly, using a reporter gene consisting of the IL-10 promoter linked to a luciferase reporter transfected into a Th1 cell line, TGF-β directly induces activation of the IL-10 promoter.[37] Together, these *in vitro* studies prove beyond question that co-induction of TGF-β and IL-10 results from a direct molecular effect of TGF-β on IL-10 synthesis. It should be noted, however, that although TGF-β induces IL-10, there is no evidence that IL-10 induces TGF-β.

The close (one-way) association of TGF-β and IL-10 production begs the question: What is the selective advantage of this association to the organism? One possibility is suggested by studies of bleomycin-induced fibrosis in which it was demonstrated that fibrosis was paradoxically reduced by intranasal TGF-β plasmid administration and that such reduction was IL-10 dependent, because it was not observed in IL-10 deficient mice.[37] Thus, IL-10 induced by TGF-β may play an important role in controlling the untoward side effects of TGF-β, such as the latter's capacity to induce excess fibrosis at inflammatory sites. Another possibility, and one more pertinent to the function of regulatory cells, is the one already discussed at some length above, namely, that IL-10 has been shown to be necessary for regulatory cell function mediated by TGF-β in the TNBS-colitis model, although it is still unclear just how IL-10 functions in this role. Relevant to this point, whereas the TGF-β–inducing plasmid is effective in reversing established Th1-mediated inflammation, suggesting that the activity of the plasmid may be less dependent on IL-10 in resisting downregulation by Th1 cytokines, the fact is that the plasmid was found to be ineffective in quelling colonic inflammation arising in IL-10 KO mice (A. Kitani, W. Strober, and B. Sartor, unpublished observation). Thus, the necessity for IL-10 in TGF-β–mediated interactions may go beyond the mere facilitation of regulatory cell expansion.

THE NATURE OF THE REGULATORY CELLS IN CELL-TRANSFER AND TNBS-COLITIS

In discussing the regulatory cells providing protection or, indeed, the treatment of either cell-transfer colitis or TNBS-colitis, a certain imbalance is apparent, in that in the former model the regulatory cell has been well defined as a $CD25^+$ $CD4^+$ T cell. Recent work has shown that this cell is dependent on TGF-β for its activity and that, in fact, it requires target cells that bear TGF-β receptors, because it does not provide protection of mice bearing a gene expressing a dominant negative TGF-βRII receptor chain.[10–12] The T cell providing regulatory activity after feeding is less well defined, although as already mentioned, it is a $CD4^+$ T cell that acts through its production of TGF-β. One of the problems associated with establishing whether or not this cell is also a $CD25^+$ T cell is that it is derived from lamina propria following feeding and thus from tissue that contains activated T cells that bear CD25 on the basis of their activation status. Thus, other approaches to the identification of this cell will be necessary to establish its identity.

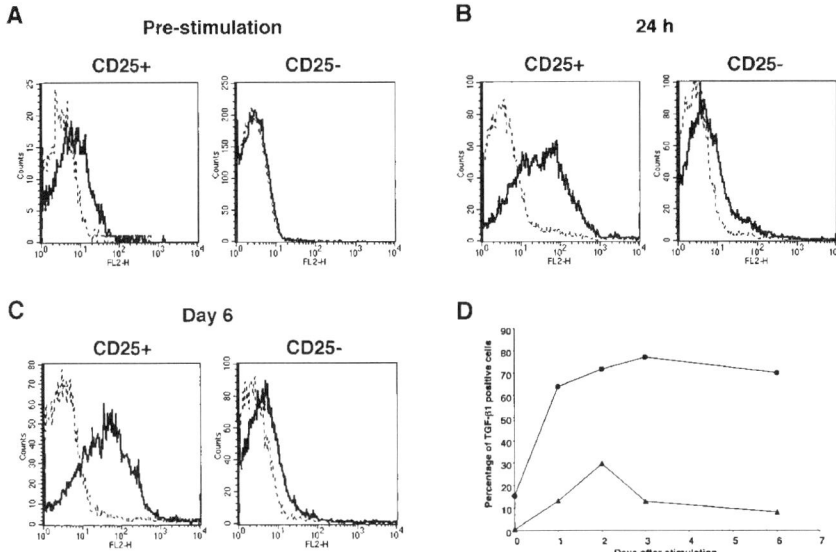

FIGURE 5. CD4+ CD25+ T cells express TGF-β1 on the cell surface. (**A**) Enriched CD4+ T cells were stained with FITC-conjugated anti-CD25, Cy-Chrome–conjugated anti-CD4, and either biotin-conjugated chicken anti–TGF-β1 or biotin-conjugated normal chicken IgG, washed, and stained with PE-conjugated streptavidin. CD4+ CD25+ and CD4+ CD25− T cells were gated, and expression of cell surface-bound TGF-β1 is shown. *Thick lines*, anti–TGF-β; *thin lines*, normal chicken IgG. The results shown are the representative of three independent experiments. (**B,C**) Purified CD4+ CD25+ and CD4+ CD25− T cells were stimulated with soluble anti-CD3 (10 μg/mL) and irradiated non–T cells in the presence of IL-2 (20 U/mL) for 24 h (**B**) or 6 d (**C**). Cells were then stained with Cy-Chrome–conjugated anti-CD4 and either biotin-conjugated chicken anti–TGF-β1 or biotin-conjugated normal chicken IgG, washed, and stained with PE-conjugated streptavidin. CD4+ cells were gated, and expression of cell surface–bound TGF-β1 is shown. *Thick lines*, anti–TGF-β; *thin lines*, normal chicken IgG. The results shown are representative of three independent experiments. (**D**) Graphic representation of the percentage of surface TGF-β1 positive cells in CD4+ CD25+ (*triangle*) and CD4+ CD25− (*circle*) T cells after stimulation.

Recently, several advances in our ability to characterize and recognize regulatory cells have been made that may help resolve this problem. One advance is the fact that CD25+ cells have been shown to express an intracellular protein known as foxP3, a fork-winged transcription factor whose absence in both mice and humans is associated with severe autoimmunity,[38,39] including an IBD-like syndrome. Thus, it should become possible to determine whether the regulatory cell that protects fed mice from TNBS-colitis is foxP3-positive and thus a bona fide CD25+ regulatory cell. Another advance concerns the fact that it has been shown that CD25+ regulatory cells bear cell surface TGF-β in an inactive form in which the TGF-β is associated with latency-associated protein (LAP)[13,14] (FIG. 5). Furthermore, it has been shown that such surface TGF-β on CD25+ T cells is biologically active in that CD25+ cells cultured with CD25− cells can induce Smad phosphorylation as well as expression

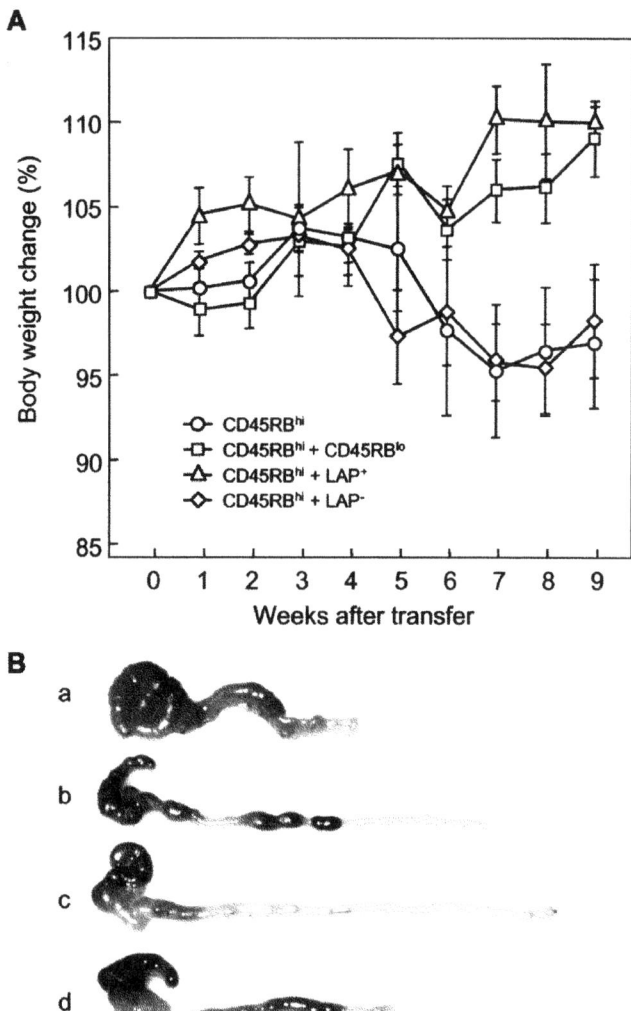

FIGURE 6. *In vivo* suppressor function of LAP$^+$ and LAP$^-$ T cells in the SCID transfer colitis. Weight curves and gross appearance of colons. (**A**) C.B.-17 SCID mice were reconstituted with CD4$^+$ CD45RB^{high} T cells (○), CD4$^+$ CD45RB^{high} and CD4CD45RB^{low} T cells (□), CD4CD45RB^{high} and CD4$^+$LAP$^+$ T cells (△), or CD4$^+$CD45RB^{high} and CD4$^+$LAP$^-$ T cells (◇). The change in weight was monitored weekly after the transfer. (**B**) The gross appearance of colons in each group. Recipients of (**a**) CD4$^+$ CD45RB^{high} T cells, (**b**) CD4$^+$ CD45RB^{high} and CD4$^+$ CD45RB^{low} T cells, (**c**) CD4$^+$ CD45RB^{high} and CD4$^+$ LAP$^+$ T cells, and (**d**) CD4$^+$ CD45RB^{high} and CD4$^+$ LAP$^-$ T cells.

of CD103, the latter a TGF-β–dependent event.[13] Finally, the biological role of surface TGF-β in regulatory events has been shown both *in vitro* and *in vivo*. Thus, it has been shown that addition of anti–TGF-β antibody or LAP inhibits $CD25^+$ suppressor cell activity in *in vitro* assays of such activity; in addition, it has been shown that LAP^+ cells, but not LAP^- cells, provide protection against the development of colitis inducted by $CD45RB^{hi}$ cells in the cell-transfer model of colitis[13] (FIG. 6). Taken together, there is little doubt that $CD25^+$ regulatory cells act, at least in part, through cell–cell interactions that involve cell surface TGF-β. The way is now open to determine whether the regulatory cell induced by feeding TNP-haptenated colonic protein is a $CD25^+$ regulatory cell on the basis of its ability to express surface TGF-β.

Finally, the view that regulatory cells mediate regulatory cell function via surface TGF-β raises the question of the role of secreted TGF-β in such function. One attractive possibility is that secreted TGF-β actually has no direct role in regulation and only serves as an expander of $CD25^+$ regulatory cells, as recently shown by a number of groups.[20–22] This would explain why anti–TGF-β is required at high concentration to inhibit the $CD25^+$ T cell regulatory *in vitro*, but not *in vivo*, because in the former situation one has to inhibit the activity of secreted TGF-β, whereas in the latter situation one has the more difficult task of inhibiting surface bound TGF-β. In addition, it would explain the activity of the plasmid encoding TGF-β discussed above, even though this plasmid encodes an active TGF-β that does not include LAP and thus is unlikely to be expressed on the cell surface: the function of this plasmid may lie in its ability to expand pre-existing (endogenous) regulatory cells rather than *de novo* regulatory cells.

CONCLUSION

In this review, we have attempted to elucidate the nature of oral tolerance using the "lens" of experimental mucosal inflammation. The data clearly support the view that regulatory cells profoundly influence the course of such inflammation in the two most commonly studied colitis models, cell-transfer colitis and TNBS-colitis. In the former case, the regulatory cells have been exceedingly well characterized, whereas in the latter case they have been clearly related to the oral tolerance process. In both cases, their relation to both TGF-β and IL-10 production has been thoroughly explored and, at least within the context of TNBS-colitis, it has been established the TGF-β plays the primary role as a suppressor cytokine whereas IL-10 plays a secondary (but still essential) role.

Overall, the accumulated data derived from these models (as well as other models) have greatly expanded our knowledge of oral tolerance mediated by regulatory cells in that they have helped define these cells and the conditions under which they operate. This being said, several key unanswered questions remain to be addressed using these models. One question that would require the use of the TNBS-colitis model involves the exploration of the cellular interactions that result in the elaboration of TGF-β–producing regulatory cells upon feeding TNP-haptenated colonic protein. Do these interactions involve particular dendritic cell types and, if they do, what are the signaling pathways used by the dendritic cells to induce the cytokines necessary for regulatory cell induction? Another unanswered question, in this case requiring study of both types of models, involves the exploration of the conditions that allow regulatory cells to overcome established inflammation. Is a critical mass of regulatory cells necessary or are critical concentrations of certain cytokines (i.e., IL-10) necessary for this to occur? We believe that studies using the models can now be designed that can provide answers to these questions and, in doing so, provide new insights on how oral tolerance may be harnessed to treat human disease.

REFERENCES

1. KRAJINA, T., F. LEITHAUSER, P. MOLLER, et al. 2003. Colonic lamina propria dendritic cells in mice with CD4+ T cell-induced colitis. Eur. J. Immunol. **33:** 1073–1083.
2. POWRIE, F., R. CORREA-OLIVEIRA, S. MAUZE, et al. 1994 Regulatory interactions between $CD45RB^{high}$ and $CD45RB^{low}$ CD4+ T cells are important for the balance between protective and pathogenic cell-mediated immunity. J. Exp. Med. **179:** 589–600.
3. OPPMANN, B., R. LESLEY, B. BLOM, et al. 2000. Novel p19 protein engages IL-12p40 to form a cytokine, IL-23, with biological activities similar as well as distinct from IL-12. Immunity **13:** 715–725.
4. MOTTET, C., H.H. UHLIG & F. POWRIE. 2003. Cutting edge: cure of colitis by CD4+CD25+ regulatory T cells. J. Immunol. **170:** 3939–3943.
5. MALLOY, K.J., L. SALAUN, R. CAHILL, et al. 2003. CD4+CD25+ T(R) cells suppress innate immune pathology through cytokine-dependent mechanisms. J. Exp. Med. **197:** 111–119.
6. SAKAGUCHI, S., N. SAKAGUCHI, J. SHIMIZU, et al. 2001. Immunologic tolerance maintained by CD25+CD4+ regulatory T cells: their common role in controlling autoimmunity, tumor immunity, and transplantation tolerance. Immunol. Rev. **182:** 18–32.
7. READ, S., V. MALMSTROM & F. POWRIE. 2000. Cytotoxic T lymphocyte-associated antigen 4 plays an essential role in the function of CD25+CD4+ regulatory cells that control intestinal inflammation. J. Exp. Med. **192:** 295–302.
8. LIU, H., B. HU, D. XU, et al. 2003. CD4+CD25+ regulatory T cells cure murine colitis: the role of IL-10, TGF-β, and CTLA-4. J. Immunol. **171:** 5012–5017.
9. MALMSTROM, V., D. SHIPTON, B. SINGH, et al. 2001. CD134L expression on dendritic cells in the mesenteric lymph nodes drives colitis in T cell-restored SCID mice. J. Immunol. **166:** 6972–6981.
10. HAHM, K.B., Y.H. IM, T.W. PARKS, et al. 2001. Loss of transforming growth factor beta signaling in the intestine contributes to tissue injury in inflammatory bowel disease. Gut **49:** 164–165.
11. BECK, P.L., I.M. ROSENBERG, R.J. XAVIER, et al. 2003. Transforming growth factor-beta mediates intestinal healing and susceptibility to injury in vitro and in vivo through epithelial cells. Am. J. Pathol. **162:** 597–608.
12. GORELIK, L. & R.A. FLAVELL. 2000. Abrogation of TGF-β signaling in T cells leads to spontaneous T cell differentiation and autoimmune disease. Immunity **12:** 171–181.
13. NAKAMURA, K., A. KITANI, I. FUSS, et al. 2004. TGF-β1 plays an important role in the mechanism of CD4+CD25+ regulatory T cell activity in both humans and mice. J. Immunol. **172:** 834–842.
14. NAKAMURA, K., A. KITANI & W. STROBER. 2001. Cell contact-dependent immunosuppression by CD4+CD25+ regulatory T cells is mediated by cell surface-bound transforming growth factor beta. J. Exp. Med. **194:** 629–644.
15. PICCIRILLO, C.A., J.J. LETTERIO, A.M. THORNTON, et al. 2002. CD4+CD25+ regulatory T cells can mediate suppressor function in the absence of transforming growth factor beta1 production and responsiveness. J. Exp. Med. **196:** 237–246.
16. BRIMNES, J., J. REIMANN, M. NISSEN, et al. 2001. Enteric bacterial antigens activate CD4+ T cells from scid mice with inflammatory bowel disease. Eur. J. Immunol. **31:** 23–31.
17. POWRIE, F. & M.W. LEACH. 1995. Genetic and spontaneous models of inflammatory bowel disease in rodents: evidence for abnormalities in mucosal immune regulation. Ther. Immunol. **2:** 115–123.
18. MACPHERSON, A.J. & T. UHR. 2004. Induction of protective IgA by intestinal dendritic cells carrying commensal bacteria. Science **303:** 1662–1665.

19. BECKER, C., S. WIRTZ, M. BLESSING, et al. 2003. Constitutive p40 promoter activation and IL-23 production in the terminal ileum mediated by dendritic cells. J. Clin. Invest. **112:** 693–706.
20. FANTINI, M.C., C. BECKER, G. MONTELEONE, et al. 2004. Cutting edge: TGF-β induces a regulatory phenotype in CD4+CD25- T cells through Foxp3 induction and down-regulation of Smad7. J. Immunol. **179:** 5149–5153.
21. OUSTROUKHOVA, M., C. SEGUIN-DEVAUX, T.B. ORISS, et al. 2004. Tolerance induced by inhaled antigen involves CD4+ T cells expressing membrane-bound TGF-β and FOXP3. J. Clin. Invest. **114:** 28–38.
22. ZHENG, S.G., J.H. WANG, J.D. GRAY, et al. 2004. Natural and induced CD4+CD25+ cells educate CD4+CD25- cells to develop suppressive activity: the role of IL-2, TGF-β, and IL-10. J. Immunol. **172:** 5213–5221.
23. NEURATH, M.F., I. FUSS, B.L. KELSALL, et al. 1995. Antibodies to interleukin 12 abrogate established experimental colitis in mice. J. Exp. Med. **182:** 1281–1290.
24. BOUMA, G., A. KAUSHIVA & W. STROBER. 2002. Experimental murine colitis is regulated by two genetic loci, including one on chromosome 11 that regulates IL-12 responses. Gastroenterology **123:** 554–565.
25. STUBER, E., W. STROBER & M. NEURATH. 1996. Blocking the CD40L-CD40 interaction in vivo specifically prevents the priming of T helper 1 cells through the inhibition of interleukin 12 secretion. J. Exp. Med. **183:** 693–698.
26. NEURATH, M.F., I. FUSS, B.L. KELSALL, et al. 1996. Experimental granulomatous colitis in mice is abrogated by induction of TGF-β-mediated oral tolerance. J. Exp. Med. **183:** 2605–2616.
27. FUSS, I.J., M. BOIRIVANT, B. LACY, et al. The interrelated roles of TGF-β and IL-10 in the regulation of experimental colitis. J. Immunol. **168:** 900–908.
28. STROBER, W., B. KELSALL & T. MARTH. 1998. Oral tolerance. J. Clin. Immunol. **18:** 1–30.
29. IWASAKI, A. & B.L. KELSALL. 1999. Freshly isolated Peyer's patch, but not spleen, dendritic cells produce interleukin 10 and induce the differentiation of T helper type 2 cells. J. Exp. Med. **190:** 229–239.
30. ASSEMAN, C., S. READ & F. POWRIE. 2003. Colitogenic Th1 cells are present in the antigen-experienced T cell pool in normal mice: control by CD4+ regulatory T cells and IL-10. J. Immunol. **171:** 971–978.
31. GROUX, H., A. O'GARRA, M. BIGLER, et al. 1997. A CD4+ T-cell subset inhibits antigen-specific T-cell responses and prevents colitis. Nature **389:** 737–742.
32. KULLBERG, M.C., D. JANKOVIC, P.L. GORELICK, et al. 2002. Bacteria-triggered CD4+ T regulatory cells suppress *Helicobacter hepaticus*-induced colitis. J. Exp. Med. **196:** 505–515.
33. COTTREZ, F. & H. GROUX. 2001. Regulation of TGF-β responses during T cell activation is modulated by IL-10. J. Immunol. **167:** 773–778.
34. NAKAO, A., M. AFRAKHTE, A. MOREN, et al. 1997. Identification of Smad7, a TGF-β-inducible antagonist of TGF-β signaling. Nature **389:** 549–551.
35. SEDER, R.A., T. MARTH, M.C. SIEVE, et al. 1998. Factors involved in the differentiation of TGF-β-producing cells from naive CD4+ T cells: IL-4 and IFNγ have opposing effects, while TGF-β positively regulates its own production. J. Immunol. **160:** 5719–5728.
36. KITANI, A., I.J. FUSS, K. NAKAMURA, et al. 2000. Treatment of experimental (Trinitrobenzene sulfonic acid) colitis by intranasal administration of transforming growth factor (TGF)-β1 plasmid: TGF-β1-mediated suppression of T helper cell type 1 response occurs by interleukin (IL)-10 induction and IL-12 receptor β2 chain down-regulation. J. Exp. Med. **192:** 41–52.
37. KITANI, A., I. FUSS, K. NAKAMURA, et al. 2003. Transforming growth factor (TGF)-β1-producing regulatory T cells induce Smad-mediated interleukin 10 secretion that facilitates coordinated immunoregulatory activity and amelioration of TGF-β1-mediated fibrosis. J. Exp. Med. **198:** 1179–1188.
38. HORI, S., T. NOMURA & S. SAKAGUCHI. 2003. Control of regulatory T cell development by the transcription factor Foxp3. Science **299:** 1057–1061.
39. HORI, S., T. TAKAHASHI & S. SAKAGUCHI. 2003. Control of autoimmunity by naturally arising regulatory CD4+ T cells. Adv. Immunol. **81:** 331–371.

Immune Regulation in the Intestine

A Balancing Act between Effector and Regulatory T Cell Responses

FIONA POWRIE

Sir William Dunn School of Pathology, University of Oxford, Oxford, United Kingdom

ABSTRACT: The immune system in the intestine must respond rapidly to invading pathogens without mounting sustained effector cell responses to the indigenous commensal bacteria. Results from this laboratory using the T cell transfer model of colitis suggest that specialized populations of regulatory T cells control the immune response in the intestine. Regulatory T (Tr) cell activity is enriched within the naturally arising $CD4^+$ $CD25^+$ Tr subset that has been shown to prevent a number of inflammatory diseases. $CD4^+$ $CD25^+$ Tr cells control intestinal inflammation induced by both innate and adaptive immune responses via IL-10– and TGF-β–dependent mechanisms. Recent results have shown that $CD4^+$ $CD25^+$ Tr cells can cure established colitis, suggesting their utility for the treatment of inflammatory bowel disease.

KEYWORDS: regulatory T cell; inflammatory bowel disease; colitis; T cell transfer; IL-10; TGF-β

INTRODUCTION

The gastrointestinal (GI) tract is the largest interface between the immune system and the outside world. It is home to a large number and diverse array of commensal bacteria and is also one of the major surfaces through which pathogens gain access to the body. Immune cells in the intestine are intimately associated with the epithelium and are continually challenged by a myriad of antigens derived from food and commensal bacteria, as well as pathogenic organisms. Specific anatomical features of the intestine and the presence of specialized immune cells ensures rapid and local responses to contain and eradicate pathogens without development of sustained inflammatory responses to harmless intestinal antigens.[1]

The intestinal bacterial complex, composed of over 400 species in humans, exists in an overall symbiotic relationship with the host, playing an important role in nutrition, host defense, and organ development.[2] Although the majority of commensal bacteria are separated from immune cells by the epithelial cell barrier, there is good

Address for correspondence: Fiona Powrie, Sir William Dunn School of Pathology, University of Oxford, South Parks Road, Oxford OX1 3RE, UK. Fax: +44-1865-275591.
fiona.powrie@path.ox.ac.uk

evidence that local immune responses are activated in response to intestinal bacteria.[3,4] Production of anti-inflammatory cytokines, such as IL-10 and TGF-β, is often dominant during immune responses at mucosal surfaces, and this may be an important adaptive mechanism to prevent the development of chronic inflammation.[1]

Inflammatory bowel disease (IBD), encompassing Crohn's disease (CD) and ulcerative colitis, is a chronic condition involving relapsing and remitting inflammation of the gastrointestinal tract.[5] Clinical and experimental studies suggest that IBD is the consequence of an aberrant inflammatory response to intestinal bacteria that occurs in genetically susceptible individuals.[6] Recently, mutations in the intracellular bacterial sensing protein, nucleotide-binding oligomerization domain 2 (NOD2), have been shown to confer susceptibility to CD.[7,8] Although it is not fully understood how alterations in the NOD2 bacterial recognition pathway predispose to IBD, the results do identify innate immune recognition pathways as important in controlling intestinal inflammation.

The complex multifactorial nature of IBD makes it difficult to dissect the role of individual components in the etiology and pathogenesis of disease. Over the last decade, a number of models of chronic intestinal inflammation have been described that share features with human IBD (reviewed in Ref. 6). Results from these studies have shown that IBD can develop as a consequence of altered intestinal barrier function, impaired innate immunity, excessive effector cell responses, or a deficiency in regulatory pathways.

Studies from this laboratory using the T cell transfer model of colitis indicate that CD4$^+$ regulatory T cells (Tr) play a key role in intestinal homeostasis. Here, we describe the properties of Tr cells that control intestinal inflammation and discuss their application for therapy in IBD.

T CELL TRANSFER MODEL OF COLITIS

In mice, transfer of primarily naive (CD45RB^{high}) CD4$^+$ T cells to T and B cell–deficient recipients leads to wasting disease and colitis.[10,11] Intestinal inflammation resembles that seen in human IBD, with transmural leukocytic infiltrates, epithelial cell hyperplasia, and goblet cell depletion. Immune pathology in this model is Th1-mediated and, accordingly, can be prevented by treatment with antibodies to IL-12p40, TNFα, or IFNγ.[12,13] As with other models, colitis is bacterially driven, as it does not occur when T cells are transferred to recipients that have been maintained in germ-free conditions, or that have reduced bacterial loads.[14,15] Colitis in the T cell transfer model has not been attributed to the presence of a common pathogen, and it seems more likely that commensal bacteria stimulate the inflammatory response. T cells reactive to antigens from the normal bacterial flora are present in mice and humans with IBD,[16] providing clear evidence that development of intestinal inflammation is accompanied by immune sensitization toward the commensal flora. Monocolonization of germ-free SCID mice with Helicobacter muridarium results in colitis following transfer of CD4$^+$ CD45RB^{high} cells, indicating that a single commensal bacterial species is sufficient to induce T cell–mediated colitis.[17]

ACTIVATED DENDRITIC CELLS DRIVE INTESTINAL INFLAMMATION

Dendritic cells (DCs) are abundant in the GI tract, in organized lymphoid structures, as well as in the lamina propria, where they may sample incoming antigens. DCs express a number of pattern recognition receptors on their surface, allowing them to detect and respond to the presence of microbes.[18] Bacteria-induced activation of DCs leads to their maturation and migration to the secondary lymphoid organs, where they are able to present antigen to naive T cells. In addition, mature, activated DCs produce a number of inflammatory cytokines and costimulatory molecules that are required for the development of sustained T cell responses.

In mice with colitis there is an accumulation of DCs in the mesenteric lymph nodes (MLNs) as well as in colonic LP.[19,20] DCs in the MLNs expressed an activated phenotype with increased expression of CD40 and the TNF-like molecule CD134L. Analysis of T cell proliferation in mice with colitis showed that up to 20 to 30% of T cells were proliferating in the MLNs, consistent with the high proportion of activated DCs present.[21] Activated T cells express the cell surface costimulatory molecules CD40 ligand (CD40L) and CD134. CD40L binds CD40 on antigen-presenting cells (APCs), inducing CD134L expression[22] leading to the transmission of further activatory signals to both the T cell and APC. The CD40-CD40L and CD134L-CD134 pathways play functional roles in the inflammatory response, as blockade of either pathway inhibits colitis.[19,23,24]

In addition to proliferating in the draining lymph nodes, colitogenic T cells also proliferated locally in the colon. Proliferating T cells were typically located adjacent to DCs in organized leukocyte clusters in the lamina propria.[21] T cells were found to home to DC clusters in the colon very early after transfer into immune-deficient recipients, prior to the onset of colitis,[20] making it tempting to speculate that colonic leukocyte clusters also contribute to the initiation and perpetuation of the inflammatory response in the intestine.

Together, the data suggest that interactions between activated DCs and activated T cells drive intestinal inflammation, and that disruption of this positive-feedback loop is sufficient to inhibit colitis.

COLITIS AS A RESULT OF SUSTAINED ACTIVATION OF THE INNATE IMMUNE SYSTEM

The activation of the innate immune system that accompanies T cell–dependent colitis suggests a causative link between innate effector mechanisms and intestinal pathology. Infection with the mouse intestinal pathogen *Helicobacter hepaticus* triggers typholocolitis in several strains of immune-deficient mice, providing direct evidence that chronic colitis can develop in the absence of T cells.[25–27] *H. hepaticus* infection of 129SvEv RAG-2$^{-/-}$ mice induces systemic and local activation of innate immune cells, with accumulation of neutrophils, macrophages, and IFNγ-producing natural killer (NK) cells in the spleen as well as in the intestine.[27] Similar to T cell–dependent colitis, the proinflammatory cytokines IL-12p40 and TNFα play functional roles in the immune pathological response, suggesting that intestinal inflammation involving adaptive or innate immune mechanisms involves common effector mechanisms.

PREVENTION OF COLITIS BY CD4$^+$ CD25$^+$ REGULATORY T CELLS

An important theme that has emerged from the T cell transfer model is that functionally specialized Tr cells capable of inhibiting intestinal inflammation are present among the CD4$^+$ T cell pool in normal mice. Initially identified as being contained within the antigen-experienced CD4$^+$ CD45RB^{low} population,[11] Tr cell activity has since been shown to be enriched within the CD4$^+$ CD25$^+$ subset.[28] These "naturally occurring" Tr cells inhibit T cell proliferation *in vitro*, and are important in the control of T cell responses to self-antigens, thus preventing the development of autoimmune disease.[29] Recent studies have shown that CD4$^+$ CD25$^+$ Tr cells also play a more general suppressive role, acting to limit immune pathology associated with chronic immune stimulation.[30]

CD4$^+$ CD25$^+$ Tr cells account for 5 to 10% of peripheral T cells in mice, rats, and humans.[29] A feature that distinguishes CD4$^+$ CD25$^+$ Tr cells from other CD4$^+$ T cells is that they adopt their effector function in the thymus.[29] Current evidence suggests that CD4$^+$ T cells bearing receptors with a high affinity for self-peptide will differentiate into CD4$^+$ CD25$^+$ Tr cells following an encounter with cognate peptide on thymic stromal cells.[31] Foxp3, from the family of forkhead/winged helix transcription factors, is differentially expressed by CD4$^+$ CD25$^+$ Tr cells and is required for their development in the thymus.[32,33] Retroviral transduction with Foxp3 leads to the development of regulatory T cells from naive precursors, indicating that Foxp3 may be a master control switch for Tr cell development.[34] Importantly, loss-of-function mutations in Foxp3 have been shown to be responsible for the lymphoproliferative disease that develops in scurfy mice, and for the human disease immune polyendocrine enteropathy X-linked (IPEX) syndrome.[35] Strikingly, patients with IPEX develop a similar spectrum of diseases that develops in animal models in the absence of regulatory T cells, including type 1 diabetes, allergy, and IBD-like enteropathy.

CD4$^+$ CD25$^+$ Tr CELLS SUPPRESS THE INNATE IMMUNE RESPONSE

Transfer of CD4$^+$CD25$^+$ Tr cells prevents the accumulation of activated DCs in immune-deficient mice transfused with CD4$^+$ CD45RB^{high} T cells, suggesting that Tr cells act to inhibit the ability of DCs to induce a sustained T cell response.[19] T cell–independent colitis that develops in 129SvEv RAG2$^{-/-}$ mice following *Helicobacter hepaticus* infection can also be inhibited by transfer of CD4$^+$ CD25$^+$ Tr cells, providing direct evidence that CD4$^+$ CD25$^+$ Tr cells suppress the innate immune response.[27,36] Tr cells were found to accumulate in the spleen, MLNs, and colon, and suppressed local and systemic innate immune pathology via IL-10– and TGF-β–dependent mechanisms. CD4$^+$ CD25$^+$ Tr cells from IL-10$^{-/-}$ mice failed to inhibit colitis, suggesting that IL-10 production is crucial for their function. Kinetic studies showed that the suppressive effects of CD4$^+$ CD25$^+$ Tr cells were most evident later in infection, suggesting that Tr cells do not inhibit the initial activation of the innate immune response but act to prevent chronic activation. Indeed, there is evidence that stimulation via the toll-like receptor (TLR) pathway breaks Tr-mediated control by a mechanism involving IL-6 production by activated DCs.[37]

The ability of CD4$^+$ CD25$^+$ Tr cells to control the innate immune response may underlie the ability of these cells to inhibit chronic immune responses to a number of infectious agents, and be an important host mechanism to prevent immune pathology during persistent microbial infection.[27,38,39]

SPECIFICITY

The specificity of CD4$^+$ CD25$^+$ Tr cells that control intestinal inflammation remains something of an enigma. CD4$^+$ CD25$^+$ Tr cells isolated from mice that had not been infected with *Helicobacter hepaticus* were capable of preventing T cell–independent colitis, indicating that Tr cells can suppress immune pathology triggered by organisms to which they have not been exposed.[27] However, the ability to control T cell–dependent colitis was enhanced in Tr populations from *Helicobacter hepaticus*–infected donors, suggesting that bacterial infection can induce antigen-specific Tr cells.[40] Furthermore, these bacteria-specific Tr cells were found to be within the CD4$^+$ CD25$^-$ T cell subset. Together, the data are compatible with the view that CD4$^+$ CD25$^+$ Tr cells able to prevent *H. hepaticus*–induced colitis occur naturally in all mice, while a further CD4$^+$ CD25$^-$ regulatory population can be primed in the presence of *H. hepaticus* infection.

OTHER SUBSETS OF Tr CELLS

In addition to naturally occurring CD4$^+$ CD25$^+$ Tr cells, antigen-induced IL-10–secreting Tr1 cells also play an important role in intestinal homeostasis. Tr1 cells inhibit Th1 and Th2 responses via IL-10–dependent mechanisms.[41] Tr1 cells develop alongside Th1 cells in a number of chronic infectious diseases and are present in the intestine of normal mice, where they regulate the response to intestinal pathogens[40] and the commensal flora.[42] Recently, pathogen-derived molecules have been shown to stimulate IL-10 production from DCs via a TLR-4–dependent mechanism.[43] DC production of IL-10 favors Tr1 cell development, illustrating that, in addition to inducing proinflammatory responses, microbial-induced activation of the innate immune system also induces anti-inflammatory cytokines and Tr cell development.

Although Tr1 cells have some properties similar to those of CD4$^+$ CD25$^+$ Tr cells, they do not express Foxp3, suggesting that they are a distinct population of cells.[9] Studies *in vitro* have shown that CD4$^+$ CD25$^+$ cells can act on naive T cells to induce their differentiation to Tr1 cells,[44] raising the possibility that CD4$^+$ CD25$^+$ Tr and Tr1 cells synergize to control inflammation.

THE ROLE OF IMMUNE SUPPRESSIVE CYTOKINES IN Tr FUNCTION

The immune suppressive cytokines IL-10 and TGF-β play nonredundant roles in intestinal homeostasis, as IL-10$^{-/-}$[45] and TGF-β1$^{-/-}$[46] mice develop chronic colitis.

Colitis in IL-10$^{-/-}$ mice may be attributable in part to deficient Tr activity, as IL-10 production by Tr cells has been shown to be essential for control of intestinal inflammation.[27,40,47] IL-10 mediates a wide range of suppressive activities on T cells, as well as innate immune cells such as myeloid cells and neutrophils.[48] Suppression of intestinal inflammation by IL-10 may be mediated primarily via effects on innate immune cells, as disruption of IL-10 signaling in myeloid cells and neutrophils, but not T cells, triggered colitis.[49]

Suppression of T cell–dependent and T cell–independent colitis by CD4$^+$ CD25$^+$ Tr cells was abrogated by anti–TGF-β treatment.[14,27] By contrast with IL-10, the effects of TGF-β may be mediated primarily via negative regulation of T cells, as mice expressing a dominant negative form of the TGF-βRII (dnTGF-βRII) restricted to T cells developed an IBD-like syndrome.[50] Recently, we have found that colitis induced by transfer of CD4$^+$ CD45RB^{high} cells isolated from dnTGF-βRII transgenic mice cannot be suppressed by CD4$^+$ CD25$^+$ Tr cells, indicating that T cells that cannot respond to TGF-β escape control by Tr cells (S. Read, L. Fahlen, and F. Powrie, unpublished data). Recent studies indicate that TGF-β can also act as a costimulatory molecule for development of Foxp3$^+$ Tr cells from naive precursors, suggesting that TGF-β may also be involved in the generation of Tr cells.[51]

There are conflicting data on whether production of TGF-β by CD4$^+$ CD25$^+$ Tr cells is required for their function.[52,53] CD4$^+$ CD25$^+$ Tr cells express membrane bound TGF-β,[52] and the ability of CD4$^+$ Tr populations to suppress colitis was found to correlate with expression of membrane-bound TGF-β or latency-associated peptide.[54,55] In addition, CD4$^+$ CD25$^+$ cells from TGF-β1$^{-/-}$ mice failed to prevent colitis in the T cell transfer model,[54] further supporting a role for TGF-β1 production by Tr cells themselves. However, in our own studies we have found that TGF-β1$^{-/-}$ CD4$^+$ CD25$^+$ Tr cells retain the ability to suppress colitis. Addition of anti–TGF-β monoclonal antibody abrogates suppression of colitis by TGF-β1$^{-/-}$ CD4$^+$ CD25$^+$ Tr cells, indicating that in some settings TGF-β from non–Tr-derived sources is sufficient to control the inflammatory response (Fahlen, Read, and Powrie, unpublished data).

CURE OF COLITIS BY CD4$^+$ CD25$^+$ Tr CELLS

The ability of various populations of Tr cells to prevent development of experimental colitis suggests that stimulation of these cells may be beneficial in patients with IBD. However, to be of use in the clinical setting, Tr cells must be able to inhibit ongoing T cell responses and reverse established pathology. In recent studies we found that a single transfusion of CD4$^+$ CD25$^+$ Tr cells into mice with established colitis led to resolution of the inflammatory response and restoration of normal intestinal architecture.[21] Others found similar results and showed, furthermore, that the therapeutic effect of CD4$^+$ CD25$^+$ Tr cells is mediated via IL-10 and TGF-β.[56]

A characteristic feature of CD4$^+$ CD25$^+$ Tr cells is their inability to undergo mitogen- or antigen-induced proliferation *in vitro*.[29] By contrast, after transfer into colitic mice, Tr cells were found to proliferate in MLN and colon, where they inhibited the proliferation of pathogenic CD4$^+$ T cells.[21] The presence of regulatory T cells in the colon was also associated with cure of colitis by Tr1 cells,[57] suggesting that suppression of established inflammation requires Tr activity in secondary lymphoid tissue and effector sites. Recently, a subset of CD4$^+$ CD25$^+$ Tr cells expressing the integrin αE (CD103) was shown to home most efficiently to inflammatory sites and to control acute inflammation. This suggests that distinct subsets of Tr cells may control responses in lymphoid organs and tissues.[58] Proliferation of CD4$^+$ CD25$^+$ Tr cells was significantly reduced following resolution of the inflammatory response, suggesting that CD4$^+$ CD25$^+$ Tr cells respond to the inflammation that they regulate.[21]

In the MLN and colon, CD4$^+$ CD25$^+$ Tr cells localized at the interface between pathogenic effector T cells and DCs and were in direct contact with both populations of cells.[21] This specific distribution *in vivo* may reflect the ability of activated DCs to induce the activation and migration of CD4$^+$ CD25$^+$ Tr cells.[59,60] Tr cells, in turn, may suppress the immune response via effects on activated DCs[1] or via direct effects on effector T cells.[62]

OUTLOOK

The balance between effector and regulatory T cell responses is a key factor in the development of intestinal inflammation. There is now a large body of evidence showing that enhancement of Tr cell activity can prevent and even cure intestinal inflammation in mouse models, suggesting novel therapeutic strategies for the treatment of IBD. IPEX patients lacking functional Foxp3 protein develop severe enteropathy, suggesting that Tr cells also control intestinal inflammation in humans. However, further studies are required to determine whether defects in Tr activity are associated with genetic susceptibility to IBD in humans.

ACKNOWLEDGMENTS

F. Powrie is funded by the Wellcome Trust.

REFERENCES

1. MOWAT, A.M. 2003. Anatomical basis of tolerance and immunity to intestinal antigens. Nat. Rev. Immunol. **3**: 331–341.
2. HOOPER, L.V. & J.I. GORDON. 2001. Commensal host-bacterial relationships in the gut. Science **292**: 1115–1118.
3. JIANG, H.Q., N.A. BOS & J.J. CEBRA. 2001. Timing, localization, and persistence of colonization by segmented filamentous bacteria in the neonatal mouse gut depend on immune status of mothers and pups. Infect. Immun. **69**: 3611–3617.
4. MACPHERSON, A.J., D. GATTO, E. SAINSBURY, *et al.* 2000. A primitive T cell-independent mechanism of intestinal mucosal IgA responses to commensal bacteria. Science **288**: 2222–2226.
5. PODOLSKY, D.K. 2002. Inflammatory bowel disease. N. Engl. J. Med. **347**: 417–429.
6. BOUMA, G. & W. STROBER. 2003. The immunological and genetic basis of inflammatory bowel disease. Nat. Rev. Immunol. **3**: 521–533.
7. HUGOT, J.P., M. CHAMAILLARD, H. ZOUALI, *et al.* 2001. Association of NOD2 leucine-rich repeat variants with susceptibility to Crohn's disease. Nature **411**: 599–603.

8. OGURA, Y., D.K. BONEN, N. INOHARA, et al. 2001. A frameshift mutation in NOD2 associated with susceptibility to Crohn's disease. Nature **411:** 603–606.
9. VIEIRA, P.L., J.R. CHRISTENSEN, S. MINAEE, et al. 2004. IL-10-secreting regulatory T cells do not express Foxp3 but have comparable regulatory function to naturally ocurring CD4+CD25+ regulatory T cells. J. Immunol. **172:** 5986–5993.
10. MORRISSEY, P.J., K. CHARRIER, S. BRADDY, et al. 1993. CD4+ T cells that express high levels of CD45RB induce wasting disease when transferred into congenic severe combined immunodeficient mice. Disease development is prevented by cotransfer of purified CD4+ T cells. J. Exp. Med. **178:** 237–244.
11. POWRIE, F., M.W. LEACH, S. MAUZE, et al. 1993. Phenotypically distinct subsets of CD4+ T cells induce or protect from chronic intestinal inflammation in C. B-17 scid mice. Int. Immunol. **5:** 1461–1471.
12. POWRIE, F., M.W. LEACH, S. MAUZE, et al. 1994. Inhibition of Th1 responses prevents inflammatory bowel disease in scid mice reconstituted with CD45RBhi CD4+ T cells. Immunity **1:** 553–562.
13. SIMPSON, S.J., S. SHAH, M. COMISKEY, et al. 1998. T cell-mediated pathology in two models of experimental colitis depends predominantly on the interleukin 12/Signal transducer and activator of transcription (Stat)-4 pathway, but is not conditional on interferon gamma expression by T cells. J. Exp. Med. **187:** 1225–1234.
14. SINGH, B., S. READ, C. ASSEMAN, et al. 2001. Control of intestinal inflammation by regulatory T cells. Immunol. Rev. **182:** 190–200.
15. ARANDA, R., B.C. SYDORA, P.L. MCALLISTER, et al. 1997. Analysis of intestinal lymphocytes in mouse colitis mediated by transfer of CD4+, CD45RBhigh T cells to SCID recipients. J. Immunol. **158:** 3464–3473.
16. LODES, M.J., Y. CONG, C.O. ELSON, et al. 2004. Bacterial flagellin is a dominant antigen in Crohn disease. J. Clin. Invest. **113:** 1296–1306.
17. JIANG, H.Q., N. KUSHNIR, M.C. THURNHEER, et al. 2002. Monoassociation of SCID mice with *Helicobacter muridarum*, but not four other enterics, provokes IBD upon receipt of T cells. Gastroenterology **122:** 1346–1354.
18. REIS E SOUSA, C. 2004. Toll-like receptors and dendritic cells: for whom the bug tolls. Semin. Immunol. **16:** 27–34.
19. MALMSTROM, V., D. SHIPTON, B. SINGH, et al. 2001. Cd134l expression on dendritic cells in the mesenteric lymph nodes drives colitis in t cell-restored scid mice. J. Immunol. **166:** 6972–6981.
20. KRAJINA, T., F. LEITHAUSER, P. MOLLER, et al. 2003. Colonic lamina propria dendritic cells in mice with CD4+ T cell-induced colitis. Early events in the pathogenesis of a murine transfer colitis. Eur. J. Immunol. **33:** 1073–1083.
21. MOTTET, C., H.H. UHLIG & F. POWRIE. 2003. Cutting edge: cure of colitis by CD4+CD25+ regulatory T cells. J. Immunol. **170:** 3939–3943.
22. BROCKER, T., A. GULBRANSON-JUDGE, S. FLYNN, et al. 1999. CD4 T cell traffic control: in vivo evidence that ligation of OX40 on CD4 T cells by OX40-ligand expressed on dendritic cells leads to the accumulation of CD4 T cells in B follicles. Eur. J. Immunol. **29:** 1610–1616.
23. DE JONG, Y.P., M. COMISKEY, S.L. KALLED, et al. 2000. Chronic murine colitis is dependent on the CD154/CD40 pathway and can be attenuated by anti-CD154 administration. Gastroenterology **119:** 715–723.
24. LIU, Z., K. GEBOES, S. COLPAERT, et al. 2000. Prevention of experimental colitis in SCID mice reconstituted with CD45RBhigh CD4+ T cells by blocking the CD40-CD154 interactions. J. Immunol. **164:** 6005–6014.
25. FOX, J.G., F.E. DEWHIRST, J.G. TULLY, et al. 1994. *Helicobacter hepaticus* sp. nov., a microaerophilic bacterium isolated from livers and intestinal mucosal scrapings from mice. J. Clin. Microbiol. **32:** 1238–1245.
26. CAHILL, R.J., C.J. FOLTZ, J.G. FOX, et al. 1997. Inflammatory bowel disease: an immunity-mediated condition triggered by bacterial infection with *Helicobacter hepaticus*. Infect. Immun. **65:** 3126–3131.
27. MALOY, K.J., L. SALAUN, R. CAHILL, et al. 2003. CD4+CD25+ T(R) cells suppress innate immune pathology through cytokine-dependent mechanisms. J. Exp. Med. **197:** 111–119.

28. READ, S., V. MALMSTROM & F. POWRIE. 2000. Cytotoxic T lymphocyte-associated antigen 4 plays an essential role in the function of CD25(+)CD4(+) regulatory cells that control intestinal inflammation. J. Exp. Med. **192:** 295–302.
29. SAKAGUCHI, S. 2004. Naturally arising CD4+ regulatory t cells for immunologic self-tolerance and negative control of immune responses. Annu. Rev. Immunol. **22:** 531–562.
30. THOMPSON, C. & F. POWRIE. 2004. Regulatory T cells. Curr. Opin. Pharmacol. **4:** 408–414.
31. JORDAN, M.S., A. BOESTEANU, A.J. REED, et al. 2001. Thymic selection of CD4+CD25+ regulatory T cells induced by an agonist self-peptide. Nat. Immunol. **2:** 301–306.
32. FONTENOT, J.D., M.A. GAVIN & A.Y. RUDENSKY. 2003. Foxp3 programs the development and function of CD4+CD25+ regulatory T cells. Nat. Immunol. **4:** 330–336.
33. KHATTRI, R., T. COX, S.A. YASAYKO & F. RAMSDELL. 2003. An essential role for Scurfin in CD4+CD25+ T regulatory cells. Nat. Immunol. **4:** 337–342.
34. HORI, S., T. NOMURA & S. SAKAGUCHI. 2003. Control of regulatory T cell development by the transcription factor FOXP3. Science **299:** 1057–1061.
35. RAMSDELL, F. & S.F. ZIEGLER. 2003. Transcription factors in autoimmunity. Curr. Opin. Immunol. **15:** 718–724.
36. ERDMAN, S.E., V.P. RAO, T. POUTAHIDIS, et al. 2003. CD4(+)CD25(+) regulatory lymphocytes require interleukin 10 to interrupt colon carcinogenesis in mice. Cancer Res. **63:** 6042–6050.
37. PASARE, C. & R. MEDZHITOV. 2003. Toll-like receptors: balancing host resistance with immune tolerance. Curr. Opin. Immunol. **15:** 677–682.
38. BELKAID, Y., C.A. PICCIRILLO, S. MENDEZ, et al. 2002. CD4+CD25+ regulatory T cells control *Leishmania major* persistence and immunity. Nature **420:** 502–507.
39. HORI, S., T.L. CARVALHO & J. DEMENGEOT. 2002. CD25+CD4+ regulatory T cells suppress CD4+ T cell-mediated pulmonary hyperinflammation driven by Pneumocystis carinii in immunodeficient mice. Eur. J. Immunol. **32:** 1282–1291.
40. KULLBERG, M.C., D. JANKOVIC, P.L. GORELICK, et al. 2002. Bacteria-triggered CD4(+) T regulatory cells suppress *Helicobacter hepaticus*-induced colitis. J. Exp. Med. **196:** 505–515.
41. RONCAROLO, M.G., S. GREGORI & M. LEVINGS. 2003. Type 1 T regulatory cells and their relationship with CD4+CD25+ T regulatory cells. Novartis Found. Symp. **252:** 115–127; discussion 127–131, 203–110.
42. CONG, Y., C.T. WEAVER, A. LAZENBY & C.O. ELSON. 2002. Bacterial-reactive T regulatory cells inhibit pathogenic immune responses to the enteric flora. J. Immunol. **169:** 6112–6119.
43. HIGGINS, S.C., E.C. LAVELLE, C. MCCANN, et al. 2003. Toll-like receptor 4-mediated innate IL-10 activates antigen-specific regulatory T cells and confers resistance to *Bordetella pertussis* by inhibiting inflammatory pathology. J. Immunol. **171:** 3119–3127.
44. JONULEIT, H., E. SCHMITT, H. KAKIRMAN, et al. 2002. Infectious tolerance: human CD25(+) regulatory T cells convey suppressor activity to conventional CD4(+) T helper cells. J. Exp. Med. 196: 255–260.
45. KUHN, R., J. LOHLER, D. RENNICK, et al. 1993. Interleukin-10-deficient mice develop chronic enterocolitis. Cell **75:** 263–274.
46. SHULL, M.M., I. ORMSBY, A.B. KIER, et al. 1992. Targeted disruption of the mouse transforming growth factor-beta 1 gene results in multifocal inflammatory disease. Nature **359:** 693–699.
47. ASSEMAN, C., S. MAUZE, M.W. LEACH, et al. 1999. An essential role for interleukin 10 in the function of regulatory T cells that inhibit intestinal inflammation. J. Exp. Med. **190:** 995–1004.
48. MOORE, K.W., R. DE WAAL MALEFYT, R.L. COFFMAN & A. O'GARRA. 2001. Interleukin-10 and the interleukin-10 receptor. Annu. Rev. Immunol. **19:** 683–765.
49. TAKEDA, K., B.E. CLAUSEN, T. KAISHO, et al. 1999. Enhanced Th1 activity and development of chronic enterocolitis in mice devoid of Stat3 in macrophages and neutrophils. Immunity **10:** 39–49.
50. GORELIK, L. & R.A. FLAVELL. 2000. Abrogation of TGFbeta signaling in T cells leads to spontaneous T cell differentiation and autoimmune disease. Immunity **12:** 171–181.

51. CHEN, W., W. JIN, N. HARDEGEN, et al. 2003. Conversion of peripheral CD4+CD25- naive T cells to CD4+CD25+ regulatory T cells by TGF-beta induction of transcription factor Foxp3. J. Exp. Med. **198:** 1875–1886.
52. NAKAMURA, K., A. KITANI & W. STROBER. 2001. Cell contact-dependent immunosuppression by CD4(+)CD25(+) regulatory T cells is mediated by cell surface-bound transforming growth factor beta. J. Exp. Med. **194:** 629–644.
53. PICCIRILLO, C.A., J.J. LETTERIO, A.M. THORNTON, et al. 2002. CD4(+)CD25(+) regulatory T cells can mediate suppressor function in the absence of transforming growth factor beta1 production and responsiveness. J. Exp. Med. **196:** 237–246.
54. NAKAMURA, K., A. KITANI, I. FUSS, et al. 2004. TGF-beta 1 plays an important role in the mechanism of CD4+CD25+ regulatory T cell activity in both humans and mice. J. Immunol. **172:** 834–842.
55. OIDA, T., X. ZHANG, M. GOTO, et al. 2003. CD4+CD25− T cells that express latency-associated peptide on the surface suppress CD4+CD45RBhigh-induced colitis by a TGF-beta-dependent mechanism. J. Immunol. **170:** 2516–2522.
56. LIU, H., B. HU, D. XU & F.Y. LIEW. 2003. CD4+CD25+ regulatory T cells cure murine colitis: the role of IL-10, TGF-beta, and CTLA4. J. Immunol. **171:** 5012–5017.
57. FOUSSAT, A., F. COTTREZ, V. BRUN, et al. 2003. A comparative study between T regulatory type 1 and CD4+CD25+ T cells in the control of inflammation. J Immunol. **171:** 5018–5026.
58. HUEHN, J., K. SIEGMUND, J.C. LEHMANN, et al. 2004. Developmental stage, phenotype, and migration distinguish naive- and effector/memory-like CD4+ regulatory T cells. J. Exp. Med. **199:** 303–313.
59. BYSTRY, R.S., V. ALUVIHARE, K.A. WELCH, et al. 2001. B cells and professional APCs recruit regulatory T cells via CCL4. Nat. Immunol. **2:** 1126–1132.
60. Yamazaki, S., T. Iyoda, K. Tarbell, et al. 2003. Direct expansion of functional CD25+ CD4+ regulatory T cells by antigen-processing dendritic cells. J. Exp. Med. **198:** 235–247.
61. OLDENHOVE, G., M. DE HEUSCH, G. URBAIN-VANSANTEN, et al. 2003. CD4+ CD25+ regulatory T cells control T helper cell type 1 responses to foreign antigens induced by mature dendritic cells in vivo. J. Exp. Med. **198:** 259–266.
62. PICCIRILLO, C.A. & E.M. SHEVACH. 2001. Cutting edge: control of CD8+ T cell activation by CD4+CD25+ immunoregulatory cells. J. Immunol. **167:** 1137–1140.

IL-10–Producing T Regulatory Type 1 Cells and Oral Tolerance

MANUELA BATTAGLIA,[a] CARMEN GIANFRANI,[b] SILVIA GREGORI,[a] AND MARIA-GRAZIA RONCAROLO[a,c]

[a]*San Raffaele Telethon Institute for Gene Therapy (HSR-TIGET), Milano, Italy*

[b]*Institute of Food Science and Technology, Consiglio Nazionale delle Ricerche, Avellino, Italy*

[c]*Vita Salute San Raffaele University, Milano, Italy*

ABSTRACT: Oral tolerance is mediated by multiple mechanisms such as anergy and/or active suppression of antigen-specific effector T cells by T regulatory (Tr) cells. Among the $CD4^+$ Tr cells, T regulatory type 1 cells (Tr1) have been shown to downmodulate immune responses through production of the immunosuppressive cytokines IL-10 and TGF-β. Human Tr1 cells can be induced to differentiate *in vitro* by IL-10 + IFN-α or after stimulation by immature dendritic cells (DCs) or DCs rendered tolerogenic by exposure to immunomodulatory compounds. Murine Tr1 cells can be induced to differentiate *in vitro* by activating naive $CD4^+$ T cells in the presence of high doses of IL-10. Several protocols for induction of oral tolerance, including oral administration of the antigen with IL-10, have been shown to induce antigen-specific Tr1 cells that suppress undesired immune responses toward self-antigens, allergens, and food antigens. Overall, these data demonstrate that IL-10–producing Tr1 cells play a central role in the induction of oral as well as systemic tolerance.

KEYWORDS: IL-10; T regulatory cells; oral tolerance

INTRODUCTION

The gut-associated lymphoid tissue (GALT) is one of the largest and most complex parts of the immune system. Not only does it encounter a larger variety of antigens than any other part of the organism, but it must also discriminate between pathogenic organisms and harmless antigens, such as food proteins and commensal bacteria. Most human pathogens enter the body through the intestine, and strong immune responses are required to protect this essential organ. By contrast, active immunity against nonpathogenic antigens would be wasteful, and hypersensitivity responses against dietary antigens or commensal bacteria can lead to inflammatory disorders, such as celiac disease and Crohn's disease, respectively. In normal conditions, immune responses to harmless gut antigens leads to the induction of local and systemic immunological tolerance, known as oral tolerance. To some extent, this

Address for correspondence: Manuela Battaglia, Via Olgettina 58 20132 Milano, Italy. Voice: +39-2-2643-4669; fax: +39-2-2643-4668.
manuela.battaglia@hsr.it

discrimination between harmful and harmless antigens also occurs in other parts of the immune system. However, it has been proposed that there are specific features of mucosal tissues that favor induction of oral tolerance.[1]

The mechanisms of immune suppression mediated by oral tolerance include anergy, which may occur when the T cell receptor (TCR) engages the MHC-antigen complex in the absence of proper costimulation[2] and/or active cellular suppression mediated by Tr cells. Many different Tr cell subsets have been shown to play a central role in intestinal immunity. A $CD8^+$ T suppressor cell subset was the first population of Tr cells identified in oral tolerance,[3,4] but its functions and features were not clearly defined. Tolerance to dietary antigen in mice has been shown to be mediated by Th_3 cells, a $CD4^+$ Tr cell subset that produces TGF-β and is involved in induction of tolerance to antigens ingested at low doses. These cells are generated in mucosal lymphoid tissues in an activation-dependent manner, and mediate bystander suppression within the gut by inhibiting activation of all surrounding lymphocytes.[5] Recently, it was shown that children with food allergies have reduced numbers of Th_3 cells in the duodenal mucosa compared with controls.[6] Several studies in knockout mice have indicated that TCR $\gamma\delta^+$ T cells also play an important role in some models of oral tolerance.[7,8] Tolerance can, indeed, be transferred to normal mice by injection of TCR $\gamma\delta^+$ T cells isolated from fed mice[9]. A well-characterized Tr cell subset is represented by the $CD4^+$ $CD25^+$ naturally occurring Tr cells.[10] Although the role of this Tr cell population in controlling auto- and alloimmunity has largely been established,[10] few studies have reported its involvement in orally induced tolerance. Generation of $CD4^+$ $CD25^+$ Tr cells *in vivo* after tolerance induction with oral antigens has been reported, but the relationship with naturally occurring $CD4^+$ $CD25^+$ Tr cells remains unclear.[11,12] Only recently, Dubois *et al.* showed that naturally occurring $CD4^+$ $CD25^+$ Tr cells are instrumental in orally induced tolerance and are essential for the control of antigen-specific $CD8^+$ T effector cells mediating skin inflammation.[13] The last, but not least, Tr cell subset that plays a role in oral tolerance is represented by the T regulatory type 1 cells (Tr1).

In the present review we will describe extensively the Tr1 cell subset that has been largely studied for several years by our group, and we will discuss its specific role in promoting oral tolerance both in mouse and human.

Tr1 CELLS: FEATURES

Tr1 cells display a unique profile of cytokine production that is distinct from that of Th_0, Th_1, or Th_2 cells. The main cytokines produced by Tr1 cells are IL-10 and TGF-β, which downregulate immune responses mediated by naive and memory T cells.[14] Interestingly, Tr1 cells produce these cytokines in the absence of significant levels of IL-2 or IL-4,[15] which are potent T-cell growth factors. The ability of Tr1 cells to produce IFN-γ is controversial, owing to differences between the Tr1 cells isolated from inbred and/or TCR-transgenic mice and humans. Tr1 cells from humans usually produce IFN-γ, although at levels that are at least one log lower than those produced by Th1 cells,[16] whereas murine Tr1 cells generally do not (M. Battaglia, unpublished data).

Tr1 cells proliferate poorly following polyclonal TCR-mediated or antigen-specific activation, and this is partially because autocrine production of IL-10, as anti–

IL-10 monoclonal antibodies, partially restores their proliferative responses.[15] The intrinsic low proliferative capacity of Tr1 cells is a major limitation in characterizing this unique cell type *in vitro*. However, we recently demonstrated that *in vitro* proliferative capacity of Tr1 cells can be significantly enhanced by exogenous IL-2 and IL-15.[17] Importantly, long-term culture in the presence of IL-15 does not significantly alter the cytokine production profile of any human Tr1-cell clone, with the exception of an increase in IFN-γ production.[17]

Despite their low proliferative capacity, Tr1 cell clones express normal levels of activation markers, such as CD25, CD40L, CD69, HLA-DR, and CTLA-4 following TCR-mediated activation.[17] The difficulties associated with identifying Tr1 cells on the basis of their cytokine production profile encouraged several studies aimed at identifying specific cell-surface markers. Tr1 cell clones in the resting state constitutively express high levels of the IL-2/IL-15R β and γ common chains.[17] In addition, Tr1 cells express several chemokine receptors, including some associated with the Th_1 or Th_2 phenotype.[18] Tr1 cells do not express T1/ST2, an IL-1R–like molecule present on Th2 cells.[19] Interestingly, it was reported that Tr1, but not Th_1 or Th_2, cell clones express CCR7, a receptor recently implicated in homing to lymph nodes.[18] Thus far, it can be concluded that neither a single cell-surface marker nor a combination of markers has been identified that can be used to track and purify Tr1 cells.

Tr1 cells regulate the responses of naive and memory T cells *in vitro* and *in vivo* owing to their ability to produce IL-10 and TGF-β, and can suppress both Th_1 and Th_2 cell–mediated pathologies.[20] The suppressive effect of Tr1 cell clones on $CD4^+$ T cells is reversed by neutralizing anti–TGF-β and/or anti–IL-10 monoclonal antibodies.[15] Human Tr1 cell clones also suppress the production of immunoglobulin by B cells[21] and the antigen-presenting capacity of monocytes and DCs.[19,22]

Tr1 CELLS: *IN VITRO* AND *IN VIVO* INDUCTION

Several protocols have been developed to obtain Tr1 cells *in vitro*. In a system where murine fibroblasts expressing high levels of hCD32, hCD58, and hCD80 are used in combination with anti-CD3 monoclonal antibodies to activate naive human $CD4^+$ T cells, addition of exogenous IL-10 results in a relatively small increase in IL-10–producing cells. IFN-α, a crucial cytokine for clearing viral infections and increasing IL-10 production by T cells,[23] combines synergistically with IL-10 *in vitro* to promote differentiation of human $CD4^+$ Tr1 cells.[16] Interestingly, TGF-β, which is clearly involved in the effector function of Tr1 cells, does not synergize with IL-10 to induce human Tr1 cells *in vitro*, but, rather, inhibits differentiation of cytokine-producing cells.

Murine Tr1 cells share most of the biological features of human Tr1 cells. However, the *in vitro* requirements for differentiation of murine Tr1 cells differ from those of human Tr1 cells. High doses of IL-10 and repeated TCR stimulation are indeed sufficient to induce a population of murine $CD4^+$ cells containing high number of Tr1 cells with the ability to suppress immune responses both *in vitro* (FIG. 1) and *in vivo* in a model of inflammatory bowel disease (IBD).[15] Moreover, T cells cultured *in vitro* with IL-10 + TGF-β become anergic, remain tolerant *in vivo*, and

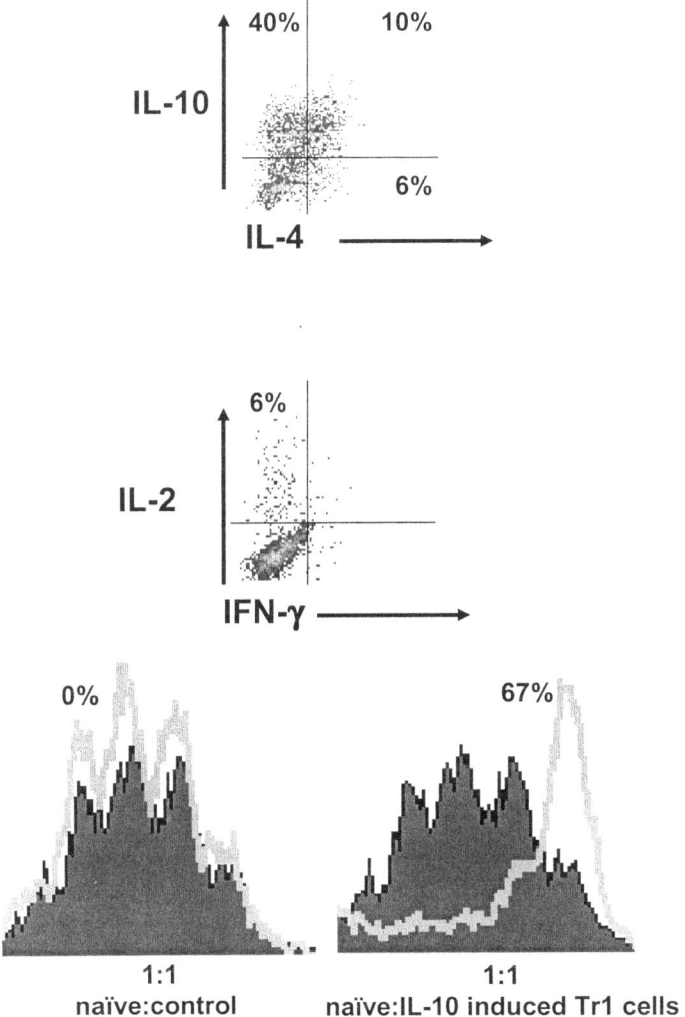

FIGURE 1. Murine Tr1 cells. (*Top*) Naive CD4$^+$ T cells from DO11.10 transgenic (tg) mice were activated with self-APCs and ovalbumin (OVA) in the presence of IL-10. Following three rounds of identical stimulation, cytokine production was evaluated by intracytoplasmic staining. Numbers indicate the percentage of positive cells for the listed cytokines. A cytokine production profile consistent with that of murine Tr1 cells was detected. (*Bottom*) Proliferative response of naive CD4$^+$ DO11.10 tg T cells to OVA was tested by CFSE dilution (*filled histogram*). CD4$^+$ DO11.10 tg T cells activated in the presence of non-polarizing agents (control) or IL-10 for three rounds of stimulation (IL-10–induced Tr1 cells) were tested for their ability to suppress proliferation of naive autologus CD4$^+$ T cells to OVA at a ratio of 1:1 (*open histogram*). After 4 days of culture, cell division was monitored by CFSE dilution. Numbers represent percentages of suppression in comparison to cell proliferation of naive cells.

do not induce graft versus host disease in a murine model of mismatched MHC class II bone marrow transplantation.[24]

Dendritic cells may control the differentiation of Tr1 cells *in vivo*.[20,25] Several types of DCs have been described so far that are able to present antigen in a tolerogenic or immunogenic form, depending on their stage of maturation and biological properties. Myeloid DCs can be rendered tolerogenic by several manipulations, including "freezing" in an immature state;[26,27] treatment with IL-10[28] or immunosuppressive agents such as vitamin D3 and dexamethasone;[29,30] and exposure to certain types of bacteria[31] or certain endogenous proteins such as heavy chain ferritin.[32] In addition, DCs can also be transduced with retroviral vectors that encode tolerogenic molecules such as IL-10, TGF-β, CTLA-4, or Serrate (one of the ligands for Notch proteins).[33] It is currently unknown whether the phenotype and function of DCs generated using all these different strategies are equivalent.

The ability of tolerogenic DCs to induce Tr1 cells is linked to inhibition of IL-12 and increased production of IL-10. However, the synthesis of IL-10 either by the T cells or by APCs is necessary for Tr1 cell differentiation *in vivo*, but it is not sufficient. Factors that act in concert with IL-10 to inhibit the expression of transcription factors that promote the production of Th_2- and Th_1-associated cytokines are probably also required.[30]

The lack of expression of costimulatory molecules does not correlate well with the capacity of DCs to induce Tr1 cells. For example, monocyte-derived DCs exposed to heavy-chain ferritin induce the differentiation of IL-10–producing T cells, despite increased expression of the costimulatory molecules CD86 and B7H1 (PD-L1).[32] Similarly, *B. pertussis*–treated DCs, which induce the differentiation of antigen-specific Tr1 cells, express normal levels of CD86 and CD40.[31] It is possible that rather than the loss of costimulatory molecules, the engagement of other molecules that act as dominant tolerogenic factors is important for the generation of Tr1 cells.[34] For example, bronchial DCs induced after nasal antigen challenge promote the differentiation of Tr1 cells via a mechanism that requires expression of ICOS-L.[35] Furthermore, CD58, the ligand for CD2, has recently been shown to determine the differentiation of human Tr1 cells.[36] Expression of soluble suppressive molecules such as the tryptophan catabolizing enzyme indoleamine 2,3-dioxygenase (IDO), which is upregulated by IL-10 and induces T cell hyporesponsiveness,[37] may also be involved. Thus, although therapeutic strategies that rely solely on blockade of costimulatory molecules may inhibit immune responses in the short term, they may be inefficient at inducing long-term tolerance mediated by Tr1 cells.

As described above, the Tr1-inducing ability of DCs may depend on their state of differentiation or on features of the microenvironment in which DC–T cell contact occurs. An alternative possibility is that specialized subsets of DCs dedicated to tolerance induction exist. A subset of $DEC205^+$ $B220^+$ CD19– DCs, isolated from the liver and activated *in vitro* by IL-3 and CD40 cross-linking, that is able to induce Tr1 cells has been described.[38] Furthermore, human plasmacytoid DCs (DC2s) have been shown to have intrinsic tolerogenic functions. Naive $CD8^+$ T cells primed with allogeneic DC2s, activated via CD40, become IL-10–producing cells and suppress proliferation of $CD8^+$ T cells.[39] In addition, human DC2s activated by viruses can induce a population of IL-10–producing $CD4^+$ T cells.[40] Interestingly, donors who undergo hematopoietic stem cell mobilization with G-CSF have a fivefold increase in DC2s in their periphery,[41] and it has recently been reported that CD4+ T cells from these donors are enriched for Tr1 cells.[42]

Identification and isolation of a source of DCs that can be used to efficiently differentiate and expand antigen-specific Tr1 cells *in vitro* and/or *in vivo* will be a major step toward their use as a cellular therapy to control undesired immune responses.

Tr1 CELLS: *IN VIVO* FUNCTION

The first suggestion that human Tr1 cells are involved in maintaining peripheral tolerance *in vivo* came from studies on severe combined immunodeficiency (SCID) patients successfully transplanted with HLA-mismatched allogeneic stem cells. Despite the HLA disparity, these patients do not develop graft versus host disease (GVHD) in the absence of immunosuppressive therapy. Interestingly, high levels of IL-10 are detected in the plasma of these patients and a significant proportion of donor-derived T cells, which are specific for the host HLA antigens and produce high levels of IL-10, can be isolated *in vitro*.[43] In addition, high spontaneous IL-10 production by peripheral blood mononuclear cells (PBMCs) before bone marrow transplantation is associated with a subsequent low incidence of GVHD and transplant-related mortality.[44,45] Studies of patients who spontaneously developed tolerance to kidney or liver allograft revealed the presence of CD4+ T cells that suppress naive T cell responses via production of IL-10 or TGF-β.[46] Together, these data indicate that Tr1 cells can naturally regulate tolerance *in vivo* in the setting of bone marrow and solid organ transplantation.

The indication that these cells can also play a role in modulating responses to self-antigens came from the studies of Kitani *et al.*, who isolated human self-reactive Tr1 cells from healthy donors.[21] A decreased frequency of IL-10–producing CD4+ T cells is observed in the inflamed synovium and peripheral blood of patients with rheumatoid arthritis,[47] indicating that a deficiency in Tr1 cells may contribute to the loss of self-tolerance in autoimmune diseases.

Tr1 cells are also important in downregulation of immune responses toward allergens such as nickel.[22]

Overall, these studies demonstrate that Tr1 cells are certainly beneficial for the induction of tolerance to self-, allo-, and nonharmful foreign antigens, such as allergens. However, Tr1 cells specific for infectious agents or tumor antigens may interfere with the host's immune response and thus be detrimental. Presumably, it is advantageous for pathogens to evolve strategies to enhance the differentiation of Tr1 cells, which would then limit the protective immune response and allow long-term infection of the host.[31] Hemagglutinin from *Bordetella pertussis* inhibits IL-12 and enhances IL-10 production from DCs in the lung and bronchial lymph nodes.[31] Priming of naive CD4+ T cells with DCs thus modulated induces the differentiation of antigen-specific Tr1 cells, which ultimately inhibits protective Th$_1$-mediated responses against *B. pertussis* both *in vitro* and *in vivo*. Similarly, in chronic helminthic infections, where patients have relatively little sign of dermatitis despite the presence of small worms in the skin, antigen-specific Tr1 cells can be obtained. These cells are able to inhibit proliferation of other T cells.[48]

Similar to the roles of Th_1 and Th_2 cells in different pathologies, the balance between beneficial and detrimental effects of Tr1 cells need to be precisely tuned.

Tr1 CELLS AND ORAL TOLERANCE

Antigen-specific Tr1 cells have been shown to be induced in Peyer's patches (PPs) and mesenteric lymph nodes (MNLs) by feeding exogenous proteins. This approach for tolerance induction has been studied for the prevention of autoimmune diseases. Several studies have shown that multiple feeding of self-antigens induce Tr1 cells that can suppress multiple sclerosis and diabetes in animal models. Oral administration of myelin basic protein (MBP) suppresses experimental autoimmune encephalomyelitis (EAE) by inducing peripheral tolerance. T cell clones isolated from the MLNs of tolerant mice were $CD4^+$ and $IL-10^+$ $TGF-\beta^+$.[49] Other reports confirmed the role of orally induced Tr1 cells in preventing multiple sclerosis-like disease.[50,51] Interestingly, treatment with low doses of oral MBP and simultaneous administration of oral IL-10 reduced the incidence and severity of EAE.[52] Similarly, suppression of diabetes development by oral insulin in NOD mice was enhanced by oral co-administration of IL-10.[52] In both systems, reductions in IL-2 and IFN-γ and increases in IL-10 and TGF-β were observed in tolerant mice resistant to autoimmunity. Oral administration of MBP or insulin in the absence of IL-10 was not effective in oral tolerance induction, highlighting the requirement for IL-10 for the *in vivo* development of Tr1 cells.

There is a large body of evidence showing that IL-10 plays a key role in modulating inflammatory responses in the intestine. IL-10 controls the immune responses to nonpathogenic enteric flora and dietary antigens, as suggested by several studies on mucosal immunity in murine models.[53,54] Importantly, IL-10 knockout mice develop a severe form of enterocolitis, a mouse model of human inflammatory bowel disease (IBD).[55] Ovalbumin-specific Tr1 cells have been shown to prevent IBD development induced by transfer of $CD4^+$ $CD45RB^{high}$ T cells in SCID mice, through bystander suppression.[15] These data support the notion that IBD in $IL-10^{-/-}$ mice is partially a result of the absence of Tr1 cells.

Orally induced Tr1 cells also play an important role in preventing undesired immune responses to food antigens. Low-dose oral tolerance against beta lactoglobulin (BLG), a potent milk allergen, is mediated by BLG-specific/IL-10–secreting cells in Peyer's patches. These cells inhibit the T cell proliferative response *in vitro* and T cell–mediated inflammation *in vivo*.[56] Celiac disease is another common disorder of the small intestine resulting from permanent intolerance to dietary wheat gluten. An abnormal T cell–mediated immune response to gliadin, together with the absence of specific immune suppression, plays a crucial role in inducing the celiac enteropathy.[57] In accordance with this observation, we found that gliadin-specific T cell activation was suppressed in celiac intestinal mucosa cultured 24 hours *ex vivo* with gliadin and IL-10. Interestingly, these gliadin-specific T cell lines generated in the presence of IL-10 were anergic in response to gliadin (Salvati *et al.*, submitted). Moreover, we recently isolated gliadin-specific Tr1 cell clones from the intestinal mucosa of a treated celiac patient. These Tr1 cell clones were anergic, produced IL-10 and TGF-β, and had a strong inhibitory effect on the gliadin-specific T cell response (C. Gianfrani, manuscript in preparation). Based on these findings, we

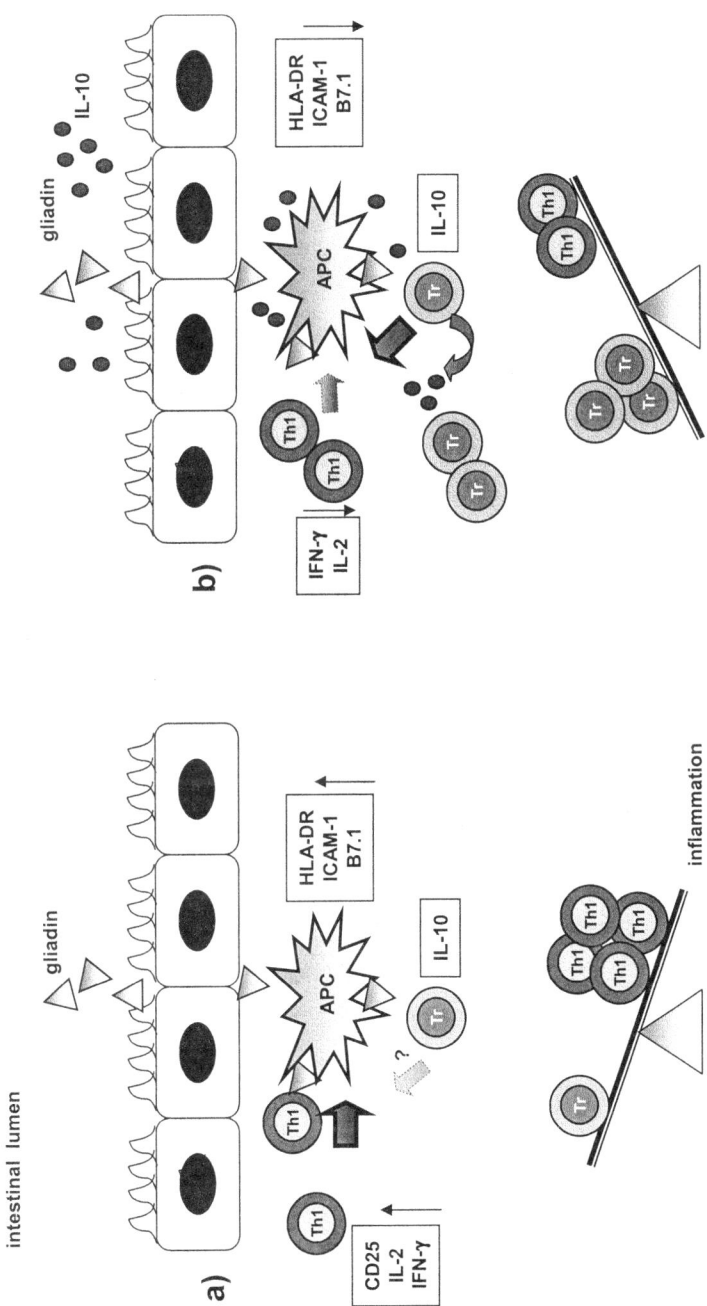

FIGURE 2. See following page for legend.

hypothesize that Tr1 cells, although present in the inflamed intestinal mucosa of celiac patients, are not able to downmodulate the massive anti-gliadin immune response. Addition of exogenous IL-10 might affect gliadin presentation by local APC and induce gliadin-specific Tr1 cells, leading to downmodulation of the adverse gliadin-specific immune response (FIG. 2). These data indicate the involvement of IL-10–producing Tr1 cells in suppressing immune responses toward antigens that are orally introduced into the organism on a daily basis.

CONCLUSIONS

Following their initial description,[15] Tr1 cells have been extensively characterized and today are considered a specialized subset of Tr cells able to prevent immune-mediated diseases and to maintain immunological tolerance. It has been shown that oral administration of antigens in combination with IL-10 is one mechanism, among many, for the *in vivo* differentiation of Tr1 cells, and this can be envisaged as a novel strategy for tolerance induction.

REFERENCES

1. MOWAT, A.M. 2003. Anatomical basis of tolerance and immunity to intestinal antigens. Nat. Rev. Immunol. **3:** 331–341.
2. VAN PARIJS, L. *et al.* 1997. Functional consequences of dysregulated B7-1 (CD80) and B7-2 (CD86) expression in B or T lymphocytes of transgenic mice. J. Immunol. **159:** 5336–5344.
3. RICHMAN, L.K. *et al.* 1978. Enterically induced immunologic tolerance. I. Induction of suppressor T lymphoyctes by intragastric administration of soluble proteins. J. Immunol. **121:** 2429–2434.
4. KE, Y. & J.A. KAPP. 1996. Oral antigen inhibits priming of CD8+ CTL, CD4+ T cells, and antibody responses while activating CD8+ suppressor T cells. J. Immunol. **156:** 916–921.
5. MILLER, A. *et al.* 1992. Suppressor T cells generated by oral tolerization to myelin basic protein suppress both in vitro and in vivo immune responses by the release of transforming growth factor beta after antigen-specific triggering. Proc. Natl. Acad. Sci. USA **89:** 421–425.

FIGURE 2. Possible mechanisms underlying suppression of immune responses to dietary gliadin mediated by gliadin-specific Tr1 cells. This model was suggested by our results in organ culture of intestinal mucosa (Salvati *et al.*, submitted). (**a**) Intestinal biopsies from celiac patients on a gluten-free diet (treated) were challenged with gliadin for 24 h. High expression of activation markers (CD25, HLA-DR), costimulatory and adhesion molecules (B7.1, ICAM-1), and inflammatory cytokines (IFN-γ, IL-2) produced by gliadin-specific Th_1 cells, were observed in intestinal mucosa after gliadin challenge. Although Tr1 cells are recruited to the inflamed intestinal mucosa during the acute disease and are still resident in the treated mucosa, they cannot downmodulate the massive inflammatory immune response. (**b**) By contrast, treated mucosa challenged with gliadin and exogenous IL-10 shows a marked decrease in T cell activation. It is likely that exogenous IL-10 both affects gliadin presentation by local APCs and enhances induction of gliadin-specific Tr1 cells, which in turn mediates their own expansion leading to downmodulation of adverse gliadin-specific Th1 responses.

6. PEREZ-MACHADO, M.A. *et al.* 2003. Reduced transforming growth factor-beta1-producing T cells in the duodenal mucosa of children with food allergy. Eur. J. Immunol. **33:** 2307–2315.
7. MCMENAMIN, C. *et al.* 1994. Regulation of IgE responses to inhaled antigen in mice by antigen-specific gamma delta T cells. Science **265:** 1869–1871.
8. MENGEL, J. *et al.* 1995. Anti-gamma delta T cell antibody blocks the induction and maintenance of oral tolerance to ovalbumin in mice. Immunol. Lett. **48:** 97–102.
9. KE, Y. *et al.* 1997. Gamma delta T lymphocytes regulate the induction and maintenance of oral tolerance. J. Immunol. **158:** 3610–3618.
10. SHEVACH, E.M. 2002. CD4+ CD25+ suppressor T cells: more questions than answers. Nat. Rev. Immunol. **2:** 389–400.
11. THORSTENSON, K.M. & A. KHORUTS. 2001. Generation of anergic and potentially immunoregulatory CD25+CD4 T cells in vivo after induction of peripheral tolerance with intravenous or oral antigen. J. Immunol. **167:** 188–195.
12. TSUJI, N.M., K. MIZUMACHI & J. KURISAKI. 2003. Antigen-specific, CD4(+)CD25(+) regulatory T cell clones induced in Peyer's patches. Int. Immunol. **15:** 525–534.
13. DUBOIS, B. *et al.* 2003. Innate CD4+CD25+ regulatory T cells are required for oral tolerance and control CD8+ T cells mediating skin inflammation. Blood **102:** 3295–3301.
14. RONCAROLO, M.G. *et al.* 2001. Type 1 T regulatory cells. Immunol. Rev. **182:** 68–79.
15. GROUX, H. *et al.* 1996. Interleukin-10 induces a long-term antigen-specific anergic state in human CD4+ T cells. J. Exp. Med. **184:** 19–29.
16. LEVINGS, M.K. *et al.* 2001. IFN-alpha and IL-10 Induce the Differentiation of Human Type 1 T Regulatory Cells. J. Immunol. **166:** 5530–5539.
17. BACCHETTA, R. *et al.* 2002. Growth and expansion of human T regulatory type 1 cells are independent from TCR activation but require exogenous cytokines. Eur. J. Immunol. **32:** 2237–2245.
18. SEBASTIANI, S. *et al.* 2001. Chemokine receptor expression and function in CD4+ T lymphocytes with regulatory activity. J. Immunol. **166:** 996–1002.
19. LECART, S. *et al.* 2001. Phenotypic characterization of human CD4+ regulatory T cells obtained from cutaneous dinitrochlorobenzene-induced delayed type hypersensitivity reactions. J. Invest. Dermatol. **117:** 318–325.
20. RONCAROLO, M.G., M.K. LEVINGS & C. TRAVERSARI. 2001. Differentiation of T regulatory cells by immature dendritic cells. J. Exp. Med. **193:** F5–9.
21. KITANI, A. *et al.* 2000. Activated self-MHC-reactive T cells have the cytokine phenotype of Th3/T regulatory cell 1 T cells. J. Immunol. **165:** 691–702.
22. CAVANI, A. *et al.* 2000. Human CD4+ T lymphocytes with remarkable regulatory functions on dendritic cells and nickel-specific Th1 immune responses. J. Invest. Dermatol. **114:** 295–302.
23. MCRAE, B.L. *et al.* 1998. Type I IFNs inhibit human dendritic cell IL-12 production and Th1 cell development. J. Immunol. **160:** 4298–4304.
24. BOUSSIOTIS, V.A. *et al.* 2001. Altered T-cell receptor + CD28-mediated signaling and blocked cell cycle progression in interleukin 10 and transforming growth factor-beta-treated alloreactive T cells that do not induce graft-versus-host disease. Blood **97:** 565–571.
25. MAHNKE, K. *et al.* 2002. Immature, but not inactive: the tolerogenic function of immature dendritic cells. Immunol. Cell Biol. **80:** 477–483.
26. JONULEIT, H. *et al.* 2000. Induction of interleukin-10-producing, nonproliferating CD4+ T cells with regulatory properties by repetitive stimulation with allogenic immature human dendritic cells. J. Exp. Med. **192:** 1213–1222.
27. DHODAPKAR, M.V. *et al.* 2001. Antigen-specific inhibition of effector T cell function in humans after injection of immature dendrtitic cells. J. Exp. Med. **193:** 233–238.
28. STEINBRINK, K. *et al.* 2002. CD4(+) and CD8(+) anergic T cells induced by interleukin-10-treated human dendritic cells display antigen-specific suppressor activity. Blood **99:** 2468–2476.
29. PENNA, G. & L. ADORINI. 2000. 1 Alpha,25-dihydroxyvitamin D3 inhibits differentiation, maturation, activation, and survival of dendritic cells leading to impaired alloreactive T cell activation. J. Immunol. **164:** 2405–2511.

30. BARRAT, F.J. *et al.* 2002. In vitro generation of interleukin 10-producing regulatory CD4(+) T cells is induced by immunosuppressive drugs and inhibited by T helper type 1 (Th1)- and Th2-inducing cytokines. J. Exp. Med. **195:** 603–616.
31. MCGUIRK, P. & K. MILLS. 2002. Pathogen-specific regulatory T cells provoke a shift in the Th1/Th2 paradigm in immunity to infectious diseases. Trends Immunol. **23:** 450–455.
32. GRAY, C.P., P. AROSIO & P. HERSEY. 2002. Heavy chain ferritin activates regulatory T cells by induction of changes in dendritic cells. Blood **99:** 3326–3334.
33. HACKSTEIN, H., A.E. MORELLI & A.W. THOMSON. 2001. Designer dendritic cells for tolerance induction: guided not misguided missiles. Trends Immunol. **22:** 437–442.
34. GREENWALD, R.J., Y.E. LATCHMAN & A.H. SHARPE. 2002. Negative co-receptors on lymphocytes. Curr. Opin. Immunol. **14:** 391–396.
35. AKBARI, O. *et al.* 2002. Antigen-specific regulatory T cells develop via the ICOS#150;ICOS- ligand pathway and inhibit allergen-induced airway hyperreactivity. Nat. Med. **8:** 1024–1032.
36. WAKKACH, A., F. COTTREZ & H. GROUX. 2001. Differentiation of regulatory T cells 1 is induced by CD2 costimulation. J. Immunol. **167:** 3107–3113.
37. MUNN, D.H. *et al.* 2002. Potential regulatory function of human dendritic cells expressing indoleamine 2,3-dioxygenase. Science **297:** 1867–1870.
38. LU, L. *et al.* 2001. Liver-derived DEC205+B220+CD19- dendritic cells regulate T cell responses. J. Immunol. **166:** 7042–7052.
39. GILLIET, M. & Y.J. LIU. 2002. Generation of human CD8 T regulatory cells by CD40 ligand-activated plasmacytoid dendritic cells. J. Exp. Med. **195:** 695–704.
40. KADOWAKI, N. *et al.* 2000. Natural interferon alpha/beta-producing cells link innate and adaptive immunity. J. Exp. Med. **192:** 219–226.
41. ARPINATI, M. *et al.* 2000. Granulocyte-colony stimulating factor mobilizes T helper 2-inducing dendritic cells. Blood **95:** 2484–2490.
42. RUTELLA, S. *et al.* 2002. Role for granulocyte colony-stimulating factor in the generation of human T regulatory type 1 cells. Blood **100:** 2562–71.
43. BACCHETTA, R. *et al.* 1994. High levels of interleukin 10 production in vivo are associated with tolerance in SCID patients transplanted with HLA mismatched hematopoietic stem cells. J. Exp. Med. **179:** 493–502.
44. BAKER, K. *et al.* 1999. High spontaneous IL-10 production in unrelated bone marrow transplant recipients is associated with fewer transplant-related complications and early deaths. Bone Marrow Transplant. **23:** 1123–1129.
45. HOLLER, E. *et al.* 2000. Prognostic significance of increased IL-10 production in patients prior to allogeneic bone marrow transplantation. Bone Marrow Transplant. **25:** 237–241.
46. VANBUSKIRK, A.M. *et al.* 2000. Human allograft acceptance is associated with immune regulation. J. Clin. Invest. **106:** 145–155.
47. YUDOH, K. *et al.* 2000. Reduced expression of the regulatory CD4+ T cell subset is related to Th1/Th2 balance and disease severity in rheumatoid arthritis. Arthritis Rheum. **43:** 617–627.
48. SATOGUINA, J. *et al.* 2002. Antigen-specific T regulatory-1 cells are associated with immunosuppression in a chronic helminth infection (onchocerciasis). Microbes Infect. **4:** 1291–1230.
49. CHEN, Y. *et al.* 1994. Regulatory T cell clones induced by oral tolerance: suppression of autoimmune encephalomyelitis. Science **265:** 1237–1240.
50. WILDBAUM, G., N. NETZER & N. KARIN. 2002. Tr1 cell-dependent active tolerance blunts the pathogenic effects of determinant spreading. J. Clin. Invest. **110:** 701–710.
51. FARIA, A.M. *et al.* 2003. Oral tolerance induced by continuous feeding: enhanced up-regulation of transforming growth factor-beta/interleukin-10 and suppression of experimental autoimmune encephalomyelitis. J. Autoimmun. **20:** 135–145.
52. SLAVIN, A.J., R. MARON & H.L. WEINER. 2001. Mucosal administration of IL-10 enhances oral tolerance in autoimmune encephalomyelitis and diabetes. Int. Immunol. **13:** 825–833.
53. CONG, Y. *et al.* 2002. Bacterial-reactive T regulatory cells inhibit pathogenic immune responses to the enteric flora. J. Immunol. **169:** 6112–6119.

54. ANNACKER, O. *et al.* 2003. Interleukin-10 in the regulation of T cell-induced colitis. J. Autoimmun. **20:** 277–279.
55. KUHN, R. *et al.* 1993. Interleukin-10-deficient mice develop chronic enterocolitis. Cell **75:** 263–274.
56. TSUJI, N.M., K. MIZUMACHI & J. KURISAKI. 2001. Interleukin-10-secreting Peyer's patch cells are responsible for active suppression in low-dose oral tolerance. Immunology **103:** 458–64.
57. TRONCONE, R. *et al.* 1998. Majority of gliadin-specific T-cell clones from celiac small intestinal mucosa produce interferon-gamma and interleukin-4. Dig. Dis. Sci. **43:** 156–161.

Natural Killer T Cells in Mucosal Homeostasis

ARTHUR KASER,[a] EDWARD E. S. NIEUWENHUIS,[a,b] WARREN STROBER,[c] LLOYD MAYER,[d] IVAN FUSS,[c] SEAN COLGAN,[a] AND RICHARD S. BLUMBERG[a]

[a]*Brigham and Women's Hospital, Harvard Medical School, Boston, Massachusetts 02115, USA*

[b]*Erasmus Medical Center, Rotterdam, the Netherlands*

[c]*National Institutes of Health, Bethesda, Maryland 20892, USA*

[d]*Mount Sinai Medical School, New York, New York 10029, USA*

ABSTRACT: The mucosal-associated lymphoid tissues (MALT), including the gut-associated lymphoid tissues, are a tightly regulated environment. In fact, it might be stated that on the basis of studies from animal models of inflammatory bowel disease (IBD), the major means of peripheral regulation of immune responses in the intestine is not necessarily from processes such as deletion or anergy, but more likely from the controls imposed upon responses due to the activities of a variety of regulatory subsets of cells. One type of regulatory cellular subset that has recently gained attention is the subset of T cells that are associated with CD1d-restricted responses. Recently, CD1d-restricted T cells have been increasingly appreciated to play a significant role in mucosal tissues of the intestine and lung, for example. Insights from these studies have clearly elevated these cells to particular importance in the regulation of a variety of infectious and inflammatory conditions, such as those associated with idiopathic IBD. In this review, we focus on recent observations on the characteristics of CD1d-restricted pathways in mucosal compartments, after a brief introduction into the biology of CD1d and CD1d-restricted T cells.

KEYWORDS: mucosal homeostasis; inflammatory bowel disease; CD1; CD1d; natural killer T (NKT) cells; epithelial cells; antigen-presenting cells

INTRODUCTION

CD1d is a member of the CD1 gene family,[1,2] which consists of five genes, CD1a to CD1e. Four of these genes (CD1a to CD1d) encode functional proteins, whereas the CD1e gene has not been associated with a detectable product to date.[3] The CD1 gene family can be divided into two groups, CD1a to CD1c and CD1d, based on sequence homology.[3] Whereas humans contain genes on chromosome 1 for CD1a to CD1d, rodents express only a CD1d homologue. In fact, the human CD1d isoform is more similar to mouse and rat CD1d than it is to the other human CD1 isoforms.[3]

Address for correspondence: Richard S. Blumberg, M.D., Division of Gastroenterology, Brigham and Women's Hospital, Harvard Medical School, 75 Francis St., Boston, MA 02115. Voice: 617-732-6917; fax: 617-264-5185.
  rblumberg@partners.org

All CD1 genes have an MHC class I–like structure both genetically and biochemically.[4] In this regard, the CD1 genes contain exons 2 to 4, encoding domains α1, α2, and α3, that generate a protein product that is associated with β2-microglobulin. The recent solution of the X-ray crystallographic structure of CD1d[5] and, more recently, CD1a,[6] have confirmed earlier predictions from cellular studies by Brenner and Porcelli that the CD1-related molecules play a role in presenting a variety of glycolipid antigens to unique subsets of T cells. In particular, the glycolipid antigens presented by the CD1a to CD1c proteins have been shown to be a variety of lipoglycan antigens that derive from mycobacteria and other bacteria.[7] The glycolipid antigens presented by CD1d are less well defined. Whereas a model glycolipid antigen derived from marine sponge, α-galactosylceramide (αGalCer), has been shown to be presented by CD1d to unique groups of CD1d-restricted T cells,[8] the endogenous antigens that are presented by CD1d to CD1d-restricted T cells, either *in vitro* or *in vivo*, are less clear but do include such molecules as the phospholipid phosphatidylethanolamine.[9] It also remains unclear whether exogenous glycolipid antigens derived from the microbial universe can also be presented by CD1d, with most information suggesting that the CD1d-specific antigens are derived from host lipids. This, in particular, emphasizes the significant autoreactivity that has been identified in the CD1 system.

The types of T cells that have been shown to be restricted by CD1d, both in mouse and human, include either those that have an invariant T cell receptor (TCR)-α chain or those that have a semidiverse group of TCR-α chains.[10]

Characteristics of the first group of T cells, the so-called invariant natural killer T (iNKT) cells, include the following: These T cells express an invariant TCR-α chain that results from the rearrangement of TCR-α gene products to contain only canonical germ line sequences. In rodents, this invariant TCR-α chain comprises a Vα14 gene product in contiguity with a Jα18 gene product.[11] The human homologue for this invariant TCR-α chain is the result of the rearrangement of a Vα24 gene segment to JαQ gene segment.[11] Because invariant T cells often carry NK cell markers on the cell surface, in addition to the TCR/CD3 complex, they are considered to be natural killer T (NKT) cells. Invariant NKT cells either express CD4 or are double negative; in fact, forced expression of CD8 in the thymus causes deletion of these particular cells. Although these cells carry an invariant TCR-α chain, the TCR-α chains pair with a wide variety of TCR-β chains that predominantly use Vβ8.2, Vβ7, or Vβ2.[11] As a result, although iNKT cells express an invariant TCR-α chain, owing to the association of this invariant TCR-α chain with a wide variety of TCR-β chains, these cells are, in fact, quite polymorphic. This may explain the wide variety of biologic processes that these cells are able to regulate, as described in more detail below. The iNKT subset is the major subset that responds to αGalCer.[8] Indeed, virtually all αGalCer reactivity maps to the iNKT subset of CD1d-restricted T cells.

In addition to iNKT cells, recent studies in both mouse and human have identified a perhaps larger group of CD1d-restricted T cells that contain a much more diverse TCR repertoire.[12–14] The so-called semidiverse NKT cells are also either CD4 or double negative in mouse and, perhaps, CD8, CD4 or double negative in humans with a preferential usage of particular TCR-α and -β chains.[12,14] Specifically, semidiverse iNKT cells use either Vα3.2 conjoined to a Jα9 gene segment or a Vα8 gene segment, together with a Vβ8 gene segment.[12] The glycolipid antigens that restrict these T cells are less clear, but they are defined as CD1d-reactive owing to the ability to detect restriction to CD1d when costimulation is provided and/or autoreactivity is evident in cellular model systems.[12]

Finally, there is a much larger number of NKT cells that are not CD1d-restricted but are restricted to either MHC class I or MHC class II.[15] These cells are considered NKT cells because of the expression of the NK1.1 marker on the cell surface, a marker that recently has come to be appreciated as one frequently associated with T cell activation.[16] These non–CD1d-restricted NKT cells have a very diverse array of TCRs and express CD4, CD8, or are double negative.[15]

The vast majority of biologic functions that have been assigned to CD1d-restricted T cells to date are those associated with the iNKT subset of cells.[10] A unique feature of the regulatory functions of iNKT cells is the fact that they are able to regulate a wide variety of cell types and, thus, subsequent cellular processes owing to their involvement at the earliest points of the immune response.[17] iNKT cells have a very special relationship with dendritic cells (DCs) through expression of CD1d on the DC.[17] This interaction between the DC and the iNKT cell leads to regulation of both subsets through secretion of IL-12 by the DC and secretion of IFN-γ, for example, by the iNKT cell that is, in turn, regulated by CD40 on the DC and CD40 ligand on iNKT.[17] Once activated by CD1d on the antigen-presenting cell (APC), the iNKT cell is able to regulate a wide variety of cell types, both through cell-cell contact and through secretion of a large number of cellular mediators.[17] In fact, the iNKT cell predominantly has a T helper 0 (Th0) phenotype when stimulated through its TCR-CD3 complex.[18–21] Recent studies with human iNKT cells suggest that there might be polarization of these cells, with IFN-γ production primarily associated with the double-negative subset, and Th0 associated with the $CD4^+$ subset.[18] Such polarization is less evident with rodent iNKT cells but may indeed be present. iNKT cells have been shown to express Fas ligand on the cell surface and to exert cytolytic activity through the secretion of perforin and granzyme,[22] and thus to regulate tumor cells and perhaps DCs, which, in turn, would have significant effects on subsequent immune responses.[23] In fact, through these cytolytic properties, iNKT cells may not only play a role in antitumor immunity but may also, through the cytolytic removal of DC1 cells, lead to potent effects on subsequent immune responses and downregulation of immune responses, in particular.[23,24] Through the secretion of MIP1, iNKT cells regulate neutrophils.[25] Through signals that are yet to be defined, iNKT cells are well known to regulate NK cells and B cells. In fact, iNKT cell activation may be the most potent mediator of NK cell mobilization during the course of an immune response.[10] Finally, through the secretion of a wide range of cytokines and chemokines, including IL-4, IL-10, IL-13, TGF-β, and IFN-γ, iNKT cells have the potent ability to immune deviate conventional T cells to Th1 or Th2.[10] With that said, it is also well known that the absence of CD1d-restricted T cells due to deletion of the CD1d gene, for example, does not abrogate a Th2 response,[26–28] indicating that CD1d is one of many regulatory pathways that are involved in immune deviation of conventional T cells.

As indicated in the introductory comments, these properties of iNKT cells are likely to be relevant to mucosal homeostasis and, perhaps more importantly, to the regulation and/or pathogenesis of a variety of disease processes. The MALT is constantly bombarded by a variety of foreign antigens, which require tight regulation of immune responses along the epithelial cell surface. Using IBD as a model, immune responses that are characterized by either Th1 or Th2 cytokine production can be associated with chronic inflammation.[29,30] Therefore, regulation of conventional T cell responses is particularly important. Given the aforementioned comments on the biology of iNKT cells, it is not surprising that iNKT cells have recently been shown to play an important role in a variety of processes related to the mucosal immune system.[31,32] In particular, a variety of cellular subsets that bear CD1d on the cell surface, including intestinal epithelial cells (IECs), DCs, and B cells, reside within these compartments. Similarly, iNKT cells have been detected in mucosal compartments, such as the epithelium, albeit at very low proportions.[32,33] Although iNKT cells have been identified in the epithelial compartments by the use of CD1d-tetramers, little information has been obtained on the semidiverse group of CD1d-restricted T cells as yet. However, recent studies in the oxazolone colitis model and in humans with ulcerative colitis (UC) suggest that this form of T cell may be particularly important, as discussed further below.[31] The next section of this chapter will focus on evidence that supports a role for CD1d-restricted pathways in the regulation of several MALTs, most notably in the intestine and in the lung.

REGULATION OF MUCOSAL INFLAMMATION BY iNKT CELLS

IBD appears to be a dysregulated mucosal immune response to a subset of bacterial antigens in a genetically susceptible host.[29,30,34] These concepts are largely based upon recent studies in a variety of animal models of colitis, which require the presence of a normal microbial ecology in conjunction with some perturbation of the MALT either through genetic manipulation or the administration of a variety of exogenous agents, including those that break down the intestinal barrier.[30] All of these models of IBD suggest that the mucosal inflammation is distilled from a final common pathway that generates either excess Th1 or excess Th2 cytokine production, either of which will cause the development of IBD-like immunopathology. Both Th1 and Th2 inflammation are, in turn, tightly regulated by cytokines derived from a variety of both B cells and T cells. The latter include both $CD4^+CD25^+$ T cells, the so-called T regulatory cells, which secrete TGF-β and/or IL-10. The recent appreciation that iNKT cells are decreased in a variety of autoimmune conditions (as well as, perhaps, IBD), and the fact that iNKT cells can regulate autoimmune diseases such as allergic autoimmune encephalitis and diabetes mellitus in animal models,[17] originally suggested that iNKT cells may have a similar regulatory effect in IBD.

One of the earliest studies to test this hypothesis was performed in the dextran sodium sulfate (DSS) colitis model.[35] In this model, the administration of DSS leads to disruption of the epithelial barrier and activation of macrophages, leading to a severe colonic inflammation that is often associated with significant mortality. DSS colitis can be established in a T cell–deficient environment, in either SCID or Rag-deficient animals. However, studies from others have shown that although the generation of colitis is T cell independent, T cells clearly play an important role in the perpetuation and possibly, as shown below, the regulation of inflammation associated with the administration of DSS.

To determine whether iNKT cells are able to regulate colitis, either C57BL/6J (wild-type), CD1d-deficient, or Rag2-deficient mice were exposed to 2.5% DSS *ad libitum* in the presence of either the agonist glycolipid antigen, αGalCer, or a nonagonist (nonfunctional) glycolipid analogue of αGalCer, αManCer.[35] These studies showed that treatment of wild-type mice with αGalCer, but not αManCer, prolonged survival after administration of DSS.[35] This was also associated with an amelioration of clinical symptoms (body weight loss) or signs (evidence of gastrointestinal bleeding).[35] The protective effect of αGalCer was dependent on iNKT cells in wild-type mice because it was abrogated by the deletion of these cells by monoclonal antibodies.[35] Moreover, the protective effect of aGalCer was iNKT cell–dependent because αGalCer activity was lost in either Rag-deficient or CD1d-deficient mice.[35] Specifically, the survival of wild-type mice was prolonged by the administration of αGalCer but not αManCer.[35] The survival score of the αManCer-treated group was identical to that of either Rag-deficient or CD1d-deficient mice administered αGalCer. Finally, to prove that these effects were due to iNKT cells, when iNKT cells were obtained from wild-type mice primed with αGalCer, they were able to adoptively transfer protection to Rag-deficient mice.[35] In contrast, iNKT cells from wild-type mice that had been primed with αManCer were unable to confer protection against DSS administration.[35] Although the basis for the amelioration of DSS colitis by iNKT cells was not determined initially, subsequent studies have shown that the regulation of DSS colitis by iNKT cells was the result of the production of Th2 and perhaps regulatory cytokines.[36] Specifically, intraperitoneal injection of a glycolipid, OCH, that has previously been shown to preferentially induce production of Th2 cytokines by iNKT cells resulted in an amelioration of colitis in wild-type mice exposed to DSS but not in Jα18-deficient mice.[36] This protection from colitis in wild-type mice was associated with induction of IL-4 and IL-10.[36] In addition, Jα18-deficient mice exhibited significantly increased colitis in comparison with wild-type mice.[36] Taken together, these studies in the DSS colitis model suggested that certain iNKT cells are associated with the intestine and have a unique ability to preferentially secrete Th2 cytokines and/or regulatory cytokines, which are able to either immune deviate away from Th1 bias or regulate colitis.

More definitive evidence that CD1d-restricted pathways are involved in mucosal regulation associated with intestinal inflammation came from the following series of studies in hapten-mediated colitis: Instillation of several different haptens is able to induce colitis. Specifically, administration of either trinitrobenzene sulfonic acid (TNBS) or oxazolone to mice, either with or without prior skin sensitization, induced colitis that is predominantly characterized by a Th1 response in certain animal strains with the former hapten, or Th2 in certain animal strains with the latter.[30] Recent studies suggest that in some strains, such as Balb/C, oxazolone-induced colitis is a process generated by both Th1 and Th2 cytokines.[30] Similarly, C57BL/6J mice develop an oxazolone-induced colitis that is a mixed Th1- and Th2-mediated process, in contrast to SJL/J mice, which, as originally described, generate a predominantly Th2-mediated colitis. With this in mind, we studied colitis induced by oxazolone in CD1d-deficient mice. These studies showed that both CD1d-deficient and Jα18-deficient mice were resistant to oxazolone-induced colitis, in comparison to wild-type C57BL/6J mice.[31] Similarly, administration of a neutralizing anti-CD1d antibody was able to achieve a similar protection of wild-type mice from the development of immunopathology associated with oxazolone administration.[31] These studies suggested that CD1d-restricted T cells acted as provocateurs in the generation of colitis. However, other studies suggested that the ability of iNKT cells to produce or drive colitis was the result of the preferential production of Th2 cytokines.[31,37] Previous studies in the SJL/J mouse strain had shown that oxazolone colitis in this genetic background is caused by the production of IL-4.[37] Studies with both lamina propria mononuclear cells (LPMCs) and mesenteric lymph nodes in the C57BL/6J strain showed that oxazolone administration was also associated with a very high production of IL-4 early in the course of colitis (days 2 to 4) and is superseded by a very large production of IL-13 (days 4 to 7).[31] This production of IL-13 was shown to be biologically important, as oxazolone colitis could be prevented by neutralization of IL-13 activity through intraperitoneal injection of an IL-13–receptor α2-Fc fusion protein.[31] Evidence that IL-13 responsible for the generation of colitis was derived from iNKT cells was obtained from observations showing that stimulation of LPMC by either anti-CD3 + CD28 or L cells transfected with CD1d, but not untransfected L cells, in the presence of αGalCer, induced significant production of IL-4 and, to a greater extent, IL-13.[31] Taken together, the observations that (1) deletion of either CD1d or iNKT cells, or neutralization of IL-13, ameliorated colitis, and (2) activation of LPMCs by CD1d-restricted antigens induced IL-13 suggest that CD1d-restricted T cells act as effector cells in the development of Th2-mediated colitis in the oxazolone model.[31] Thus, it would appear that Th2-associated colitis is driven by iNKT cells. This is consistent with recent studies in Th2-associated inflammation of the lungs such as asthma, which is also iNKT cell mediated.[32]

Recent studies have advanced the notion that iNKT cells are protagonists in the development of Th2-associated inflammation and have provided additional insights into the regulation of these processes. Specifically, whereas the Th1-associated IBD-like inflammation characteristic of Crohn's disease is the result of DC-mediated production of IL-12, which functions as a master cytokine in driving Th1 responses, the factors presumably secreted by DCs in response to iNKT cells in Th2-associated immunopathology are less well defined.[38] One possibility is that, like the Th1 inflammation caused by DC production of IL-12, DCs secrete an IL-12–related factor that drives iNKT cells to regulate conventional T cell production of excess Th2 cytokines. This particular notion has, in fact, been investigated and a novel IL-12 p40-like molecule, Epstein-Barr virus–induced gene 3 (EBI3), has been identified as a potential factor in this effect.[39]

In addition to the IL-12 molecule, a heterodimer that consists of a p40 chain and a p35 chain,[40] recent studies have identified a variety of other IL-12 family members. These include IL-23, a heterodimer consisting of the p40 chain, IL-12, and a novel p19 chain, and IL-27, a novel heterodimer formed by EBI3 and p28.[40,41] Recent studies suggest that whereas IL-27 acts very early in the immune response to support the development of Th1 responses through interactions with an orphan cytokine receptor, WSX-1, the subsequent perpetuation of the Th1 response is mediated by IL-12, and its maintenance through effects on T memory cells by IL-23.[40–42] However, in addition to the association between EBI3 and p28, it is clear from other studies that EBI3 may associate either with itself as a homodimer or with other factors, as yet to be defined, to produce other effects such as the possible induction of Th2 responses. These effects have recently been suggested by investigations in models of mucosal inflammation, and may include a role for EBI3 in regulating Th2 pathways (in addition to Th1 pathways) through effects on the iNKT cell.[39]

Recently, EBI3-deficient mice have been generated.[39] Although these mice have normal numbers of conventional T cells and B cells and have no obvious immunopathology, they maintain a reduced number of iNKT cells in the liver as well as in the spleen in comparison with control mice, as evidenced by CD1d tetramer staining of CD3-positive cells.[39] Moreover, CD1d-restricted iNKT cells from EBI3-deficient mice secrete lower levels of the Th2 cytokine, IL-4, but not the Th1 cytokine, IFN-γ, when stimulated with a model glycolipid antigen, αGalCer.[39] Specifically, when iNKT cells were obtained from EBI3-deficient animals, low levels of IL-4 secretion were stimulated, in comparison with quantities of IFN-γ secreted, when these cells were exposed to CD1d-transfected B cells in the presence of αGalCer.[39] Similarly, serum IL-4 was lower in EBI3 mice that received αGalCer intravenously than in comparable wild-type mice.[39] In other studies, it was shown that these defects in IL-4 production by iNKT cells were due not only to the quantitative defect in iNKT cells, but presumably also to a defect in DC regulation of iNKT cell responses (unpublished observations). This defect in Th2 cytokine production by iNKT cells was clinically meaningful in that EBI3-deficient mice were protected from the development of oxazolone-associated colitis.[39] In contrast, the response of EBI3-deficient mice to TNBS was similar to that of wild-type mice.[39] These results further support the concept that iNKT cells are major drivers in the development of oxazolone-associated colitis. Moreover, the results in the EBI3-deficient environment suggest that EBI3 is a major regulator of this iNKT cell-mediated response and, ultimately, colitis.[39] This protection from pathologic injury to oxazolone in the context of EBI3 deficiency was, importantly, associated with diminution in not only clinical scores as defined by body weight loss, but also the degree of pathology and the production of IL-4, but not IFN-γ, in the EBI3-deficient mice.[39] Specifically, the absence of EBI3 was associated with decreased IL-4 production by the LPMCs and diminished nuclear translocation of GATA-3, a major nuclear transcription factor associated with Th2 cytokine production.[39]

These studies suggest that the CD1d-restricted T cell, notably the iNKT cell subset, is a major effector cell in the development of Th2-associated colitis. This, in turn, suggests that an EBI3-secreting APC, such as a DC, (1) regulates both the quantity and function of iNKT cells that may directly cause colitis through the secretion of Th2 cytokines, or (2) regulates the ability of the iNKT cell to cause cytolysis at target cells such as intestinal epithelial cells (IEC), or (3) modulates the quantities of Th2 cytokine production by conventional T cells. This contrasts with the ability of DCs, through the production of IL-12, to regulate Th1-mediated colitis and, ultimately, production of IFN-γ and TNF-α. The molecular form of EBI3 that is associated with this biologic response remains undefined. It is unlikely to be IL-27, based on the major role of this cytokine in regulating proliferation of naive T cells and promoting Th1 cytokine production.[41] It may very well be the case that the proliferative effect of IL-27 on iNKT cells may play such a role. It is possible, however, that EBI3 causes these effects in Th2 cytokine production either through its molecular association with itself as a homodimer or with other molecules, such as either the p35 chain of IL-12 or other as yet to be defined molecules. Nonetheless, these studies show how CD1d-restricted pathways can regulate mucosal inflammation and prove the biologic importance of CD1d-restricted T cells in the generation of mucosal inflammation. These concepts derived from studies in Th2-deviated animals may apply to analogous human disease, namely, ulcerative colitis (UC).[43] Increased EBI3 expression has been found in patients with active UC.[43,44] In contrast, EBI3 expression is relatively normal in Crohn's disease (CD), similar to that in normal subjects, as evidenced by several different quantitative RT PCR analyses.[43,44] This contrasts again with the production of IL-12 in humans, where the expression is increased in CD but not in UC.[45] The production of EBI3 in human UC appears also to be primarily associated with DCs. Moreover, recent preliminary studies have shown that LP-MCs from patients with CD secrete significant quantities of IFN-γ, in contrast to UC patients who secrete very high concentrations of IL-13 and IL-5 but, interestingly, not IL-4, suggesting a modified Th2 response in human UC. This production of IL-13 and IL-5 is derived from CD1d-restricted T cells and, perhaps, predominantly from the semidiverse subset of human CD1d-restricted T cells within the LP (I.F. and W.S., unpublished observation). This contrasts somewhat with studies in mouse models and deserves further investigation. Nonetheless, this does suggest that CD1d-restricted T cell pathways play a role not only in mouse models of colitis, but also in the human condition.

REGULATION OF MUCOSAL COLONIZATION BY BACTERIAL PATHOGENS

A characteristic feature of iNKT cells is their ability to secrete both Th1 and Th2 cytokines. This property is presumably due to the heterogeneity of these cells and/or the variation in glycolipid antigens to which they respond, as well as other factors, including the characteristics of costimulatory molecules on the cell surface of the stimulating APC at the time of activation. This may also account for the ability of iNKT cells to both promote and downregulate inflammation, and to participate in such disparate biologic processes as regulation of Th1 and/or Th2 inflammation.[10] Further evidence that iNKT cells and, thus, CD1d-restricted antigen presentation pathways are operative in mucosal tissues has been obtained from studying clearance of *Pseudomonas aeruginosa* from the lungs.[46]

Previous studies on the pathogenesis of *Pseudomonas* airway infection have identified alveolar macrophages and their products as well as neutrophils as important mediators of anti-*Pseudomonas* immunity.[47] Alveolar macrophages have been shown to secrete chemokines such as MIP-2 and KC, which activate neutrophils through the CXCR2 receptor.[47] Depletion of macrophages, neutralization of MIP-2, or neutralization of CXCR2 have all been shown to abrogate *Pseudomonas* infection within the the lung.[47]

The importance of CD1d-restricted T cells in these processes was recently established through experiments in a *P. aeruginosa* model lung system.[46] In these experiments, Balb/C or C57BL/6J mice, Rag-deficient mice, or CD1d-deficient mice were inoculated with a clinical strain of *P. aeruginosa* (strain D4) and the lung tissues, blood and peritoneal macrophages examined before or after different experimental manipulations, including administration of αGalCer (or the nonfunctional glycolipid analogue, αManCer) or neutralizing anti-CD1d antibody.[46] Studies showed that CD1d-deficient animals exhibited reduced clearance of *P. aeruginosa* from lung tissues.[46] Similar observations were made when wild-type Balb/C mice were treated with an anti-CD1d monoclonal antibody 24 h after inoculation with the bacterial pathogen.[46] The reduced ability of CD1d-deficient animals to clear *P. aeruginosa* was observed in mice from both a C57BL/6J or Balb/C background, consistent with the nonpolymorphic nature of CD1d. It was associated with a decrease in MIP-2 production and, as a corollary, neutrophil recruitment into bronchoalveolar lavage fluid (BALF) at 6 h after induction of the *Pseudomonas* infection.[46] These studies indicate that *P. aeruginosa* clearance is CD1d-dependent and is mediated through macrophage regulation of MIP-2 production, which results in neutrophil recruitment. In the absence of CD1d, MIP-2 production and neutrophil recruitment are abrogated.[46]

To confirm and extend these results, wild-type mice were treated with αGalCer or the nonfunctional glycolipid analogue, αManCer.[46] In these studies, activation of CD1d and NKT cell pathways by αGalCer enhanced *P. aeruginosa* clearance in the lungs.[46] Interestingly, in the setting of activation of the CD1d-restricted pathway by αGalCer, clearance of *P. aeruginosa* was shown to be independent of neutrophil recruitment into the BALF.[46] The rapid clearance of *P. aeruginosa* in these circumstances was associated with rapid recovery from pneumonia, despite evidence of tissue inflammation within hours of infection. In contrast to the rapid resolution of inflammation seen in αGalCer-treated mice, similar animals that received αManCer had very severe pneumonia by 24 h after *P. aeruginosa* infection.[46] In addition, αGalCer treatment of wild-type mice was noted to activate peritoneal macrophages within 30 min of αGalCer administration.[46] This effect was presumably based on the ability of αGalCer to activate iNKT cells, in that direct treatment of peritoneal macrophages with αGalCer did not result in increased peritoneal macrophage activation and, thus, clearance of *P. aeruginosa* through phagocytosis.[46] As shown by

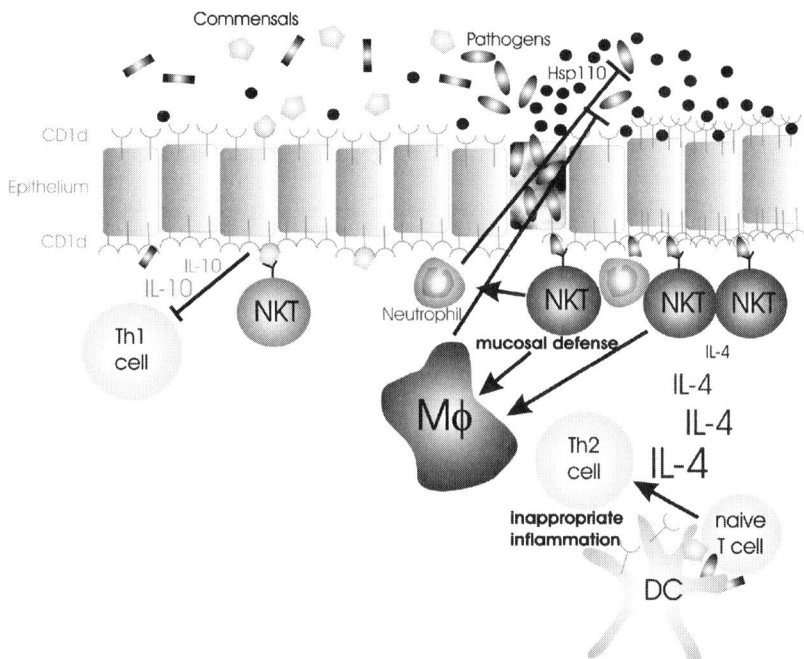

FIGURE 1. Proposed model of CD1d function in the intestinal epithelium.

CD1d tetramer staining in BALF, αGalCer also caused significant augmentation of CD1d-restricted T cells.[46] Interestingly, normal BALF contained a small number of iNKT cells that increased dramatically by almost a thousandfold after αGalCer treatment in direct proportion to the number of conventional T cells after *P. aeruginosa* instillation.[46] This was associated with high levels of IFN-γ and TNF-α in BALF after αGalCer treatment.[46] In addition, alveolar macrophages of αGalCer-treated mice had strongly enhanced phagocytosis of *P. aeruginosa* within one hour of colonization.[46]

Taken together, these studies indicate that CD1d-restricted T cells play a key role as sentinels within mucosal tissues monitoring and reacting to mucosal colonization by bacterial pathogens. Specifically, observations in CD1d-deficient animals suggest that CD1d-restricted pathways are an endogenous antimicrobial defense in the lung and perhaps other mucosal tissues. In animals given αGalCer, these observations suggest that once activated, the CD1d-restricted T cell arms the mucosal immune system by regulating macrophage phagocytosis of microbial pathogens. These studies further indicate that iNKT cells activated early during the immune response regulate downstream effector cells, such as macrophages and neutrophils, critical to mucosal defense. These observations in αGalCer-treated animals may present a paradigm for the role of mucosal immunity in preventing colonization of the intestine by *P. aeruginosa*, in the absence of alterations in either intestinal morphology or epithelial barrier function. Consistent with this, CD1d-deficient mice exhibit a decreased ability to clear mucosal colonization by *P. aeruginosa* from the intestine (E.E.S.N. & R.S.B., unpublished observations).

THE INTESTINAL EPITHELIAL CELL, A NOVEL ANTIGEN-PRESENTING CELL TYPE IN MUCOSAL TISSUES

The comments above show that CD1d and CD1d-restricted pathways are operative in both promoting inflammation and providing defense. A number of different cell populations expressing CD1d that might provide these functions are present at mucosal surfaces. These include dendritic cells, macrophages, B lymphocytes and, importantly, epithelial cells.[48] Over the past decade, increasing evidence has suggested that epithelial cells in the intestine and, it is likely, other organ systems may very well play an important role in regulating CD1d-restricted pathways. The remainder of this review will focus on evidence to support a role for CD1d-restricted antigen presentation by epithelial cells (FIG. 1).

Immunohistochemical studies have shown that CD1d is expressed by intestinal epithelial cells in both humans[49] and rodents (mice and rats).[50] In rats, CD1d protein expression occurs primarily in the villous epithelial cells, with transcription most evident in the crypt cells. Recent studies have confirmed these results in humans (personal observation, L. M.). In addition to IECs, CD1d has been found to be expressed on epithelial cells of the bile ducts and skin.[51] Additional morphologic evidence that IECs express CD1d is derived from an observation that when αGalCer is injected into mice, it localizes very specifically to IECs; such localization is not observed in CD1d-deficient animals.[35]

The biochemical expression of CD1d on IECs is unique.[4,48] Two isoforms have been identified. The major isoform is a bona fide 48-kDa glycoprotein, consistent with the known molecular weight of CD1d, that consists of a polypeptide backbone of approximately 35 kDa with four N-linked carbohydrate side chain modifications.[48,49,52] This 48-kD glycoprotein is associated with β_2-microglobulin (β2M) and has been shown by selective cell surface biotinylation to be localized to both apical and basal cell surfaces.[48] A smaller proportion of CD1d, approximately 10% or less of the CD1d associated with the IEC, has been identified as a novel, 37-kDa isoform that is not associated with β2M and is nonglycosylated.[48,53–55] This isoform of CD1d is restricted to the apical cell surface of the IEC; there is no evidence of expression on the basal cell surface. The 37-kDa isoform is characterized by a novel posttranslational modification that consists of hydroxylation of proline residues.[55] This is consistent with the observed association of CD1d with protein disulfide isomerase (PDI), an endoplasmic reticulum resident protein that itself associates with prolyl-4 hydroxylase and other ER proteins.[55]

CD1d on the IEC is functional, as neutralization of CD1d neutralizes the activation of peripheral blood T cells by mouse and human IEC lines, and freshly isolated IECs are capable of CD1d-restricted antigen presentation. This was shown by the following observations: The IEC line MODE-K, which is an immortalized but not transformed mouse cell line derived from normal mouse small intestine, exhibits dose-dependent presentation of αGalCer but not βGalCer, as interpreted by the production of murine IL-2 by the iNKT cell hybridoma, DN32.D3.[56] Similarly, freshly isolated human IECs and the human IEC line T84 transfected with human CD1d exhibit dose-dependent presentation of αGalCer to the DN32 cell line.[56] This presentation of αGalCer is CD1d restricted because it is inhibited by a monoclonal antibody specific for human CD1d.[56] The CD1d-restricted antigen presentation also exhibits polarity: when T84 cells transfected with CD1d are grown in polarized monolayers, CD1d-restricted antigen presentation is evident primarily on the basal cell surface and less so on the apical cell surface.[56] This is consistent with the normal localization of intestinal intraepithelial lymphocytes (iIEL) to this anatomic space. However, in contrast to CD1d-restricted antigen presentation by specialized APCs, IECs are incapable of processing glycolipid antigens, as shown by modeling with glycolipid analogues of αGalCer. Whereas Gal(α1–6)GalCer does not require processing for presentation on CD1d, Gal(α1–2)GalCer requires processing by lysosomal galactosidases.[57] Unlike B cells, which are capable of processing and presenting these modified glycolipid antigens, IECs cannot present such glycolipid antigens that require processing.[56] These studies indicate that CD1d on IECs is functional and capable of CD1d-restricted antigen presentation.

Altogether, it is likely that IECs are a novel, CD1d-restricted APC type. A characteristic feature of specialized APCs that express CD1d is their ability to communicate in a bidirectional fashion with the CD1d-restricted T cell through the expression of ligands on the APC, such as CD40, and counter-ligands on the CD1d-restricted T cells, such as CD40 ligand.[10,17] Such interactions lead to the expression of IL-12, for example. A similar attribute is likely to be ascribed to IECs as a CD1d-restricted APC, in view of the observation that when CD1d is ligated on the IEC, it is able to induce significant IL-10 secretion by the IEC.[58] The quantities of IL-10 that are secreted by the IEC are sufficient to abrogate the permeability defect induced by IFN-γ.[58] Because IFN-γ is a major proinflammatory cytokine secreted by iIELs and is a potent cytokine upregulating CD1d on the IEC,[59] IL-10 induced by CD1d ligation on IECs may promote the preservation of epithelial barrier function during the course of proinflammatory events, as in IBD and mucosal infections. CD1d may function together with a novel CEA-like molecule, gp180, to provide these effects.[60,61]

Finally, CD1d on IECs seems to be uniquely regulated. Very little is known about the regulation of CD1d on any cell type. However, recent studies in IECs have shed important light on IECs and perhaps other CD1d-restricted APCs. Earlier studies indicated that IFN-γ, but not other cytokines, is capable of regulating CD1d on IECs.[59] A notable characteristic of CD1d expression in the intestine is the increased expression with freshly isolated epithelial cells versus epithelial cell lines.[62] This suggests that factors are present *in vivo* that are uniquely capable of regulating CD1d expression. Recently, in testing this hypothesis, it was discovered that IEC expression of CD1d is induced by aqueous components from the normal human and murine milieu.[62] These factors were shown to be proteinaceous in character, and thus sensitive to heat denaturation, and to be of large molecular weight (>100 kDa).[62] It was shown that these components exhibited activity within the intestinal lumen on multiple IEC lines and could be identified in the luminal milieu of germ-free mice, indicating a likely eukaryotic origin, rather than a prokaryotic one. This was confirmed when purification and tryptic digest sequencing identified the biologic activity as heat shock protein (HSP)-110.[62] Indeed, HSP-110 could be identified in the luminal aqueous milieu, the biologic activity of the luminal components could be neutralized by an antibody specific for HSP-110, and recombinant HSP-110 added to epithelial cell lines was able to induce CD1d expression.[62] Perhaps most interestingly, the cellular origin of the HSP-110, as shown by immunohistochemistry, appears to be the IEC itself.[62] IECs of the human small and large intestine express significant amounts of HSP-110.[62] These studies indicate an autocrine pathway of CD1d regulation controlled by the release into the luminal milieu of HSP-110, which is able to act upon a cellular receptor, presumably apical in origin, to induce CD1d. The molecular nature of this putative apical receptor remains to be defined. However, it is well known that several heat shock proteins, including HSP-70 and HSP-90, are able to bind a variety of putative HSP receptors, potentially including CD36, CD40, and Toll-like receptors (TLR)-4 and TLR-2, among others. Ligation of these receptors induces an activation pathway that upregulates cell surface molecules and induces the secretion of cytokines such as IL-12, TNF-α, and IL-1β. Presumably, HSP-110 acts similarly on IECs and includes in its repertoire the upregulation of CD1d.[62] Thus, CD1d expression on the epithelial cell may very well be involved in the maintenance of mucosal homeostasis as well as the regulation of mucosal inflammation and antimicrobial defense through its ability to regulate and/or be regulated by HSP-110.

CONCLUSION

The MALTs in intestine and lung are uniquely responsible for managing a variety of environmental antigenic exposures, including exposure to microbial pathogens. A unique feature of these mucosal surfaces is the expression of CD1d on novel APCs, such as epithelial cells, and the presence of CD1d-restricted T cells that are operative in managing a variety of events by promoting mucosal inflammation and, at the same time, providing resistance against pathogenic microbial exposure. The relationship between CD1d-restricted pathways and a variety of different mucosal-related immunopathologies may, on the one hand, appear paradoxical. On the other hand, however, they are consistent with the pleiotropic functions of these novel antigen-presenting pathways in managing a variety of biologic processes, and with the cell types associated with these pathways. The association of CD1d-restricted pathways in promoting IBD, in particular, may illustrate their role in mucosal infections that cause inappropriate inflammation. Providing insights and defining additional molecular details of these CD1d-restricted pathways on epithelial surfaces will likely be extremely informative for understanding mucosal immunobiology and for designing novel therapeutic strategies for treating numerous clinical conditions of these organs.

REFERENCES

1. CALABI, F. & C. MILSTEIN. 1986. A novel family of human major histocompatibility complex-related genes not mapping to chromosome 6. Nature **323:** 540–543.
2. MARTIN, L.H., F. CALABI & C. MILSTEIN. 1986. Isolation of CD1 genes: a family of major histocompatibility complex-related differentiation antigens. Proc. Natl. Acad. Sci. USA **83:** 9154–9158.
3. DASCHER, C.C. & M.B. BRENNER. 2003. Evolutionary constraints on CD1 structure: insights from comparative genomic analysis. Trends Immunol. **24:** 412–418.
4. BLUMBERG, R.S., D. GERDES, A. CHOTT, et al. 1995. Structure and function of the CD1 family of MHC-like cell surface proteins. Immunol. Rev. **147:** 5–29.
5. ZENG, Z., A.R. CASTANO, B.W. SEGELKE, et al. 1997. Crystal structure of mouse CD1: An MHC-like fold with a large hydrophobic binding groove. Science **277:** 339–345.
6. ZAJONC, D.M., M.A. ELSLIGER, L. TEYTON & I.A. WILSON. 2003. Crystal structure of CD1a in complex with a sulfatide self antigen at a resolution of 2.15 A. Nat. Immunol. **4:** 808–815.
7. GUMPERZ, J.E. & M.B. BRENNER. 2001. CD1-specific T cells in microbial immunity. Curr. Opin. Immunol. **13:** 471–478.
8. KAWANO, T., J. CUI, Y. KOEZUKA, et al. 1997. CD1d-restricted and TCR-mediated activation of valpha14 NKT cells by glycosylceramides. Science **278:** 1626–1629.
9. GUMPERZ, J.E., C. ROY, A. MAKOWSKA, et al. 2000. Murine CD1d-restricted T cell recognition of cellular lipids. Immunity **12:** 211–221.
10. KRONENBERG, M. & L. GAPIN. 2002. The unconventional lifestyle of NKT cells. Nat. Rev. Immunol. **2:** 557–568.
11. LANTZ, O. & A. BENDELAC. 1994. An invariant T cell receptor alpha chain is used by a unique subset of major histocompatibility complex class I-specific CD4+ and CD4-8- T cells in mice and humans. J. Exp. Med. **180:** 1097–1106.
12. BEHAR, S.M., T.A. PODREBARAC, C.J. ROY, et al. 1999. Diverse TCRs recognize murine CD1. J. Immunol. **162:** 161–167.
13. RIESE, R.J., G.P. SHI, J. VILLADANGOS, et al. 2001. Regulation of CD1 function and NK1.1(+) T cell selection and maturation by cathepsin S. Immunity **15:** 909–919.
14. PARK, S.H., A. WEISS, K. BENLAGHA, et al. 2001. The mouse CD1d-restricted repertoire is dominated by a few autoreactive T cell receptor families. J. Exp. Med. **193:** 893–904.
15. EBERL, G., R. LEES, S.T. SMILEY, et al. 1999. Tissue-specific segregation of CD1d-dependent and CD1d-independent NK T cells. J. Immunol. **162:** 6410–6419.
16. SLIFKA, M.K., R.R. PAGARIGAN & J.L. WHITTON. 2000. NK markers are expressed on a high percentage of virus-specific CD8+ and CD4+ T cells. J. Immunol. **164:** 2009–2015.
17. WILSON, S.B. & T.L. DELOVITCH. 2003. Janus-like role of regulatory iNKT cells in autoimmune disease and tumour immunity. Nat. Rev. Immunol. **3:** 211–222.

18. GUMPERZ, J.E., S. MIYAKE, T. YAMAMURA & M.B. BRENNER. 2002. Functionally distinct subsets of CD1d-restricted natural killer T cells revealed by CD1d tetramer staining. J. Exp. Med. **195:** 625–636.
19. KADOWAKI, N., S. ANTONENKO, S. HO, et al. 2001. Distinct cytokine profiles of neonatal natural killer T cells after expansion with subsets of dendritic cells. J. Exp. Med. **193:** 1221–1226.
20. MATSUDA, J.L., L. GAPIN, J.L. BARON, et al. 2003. Mouse V alpha 14i natural killer T cells are resistant to cytokine polarization in vivo. Proc. Natl. Acad. Sci. USA **100:** 8395–8400.
21. LEE, P.T., K. BENLAGHA, L. TEYTON & A. BENDELAC. 2002. Distinct functional lineages of human V(alpha)24 natural killer T cells. J. Exp. Med. **195:** 637–641.
22. KANEKO, Y., M. HARADA, T. KAWANO, et al. 2000. Augmentation of Valpha14 NKT cell-mediated cytotoxicity by interleukin 4 in an autocrine mechanism resulting in the development of concanavalin A-induced hepatitis. J. Exp. Med. **191:** 105–114.
23. YANG, O.O., F.K. RACKE, P.T. NGUYEN, et al. 2000. CD1d on myeloid dendritic cells stimulates cytokine secretion from and cytolytic activity of V alpha 24J alpha Q T cells: a feedback mechanism for immune regulation. J. Immunol. **165:** 3756–3762.
24. STROMINGER, J.L., M.C. BYRNE & S.B. WILSON. 2003. Regulation of dendritic cell subsets by NKT cells. C. R. Biol. **326:** 1045–1048.
25. KAWAKAMI, K., N. YAMAMOTO, Y. KINJO, et al. 2003. Critical role of Valpha14+ natural killer T cells in the innate phase of host protection against *Streptococcus pneumoniae* infection. Eur. J. Immunol. **33:** 3322–3330.
26. SMILEY, S.T., M.H. KAPLAN & M.J. GRUSBY. 1997. Immunoglobulin E production in the absence of interleukin-4-secreting CD1-dependent cells. Science **275:** 977–979.
27. CHEN, Y.H., N.M. CHIU, M. MANDAL, et al. 1997. Impaired NK1+ T cell development and early IL-4 production in CD1-deficient mice. Immunity **6:** 459–467.
28. MENDIRATTA, S.K., W.D. MARTIN, S. HONG, et al. 1997. CD1d1 mutant mice are deficient in natural T cells that promptly produce IL-4. Immunity **6:** 469–477.
29. BLUMBERG, R.S., L.J. SAUBERMANN & W. STROBER. 1999. Animal models of mucosal inflammation and their relation to human inflammatory bowel disease. Curr. Opin. Immunol. **11:** 648–656.
30. STROBER, W., I.J. FUSS & R.S. BLUMBERG. 2002. The immunology of mucosal models of inflammation. Annu. Rev. Immunol. **20:** 495–549.
31. HELLER, F., I.J. FUSS, E.E. NIEUWENHUIS, et al. 2002. Oxazolone colitis, a Th2 colitis model resembling ulcerative colitis, is mediated by IL-13-producing NK-T cells. Immunity. **17:** 629–638.
32. AKBARI, O., P. STOCK, E. MEYER, et al. 2003. Essential role of NKT cells producing IL-4 and IL-13 in the development of allergen-induced airway hyperreactivity. Nat. Med. **9:** 582–588.
33. PARK, S.H., K. BENLAGHA, D. LEE, et al. 2000. Unaltered phenotype, tissue distribution and function of Valpha14(+) NKT cells in germ-free mice. Eur. J. Immunol. **30:** 620–625.
34. BLUMBERG, R.S. & W. STROBER. 2001. Prospects for research in inflammatory bowel disease. JAMA **285:** 643–647.
35. SAUBERMANN, L.J., P. BECK, Y.P. DE JONG, et al. 2000. Activation of natural killer T cells by alpha-galactosylceramide in the presence of CD1d provides protection against colitis in mice. Gastroenterology **119:** 119–128.
36. UENO, Y., M. SUMII, S. TANAKA, et al. 2003. OCH, a newly synthetic glycolipid, enhances protective immunity against mouse DSS-induced colitis in the presence of Valpha14 natural killer T cells [abstract]. Gastroenterology **124:** A-36.
37. BOIRIVANT, M., I.J. FUSS, A. CHU & W. STROBER. 1998. Oxazolone colitis: A murine model of T helper cell type 2 colitis treatable with antibodies to interleukin 4. J. Exp. Med. **188:** 1929–1939.
38. NEURATH, M.F., S. FINOTTO & L.H. GLIMCHER. 2002. The role of Th1/Th2 polarization in mucosal immunity. Nat. Med. **8:** 567–573.
39. NIEUWENHUIS, E.E., M.F. NEURATH, N. CORAZZA, et al. 2002. Disruption of T helper 2-immune responses in Epstein-Barr virus-induced gene 3-deficient mice. Proc. Natl. Acad. Sci. USA **99:** 16951–16956.

40. TRINCHIERI, G., S. PFLANZ & R.A. KASTELEIN. 2003. The IL-12 family of heterodimeric cytokines: new players in the regulation of T cell responses. Immunity. **19:** 641–644.
41. PFLANZ, S., J.C. TIMANS, J. CHEUNG, *et al.* 2002. IL-27, a heterodimeric cytokine composed of EBI3 and p28 protein, induces proliferation of naive CD4(+) T cells. Immunity **16:** 779–790.
42. PFLANZ, S., L. HIBBERT, J. MATTSON, *et al.* 2004. WSX-1 and glycoprotein 130 constitute a signal-transducing receptor for IL-27. J. Immunol. **172:** 2225–2231.
43. OMATA, F., M. BIRKENBACH, S. MATSUZAKI, *et al.* 2001. The expression of IL-12 p40 and its homologue, Epstein-Barr virus-induced gene 3, in inflammatory bowel disease. Inflamm. Bowel. Dis. **7:** 215–220.
44. CHRIST, A.D., A.C. STEVENS, H. KOEPPEN, *et al.* 1998. An interleukin 12-related cytokine is up-regulated in ulcerative colitis but not in Crohn's disease. Gastroenterology **115:** 307–313.
45. PODOLSKY, D.K. 2002. Inflammatory bowel disease. N. Engl. J. Med. **347:** 417–429.
46. NIEUWENHUIS, E.E., T. MATSUMOTO, M. EXLEY, *et al.* 2002. CD1d-dependent macrophage-mediated clearance of Pseudomonas aeruginosa from lung. Nat. Med. **8:** 588–593.
47. CHEUNG, D.O., K. HALSEY & D.P. SPEERT. 2000. Role of pulmonary alveolar macrophages in defense of the lung against *Pseudomonas aeruginosa*. Infect. Immun. **68:** 4585–4592.
48. BALK, S.P., S. BURKE, J.E. POLISCHUK, *et al.* 1994. Beta 2-microglobulin-independent MHC class Ib molecule expressed by human intestinal epithelium. Science **265:** 259–262.
49. BLUMBERG, R.S., C. TERHORST, P. BLEICHER, *et al.* 1991. Expression of a nonpolymorphic MHC class I-like molecule, CD1D, by human intestinal epithelial cells. J. Immunol. **147:** 2518–2524.
50. BLEICHER, P.A., S.P. BALK, S.J. HAGEN, *et al.* 1990. Expression of murine CD1 on gastrointestinal epithelium. Science **250:** 679–682.
51. CANCHIS, P.W., A.K. BHAN, S.B. LANDAU, *et al.* 1993. Tissue distribution of the nonpolymorphic major histocompatibility complex class I-like molecule, CD1d. Immunology **80:** 561–565.
52. BALK, S.P., P.A. BLEICHER & C. TERHORST. 1989. Isolation and characterization of a cDNA and gene coding for a fourth CD1 molecule. Proc. Natl. Acad. Sci. USA **86:** 252–256.
53. KIM, H.S., J. GARCIA, M. EXLEY, *et al.* 1999. Biochemical characterization of CD1d expression in the absence of beta2-microglobulin. J. Biol. Chem. **274:** 9289–9295.
54. SOMNAY-WADGAONKAR, K., A. NUSRAT, H.S. KIM, *et al.* 1999. Immunolocalization of CD1d in human intestinal epithelial cells and identification of a beta2-microglobulin-associated form. Int. Immunol. **11:** 383–392.
55. KIM, H.S., S.P. COLGAN, R. PITMAN, *et al.* 2000. Human CD1d associates with prolyl-4-hydroxylase during its biosynthesis. Mol. Immunol. **37:** 861–868.
56. VAN DE, W.Y., N. CORAZZA, M. ALLEZ, *et al.* 2003. Delineation of a CD1d-restricted antigen presentation pathway associated with human and mouse intestinal epithelial cells. Gastroenterology **124:** 1420–1431.
57. PRIGOZY, T.I., O. NAIDENKO, P. QASBA, *et al.* 2001. Glycolipid antigen processing for presentation by CD1d molecules. Science **291:** 664–667.
58. COLGAN, S.P., R.M. HERSHBERG, G.T. FURUTA & R.S. BLUMBERG. 1999. Ligation of intestinal epithelial CD1d induces bioactive IL-10: critical role of the cytoplasmic tail in autocrine signaling. Proc. Natl. Acad. Sci. USA **96:** 13938–13943.
59. COLGAN, S.P., V.M. MORALES, J.L. MADARA, *et al.* 1996. IFN-gamma modulates CD1d surface expression on intestinal epithelia. Am. J. Physiol. **271:** C276–C283.
60. CAMPBELL, N.A., H.S. KIM, R.S. BLUMBERG & L. MAYER. 1999. The nonclassical class I molecule CD1d associates with the novel CD8 ligand gp180 on intestinal epithelial cells. J. Biol. Chem. **274:** 26259–26265.
61. YIO, X.Y. & L. MAYER. 1997. Characterization of a 180-kDa intestinal epithelial cell membrane glycoprotein, gp180. A candidate molecule mediating t cell-epithelial cell interactions. J. Biol. Chem. **272:** 12786–12792.
62. COLGAN, S.P., R.S. PITMAN, T. NAGAISHI, *et al.* 2003. Intestinal heat shock protein 110 regulates expression of CD1d on intestinal epithelial cells. J. Clin. Invest **112:** 745–754.

Mechanisms of Oral Tolerance: Regulatory T Cells

Summary of Part III

MODERATORS: CATHRYN NAGLER-ANDERSON[a] AND WARREN STROBER[b]

[a]*Mucosal Immunology Laboratory, Massachusetts General Hospital East, Charlestown, Massachusetts 02129-4402, USA*

National Institutes of Health, Bethesda, Maryland 20892, USA

This discussion followed talks by Andrew Caton, Warren Strober, Fiona Powrie, Manuela Battaglia, and Richard Blumberg on various aspects of regulatory cell function.

Meeting organizer Lloyd Mayer kicked off the session by pointing out that regulatory cells form a large grouping. Rather than comprising just one population, there is a wide panoply of regulatory cells in the body. Mayer posed a series of questions to the panel: Is there crosstalk between different types of regulatory cells? Which are most important? Are there organ specificities? Are there unique features about the ways in which investigators are activating/isolating regulatory cells *in vitro* or *in vivo* that obscure their real function *in vivo*? Although much current interest is focused on regulatory $CD4^+CD25^+$ T cells, Mayer pointed out that depletion of these "natural" $CD4^+CD25^+$ regulatory T (Treg) cells by neonatal thymectomy leads to autoimmune gastritis, not colitis or other forms of autoimmunity, suggesting organ specificity in Treg cell generation and/or function. Mayer asked each of the session's speakers to attempt to describe their view of the particular type of regulatory cell they study in its *in vivo* context.

Manuela Battaglia said that Tr1 are antigen specific, and are induced in the periphery after chronic exposure to antigen in the presence of IL-10. Tr1 can be generated from $CD25^-$ T cells but it is not known if they talk to, or are dependent on, $CD25^+$ T cells. By contrast, $CD4^+CD25^+$ T cells are natural noninduced Treg cells that are present at birth.

Warren Strober agreed with Dr. Battaglia and emphasized that, in most instances, Tr1 cells are induced by exogenous microbial antigen and generated locally, not at the level of the thymus. By contrast, $CD4^+CD25^+$ Treg cells are directed at self-

---

Address for correspondence: Cathryn Nagler-Anderson, Ph.D., Associate Professor of Pediatrics (Immunology), Mucosal Immunology Laboratory, Massachusetts General Hospital East, Building 114, 16th St. (Mail Stop 114-3503), Charlestown, Massachusetts 02129-4402. Voice: 617-726-4161; fax: 617-726-4172.

cnagleranderson@partners.org

antigens and may, therefore, be more in the realm of innate immunity. How Treg cells are induced in the periphery is not understood. For example, is it not yet clear whether activation of particular types of dendritic cells (DCs), like the plasmacytoid DCs described by Jo Viney in an earlier session, are required for the generation of Treg cells.

Mayer pointed out that both types of Treg cells have been reported to suppress inflammation in transfer models, such that any source of a regulatory cell can shut down inflammation. Is this relevant in the "real world" where Treg cells must function locally in a specific microenvironment? Is information obtained about Treg cells induced in inflammatory sites applicable to Treg cell function in healthy individuals or in homeostatic immunoregulation? Which types of regulatory cells are most important?

Fiona Powrie cautioned that labeling one regulatory cell as more important than another may not be the central question, although this may ultimately become important therapeutically. It seems likely that multiple layers of immunoregulation are required in the unique microenvironment of the intestine. B cell responses and the penetrance of intestinal microbes may be very different in immunodeficient systems, where there may be a higher density of mature, activated DCs that move the system on in a way not seen when there are other types of immune cells that play a role in modulating the exposure of the mucosa to commensal bacteria. This may explain why depletion of just $CD4^+CD25^+$ Treg cells does not lead to IBD in mice. Powrie pointed out that individuals that lack Foxp3 (the transcription factor required for the development of $CD25^+$ Treg cells) do develop an IBD-like syndrome.

Cathryn Nagler-Anderson asked about Treg cell generation in healthy individuals. Treg cells are believed to accumulate in the GALT to prevent responsiveness to dietary antigens and commensal flora. But how do these Treg cells get to the gut and accumulate in this site?

Powrie said that it seems clear that antigen-induced IL-10–secreting Treg cells can be generated by a process like immune deviation, owing to features of antigen-presenting cells in a particular microenvironment. Distinguishing these antigen-induced Treg cells from $CD4^+CD25^+$ natural Treg cells is very difficult *in situ*. Foxp3 may be very helpful in mice in making this distinction and in examining division at the site of differentiation. Examination of Foxp3 expression in mice with intact immune systems, and comparisons to Treg cell generation and function in lymphopenic models, may help to settle questions related to the physiological relevance of different Treg cell subpopulations *in vivo*.

Andrew Caton pointed out that self-reactive cells are generated as part of the process of generating a healthy immune repertoire. The big question is whether, when these Treg cells are used in the periphery, they are reacting with self-antigens or with foreign or food antigens. The relative contributions of expansion and *de novo* generation to the accumulation of Treg cells in the GALT are not yet clear.

Howard Weiner agreed that most types of Treg cells appear to be generated in the GALT. Weiner pointed out that $CD4^+CD25^+$ T cells appear to act in a non–antigen-specific way, particularly in their ability to transfer suppression of various autoimmune diseases.

Andrew Caton countered that, although this lack of antigen specificity is true *in vitro*, it is not yet clear whether these cells are also non–antigen specific *in vivo*. TCR signaling seems to be required. In an inflammatory environment Treg cell function may be generated through cross-reactivity to self-antigens. Suppressor function may be degenerate at high doses of antigen, where TCR signaling could play a role in heightening, and then damping down, suppressive activity.

Mitchell Kronenberg commented on the interrelationships between different regulatory cell types. He saw a common theme in their recognition of self-antigen in the thymus. $CD25^+$ T cells, as well as $CD8\alpha\alpha$ IEL in the intestine, are generated through recognition of self-agonist in the thymus. NKT cells are also generated by recognition of self-agonist in the thymus. However, he pointed out that, if this theme is correct, it presents a problem. If these various types of Treg cells are united by their recognition of self-antigen, why do some become gut seeking? And why, with all the CD1 in the gut epithelium, don't we see NKT cells in gut?

Richard Blumberg said that NKT cells might be present at very low numbers in the gut. Their detection is hampered by the lack of marker for noninvariant CD1-restricted T cells. NKT cells are present at very high levels in the liver and less so in MLNs. We do not know whether CD1d presents antigen in the gut epithelium; it may also have other functions. It is also not clear whether CD1-restricted T cells in MLNs express gut-homing integrins. Strober, however, pointed out that, in his view, NKT cells do not see self-antigens. He said that the lipids that these cells recognize inherently have little variability. The presence of NK inhibitory receptors functions to ensure that we don't overreact to our own glycolipids.

Kronenberg disagreed. He contended that endogenous antigens keep NKT cells in a memory-like, semiactivated state. Phenotypically, they resemble recently activated cells. NKT cells may be viewed as "facilitators" of immunologic responses, and not classic regulatory cells per se.

Blumberg pointed out that oral tolerance is induced normally in $CD1^{-/-}$ mice, leading Allan Mowat to remark on how little we had actually heard about antigen-specific regulatory cells for a meeting on oral tolerance! Perhaps by the time we next meet we will have enough information on the generation and function of the various regulatory cell populations discussed to be able to better understand their specific roles in the induction of nonresponsiveness to dietary antigens.

Regulation of Autoreactive T Cell Function by Oral Tolerance to Self-Antigens

CAROLINE C. WHITACRE, FEI SONG, RICHARD M. WARDROP III,
KIM CAMPBELL, MELANIE McCLAIN, JACQUELINE BENSON,
ZHEN GUAN, AND INGRID GIENAPP

Department of Molecular Virology, Immunology and Medical Genetics,
Ohio State University College of Medicine and Public Health,
Columbus, Ohio 43210, USA

ABSTRACT: The oral administration of neuroantigens can suppress as well as treat autoimmune disease. Using EAE as a model system, we examined the antigen-presenting cell in oral tolerance. Expansion of dendritic cells (DCs) prior to or after disease is established facilitated oral tolerance. Transfer of oral antigen–loaded DCs resulted in protection from EAE by induction of IL-4 and IL-5 in recipient animals. LPS treatment of donors abrogated the ability of DCs to transfer protection from EAE, emphasizing the importance of the DC activation state. T cells exposed to orally administered antigen were monitored in TCR transgenic mice and found to undergo activation followed by deletion. The thymus plays a critical role in oral tolerance since thymectomized mice could not be tolerized. The thymus is postulated to be a site for deletion of autoreactive T cells or a site for generation of regulatory T cells.

KEYWORDS: experimental autoimmune encephalomyelitis; myelin basic protein, myelin proteolipid protein, myelin oligodendrocyte glycoprotein, myelin peptides

INTRODUCTION

The oral introduction of antigen has proven to be an effective means to suppress subsequent immune responses to the same antigen given parenterally, even when the antigen is administered together with strong adjuvants. This strategy for immunotherapy, termed oral tolerance, has been used successfully to suppress autoimmune disease in animals. We and others have reported that the oral administration of a variety of neuroantigens is effective in suppressing the T cell–mediated autoimmune disease experimental autoimmune encephalomyelitis (EAE) in acute as well as chronic relapsing-remitting disease models.[1,2] Oral or nasal administration of proteins, such as myelin basic protein (MBP), myelin proteolipid protein (PLP), myelin oligodendrocyte glycoprotein (MOG), as well as myelin peptides has been effective in decreasing the clinical as well as histological manifestations of EAE. The major-

---

Address for correspondence: Caroline C. Whitacre, Department of Molecular Virology, Immunology and Medical Genetics, Ohio State University College of Medicine and Public Health, Columbus, Ohio 43210, USA. Voice: 614-292-2595; fax: 614-292-9805.
  whitacre.3@osu.edu

Ann. N.Y. Acad. Sci. 1029: 172–179 (2004). © 2004 New York Academy of Sciences.
doi: 10.1196/annals.1309.033

ity of the work on mucosal tolerance in autoimmune diseases has been directed at disease prevention, and it is clear that disease prevention is more easily attainable than treatment of ongoing disease.

Several mechanisms have been proposed to explain oral tolerance, with the operative mechanism dependent upon the dose of antigen administered. Low doses of antigen have been shown to induce immune deviation as well as the generation of regulatory cells, either TGF-β–producing Th3 cells or $CD4^+CD25^+$ T cells that act to suppress encephalitogenic self-antigen–reactive T cells.[1,3] In contrast, high or dietary doses of antigen have been shown to result in anergy of antigen-reactive T cells and subsequent deletion.[2]

OBJECTIVES OF THE STUDY

In this series of studies, our aims were directed at answering three questions that represent current areas of inquiry in oral tolerance and for which answers are either not available or unclear. What is the nature of the cell presenting antigen when a self-protein is orally administered? Following the oral administration of antigen and uptake by antigen-presenting cells (APCs), what is the fate of T cells that recognize the antigen? Does the thymus play a role in the induction of oral tolerance?

ANTIGEN-PRESENTING CELLS IN ORAL TOLERANCE

There is much interest in the early events in oral tolerance induction, namely, which particular cell is responsible for presentation of orally administered antigen, as the state of the APC may play an important role in the ultimate outcome of the immune response.[4] It was shown by Alpan *et al.*[5] that mice lacking B cells and Peyer's patches (uMT mice) were still capable of being tolerized by antigen feeding. These results argued that B cells and Peyer's patch M cells did not constitute the APC important in oral tolerance. Work by Viney *et al.*,[6] however, pinpointed the dendritic cell (DC) as the likely APC following oral administration of antigen. These studies, carried out in animals treated with the Fms-like tyrosine kinase-3 ligand (Flt3L) to increase the number of DCs, showed that oral tolerance to ovalbumin (OVA) was enhanced following DC expansion. In further studies by Williamson *et al.*,[7] enhancement of oral tolerance in Flt-3L treated mice was accompanied by an enhancement in the activation of T cells specific for the fed antigen, OVA. Thus, under conditions of OVA feeding and in a nondisease setting, it is the DC and not the B cell, M cell, intestinal epithelial cell, or macrophage that has emerged as the likely APC important in oral tolerance.

We investigated the role of the DCs in presenting orally administered MBP to encephalitogenic T cells and the outcome on EAE induction. B10.PL mice were injected with the hematopoietic growth factor Flt3L daily for nine days. Control mice received mouse serum albumin (MSA) injections to control for the stress of multiple injections and any effects of the vehicle alone. At the end of the treatment period, mice were fed MBP or PBS as a vehicle control and challenged for EAE seven days after a single MBP feeding. It is notable that Flt3L treatment of B10.PL mice results in a massive increase in the numbers of CD11c + DCs (from 3- to 20-fold) in all lymphoid organs examined (spleen, peripheral lymph node, mesenteric lymph node, Peyer's patch, and lamina propria). Characterization of the expanded DC populations revealed that they are MHC Class II$^+$, yet express low levels of CD80 and CD86. The results showed that mice treated with Flt3L to expand their DCs and fed MBP were significantly protected from EAE relative to those not treated with Flt3L and fed MBP. Control groups that had expanded DCs but were not fed MBP had a pattern of disease no different from non–DC expanded mice, indicating that Flt3L treatment did not alter the clinical course of EAE. We also examined several different feeding regimens to determine whether expansion of DCs differentially affected low-dose or high-dose oral tolerance. In these experiments, Flt3L-treated or control mice were fed 0.1 mg MBP four times (low-dose tolerance), 0.5 mg MBP four times (low-dose tolerance), 2 mg MBP once (low-dose tolerance), or 20 mg MBP once (high-dose tolerance). Regardless of amount or frequency of the MBP feeding, the results were the same: mice with increased numbers of DCs were significantly protected from EAE following feeding of MBP. Cytokine levels (IL-2, IFN-γ, IL-4, IL-5) in response to *in vitro* stimulation with MBP were examined by Elispot in the 2 mg and 20 mg MBP-fed groups. In general, feeding either 2 or 20 mg MBP reduced the levels of IL-2, IL-4, and IL-5, with Flt3L treatment causing a further reduction in the fed groups. Interferon gamma levels were observed to increase with feeding, a trend that was reversed with Flt3L treatment. Thus, in maximally suppressed mice, that is, those treated with Flt3L and fed 20 mg MBP, we observed significantly decreased levels of IL-2, IFN-γ, and IL-4 relative to either nonfed mice or mice whose DCs were not expanded.

One area of increasing interest in EAE is the role of APCs in the re-presentation of self-antigen in the target organ or in the periphery. We explored the role of DCs in EAE that was already established. The primary question to be addressed was whether Flt3L treatment after disease was ongoing could enhance oral tolerance induced by MBP feeding. To conduct these experiments, B10.PL mice were immunized with MBP and adjuvants to induce EAE. After the initial acute phase of disease (during the lull between acute disease and the first relapse), daily injections of Flt3L were begun together with MBP feedings (twice per week). Flt3L injections were continued intermittently together with MBP feedings (two times per week) for seven weeks in a feeding regimen shown previously to induce tolerance.[8] The results showed that mice receiving both Flt3L and MBP orally exhibited significant suppression of EAE relative to all control groups. Particularly noteworthy, Flt3L treatment dramatically enhanced the suppression of disease induced by MBP feeding alone. Thus, DCs were shown to be the operative APC in oral tolerance induced by feeding self-antigens, and expansion of tolerogenic DCs before or even after disease induction proved to suppress EAE.

CAN DENDRITIC CELLS TRANSFER TOLERANCE AND PROTECT AGAINST EXPERIMENTAL AUTOIMMUNE ENCEPHALOMYELITIS?

The role of DCs in suppression of EAE was further explored by examining whether tolerance could be transferred with antigen-loaded DC populations. To conduct these experiments, B10.PL mice were injected daily with Flt3L for nine days to expand DC. At the end of the DC expansion period, mice were fed 100 mg MBP or OVA to load the DCs. Six hours later, DCs (whose only exposure to MBP had been an *in vivo* pulse delivered orally) were purified by positive selection (using CD11c columns) from spleen or mesenteric lymph node and transferred to naive recipients. The DC recipients were challenged for EAE one day later and clinical signs of disease monitored. The recipients of splenic as well as mesenteric lymph node DCs from mice fed MBP but not OVA were significantly protected from EAE. To determine whether the activation state of the DC played a significant role in disease protection, Flt3L-treated DC donors were fed MBP and injected with lipopolysaccharide (LPS) or not prior to harvest. Interestingly, mice receiving DCs from MBP-fed mice treated with LPS showed no protection from EAE but rather showed increased disease relative to animals only challenged for EAE. Thus, quiescent DCs loaded with the MBP self-antigen could transfer protection from EAE, but this effect was reversed when DCs were activated with LPS prior to transfer.

The cytokine environment in the recipients of antigen-pulsed DCs was characterized. Interestingly, lymph node cells draining the sites of MBP challenge, when re-exposed to MBP *in vitro*, showed enhanced numbers of IL-4– and IL-5–secreting cells and significantly greater levels of IL-10 production than other groups.

Thus, these studies showed that expansion of DCs prior to feeding and challenge resulted in enhanced protection from EAE. Importantly, expanding DCs combined with MBP feeding even after EAE has begun resulted in markedly enhanced disease suppression. The contribution of DCs toward protection was shown by transferring this purified population to naive recipients. DCs derived from the spleen or mesenteric lymph nodes of MBP-fed mice proved capable of transferring protection from EAE. This protection was accompanied by the induction of IL-4, IL-5, and IL-10 in protected recipients. The activation state of the DCs was shown to be important as quiescent antigen-loaded DCs transferred tolerance, whereas antigen-loaded DCs activated by LPS treatment did not.

THE FATE OF T CELLS EXPOSED TO ORALLY ADMINISTERED ANTIGEN

A number of studies have examined the fate of T cells specific for OVA following administration of low or high doses of antigen. The experimental systems used to follow these T cells have included direct feeding of OVA T cell receptor (TCR) transgenic (Tg) mice or transfer of Tg T cells to nontransgenic mice and feeding of the recipients. These studies have shown that oral feeding of low doses of antigen results in an alteration of cytokine profiles, with induction of Th3 cells producing high levels of TGF-β or immune deviation to Th2 cells (producing IL-4 and IL-10).[1] Recently, CD4$^+$CD25$^+$ T cells have been shown to result from feeding either low or high doses of OVA.[3] Feeding of high doses of OVA has been shown to result in clonal anergy or deletion of antigen-reactive T cells.[9,10]

We investigated the fate of T cells following feeding of MBP to MBP TCR Tg mice using a model system in which *in vivo* tolerance can be assessed by suppression of disease. The goal of these studies was to monitor MBP-specific T cells at early and late time points after MBP feeding to assess the dynamic interactions taking place between APC and T cells and to assess where the interactions were taking place. Vα4Vβ8.2 TCR Tg mice[11] were fed various doses of MBP either in a single feeding regimen or in multiple doses and the expression of the Tg TCR was assessed one day later. The results showed that feeding 100 mg MBP produced a marked decrease in transgene bearing T cells in the blood stream and in the peripheral lymphoid tissue (lymph nodes and spleen). The decrease in transgene expression was transient, as TCR expression returned by three days after feeding. Challenge of MBP-fed Tg mice for EAE showed that mice were protected when immunized one day after feeding (when transgenic TCR expression was lowest). In contrast, mice challenged three days after MBP feeding (when transgenic TCR expression had returned) were not protected. The association between lack of Tg TCR expression and disease protection prompted us to examine the T cell population from fed mice to determine the cause for the disappearance of the Tg TCR. Flow cytometric analysis revealed that upon exposure to oral antigen, antigen-reactive T cells internalize their TCR, a feature observed in both peripheral as well as mesenteric lymph nodes. This internalization of the TCR correlated with T cell activation as large increases in IL-

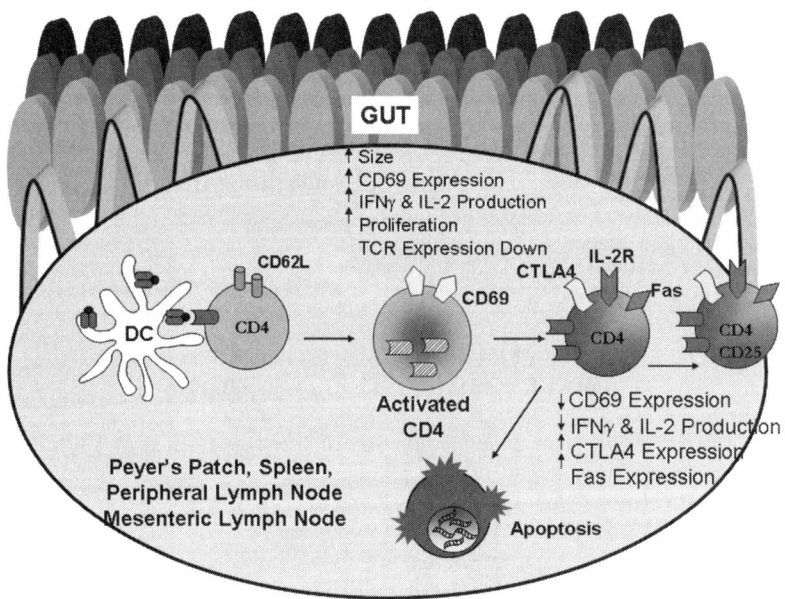

FIGURE 1. Postulated mechanism for induction of high-dose oral tolerance in Peyer's patch, spleen, peripheral lymph node, and mesenteric lymph node. Antigen is taken up by dendritic cells and presented to CD4$^+$ T cells, which then become activated (as measured by increases in size, CD69 expression, production of IFN-γ and IL-2, proliferation, and internalization of the TCR). T cell activation is decreased over the ensuing two to three days and T cells enter an anergic state. These anergic T cells go on to experience apoptosis. Alternatively, CD4$^+$CD25$^+$ cells also emerge as a result of antigen feeding, which can downregulate self-reactive immune responses.

2 and IFN-γ were also observed on one day after feeding. Analysis of the mesenteric lymph nodes at later times after feeding (days 5 to 7) showed that there were significant numbers of apoptotic cells (by TUNEL staining) in this location.

Thus, the sequence of events after feeding that takes place in the Peyer's patch, spleen, peripheral lymph node, and mesenteric lymph node, depicted in FIGURE 1, is as follows: fed antigen either absorbed through M cells in the Peyer's patch or delivered via the blood stream or lymph to the spleen or lymph node is taken up by dendritic cells and presented to antigen-specific naive T cells in these locales. These T cells undergo activation, as measured by an increase in size, increased CD69 expression, increased production of IL-2 and IFN-γ, increased proliferation, and internalization of the TCR. The activation events all occur within 1 to 2 d after antigen feeding. After 48 h, the cells lose CD69 expression, gain CTLA-4 expression, gain Fas expression, and production of IFN-γ and IL-2 is decreased. The acquisition of CD25 during the intermediate anergy stage suggests that $CD4^+CD25^+$ T cells may play a role in this form of high-dose tolerance. This intermediate stage of anergy is followed by cell apoptosis.[12]

DOES THE THYMUS PLAY A ROLE IN THE INDUCTION OF ORAL TOLERANCE?

In searching for the sites where antigen presentation and T cell activation take place following the oral administration of antigen, it became apparent that in addition to Peyer's patches, mesenteric lymph nodes, peripheral lymph nodes, and spleen, the thymus also plays an important role in oral tolerance induction. This was proven by the removal of the thymus and subsequent ablation of oral tolerance. Specifically, adult MBP TCR Tg mice were thymectomized or not (euthymic) and fed MBP or vehicle followed one day later by immunization for EAE. Euthymic mice fed MBP were protected, whereas thymectomized mice fed MBP showed clinical signs of EAE no different from nonfed controls. We hypothesized that the thymus could be serving one of two possible functions among others—as a site for deletion of possible encephalitogenic cells or as a source for T regulatory cells. Both functions proved to be true.

In assessing deletion, we examined the level of transgenic T cells in the thymus at various times after feeding. Significant decreases in the overall number of Tg T cells in the thymus was observed at days 3 and 5 after MBP feeding, which correlated with a significant increase in the number of apoptotic Tg cells in this site as measured by TUNEL staining of clonotype-bearing cells. To probe a regulatory cell function for the thymus, we focused on $CD4^+CD25^+$ cells. These cells did not increase in the thymus following MBP feeding, but we did observe an increase of $CD4^+CD25^+$ cells in the lymph node one day after feeding. At this same time, there was a large increase in mRNA for IL-4 and TGF-β in the lymph node. In the absence of a thymus, there were significantly fewer $CD4^+CD25^+$ cells generated in the lymph node, a finding that correlated with increased T cell activation. Thus, the function of the thymus in oral tolerance is to serve as a site for deletion of autoreactive cells, as well as a site for generation of regulatory T cells that are distributed to the periphery.

CONCLUSIONS AND FUTURE DIRECTIONS

It is clear that mucosal tolerance in general and oral/nasal tolerance in particular have been immensely successful in the prevention and treatment of a variety of animal disease models, including EAE, arthritis models (including those induced by collagen, adjuvants, or pristane), experimental autoimmune neuritis, experimental autoimmune thyroiditis, experimental autoimmune myasthenia gravis, diabetes, lupus, as well as transplantation.[13] However, when clinical trials have been conducted in MS, rheumatoid arthritis, uveoretinitis, diabetes, allergy, Crohn's disease, ulcerative colitis or chronic hepatitis, the results have been largely negative, with oral antigen–treated groups showing no significant improvement in outcome relative to placebo-treated controls. Given the success in animal models, why has oral tolerance not worked better when applied to the treatment of human disease? Theories have included suggestions that oral tolerance is not inducible in humans, the wrong antigens have been administered, the wrong dose of antigens have been used, or the timing of antigen administration has been wrong. It is clear that oral tolerance is inducible in humans, at least at the T cell level when novel antigens have been orally administered.[14] Perhaps, however, the answer lies in the difficulty inherent in reversing an ongoing chronic and aggressive immune response, active in a proinflammatory environment. Success in reversing such a strong response will likely take a combination of approaches, such as cytotoxic/depletion regimens to stop ongoing damage, followed by mucosal tolerance approaches to shape the returning repertoire. It will be key in the future to focus on approaches and models to treat ongoing autoimmune disease and to thoroughly assess in humans the ability to intervene in an ongoing immune response using mucosal tolerance approaches.

ACKNOWLEDGMENTS

The authors would like to acknowledge Immunex Corporation (now Amgen) for supplying Flt3L for these studies. This work was supported by NIH Grants AI35960 and AI43376, and National Multiple Sclerosis Society Grants RG2302, RG3272, and PP0904.

REFERENCES

1. FARIA, A.M. & H.L. WEINER. 1999. Oral tolerance: Mechanisms and therapeutic applications. Adv. Immunol. **73:** 153–264.
2. WHITACRE, C.C. & K.A. CAMPBELL. 2000. Oral tolerance as a treatment modality for autoimmune diseases. *In* Current Directions in Autoimmunity, Vol. 2: Biologic and Gene Therapy of Autoimmune Disease. C.G. Fathman, Ed.: 1–23. S. Karger AG. Basel.
3. ZHANG X., L. IZIKSON, I. LIU & H.L. WEINER. 2001. Activation of CD25(+)CD4(+) regulatory cells by oral antigen administration. J. Immunol. **167:** 4245–4253.
4. WARDROP, R.M. & C.C. WHITACRE. 1999. Oral tolerance in the treatment of inflammatory autoimmune diseases. Inflamm. Res. **48:** 106–119.
5. ALPAN, O., G. RUDOMEN & P. MATZINGER. 2001. The role of dendritic cells, B cells and M cells in gut-oriented immune responses. J. Immunol. **166:** 4843–4852.
6. VINEY, J.L., A.M. MOWAT, J.M. O'MALLY, *et al.* 1998. Expanding dendritic cells in vivo enhaces the induction of oral tolerance. J. Immunol. **160:** 5815–5825.

7. WILLIAMSON, E., J.N. O'MALLY & J.L. VINEY. 1999. Visualizing the T-cell response elicited by oral administration of soluble protein antigen. Immunol. **97:** 565–572.
8. BENSON, J.M., S.S. STUCKMAN, K.L. COX, *et al.* 1999. Oral administration of MBP is superior to myelin in suppressing established relapsing experimental autoimmune encephalomyelitis. J. Immunol. **162:** 6247–6254.
9. SUN, J., B. DIRDEN-KRAMER, K. ITO, *et al.* 1999. Antigen-specific T cell activation and proliferation during oral tolerance induction. J. Immunol. **162:** 5868–5875.
10. CHEN, Y., J. INOBE, F. MARKS, *et al.* 1995. Peripheral deletion of antigen-reactive T cells in oral tolerance. Nature **376:** 177–180.
11. LAFAILLE, J.J., K. NAGASHIMA, M. KATSUKI & S. TONEGAWA. 1994. High incidence of spontaneous EAE in immunodficient anti-MP TCR Tg mice. Cell **78:** 399–408.
12. BENSON, J.M., Z. GUAN, K.A. CAMPBELL, *et al.* 2000. T cell activation and receptor downmodulation precede deletion induced by orally administered antigen. J. Clin. Invest. **106:** 1031–1038.
13. Wu, H.Y. & H.L. Weiner. 2003. Oral tolerance. Immunol. Res. **28:** 265–284.
14. HUSBY, S., J. MESTECKY, Z. MOLDOVEANU, *et al.* 1994. Oral tolerance in humans. T cell but not B cell tolerance after antigen feeding. J. Immunol. **152:** 4663–4670.

Natural and Induced Regulatory T Cells

EMMA J. O'NEILL,[a] ANETTE SUNDSTEDT,[b] GRAZIELLA MAZZA,
KIRSTY S. NICOLSON, MARY PONSFORD, LESLIE SAURER,
HEATHER STREETER, STEVE ANDERTON,[c] AND DAVID C. WRAITH

Department of Pathology and Microbiology, University of Bristol Medical School, University Walk, Bristol BS8 1TD, United Kingdom

ABSTRACT: Mucosal antigen delivery can induce tolerance, as shown by suppression of subsequent responses to antigen. Our previous work showed that both intranasal and oral routes of antigen delivery were effective but indicated that the intranasal route might be more reliable. Intranasal peptide administration induced cells that could mediate bystander suppression of responses to associated antigenic epitopes. Here, we discuss further investigation into the nature of intranasal, peptide-induced tolerance. Cells from mice treated with intranasal peptide became anergic and shut down secretion of cytokines such as IL-2, but still secreted IL-10. This latter cytokine was required for suppression of immune responses *in vivo* even though suppression of responses *in vitro* was IL-10 independent. Intranasal peptide induced a subset of $CD25^-$, $CTLA-4^+$ regulatory cells that suppressed naive cell function *in vitro* and *in vivo*. We provide evidence that these cells arise from $CD25^-$ precursors and differentiate independently from natural $CD25^+$ regulatory cells. IL-10–secreting regulatory cells are also found in the peripheral blood of humans and can be induced by soluble peptide administration. This route of tolerance induction offers promise as a means of antigen-specific immunotherapy of allergic and autoimmune conditions in humans.

INTRODUCTION

The immune system is designed to combat infection. The innate immune system was clearly sufficient to ensure the survival of invertebrates, as evidenced by their successful colonization of countless environments. Vertebrates have been forced, however, to evolve an increasingly complex immune system. With the evolution of an adaptive immune system, the challenge of discriminating between self and nonself antigens has arisen. For much of the modern era of cellular immunology, scientists were comfortable with the concept of a balance between immune effector and

---

[a]Current address: Department of Small Animal Clinical Studies, Veterinary College, University College Dublin, Ireland.
[b]Current address: Active Biotech Research, P.O. Box 724, S.-22007, Lund, Sweden.
[c]Current address: Institute of Cell, Animal and Population Biology, University of Edinburgh, King's Buildings, West Mains Road, Edinburgh EH9 3JT, Scotland.
Address for correspondence: D.C. Wraith, Department of Pathology and Microbiology, University of Bristol Medical School, University Walk, Bristol BS8 1TD, UK. Voice: +44-117-928-7581; fax: +44-117-928-7896.
  d.c.wraith@bris.ac.uk

Ann. N.Y. Acad. Sci. 1029: 180–192 (2004). © 2004 New York Academy of Sciences.
doi: 10.1196/annals.1309.034

immune suppressor mechanisms.[1] This belief fell from favor in the 1980s, largely through lack of molecular evidence to support the existence of suppressor cells. The concept of immune regulation and suppression has been firmly re-established, however, thanks to work arising from many laboratories, including those of Mason,[2] Sakaguchi,[3] and Shevach.[4] It is now widely acknowledged that regulatory/suppressor CD4+ cells serve to maintain homeostasis in the immune system and to limit autoimmune pathology.[5,6] Among the naturally occurring regulatory T cells, most studies have focused on CD4+, CD25+ cells. These cells make up 5 to 10% of the adult CD4 T cell population and most probably arise in the thymus.[7] Certainly, neonatal thymectomy in mice, before these cells are generated in significant numbers, inevitably results in widespread autoimmune pathology.[8] Healthy mice, therefore, normally maintain a balance between naive effector cells and regulatory subsets, including CD25+ and additional less well characterized subsets of regulatory T cells. Similar regulatory subsets undoubtedly exist in humans.[9]

Physicians and scientists have known for at least 150 years that mucosal encounters with antigen can generate a state of tolerance.[10] The fact that the phenomenon of mucosal tolerance can be transferred from tolerant to naive animals by transfer of T cells indicates that regulatory T cells not only exist naturally but that they may also be induced by antigen administration.[11] The study of experimental models has revealed that induced regulatory cells fall into various categories or subsets. The nature of αβ regulatory T cells depends on the nature of the antigen, the route of antigen administration, and the type of immune response being measured[12] (TABLE 1). Thus, cells secreting Th2 cytokines can inhibit Th1 cell responses and vice versa.[13] Furthermore, mucosal administration of protein antigen tends to elicit transforming growth factor beta–secreting Th3 cells,[14] whereas similar administration of peptide antigen leads to generation of IL-10–secreting regulatory T cells.[15] IL-10–secreting regulatory cells have been induced by repeated administration of either peptide antigen[16] or bacterial superantigen.[17,18] Homogenous populations of these cells can also be generated *in vitro* by repeated activation of naive cells in the presence of either anti-inflammatory cytokines, such as IL-10,[19] or drugs, including dexamethasone and vitamin D3.[20] Here, we describe the use of peptide antigens to elicit mucosal tolerance. We discuss the design of tolerogenic peptides, their mode of action, the nature of the resulting regulatory cells, and evidence that such cells exist in humans.

TABLE 1. T cells induced to protect against inflammatory conditions

Regulatory Subset	Th2	Th3	IL-10–secreting regulatory T cells
How Raised	Antigen *in vivo*	Mucosal Antigen	Antigen *in vitro* with IL-10 or dexamethasone and vitamin D3. Repeated superantigen or peptide *in vivo*.
Mechanism	IL-4	TGF-β	IL-10
Reference	Liblau et al.[13]	Faria & Weiner[14]	Groux et al.[30] Sundstedt et al.[17] Miller et al.[18] Burkhart et al.[16]

TABLE 2. Hierarchy of intranasal tolerance induction in H-2^{uxs} f1 mouse

Tolerogenic Peptide[a]	Linked Suppression[b]	Bystander Suppression[b]
MBP Ac1-9[4Y]	++	–
MBP 89–101	–	–
PLP 139–151	++	++

[a]The tolerogenic peptide was administered intranasally prior to antigenic challenge with intact myelin.
[b]Mice were challenged with intact myelin, and then the response to individual peptides was measured from draining lymph nodes.

DESIGNING PEPTIDES FOR TOLERANCE INDUCTION

We have used the H-2^{uxs} f1 mouse model of experimental autoimmune encephalomyelitis (EAE) to study the requirements for peptide-induced tolerance. Peptides from myelin basic protein (MBP) (Ac1–9, 35–47, and 89–101) and proteolipid protein (PLP) (139–151 and 178–191) are all encephalitogenic in this f1 strain, allowing us to investigate whether peptides can induce linked (MBP ↔ MBP) or bystander (MBP ↔ PLP) suppression. Intranasal administration of the N-terminal peptide of MBP (Ac1–9) or its high-affinity analogue (Ac1–9[4Y]) induced suppression of the response to both Ac1–9 and 89–101 (linked suppression)[21] (TABLE 2). This peptide failed, however, to mediate bystander suppression of the response to PLP 139–151. Intranasal administration of PLP 139–151, on the other hand, suppressed subsequent responses to T cell epitopes from MBP following immunization with whole myelin. This raises the question of why one T cell epitope should mediate linked and another bystander suppression. We believe that this relates to the precursor frequency of different T cell populations. It is fair to assume that there will be a lower limit in terms of the ratio at which regulatory cells will mediate suppression. A number of studies have indicated that regulatory cells can function at a ratio as low as 1:16 naive cells, at least *in vitro*. The higher the frequency of regulatory cells, the more likely they are to mediate bystander suppression of naive cells. There is evidence that precursor cells specific for 139–151 exist in H-2^s mice at between 10- and 100-fold higher frequency when compared with precursors specific for epitopes from myelin basic protein (V. Kuchroo and S. Miller, personal communication). As such, tolerant MBP-specific cells may not be frequent enough to suppress the response to 139–151. If all 139–151 specific precursors were rendered tolerant, they would be likely to suppress the less frequent MBP-specific cells. This might well explain why it is difficult for MBP-specific regulatory cells to suppress the response to 139–151 in the H-2^{uxs} f1 mouse model.

Of all the peptides tested in the f1 mouse model, only 89–101 failed to induce either linked or bystander suppression.[21] We speculated that this might relate to the complexity of this region of the protein, as it is believed to contain a number of T cell epitopes.[22] We therefore dissected this region of MBP and identified at least three clearly distinct epitopes cross-reacting with 89–101[23] (FIG. 1). Most notably, the response to the 89–101 peptide itself was dominated by the response to a cryptic epitope. That is, the majority of T cells elicited by immunization with the 89–101 epitope responded to the 92–98 core region of the peptide. These T cells did not,

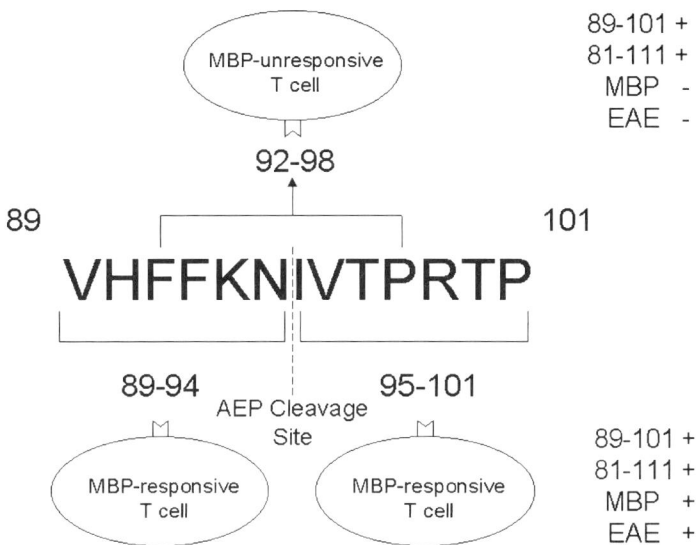

FIGURE 1. Characteristics of T cell epitopes within MBP 89–101. The 89–101 region of MBP contains three distinct epitopes. The core residues of the N- and C-terminal peptides include residues 89–94 and 95–101, respectively. T cells specific for these epitopes also respond to MBP, indicating that they recognize naturally processed epitopes. T cell clones specific for these epitopes induce EAE on passive transfer into naive mice. The core residues of the third epitope include residues 92–98. This is a cryptic epitope, as T cells specific for this region respond to peptide but not protein; these T cells are unable to respond to the naturally processed epitopes of MBP. T cell clones specific for 92–98 fail to induce EAE. The 92–98 epitope is dominant for both T cell priming and tolerance induction, because the majority of T cells from mice primed with 89–101 respond to this epitope alone. Furthermore, intranasal tolerance induction with 89–101 leads to tolerance among T cells specific for 92–98, but not cells specific for the N- and C-terminal epitopes. As a result, 89–101 fails to suppress the induction of EAE in H-2^s mice.

however, respond to the naturally processed epitopes of MBP from this region. T cells responding to naturally processed epitopes mapped to peptides 89–94 and 95–101 representing the N- and C-terminal flanking regions of the 89–101 peptide. Why should the 92–98 region of MBP contain a dominant cryptic epitope? Recent studies have revealed that the proteolytic enzyme asparagine endopeptidase cleaves a crucial peptide (Asn–Ile) bond within this peptide.[24] Most importantly, while 89–101 was capable of inducing tolerance to itself, it was unable to induce tolerance to the naturally processed epitopes. On the other hand, 87–96 induced tolerance both to itself and MBP.[23] These results show that peptide epitopes must mimic naturally processed epitopes in order to induce tolerance to self-antigens. Peptides that stimulate encephalitogenic T cell clones *in vitro* may not induce tolerance if they also contain a dominant cryptic epitope.

TABLE 3. Effect of intranasal peptide (MOG 35-55) on induction of EAE in C57BL/6 (B6) and B6.IL-10$^{-/-}$ mice

Mouse	Intranasal Treatment	Clinical Disease
B6	PBS	+++
B6	MOG 35–55	–
B6.IL-10$^{-/-}$	PBS	+++
B6.IL-10$^{-/-}$	MOG 35–55	+++

NOTE: This table shows EAE induction for groups of IL-10 knockout and wild-type C57Bl/6 mice treated with intranasal peptide compared to control mice treated with PBS alone. Each experiment comprised two main groups of age-matched female mice: one group, C57Bl/6 wild-type mice, and the other, C57Bl/6 IL-10$^{-/-}$ mice. Soluble MOG 35–55 peptide was administered on three occasions (days -7, -5, -3) to the intranasal group. The control mice received only PBS on three occasions. Disease was induced on day 0 in all groups with MOG 35–55, CFA, and Pertussis toxin (days 0 and 2). EAE was scored daily in individual mice. This table shows that although clear disease protection was provided by intranasal peptide in the wild-type mice, this effect was lost in the IL-10 knockout mice.

THE MECHANISM OF PEPTIDE-INDUCED REGULATORY T CELL FUNCTION

Previous work from our laboratory demonstrated that intranasal administration of peptide could induce linked and bystander suppression.[21,25–27] The role of the cytokine IL-10 was indicated by the fact that prior intranasal administration of peptide 35–55 of myelin oligodendrocyte glycoprotein suppressed the subsequent induction of autoimmune encephalomyelitis in the B6 mouse, but failed to have the same effect in IL-10 knockout B6 mice[28] (TABLE 3).

The role of IL-10 was further investigated in the Tg4 transgenic mouse. This mouse is transgenic for the T cell receptor specific for the Ac1–9 peptide of MBP.[29] Repeated intranasal administration of Ac1–9[4Y] rendered the Tg4 mouse resistant to the induction of EAE.[16] This required the administration of at least five doses of peptide. T cells from mice treated with soluble peptide were profoundly unresponsive *in vitro* (FIG. 2). This effect was due to CD4 T cells from tolerant mice and was reproducible, whether or not antigen-presenting cells (CD4$^-$ cells) were derived from tolerant mice. Furthermore, the cells failed to secrete IL-2, IL-4, or interferon gamma in response to antigen.[16] They did, however, secrete IL-10. The phenotype of these cells, therefore, resembles Tr1 cells grown *in vitro* in the presence of IL-10[30] and, similarly, regulatory T cells grown in the presence of vitamin D3 and dexamethasone.[20] We therefore predicted that these cells would suppress the response of naive T cells *in vitro*. This was confirmed (FIG. 2) and the mechanism investigated further.[31] Peptide-induced regulatory cells suppressed naive CD4$^+$ T cell proliferation *in vitro*. This effect was cell–cell contact dependent and could not be inhibited *in vitro* by addition of an antibody directed to the IL-10 receptor.[31] In this way, peptide-induced regulatory cells resemble natural CD25$^+$ cells that also suppress in a cell–cell contact and cytokine independent fashion *in vitro*.[4] The role of IL-10 was further investigated through the use of a proliferation assay *in vivo*. Carboxy-fluorescein acetate, succinimidyl ester (CFSE)-labeled Tg4 cells transferred into naive mice proliferated rapidly when challenged with antigen (FIG. 3). Almost 90% of cells underwent cell division in the first 48 hours. Cells transferred into tolerant Tg4 mice were suppressed, with only some 40% of cells proliferating. Importantly, however, suppression of proliferation was reversed by co-administration of an anti–IL-10 receptor antibody.[31] These results are important, because they show a divergence between the *in vitro* and *in vivo* models. The *in vivo* suppression of responses was IL-10 dependent, whereas *in vitro* suppression was completely IL-10 independent. Similarly, Belkaid and colleagues have used a cell transfer model to study the role of regulatory T cells in the persistence of infection and immunity to *Leishmania major*.[32] They were able to demonstrate that CD25$^+$ cells, derived from skin lesions of

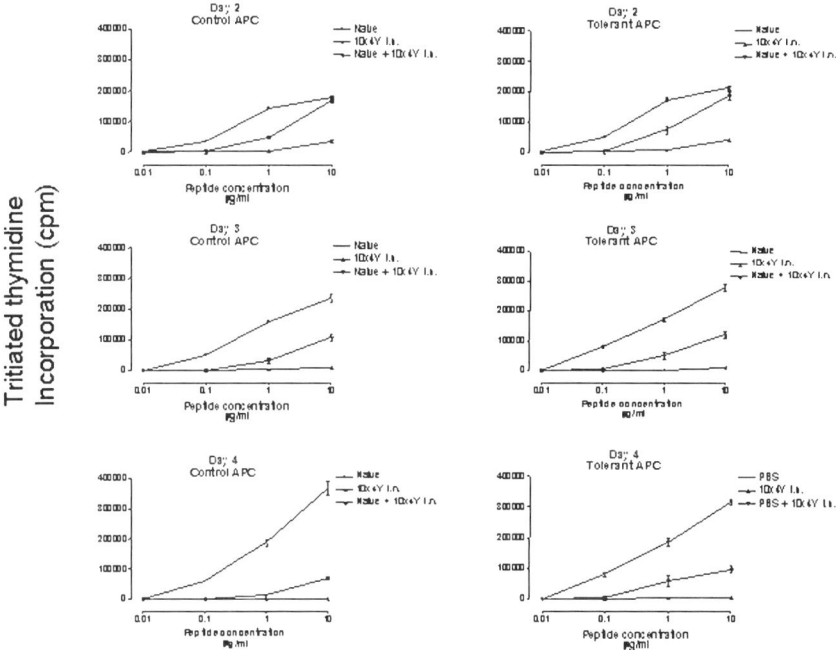

FIGURE 2. Peptide-induced regulatory cells from Tg4 mice suppress naive cell proliferation *in vitro*. This figure shows two proliferation time courses of CD4$^+$ T cells from Tg4 mice cultured *in vitro* with either naive, control APC (*left*), or tolerant APC (*right*). Two mouse treatment groups were established: intranasal peptide-treated, tolerant mice (10×4Y in) that received ten intranasal doses of Ac1–9[4Y], and PBS-treated, control mice (naive). Splenocytes from each treatment group were harvested three days after the final treatment, and CD4$^+$ T cells were obtained by positive selection using the MACS system (Milltenyi-Biotech). CD4$^+$ T cells were cultured at 5×10^4 cells per well *in vitro* in round-bottomed wells along with 1×10^5 cells per well of the CD4$^-$ fraction as APC and varying concentrations of Ac1–9[4K]. An additional group was established (naive + 10×4Y in) in which 5 × 10^4 tolerant CD4$^+$ T cells and 5 × 10^4 naive CD4$^+$ T cells were cocultured under the same conditions. Cultures were pulsed with ^{3}H-thymidine at 24-h intervals to allow measurement of cell proliferation. The lines show the mean proliferative response (±SEM) for each cell population. Inhibition of naive CD4$^+$ T cell proliferation when cocultured with tolerant cells is clearly demonstrated. Equivalent responses occurred with naive and tolerant APC.

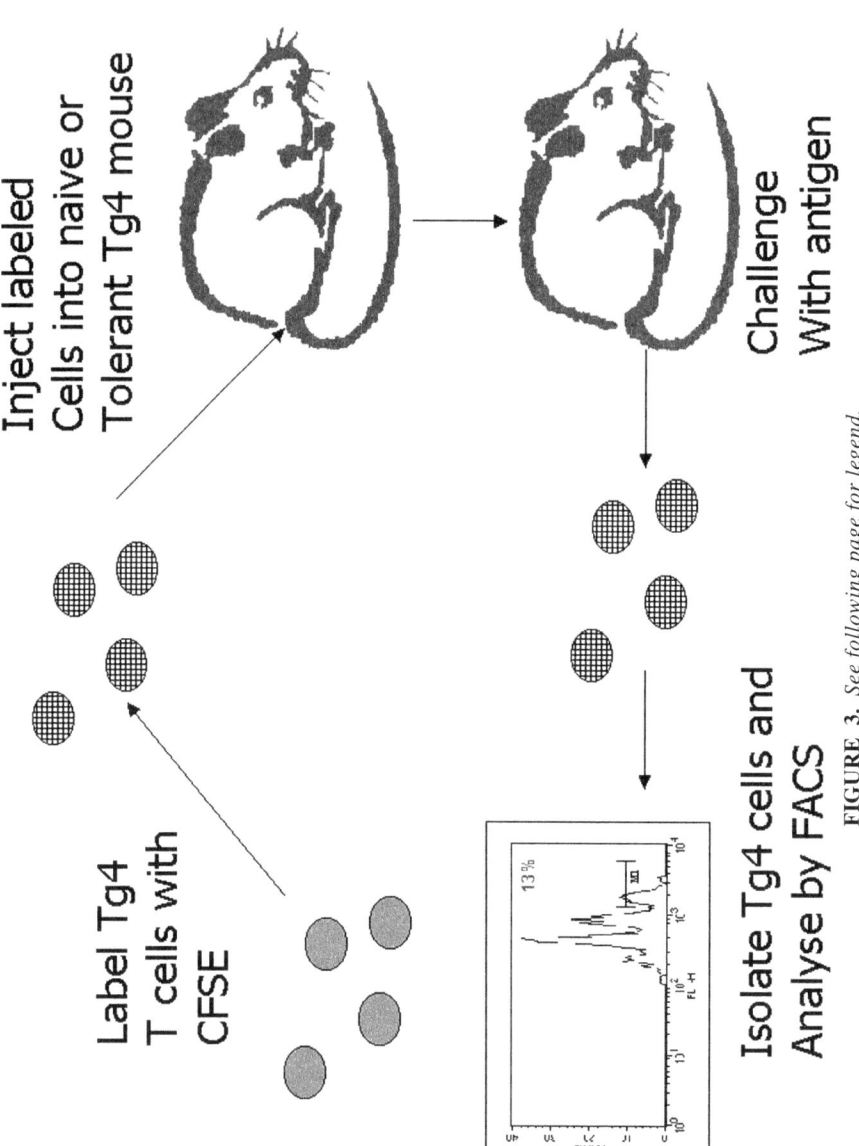

FIGURE 3. *See following page for legend.*

persistently infected mice, suppress the proliferation of naive T cells to antigen *in vitro* and were IL-10 independent. Interestingly, the lesion-derived $CD25^+$ cells secreted high levels of IL-10 in response to antigen. Belkaid *et al.* therefore tested whether such $CD25^+$ cells, derived from wild-type or IL-10 deficient mice, would mediate suppression *in vivo*. They found that suppression of immunity to *Leishmania major*, resulting in maintenance of a persistent infection, was dependent on the presence of $CD25^+$ cells and that these cells needed to be able to produce IL-10 in order to function. These two independent models, therefore, demonstrate that IL-10 may play a more important role in the function of regulatory T cells *in vivo* than the associated *in vitro* studies might lead us to believe. The most likely explanation is that IL-10 controls the expression of costimulatory molecules on antigen-presenting cells (APC).

Analysis of the cell surface phenotype of peptide-induced regulatory cells revealed that the cells are $CTLA-4^+$ and predominantly $CD25^-$.[31] We therefore investigated the relationship between these cells and natural $CD25^+$ cells. $CD25^+$ cells, purified by flow cytometry, suppressed naive T cell responses at least as well as peptide-induced regulatory cells. The possibility, therefore, remained that suppression by peptide-induced regulatory cells was mediated by cells from the $CD25^+$ population, despite their low frequency in tolerant mice. This possibility was excluded by two distinct approaches. First, a population of peptide-induced tolerant cells was enriched for $CD25^-$ cells by negative selection of $CD25^+$ cells. The $CD25^-$ population was equally suppressive when compared with the mixed population, implying that $CD25^+$ cells are not required for the suppressive phenotype of peptide-induced regulatory cells (FIG. 4). It could be, however, that $CD25^+$ cells are nevertheless required for the generation of regulatory T cells *in vivo*. This was investigated in recombination-activating gene (RAG)-deficient Tg4 mice that fail to generate $CD25^+$ cells. As previously noted, RAG-deficient mice expressing T cell receptors specific for CNS antigens suffer spontaneous autoimmune disease.[33] RAG-deficient Tg4 mice were, however, equally susceptible to peptide-induced tolerance. Furthermore, the resulting tolerant cells were potent IL-10 secretors and could suppress proliferation both *in vitro* and *in vivo* (data not shown). These results clearly demonstrate that $CD25^+$ cells are not required for either the function of peptide-induced regulatory cells or their induction *in vivo*. The peptide-induced regulatory cells are evidently a distinct subset of cells derived from naive $CD4^+$ precursors (FIG. 5).

FIGURE 3. Measuring T cell proliferation *in vivo* using CFSE-stained Tg4 cells. Splenocytes obtained from naive Tg4 mice were incubated *in vitro* with CFSE for 30 min before being washed and then adoptively transferred on day zero into either naive or peptide-treated, tolerant recipients by iv injection (5×10^6 cells in 0.25 mL PBS). On day one post–cell transfer, the recipient mice were challenged with a single dose of Ac1–9[4Y] intranasally. A single mouse in each group was retained without peptide treatment to allow determination of the baseline premitosis cell-CFSE levels. The spleens from these recipient mice were harvested on day three, disaggregated to yield a single-cell suspension and counter-stained with anti–CD4-tricolor antibody. FACS analysis of these splenocyte populations was performed gating on the $CD4^+$-tricolor, CFSE double-positive cells. In total, 10,000 events were counted for each sample. A histogram of Fl-3 positive cells within the double-positive gated area of cells transferred to naive mice and challenged with antigen is shown as an example.

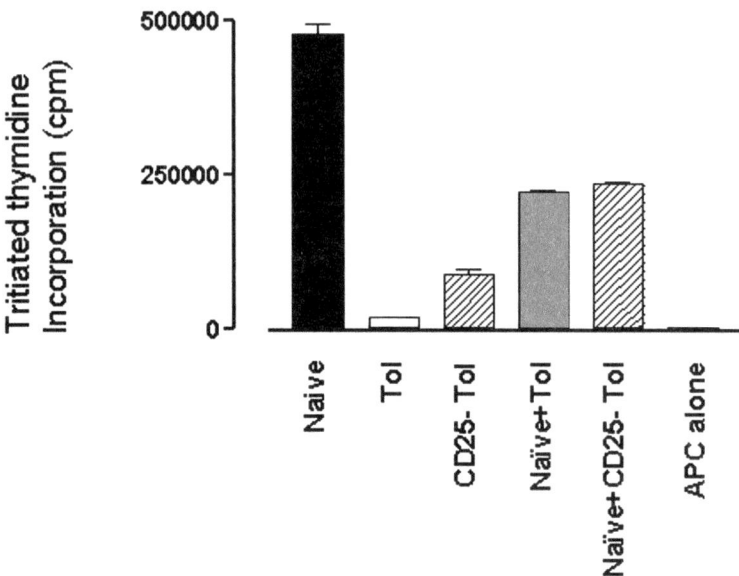

FIGURE 4. The role of CD25$^+$ cells in coculture suppression of naive CD4$^+$ T cells by peptide-induced tolerant T cells. This figure shows the proliferative responses of naive CD4$^+$ T cells from Tg4 mice cocultured *in vitro* with tolerant CD4$^+$ T cells depleted of CD25$^+$ cells. Two mouse treatment groups were established; intranasally treated, tolerant mice that received 10 intranasal doses of Ac1-9[4Y], and naive control mice. Splenocytes from each treatment group were harvested three days after the final treatment, and CD25$^+$ cells were depleted from half of the tolerant cell population by positive selection, using the MACS system (Milltenyi-Biotech). Following this, CD4$^+$ T cells were obtained by positive selection, again employing the MACS system. The remainder of the tolerant cell population underwent no initial depletion process. Tolerant or naive CD4$^+$ T cells were cultured at 5×10^4 cells per well *in vitro* in round-bottomed wells together with 1×10^5 cells per well of the CD4$^-$ fraction as APC and 10 mg/mL of Ac1-9[4K]. An additional group was established in which 5×10^4 tolerant CD4$^+$ T cells and 5×10^4 naive CD4$^+$ T cells were cocultured under the same conditions. In addition, the tolerant CD25$^-$ population was cultured alone or in a coculture with naive cells. The results gained from APC cultured alone are also shown. On day 3 of culture, cultures were pulsed with ^{3}H-thymidine to allow measurement cell proliferation. The *bars* depict the mean proliferative response for each group ($\pm$SEM). This figure demonstrates that equivalent levels of coculture inhibition were apparent in the CD25-depleted tolerant cocultures compared with the CD25-containing cocultures.

HUMAN REGULATORY T CELLS

Evidence to date suggests that human IL-10–secreting cells can be generated *in vitro* from CD25$^-$ cells, implying that human CD25$^+$, CD4$^+$ T cells are also distinct from IL-10 producing regulatory cells.[34] Recently, we have investigated whether IL-10–secreting cells exist in humans and have begun to investigate their phenotype. IL-10–secreting cells were isolated by selective magnetic bead separation (Miltenyi Biotech) and were shown to be weak IL-10 secretors. These cells were predominantly

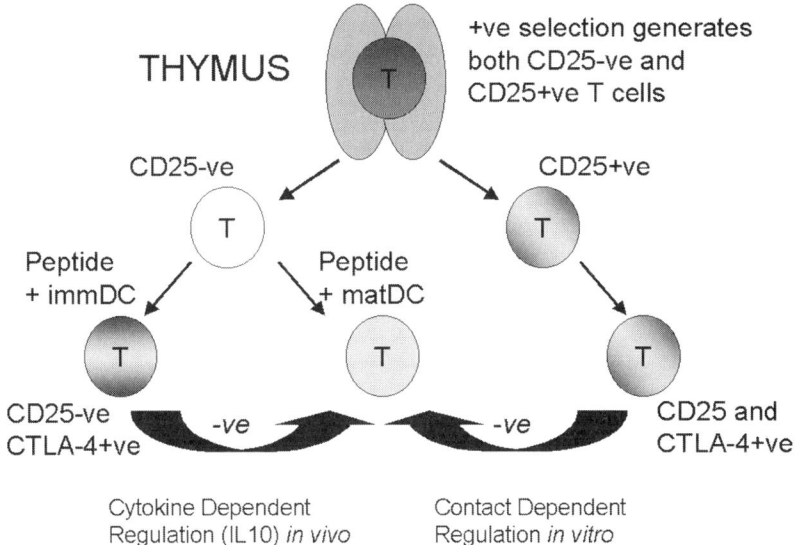

FIGURE 5. Regulatory cells induced by intranasal peptide are distinct from the $CD25^+$ subset of regulatory cells. Both $CD25^-$ and $CD25^+$ cells are generated in the thymus. $CD25^+$ cells are unique in that they constitutively express CTLA-4 and CD25. Naive cells can differentiate into various subsets of $CD4^+$ cells, depending on the nature of the antigen and the site of antigen presentation. Previous work has shown that antigen-presenting cells, such as immature dendritic cells from mice treated with intranasal peptide, can present the peptide to naive T cells.[42] Our working hypothesis is that naive T cells receive a suboptimal signal from immature/semimature dendritic cells and become anergic after transient activation. The anergic cells fail to secrete cytokines, such as IL-2, but retain the capacity to secrete IL-10 and differentiate into $CD25^-$, $CTLA-4^+$ regulatory cells.

$CTLA-4^+$ and $CD25^-$. Most importantly, these cells were potent suppressors of naive cell proliferation *in vitro*. The cells could be isolated from peripheral blood without antigenic challenge *in vitro* and were potent suppressors of immune responses to both self (MBP) and foreign (PPD) antigens.

The analysis of regulatory cells in mouse and humans has revealed an increasing variety of cell types. Much work has focused on $CD25^+$ cells. These cells are generated during thymic development in mice, although there is evidence that similar cells may be generated from mature lymphocytes in humans.[35] Transfer experiments in mice have revealed that both $CD25^+$ and $CD25^-$ populations contain regulatory cells.[36] As yet, however, little attention has been given to the natural $CD25^-$ population of cells. We have recently focused on cells of this type in humans. An important observation is that the majority of spontaneously IL-10–secreting cells in human peripheral blood are $CTLA-4^+$, $CD25^-$ cells. These cells surprisingly constitute the majority of $CTLA-4^+$ expressing cells found in peripheral blood and are highly effective suppressor cells *in vitro*. The predominance of this subset of cells in adult peripheral blood suggests that these cells play at least as important a role in immune regulation as the CTLA-4$^+$, CD25$^+$ population. It will be interesting to analyze the properties of these cells in patients suffering from autoimmune conditions.

In addition to the naturally occurring regulatory cells, it is clear that regulatory cells can be induced by antigen administration. The phenotype of the resulting cells depends on the nature of the antigen and route of administration (see above). Two recent studies have indicated that IL-10–secreting regulatory T cells may be induced in humans by soluble peptide administration by either the intradermal[37] or subcutaneous[38] route. Administration of peptides derived either from bee venom or cat dander led to the generation of IL-10–secreting cells that appeared in peripheral blood and whose appearance correlated with protection from allergic responses. The fact that IL-10–secreting regulatory T cells can be induced in both mouse and humans by soluble peptide administration suggests a common pathway for their induction. Our working hypothesis is that short peptides may be presented to T cells by immature dendritic cells. Short peptides can bind directly to empty MHC at the surface of such cells[39] and hence induce the differentiation of regulatory T cells. Recent reports have shown that CD4 regulatory T cells, induced by immature dendritic cells, resemble Tr-1 cells in that they secrete high levels of IL-10 but no IL-4 or IL-2.[40,41] The induction of IL-10–secreting regulatory cells by soluble peptide administration would, therefore, appear to be a rational approach to the induction of bystander suppression for the prevention and treatment of autoimmune and allergic conditions.

ACKNOWLEDGMENTS

D. C. Wraith is supported by a Wellcome Trust Programme Grant. Anette Sundstedt was supported by a fellowship from STINT (The Swedish Foundation for International Cooperation in Research and Higher Education). Emma O'Neill was supported by a Wellcome Trust Veterinary Studentship. Leslie Saurer was supported by a fellowship from the Swiss National Foundation.

REFERENCES

1. GERSHON, R.K. & K. KONDO. 1970. Cell interactions in the induction of tolerance: the role of thymic lymphocytes. Immunol. **18:** 723–737.
2. FOWELL, D. *et al.* 1991. Subsets of CD4+ T cells and their roles in the induction and prevention of autoimmunity. Immunol. Revs. **123:** 37–64.
3. SAKAGUCHI, S. *et al.* 1995. Immunologic self-tolerance maintained by activated T cells expressing IL-2 receptor alpha-chains (CD25). Breakdown of a single mechanism of self-tolerance causes various autoimmune diseases. J. Immunol. **155:** 1151–1164.
4. THORNTON, A.M. & E.M. SHEVACH. 1998. CD4+CD25+ immunoregulatory T cells suppress polyclonal T cell activation in vitro by inhibiting interleukin 2 production. J. Exp. Med. **188**: 287–296.
5. ANNACKER, O. *et al.* 2001. CD25+ CD4+ T cells regulate the expansion of peripheral CD4 T cells through the production of IL-10. J. Immunol. **166:** 3008–3018.
6. SHEVACH, E.M. 2001. Certified professionals: CD4$^+$CD25$^+$ suppressor T cells. J. Exp. Med. **193:** 41–45.
7. ITOH, M. *et al.* 1999. Thymus and autoimmunity: production of CD25+CD4+ naturally anergic and suppressive T cells as a key function of the thymus in maintaining immunologic self-tolerance. J. Immunol. **162:** 5317–5326.

8. SAKAGUCHI, S., T. TAKAHASHI & Y. NISHIZUKA. 1982. Study on cellular events in post-thymectomy autoimmune oophoritis in mice. II. Requirement of Lyt-1 cells in normal female mice for the prevention of oophoritis. J. Exp. Med. **156:** 1577–1586.
9. READ, S. & F. POWRIE. 2001. CD4(+) regulatory T cells. Curr. Opin. Immunol. **13:** 644–649.
10. DAKIN, R. 1829. Remarks on a cutaneous affection produced by certain poisonous vegetables. Am. J. Med. Sci. **4:** 98–100.
11. CHEN, Y. et al. 1994. Regulatory T cell clones induced by oral tolerance: suppression of autoimmune encephalomyelitis. Science **265:** 1237–1240.
12. WRAITH, D.C. 2003. Vaccines for the treatment of autoimmune diseases. In New Generation Vaccines, 3rd edit. Myron M. Levine, J.B. Kaper, Rino Rappuoli, Margaret A. Liu & Michael F. Good, Eds.: Chapter 86. M. Dekker. New York.
13. LIBLAU, R.S., S.M. SINGER & H.O. MCDEVITT. 1995. Th1 and Th2 CD4+ T-cells in the pathogenesis of organ-specific autoimmune diseases. Immunol. Today **16:** 34–38.
14. FARIA, A.M. & H.L. WEINER. 1999. Oral tolerance: Mechanisms and therapeutic applications. Adv. Immunol. **73:** 153–264.
15. MARON, R., N.S. MELICAN & H.L. WEINER. 1999. Regulatory Th2-type T cell lines against insulin and GAD peptides derived from orally- and nasally-treated NOD mice suppress diabetes. J. Autoimmun. **12:** 251–258.
16. BURKHART, C. et al. 1999. Peptide-induced T cell regulation of experimental autoimmune encephalomyelitis: a role for interleukin-10. Int. Immunol. **11:** 1625–1634.
17. SUNDSTEDT, A. et al. 1997. Immunoregulatory role of IL-10 during superantigen-induced hyporesponsiveness in vivo. J. Immunol. **158:** 180–186.
18. MILLER, C., J.A. RAGHEB & R.H. SCHWARTZ. 1999. Anergy and cytokine-mediated suppression as distinct superantigen-induced tolerance mechanisms in vivo. J. Exp. Med. **190:** 53–64.
19. GROUX, H. et al. 1996. Interleukin-10 induces a long-term antigen-specific anergic state in human CD4+ T cells. J. Exp. Med. **184:** 19–29.
20. BARRAT, F.J. et al. 2002. In vitro generation of interleukin 10-producing regulatory CD4(+) T cells is induced by immunosuppressive drugs and inhibited by T helper type 1 (Th1)- and Th2-inducing cytokines. J. Exp. Med. **195:** 603–616.
21. ANDERTON, S.M. & D.C. WRAITH. 1998. Hierarchy in the ability of T cell epitopes to induce peripheral tolerance to antigens from myelin. Eur. J. Immunol. **28:** 1251–1261.
22. KONO, D.H., J.L. URBAN, S.J. HORVATH, et al. 1988. Two minor determinants of myelin basic protein induce experimental allergic encephalomyelitis in SJL/J mice. J. Exp. Med. **168:** 213–227.
23. ANDERTON, S.M. et al. 2002. Influence of a dominant cryptic epitope on autoimmune T cell tolerance. Nat. Immunol. **3:** 175–181.
24. MANOURY, B. et al. 2002. Destructive processing by asparagine endopeptidase limits presentation of a dominant T cell epitope in MBP. Nat. Immunol. **3:** 169–174.
25. METZLER, B. & D.C. WRAITH. 1993. Inhibition of experimental autoimmune encephalomyelitis by inhalation but not oral administration of the encephalitogenic peptide: Influence of MHC binding affinity. Int. Immunol. **5:** 1159–1165.
26. METZLER, B. & D.C. WRAITH. 1996. Mucosal tolerance in a murine model of experimental autoimmune encephalomyelitis. Ann. N.Y. Acad. Sci. **778:** 228–242.
27. METZLER, B. & D.C. WRAITH. 1999. Inhibition of T cell responsiveness by nasal peptide administration: Influence of the thymus and differential recovery of T cell-dependent functions. Immunology **97:** 257–263.
28. MASSEY, E.J. et al. 2002. Intranasal peptide-induced peripheral tolerance: the role of IL-10 in regulatory T cell function within the context of experimental autoimmune encephalomyelitis. Vet. Immunol. Immunopathol. **87:** 357–372.
29. LIU, G.Y. et al. 1995. Low avidity recognition of self-antigen by T cells permits escape from central tolerance. Immunity **3:** 407–415.
30. GROUX, H. et al. 1997. A CD4+ T-cell subset inhibits antigen-specific T-cell responses and prevents colitis. Nature **389:** 737–742.
31. SUNDSTEDT, A. et al. 2003. Role for IL-10 in suppression mediated by Peptide-induced regulatory T cells in vivo. J. Immunol. **170:** 1240–1248.

32. BELKAID, Y. *et al.* 2002. CD4+CD25+ regulatory T cells control *Leishmania major* persistence and immunity. Nature **420:** 502–507.
33. LAFAILLE, J.J. *et al.* 1994. High incidence of spontaneous autoimmune encephalomyelitis in immunodeficient anti-myelin basic protein T cell receptor transgenic mice. Cell **78:** 399–408.
34. LEVINGS, M.K. *et al.* 2002. Human CD25+CD4+ T suppressor cell clones produce transforming growth factor beta, but not interleukin 10, and are distinct from type 1 T regulatory cells. J. Exp. Med. **196:** 1335–1346.
35. TAAMS, L.S. *et al.* 2002. Antigen-specific T cell suppression by human CD4+CD25+ regulatory T cells. Eur. J. Immunol. **32:** 1621–1630.
36. FURTADO, G. C. *et al.* 2001. Regulatory T cells in spontaneous autoimmune encephalomyelitis. Immunol. Rev. **182:** 122–134.
37. LARCHE, M. 2001. Inhibition of human T-cell responses by allergen peptides. Immunology **104:** 377–382.
38. AKDIS, C.A. *et al.* 1998. Role of interleukin 10 in specific immunotherapy. J. Clin. Invest. **102:** 98–106.
39. SANTAMBROGIO, L. *et al.* 1999. Abundant empty class II MHC molecules on the surface of immature dendritic cells. Proc. Natl. Acad. Sci. USA **96:** 15050–15055.
40. RONCAROLO, M.-G., M.K. LEVINGS & C. TRAVERSARI. 2001. Differentiation of T regulatory cells by immature dendritic cells. J. Exp. Med. **193:** 5–9.
41. JONULIET, H. *et al.* 2000. Induction of interleukin10-producing, nonproliferating CD4+ T cells with regulatory properties by repetitive stimulation with allogeneic immature human dendritic cells. J. Exp. Med. **192:** 1213–1222.
42. METZLER, B. *et al.* 2000. Kinetics of peptide uptake and tissue distribution following a single tolerogenic intranasal dose of peptide. Immunol. Invest. **29:** 61–70.

ADP-Ribosylating Bacterial Enzymes for the Targeted Control of Mucosal Tolerance and Immunity

NILS LYCKE

Department of Clinical Immunology, University of Göteborg, Sweden

ABSTRACT: The questions of whether mucosal tolerance and IgA immunity are mutually exclusive or can coexist and whether they represent priming of the local immune system through the same or different activation pathways are addressed. Two strategies were attempted: the first using cholera toxin (CT) or the enzymatically inactive receptor-binding B subunit of CT (CTB), and the second using CTA1-DD or an enzymatically inactive mutant thereof, CTA1R7K-DD. The CTA1-DD adjuvant is a fusion protein composed of the ADP-ribosylating part of CT, CTA1, and DD, which is derived from *Staphylococcus areus* protein A and targets the molecule to B cells. Here, we provide compelling evidence that delivery of antigen in the absence of ADP ribosylation can promote tolerance, whereas ADP-ribosyltransferase activity induces IgA immunity and prevents tolerance. By linking antigen to the ADP-ribosylating enzymes we could show that CT, although potentially binding to all nucleated cells, in fact, bound preferentially to dendritic cells (DCs) *in vivo*. On the other hand, DD-bound antigen was distinctly targeted to B cells and probably also to follicular dendritic cells (FDCs) *in vivo*. Interestingly, the CT and CTA1-DD adjuvants gave equally enhancing effects on mucosal and systemic responses, but appeared to target different APCs *in vivo*. CT- or CTB-conjugated antigen accumulated in mucosal and systemic DCs. Whereas only CT promoted an active IgA response, CTB induced tolerance to the conjugated antigen. Following intravenous injection of CT-conjugated antigen, DCs in the marginal zone (MZ) of the spleen were selectively targeted. Interestingly, CTB delivered antigen to the same MZ DCs, but failed to induce maturation and upregulation of costimulatory molecules in these cells. Thus, ADP-ribosylation was necessary for a strong enhancing effect of immune responses following CT/CTB-dependent delivery of antigen to the MZ DCs. Moreover, using CTA1-DD, antigen was targeted to the B cell follicle and FDC in the spleen after intravenous injection. Only active CTA1-DD, but not the inactive mutant CTA1R7K-DD, provided enhancing effects on immune responses. By contrast, antigen delivered by the CTA1R7K-DD stimulated specific tolerance in adoptively transferred T cell receptor transgenic CD4[+] T cells. Whether targeting of B cells suffices for tolerance induction or requires participation of DCs remains to be investigated. With CT we found that enzyme-dependent modulation of DCs affects migration, maturation, and differentiation of DCs, which resulted in CD4[+] T cell help for IgA B cell development. On the contrary, antigen presen-

Address for correspondence: Nils Lycke, M.D. Ph.D., Department of Clinical Immunology, University of Göteborg, S413 46 Göteborg, Sweden. Voice: +46-31-3424936; fax: +46-31-3424721.

nils.lycke@microbio.gu.se

tation in the absence of ADP-ribosylating enzyme, as seen with CTB or CTA1R7K-DD, appears to expand specific T cells to a similar extent as enzymatically active CT or CTA1-DD, but fails to recruit help for germinal center (GC) formation and the necessary expansion of activated B cells. Also, the $CD4^+$ T cells that are primed in a suboptimal, tolerogenic, fashion do not migrate to the B cell follicle to provide T cell help. Thus, ADP-ribosylating enzymes may be used to selectively control the induction of an active IgA response or promote the development of tolerance. In particular, on the targeted APC, modulation of the expression of costimulatory molecules, CD80, CD86, CD83, and B7RP-1, plays an important role in the effect of the ADP-ribosylating CTA1-based adjuvants on the development of tolerance or active IgA immunity. For example, the expression of CD86 *in vivo* was a prominent feature of the enzymatically active CT or CTA1-DD adjuvants. By contrast, CD80 expression appeared not to be important in CTA1-augmented APCs for an adjuvant function.

KEYWORDS: tolerance; mucosal; adjuvant; cholera toxin; ADP-ribosylation; IgA; CTA1-DD

INTRODUCTION

Activation at mucosal membranes of tolerance or IgA immunity against most protein antigens rests heavily on the presentation of antigen to $CD4^+$ T cells in a cognate fashion, that is, involving the direct interaction between the T cells and antigen-presenting cells (APCs), including B cells, in an MHC-restricted manner. Two signals are required for induction of immune responses, the first being the T cell receptor (TCR) recognition of MHC class II plus peptide, and the second the requirement for costimulation. Although it is still incompletely known to what extent costimulation is required for tolerance induction, strong evidence has accumulated indicating that costimulation is essential for an active IgA response.[1] However, the precise role of, for example, CD28, CTLA4, or ICOS on IgA antibody production still awaits to be worked out in detail. We have provided data to indicate that CD28 signaling is not essential for specific IgA responses in the intestinal lamina propria (LP), albeit we also found that blocking CD80/86 with CTLA4 immunoglobulin abrogated the specific IgA response completely.[2] Moreover, using TCR transgenic mice it has been clearly demonstrated that both mucosal tolerance and IgA immunity depend on the initial expansion and differentiation of $CD4^+$ T cells, rather than the induction of anergy at the level of the individual T cell.[3,4] However, the dichotomy between a tolerogenic or an IgA immunogenic presentation of antigen is not fully understood at present. A growing number of studies indicate that costimulation may be key to explaining the dichotomy, but insufficient knowledge as to the relative importance of CD40, OX40L, CD80, or CD86, for example, still pertains. Given that costimulation may involve many different membrane-expressed molecules, and that these may appear simultaneously or in sequence, there could be complex interactions between APCs and T and B cells in the gut-associated lymphoid tissues (GALT) that constitute a tolerogenic or an IgA immunogenic outcome of antigen presentation. We have addressed this problem by exploiting the impact on immune responses following intranasal or systemic administration of an active or inactive ADP-ribosylating cholera toxin A1 subunit as part of the CT holotoxin or as part of the CTA1-DD adjuvant system.

Most antigens recognized in the mucosal immune system are poorly associated with microbial pathogen-associated molecular patterns (PAMPs) and, thus, incompletely activate innate immunity and the APC. This results in low expression of costimulatory molecules; it is thought that immune tolerance is induced secondarily to this. This would apply, in particular, to food antigens and the gut microbial flora, which largely fail to stimulate active IgA responses, but, rather, promote tolerance. Vaccine developers have focused on the growing understanding of the importance of activation of innate immunity to obtain strong adaptive immune responses and long-term memory. What were previously regarded as "danger signals" are today recognized as defined molecules with distinct chemical and genetic properties.[5] Behind the activation of innate immunity by "danger signals" we find a series of reactions strictly controlled by specific receptors, so-called pattern-recognition receptors (PRRs), that bind microbial products, such as endotoxin or other microbial membrane products or DNA. One family of such receptors is the Toll-like receptors (TLR) that bind lipopolysaccharide (LPS), flagellin, HSP60, CpG DNA, dsRNA, or peptidoglycans, each with unique and distinct receptors.[6,7] These receptors are located on the membranes or in the intracellular compartments of many types of cells, among them DCs, macrophages, and B cells, which represent innate immunity The aforementioned cells are also the most important cells for antigen presentation and stimulation of an adaptive immune response.[8] In the case of DCs, binding to PRRs will cause the migration of DCs to regional lymph nodes and their maturation into effective APCs expressing costimulatory molecules required for optimal T cell priming.[9]

Because of a more detailed understanding of how to trigger innate immunity through specific receptor recognition, adjuvant research is increasingly focused on vaccine targeting of the innate immune system. Targeting is also a way to reduce side effects, to reduce the dose of antigen, and to limit the risk of adverse reactions to vaccination. Adjuvants can be live vectors, such as *Salmonella* and adenovirus, that have been modified by gene recombination techniques to express relevant proteins.[10] The live vector adjuvant can act both as an antigen delivery system and as an immunomodulator, for example, via TLR binding. However, live vectors are often unstable and few vaccines based on this technology have reached the state of clinical use. Nonliving adjuvants can be formulations of lipid or gel (alum) to create a depot effect of the vaccine following injection. Nonliving adjuvants can also act as delivery systems, such as liposomes and polylactide/polyglycolide microspheres, or as modulators, such as muramyl dipeptide (MDP) and monophosphoryl lipid A (MPL).[11]

CHOLERA TOXIN: FROM TOXIN TO ADJUVANT

Mucosal vaccines for nasal administration are highly warranted.[12] However, the choice of adjuvant has proven crucial for the development of nonliving mucosal vaccines. Cholera toxin (CT) and the closely related *Escherichia coli* heat-labile toxin (LT) are perhaps the most powerful and best studied mucosal adjuvants in experimental use today, but when exploited in the clinic their potential toxicity and association with cases of Bell's palsy (paralysis of the facial nerve) have led to their withdrawal from the market.[13–17] The bacterial enterotoxins CT and LT have proven to be effective immunoenhancers in experimental animals as well as in humans.[18] Structurally these enterotoxins are AB_5 complexes and consist of one ADP-ribosyltransferase active A1 subunit and an A2 subunit that links the A1 to a pentamer of B subunits. The holotoxins bind to most mammalian cells via the B subunit (CTB), which specifically interacts with the GM1-ganglioside receptor in the cell membrane. Whereas the holotoxins have been found to enhance mucosal immune responses, conjugates between CTB and antigen have been used to specifically tolerize the immune system.[19]

Studies in mice have shown that CT and LT can accumulate in the olfactory nerve and bulb when given intranasally, a mechanism that is dependent on the ability of the B subunits of CT or LT to bind GM1-ganglioside receptors, present on all nucleated mammalian cells.[20–22] Because we do not know whether such interactions occur in humans, there is great need to identify alternative ways that circumvent toxicity, but that have retained the potent adjuvant functions of CT or LT. Although less toxic mutants of CT and LT have been engineered with substantial adjuvant function, we believe that such molecules still carry a significant risk of causing adverse reactions,[23–25] especially when considering that the adjuvanticity of CT and LT appears to be a combination of the ADP-ribosyltransferase activity of the A subunit and the ability to bind ganglioside receptors on the target cells.[14,26,27] These observations and others preclude the use of CT or LT holotoxins in vaccines for humans. On the other hand, recent observations have demonstrated that it is possible to retain adjuvant functions of these molecules with no toxicity or greatly reduced toxicity by introducing site-directed mutations in the gene coding for the A1 subunit. Examples of mutant molecules that have proven to be effective adjuvants are LTK63 and LTR72,[24] the former with no enzymatic activity and the latter with significantly reduced ADP-ribosylating ability. Notwithstanding this, the GM1-ganglioside receptor–dependent binding remains a problem in these mutants and, thus, may still cause nerve cell accumulation and neurotoxicity. Thus, identifying a dose of mutant holotoxin that meets with the need for a desired immunoenhancing effect in the clinic without toxic side effects may prove a cumbersome and difficult task.

THE TARGETED CTA1-DD ADJUVANT, A NONTOXIC AND SAFE ALTERNATIVE

A better solution to this dilemma of efficacy versus toxicity is the CTA1-DD molecule that we have developed and that has proven to be a highly effective mucosal and systemic adjuvant.[28,29] This unique adjuvant is based on the enzymatically active A1-subunit of cholera toxin (CT), combined with a dimer of an immunoglobulin-binding element from *Staphylococcus areus* protein A.[30,31] The molecule thereby avoids binding to all nucleated cells, which could result in unwanted reactions, and exploits fully the CTA1-enzyme in the holotoxin. Accordingly, all studies to date have found that CTA1-DD is nontoxic and has retained excellent immunoenhancing functions.[28,32,33] When given systemically, CTA1-DD provides comparable adjuvant effect to that of intact CT, greatly augmenting both cellular and humoral immunity against specific immunogens coadministered with the adjuvant. It also functions as a mucosal adjuvant and should be safe, as it is devoid of the B subunit that is a prerequisite of CT holotoxin toxicity. CTA1-DD cannot bind to ganglioside receptors; rather, it targets B cells, limiting the CTA1-DD adjuvant to a restricted repertoire of cells that it can interact with. However, no doubt DCs could also be influenced by this ADP-ribosylating adjuvant, as seen in studies that have used CTA1-DD incorporated into ISCOMs (see below).

In a recent study, we compared the safety aspects of CT with those of CTA1-DD and found several benefits to the latter system. We found that lack of GM1-ganglioside receptor binding did not impinge on the efficacy and quality of the CTA1-DD adjuvant function following intranasal immunizations. The CTA1-DD molecule binds exclusively to the immunoglobulin receptor on both naive and memory type B cells; Fc receptors are not necessary for the adjuvant function. By contrast, CT could potentially bind to most nucleated cells, including specialized microfold (M) and dendritic cells, located in close proximity to the lumen of the nasal-associated lymphoid tissue (NALT), a property that would appear to favor efficacy and function in CT above that of CTA1-DD. However, we found that the efficacy of CTA1-DD as a mucosal adjuvant was not influenced by the lack of GM1-ganglioside binding ability. Rather, we observed a potent enhancing effect of CTA1-DD on mucosal IgA as well as serum IgG responses following intranasal immunizations, equal to that of CT.[34]

To rule out simple confounding elements that could explain the strong adjuvant effect of CTA1-DD we considered several factors. First, we asked whether endotoxin contamination in intranasal vaccines affects the immune response or could be a confounding factor in the evaluation of the immunomodulating effect of mucosal adjuvants. Furthermore, whether inflammation is part of the mechanism by which intranasal adjuvants work has been poorly investigated.[35] This is particularly interesting in the light of recent findings with DC,s that clearly ascribe both pro- and anti-inflammatory functions to CT,[36] and our previous finding that CTA1-DD does not cause inflammation.[28,37] Inflammation and a barrier disruption of the nasal mucosal membrane could have negative effects, for example, augmenting the risk of toxic side effects, such as the accumulation of ganglioside-binding adjuvants and coadministered proteins in the olfactory nerve and brain following intranasal immunization.[21,38–40] We explored the efficacy of the CTA1-DD adjuvant for its ability to enhance nasal immune responses in mice. We found that despite the lack of a mucosal binding element, the B cell–targeted CTA1-DD molecule was an equally strong adjuvant as CT. Moreover, the potency of CTA1-DD as a mucosal adjuvant was not a result of endotoxin contamination, as more than a 50-fold higher dose of LPS was needed to achieve a similar enhancement. Additionally, the adjuvant effect was TLR4-independent and absent in mutant CTA1E112K-DD, lacking enzymatic activity. The CTA1-DD adjuvant augmented GC formations and T cell priming in the draining lymph nodes and, contrary to CT, promoted a balanced Th1/Th2 response with little effect on serum IgE antibody production.[34] CTA1-DD did not induce inflammatory changes in the nasal mucosa and, most importantly, did not bind to or accumulate in the nervous tissues of the olfactory bulb, whereas CT bound avidly to the nervous tissues (FIG.1). Therefore, the nontoxic CTA1-DD adjuvant is an attractive solution to the current dilemma between efficacy and toxicity encountered in CT- or LT-holotoxin adjuvant strategies and provides a safe and promising candidate to be included in future vaccines for intranasal administration.

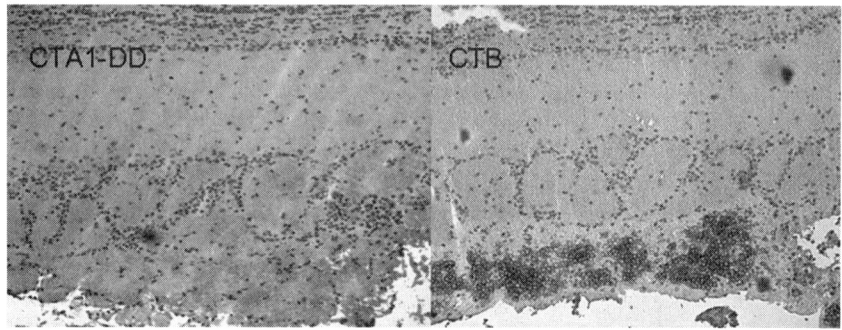

FIGURE 1. The accumulation of GM1-ganglioside receptor-binding adjuvants in the olfactory nerve and bulb. Mice were given biotinylated CTB or CTA1-DD intranasally, and the deposition of adjuvant 24 h later was investigated in the olfactory nerve and bulb. We found that CTA1-DD does not accumulate in the nervous tissues and appears not to influence nerve function. By contrast, CTB accumulated in the nervous tissues, a function that was dependent on the GM1-ganglioside receptor-binding ability of CTB.

TOLERANCE OR IgA IMMUNITY AFTER MUCOSAL ANTIGEN EXPOSURE

Recent studies have suggested that DCs are particularly important for induction of mucosal immune responses, albeit a substantial body of evidence indicates that B cells, macrophages, and epithelial cells also function as mucosal APCs.[41] Whether these latter cells have distinct functional roles in the induction and maintenance of mucosal immunity and tolerance is currently poorly understood. However, both DCs and B cells have been associated with induction of secretory IgA responses as well as with tolerance, whereas epithelial cells may, primarily, act to tolerize local responses. Mucosal DCs represent all major subgroups of DCs, myeloid ($CD11b^+$), lymphoid ($CD8\alpha^+$), and plasmacytoid ($B220^+$) DCs.[42] The phenotypic distinctions between the subgroups is based on the surface expression of CD11b, CD8α, CD4, and B220, with $CD11c^+$ DCs being negative, single- or double-positive for these surface markers.[43] Whereas the phenotypic subdivision of DCs in Peyer's patches (PPs) has been carefully investigated by Kelsall and coworkers, much less is known about the DC populations in the LP.[44] CT has been reported to induce activation and migration of DCs from the subepithelial dome of the PP to T and B cell areas of the PP[45]; the influence of other adjuvants, such as ISCOMs, on migration and activation of mucosal DCs remains to be investigated.

The functions of LP DCs have only recently attracted the attention of researchers in the field. Unpublished observations in our laboratory have indicated that luminal CT attracts DCs to gut mucosal membranes, where DCs appear to take up luminal antigens into the LP (Grdic *et al.*, unpublished observation). Whether these DCs have a particular phenotype awaits to be determined, but preliminary investigations in our laboratory ascribe the targeting of CT to $CD8\alpha^+$ DCs, the lymphoid subset of $CD11c^+$ cells in the GALT. Rescigno *et al.* have documented an intricate mechanism for DC sampling of antigen through the epithelial lining, involving breaking the tight junctions of the mucosal epithelial barrier.[46] As mentioned previously, an often overlooked problem with mucosal immunization is the potential risk of developing tolerance.[47] Therefore, in the context of mucosal vaccines, the role of the various mucosal APCs with regard to induction of protective immunity or tolerance is particularly important to investigate. Antigen sampling in the absence of a strong activator can lead to tolerance, whereas uptake in the presence of an adjuvant can result in active immune responses. Expanding the mucosal DC population with Flt3L *in vivo*, followed by oral immunizations with or without CT adjuvant, has demonstrated that induction of tolerance, as well as gut IgA immunity (in the presence of CT), is greatly facilitated by increasing the DC density in the GALT.[48,49]

CT-CONJUGATED ANTIGEN AUGMENTS IgA IMMUNITY, WHEREAS CTB-CONJUGATED ANTIGEN PROMOTES TOLERANCE

Although B cells and macrophages are known to act as APCs, dendritic cells are considered the key APC for priming of naive T cells.[8,50,51] The difficulty in targeting DCs *in vivo* has limited our knowledge about the priming events that determine whether antigen stimulation will result in a tolerogenic or immunogenic outcome.[52,53] Immature DCs that reside in tissues are known to take up antigen and, if maturation occurs, migrate to regional lymph nodes or the spleen. In the secondary lymphoid tissues, the DC immigrants, expressing strong costimulation, may be inherently stimulatory, but whether resident or poorly activated immigrants are tolerogenic is currently a much-debated issue. In particular, we lack *in vivo* information about DCs at specific anatomical sites, such as the marginal zone (MZ) of the spleen, the lamina propria of the mucosal membranes, or the conduit system in the peripheral lymph nodes.

Recent experiments using DC targeting *in vivo* have indicated that DCs can be modulated to direct tolerogenic or immunogenic priming of naive T cells depending on the degree of inflammatory signals released at the site of antigen exposure or as a result of antigen dose.[41,48,49,52,53] A proinflammatory environment would license the naive T cells to develop into effective helper cells for B cell immunity, whereas an anti-inflammatory environment would support the development of regulatory T cells. Relatively few studies have investigated the functions of APCs exposed to adjuvants *in vivo*, and little is known about the maturation and migration of specific APCs following exposure to immunomodulators. Using an adoptive transfer model of TCR transgenic T cells it was recently shown that oral feeding of protein leads to clonal expansion of naive T cells. In the absence of adjuvant, feeding fails to generate B cell help, whereas in the presence of adjuvant strong B cell help develops.[4] Thus, both the tolerogenic and the productive T cell response to fed antigen involved clonal expansion, but the quality of the primed T cells was different from that of T cells in adjuvant-exposed mice. Following priming, the tolerized T cells failed to enter B cell follicles; upon challenge with antigen they entered follicles, but still failed to provide adequate B cell help.

Previous reports have documented both a proinflammatory and an anti-inflammatory effect of CT.[49,54] From several studies, including our own work, exposure of APCs to CT has an augmenting effect on IL-1 and IL-6 production, whereas in other studies a down regulating effect on IL-12 and promoting effect on IL-10 production have been reported and would have an anti-inflammatory effect.[49,54–58] In fact, investigators have used the CT adjuvant to generate Th1 cells, but most reports have shown a bias for Th2 cells, and recently also regulatory Tr 1 cells.[54,59–61] Although data reported by different groups on the effects of CT-targeted cells on production of cytokines, especially IL-1 and IL-12, are not consistent, it is clear that CT is a strong adjuvant and may induce both a pro- and anti-inflammatory effect *in vivo*. How this dual ability of CT is regulated is still debated, but a different cytokine release and milieu might explain the observed dual behavior. Interestingly, the B subunit of CT (CTB) is a well-documented carrier for the induction of mucosal antigen-specific tolerance[62] and, thus, CT and its derivatives have the capacity to be used both as a vehicle for tolerance as well as for productive immunity. Although still controversial, it appears that oral tolerance and productive mucosal IgA immunity are reciprocally regulated and even mutually exclusive. The balance is determined, in part, by the nature and dose of the antigen, the antigen formulation, and the APC at the mucosal surfaces and the corresponding draining lymph nodes.

Recent reports on the effect of CT on DCs *ex vivo* have indicated that both migration and maturation of DCs could be stimulated by CT, thereby promoting strong T cell priming.[56,57] Previous studies by Holmgren *et al.* and Czerkinsky *et al.* using CTB-conjugated antigens have demonstrated that oral delivery of these conjugates causes systemic tolerance; this has subsequently been used as a strategy to treat autoimmune and allergic conditions.[63] Based on this information, we compared conjugates made with CTB or CT holotoxin with ovalbumin (OVA) for their effects on DCs *ex vivo*. We found that although CTB and CT delivered the same amount of antigen to DCs, CT matured DCs, whereas CTB failed to do so. When injected intravenously, OVA accumulated in DCs in the marginal zone (MZ) in the spleen after both CT and CTB conjugates were used. However, the enhancing effect of CT on antibody stimulation was more than 1000-fold stronger than that of CTB, clearly demonstrating that the immunomodulating capacity of CT greatly exceeded that of CTB, although the ability to deliver OVA to MZ DCs was similar. Importantly, it appears that CTB and CT target DCs *in vivo*, despite the presence of the GM1-ganglioside receptor on most nucleated cells. OVA was found in high concentrations in MZ DCs, but not in neighboring cells (FIG. 2). The targeted MZ DCs were unique in their phenotype, being $CD11c^+$, $CD8\alpha^-$, $CD11b^-$, $B220^-$, and expressing intermediate or low levels of MHC class II and DEC205. Whereas CTB only delivered the antigen to MZ DCs, the ADP-ribosyltransferase activity of CT was required for the maturation and migration of DCs to the T cell zone, where these cells distinctly upregulated CD86, but not CD80. This interaction appeared to instruct antigen-specific $CD4^+$ T cells to move into the B cell follicle and strongly support germinal center formation. These events may explain why CT-conjugated antigen is substantially more immunogenic than antigen admixed with soluble CT, and why CTB-conjugated antigen can tolerize immune responses when given orally or at other mucosal sites. The most obvious molecular difference between CTB and CT lies in the CTA1 moiety and its ADP-ribosylating ability, which is responsible for the adjuvant function, as is clearly demonstrated by the adjuvant function of the CTA1-DD fusion protein. Ongoing research in our laboratory using Affymetrix global gene transcriptional analysis has revealed substantial differences between CT and CTB with regard to the type and number of genes that are regulated following exposure to these molecules. In partic-

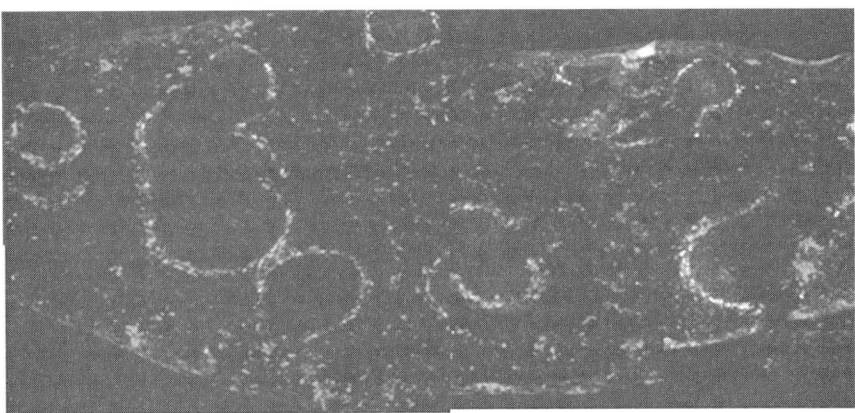
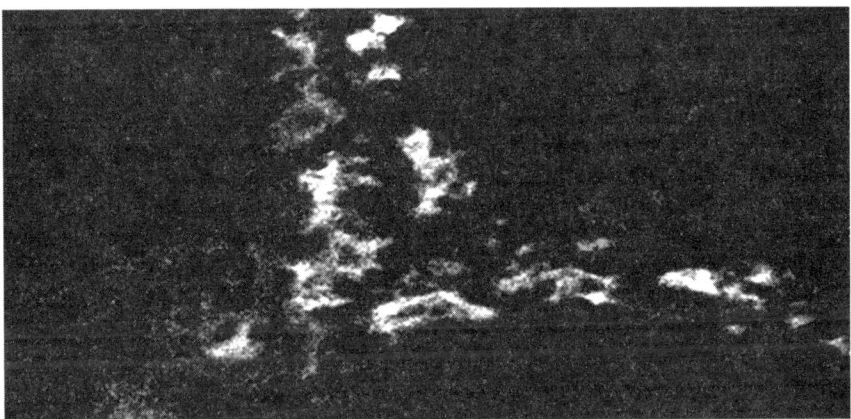

FIGURE 2. Targeting of dendritic cells in the marginal zone. Following intravenous injection of CT-OVA conjugates, high concentrations of antigen accumulate in CD11c$^+$ DCs in the marginal zone (MZ) of the spleen (*ring formations, top panel*). The MZ cells that contain OVA double label with anti-CD11c monoclonal antibodies and anti-OVA, as shown in this closeup (*bottom panel*).

ular, effects on gene transcription of the CD80, CD86, and CD83 genes were evident with CT, but absent with CTB.

THE CTA1-DD ADJUVANT SYSTEM

The novel CTA1-DD system, which exploits the full enzymatic activity of the A1 subunit in a B cell–targeted fusion protein, was found to be nontoxic when given to mice, even in very high doses (i.e., 100- to 1000-fold the toxic dose of CT holotoxin). Preliminary histopathological investigations of doses ranging from 1 to 500 µg of CTA1-DD given intraperitoneally have not shown any toxic effects on liver, kidney, or spleen. A detailed analysis of the mechanisms responsible for adjuvanticity of the targeted fusion protein has been a key element in our understanding of how safe and effective vaccine adjuvants may be constructed. Lacking the A2 and B subunits of CT and consequently devoid of the ability to bind to the GM1-ganglioside receptor, the CTA1-DD fusion protein has a more restricted repertoire of cellular interactions than the holotoxins. The DD dimer binds to surface immunoglobulin on naive and antigen-experienced B cells of all isotypes and, most importantly, CTA1-DD has adjuvant effects comparable to those of the intact CT holotoxin.[64] A mechanistically important asset to this adjuvant is that it combines cell targeting with enzymatic immunomodulation, allowing us to dissect the molecular mechanisms underlying adjuvanticity. Both CT and CTA1-DD have been shown to augment antibody responses as well as cell-mediated immune responses following mucosal immunization. With regard to B cell responses, a striking effect of both CT and CTA1-DD adjuvants is seen i n the increased number and size of germinal center formations following immunization.[64] Interestingly, MHC class II–restricted $CD4^+$ T cell responses as well as class I–restricted CTL responses are also greatly augmented by both CT and CTA1-DD, despite that the fact that the latter adjuvant appears to act primarily through B cells.[65,66] The CTA1-DD adjuvant has been shown to be effective for the stimulation of immune protection against microbial infections at mucosal surfaces. For example, in the rotavirus mouse model, CTA1-DD adjuvant gave almost as good protection as LTR192 and better than CpG ODN when used with chimeric VP6 protein.[67] CTA1-DD has also been compared with other mutant toxin adjuvants, such as LTK63 and LTR72.[24] We found that CTA1-DD was better than LTK63 and comparable or better than LTR72 when equimolar concentrations were tested for adjuvant function with OVA or tetanus toxin (TT) for intranasal immunization (FIG. 3).

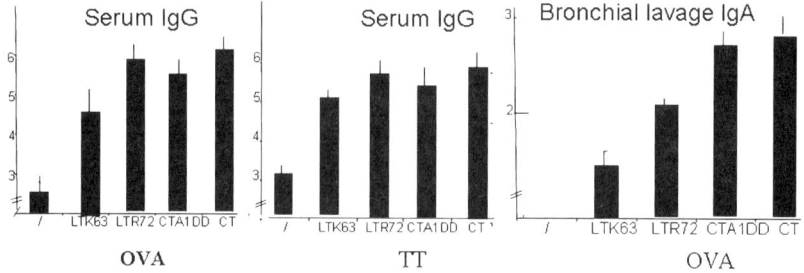

FIGURE 3. Effective augmentation of immune responses using CTA1-DD adjuvant. Mice were immunized intranasally three times with 2 μg of OVA or TT together with CTA1-DD, LTK63, or LTR72 (5 μg/dose). The antigen-specific antibody responses in serum and bronchial lavage were assessed by ELISA 8 d after the final dose. Results are given as $\log_{10}$ titers ± SD (n = 5 mice per group). Data shown are representative of three experiments giving similar results.

THE COMBINED CTA1-DD/ISCOM VECTOR

Because CTA1-DD was found to have reduced adjuvant function when given orally, we initiated attempts to protect the molecule against degradation or inactivation by incorporating the fusion protein into immune-stimulating complexes (ISCOMs). ISCOMs are structurally and chemically completely different from CT or CTA1-DD. Whereas the latter two molecules both exert ADP-ribosylation and bind to separate but distinct cell receptors, ISCOMs are enzymatically inactive and are not known to bind to a specific receptor. Nevertheless, ISCOMs are thought to interact most actively with DCs, and perhaps macrophages, *in vivo*. ISCOM s induce a wide range of immune responses to coadministered antigens, including antibody production, CD4 T cell priming, and class I–restricted CTL responses.[68–70] The two adjuvant systems also appear to share the ability to activate certain components of the innate immune system, such as upregulating costimulatory molecules CD80 and CD86 or enhancing the production of IL-1 and IL-6 by DCs, macrophages, and/or epithelial cells.

Therefore, we developed the first rationally designed targeted vaccine adjuvant vector by combining CTA1-DD with ISCOMs, which we hoped would greatly surpass the effectiveness of either system used alone. The combined CTA1-DD/ISCOM vector truly represents a novel form of adjuvant vector. It is based on the principles of targeting and immunomodulation. The targeting is achieved by the ISCOM structure and the DD element, whereas Quil-A/saponin and the ADP-ribosylating enzyme CTA1 constitute the immunomodulating components. The CTA1-DD/ISCOMs vector has proven particularly effective for mucosal immunization, stimulating strong cell-mediated and humoral, systemic, and local mucosal immunity.[71,72] In particular, we succeeded in protecting the CTA1-DD system from inactivation and, thus, could show that ADP-ribosylation greatly potentiated the function of ISCOMs given orally. Both humoral and cell-mediated immunity, as defined by antigen-specific DTH and T cell proliferation in draining lymph nodes, were significantly enhanced above that seen with ISCOMs alone or inactive CTA1R7K-DD/ISCOM immunizations (FIG. 4).

Whereas ISCOMs are taken up by DCs, CTA1-DD is targeted to B cells. The combined vector could have improved the targeting via the DD fragment to additional APC populations or enhancing the uptake in DCs, through, for example, Fc receptors. It may be that the combined vector can be taken up not only by DCs, but also by B cells *in vivo*. In fact, preliminary results in our laboratory suggest that B cells can present antigen in CTA1-DD/ISCOMs, at least *in vitro*, whereas normally only DCs present antigens incorporated into ISCOMs. A second, theoretical advantage of the intact CTA1-DD/ISCOM adjuvant is that it may also activate the targeted APCs. This could be an effect of targeting of ISCOMs and the promotion of ADP-ribosylation in B cells. If, however, the effect is restricted to DCs, then the interpretation must be that CTA1-DD can also act on DCs and not only on B cells, provided access is allowed to the DCs via uptake of the ISCOM vector. In fact, our most recent experience with the combined vector confirms this latter aspect. In addition, B cell APC functions are augmented by the combined vector, clearly arguing that CTA1-DD/ISCOMs access both DCs and B cells as APCs *in vivo*. This is a challenging field of possibilities in immune regulation that may be exploited further by this rationally designed vaccine adjuvant vector.

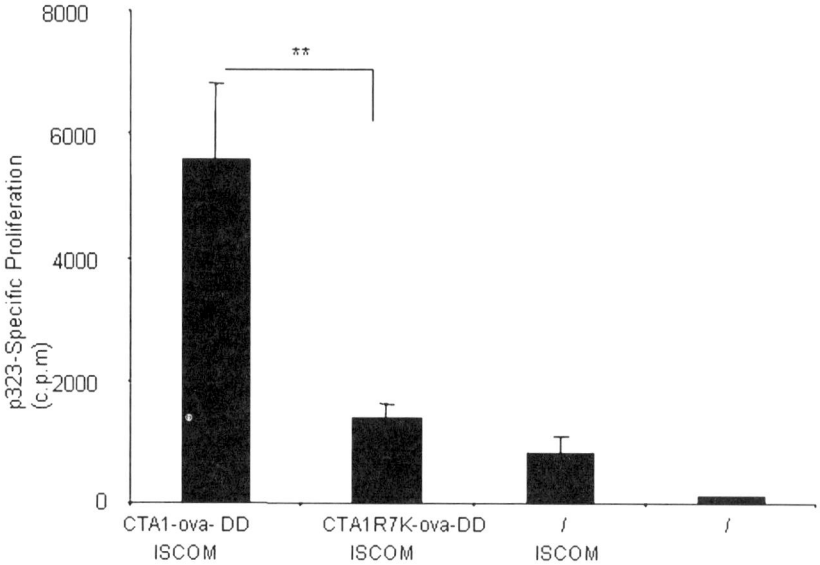

FIGURE 4. The combined CTA1-DD/ISCOM vector is a highly effective mucosal adjuvant. Mice were immunized twice intranasally with 2 μg of CTA1-ova-DD/ISCOM, mutant CTA1R7K-ova-DD/ISCOM, OVA/ISCOM, or OVA alone. Eight days after the final immunization, cervical lymph nodes were excised and single cell suspensions were cultured with 1 μM of ova-peptide p323, and 3 d later T cell proliferation was assessed by [^{3}H]thymidine incorporation. CTA1-DD and the mutant fusion protein were constructed with the ova peptide p323 inserted in frame in the protein. OVA/ISCOM and OVA represent whole ovalbumin at 4 and 100 μg, respectively. Data shown are representative of three separate experiments ($n = 5$ mice per group).

CONCLUSION

The present paper reports on encouraging results with CTA1-DD used alone or in combination with ISCOMs. It illustrates how it may be possible to construct effective, safe, and stable subunit vaccines, which are active by mucosal routes. The use of the combined vector for relevant vaccine candidates is now being tested, with progress being made for mucosal vaccines against influenza virus, rota virus, *Helicobacter pylori*, and tuberculosis, respectively. CTA1-DD or CTA1-DD/ISCOMs represent a conceptually important step in the construction of novel, rationally designed mucosal vaccine adjuvants that are both safe and efficacious. Control over the priming process by the use of ADP-ribosylating enzymes leading to tolerance or an active IgA response appears to be a powerful instrument in the future development of anti-infectious vaccines or therapeutic vaccines inducing tolerance against autoimmune diseases.

ACKNOWLEDGMENTS

I would like to thank members of my group and former colleagues for invaluable contributions to the work on the adjuvants. In particular, I would like to mention my coinventor Dr. Björn Löwenadler (Arexis AB); Prof. Allan Mowat, Glasgow; Prof. Kristian Dalsgaard, Copenhagen; and Dr. Karin Lövgren (ISCONOVA AB). I am also grateful to Dubravka Grdic, Anja Helgeby, Karin Schön, Lena Ågren, and Lena Ekman. These studies would not have been possible without generous grant support from the European Commission (Grants QLK2-CT-2001-01702 and QLK2-CT-1999-00228), Vetenskapsrådet, SAREC, LUA, and Cancerfonden.

REFERENCES

1. GARDBY, E. et al. 2003. Strong differential regulation of serum and mucosal IgA responses as revealed in CD28-deficient mice using cholera toxin adjuvant. J. Immunol. **170:** 55–63.
2. GARDBY, E., P. LANE & N.Y. LYCKE. 1998. Requirements for B7-CD28 costimulation in mucosal IgA responses: paradoxes observed in CTLA4-H gamma 1 transgenic mice. J. Immunol. **161:** 49–59.
3. SMITH, K.M. et al. 2003. Inducible costimulatory molecule-B7-related protein 1 interactions are important for the clonal expansion and B cell helper functions of naive, Th1, and Th2 T cells. J. Immunol. **170:** 2310–2315.
4. SMITH, K.M., F. MCASKILL & P. GARSIDE. 2002. Orally tolerized T cells are only able to enter B cell follicles following challenge with antigen in adjuvant, but they remain unable to provide B cell help. J. Immunol. **168:** 4318–4325.
5. MATZINGER, P. & S. GUERDER. 1989. Does T-cell tolerance require a dedicated antigen-presenting cell? Nature **338:** 74–76.
6. UNDERHILL, D.M. & A. OZINSKY. 2002. Toll-like receptors: key mediators of microbe detection. Curr. Opin. Immunol. **14:** 103–110.
7. BARTON, G.M. & R. MEDZHITOV. 2002. Control of adaptive immune responses by Toll-like receptors. Curr. Opin. Immunol. **14:** 380–383.
8. RICCIARDI-CASTAGNOLI, P. & F. GRANUCCI. 2002. Opinion: Interpretation of the complexity of innate immune responses by functional genomics. Nat. Rev. Immunol. **2:** 881–889.
9. SHARPE, A. 1995. Analysis of costimulation in vivo using transgenic and knockout mice. Curr. Opin. Immunol. **7:** 389–395.
10. EDELMAN, R. 1997. Adjuvants for the future. In New Generation Vaccines. G.C. Woodrow et al., Eds.: 173–192. Marcel Dekker, Inc. New York.
11. VOGEL, F.R. 1995. Immunologic adjuvants for modern vaccine formulations. Ann. N.Y. Acad. Sci. **754:** 153–160.
12. LEVINE, M.M. 2003. Can needle-free administration of vaccines become the norm in global immunization? Nat. Med. **9:** 99–103.
13. LEVINE, M.M. & G. DOUGAN. 1998. Optimism over vaccines administered via mucosal surfaces. Lancet **351:** 1375–1376.
14. RAPPUOLI, R. et al. 1999. Structure and mucosal adjuvanticity of cholera and *Escherichia coli* heat-labile enterotoxins. Immunol. Today **20:** 493–500.
15. GLUCK, R. et al. 2000. Safety and immunogenicity of intranasally administered inactivated trivalent virosome-formulated influenza vaccine containing Escherichia coli heat-labile toxin as a mucosal adjuvant. J. Infect. Dis. **181:** 1129–1132.
16. GLUECK, R. 2001. Pre-clinical and clinical investigation of the safety of a novel adjuvant for intranasal immunization. Vaccine **20**(Suppl. 1): S42–44.
17. MUTSCH, M. et al. 2004. Use of the inactivated intranasal influenza vaccine and the risk of Bell's palsy in Switzerland. N. Engl. J. Med. **350:** 896–903.

18. FREYTAG, L.C. & J.D. CLEMENTS. 1999. Bacterial toxins as mucosal adjuvants. Curr. Top. Microbiol. Immunol. **236:** 215–236.
19. HOLMGREN, J., C. CZERKINSKY, N. LYCKE & A. M. SVENNERHOLM. 1994. Strategies for the induction of immune responses at mucosal surfaces making use of cholera toxin B subunit as immunogen, carrier and adjuvant. Am. J. Trop. Med. Hyg. **50:** 42–54.
20. VAN GINKEL, F.W. *et al.* 2003. Pneumococcal carriage results in ganglioside-mediated olfactory tissue infection. Proc. Natl. Acad. Sci. USA **100:** 14363–14367.
21. VAN GINKEL, F.W. *et al.* 2000. Cutting edge: the mucosal adjuvant cholera toxin redirects vaccine proteins into olfactory tissues. J. Immunol. **165:** 4778–4782.
22. FUJIHASHI, K. *et al.* 2002. A dilemma for mucosal vaccination: efficacy versus toxicity using enterotoxin-based adjuvants. Vaccine **20:** 2431–2438.
23. DOUCE, G. *et al.* 1998. Mucosal immunogenicity of genetically detoxified derivatives of heat labile toxin from *Escherichia coli.* Vaccine **16:** 1065–1073.
24. GIULIANI, M.M. *et al.* 1998. Mucosal adjuvanticity and immunogenicity of LTR72, a novel mutant of *Escherichia coli* heat-labile enterotoxin with partial knockout of ADP-ribosyltransferase activity. J. Exp. Med. **187:** 1123-1132.
25. YAMAMOTO, S. *et al.* 1997. Mutants in the ADP-ribosyltransferase cleft of cholera toxin lack diarrheagenicity but retain adjuvanticity. J. Exp. Med. **185:** 1203–1210.
26. SORIANI, M., L. BAILEY & T.R. HIRST. 2002. Contribution of the ADP-ribosylating and receptor-binding properties of cholera-like enterotoxins in modulating cytokine secretion by human intestinal epithelial cells. Microbiology **148:** 667–676.
27. KAWAMURA, Y.I. *et al.* 2003. Cholera toxin activates dendritic cells through dependence on GM1-ganglioside which is mediated by NF-kappaB translocation. Eur. J. Immunol. **33:** 3205–3212.
28. AGREN, L.C. *et al.* 1997. Genetically engineered nontoxic vaccine adjuvant that combines B cell targeting with immunomodulation by cholera toxin A1 subunit. J. Immunol. **158:** 3936–3946.
29. LYCKE, N. 2001. The B-cell targeted CTA1-DD vaccine adjuvant is highly effective at enhancing antibody as well as CTL responses. Curr. Opin. Mol. Ther. **3:** 37–44.
30. LJUNGBERG, U.K. *et al.* 1993. The interaction between different domains of staphylococcal protein A and human polyclonal IgG, IgA, IgM and F(ab′)2: separation of affinity from specificity. Mol. Immunol. **30:** 1279–1285.
31. UHLEN, M. *et al.* 1984. Complete sequence of the staphylococcal gene encoding protein A. A gene evolved through multiple duplications. J. Biol. Chem. **259:** 1695–1702.
32. AGREN, L. *et al.* 2000. The ADP-ribosylating CTA1-DD adjuvant enhances T cell-dependent and independent responses by direct action on B cells involving anti-apoptotic Bcl-2- and germinal center-promoting effects. J. Immunol. **164:** 6276–6286.
33. AGREN, L.C. *et al.* 1999. Adjuvanticity of the cholera toxin A1-based gene fusion protein, CTA1-DD, is critically dependent on the ADP-ribosyltransferase and Ig-binding activity. J. Immunol. **162:** 2432–2440.
34. ERIKSSON, A.M., K.M. SCHON & N.Y. LYCKE. 2004. The cholera toxin-derived CTA1-DD vaccine adjuvant administered intranasally does not cause inflammation or accumulate in the nervous tissues. J. Immunol. **173:** 3310–3319.
35. HODGE, L.M. *et al.* 2001. Immunoglobulin A (IgA) responses and IgE-associated inflammation along the respiratory tract after mucosal but not systemic immunization. Infect. Immun. **69:** 2328–2338.
36. LAVELLE, E.C. *et al.* 2004. Effects of cholera toxin on innate and adaptive immunity and its application as an immunomodulatory agent. J. Leukoc. Biol. **75:** 756–763.
37. AGREN, L., B. LOWENADLER & N. LYCKE. 1998. A novel concept in mucosal adjuvanticity: the CTA1-DD adjuvant is a B cell-targeted fusion protein that incorporates the enzymatically active cholera toxin A1 subunit. Immunol. Cell Biol. **76:** 280–287.
38. HAGIWAR, Y. *et al.* 2001. Effectiveness and safety of mutant *Escherichia coli* heat-labile enterotoxin (LT H44A) as an adjuvant for nasal influenza vaccine. Vaccine **19:** 2071–2079.
39. GIZURARSON, S. *et al.* 1992. Stimulation of the transepithelial flux of influenza HA vaccine by cholera toxin B subunit. Vaccine **10:** 101–106.

40. LYCKE, N. et al. 1991. The adjuvant action of cholera toxin is associated with an increased intestinal permeability for luminal antigens. Scand. J. Immunol. **33:** 691–698.
41. PALUCKA, K. & J. BANCHEREAU. 2002. How dendritic cells and microbes interact to elicit or subvert protective immune responses. Curr. Opin. Immunol. **14 :** 420–431.
42. GRANUCCI, F. & P. RICCIARDI-CASTAGNOLI. 2003. Interactions of bacterial pathogens with dendritic cells during invasion of mucosal surfaces. Curr. Opin. Microbiol. **6:** 72–76.
43. SUNDQUIST, M., C. JOHANSSON & M.J. WICK. 2003. Dendritic cells as inducers of antimicrobial immunity in vivo. APMIS **111:** 715–724.
44. KELSALL, B.L. & W. STROBER. 1996. Distinct populations of dendritic cells are present in the subepithelial dome and T cell regions of the murine Peyer's patch. J. Exp. Med. **183:** 237–247.
45. SHREEDHAR, V.K., B.L. KELSALL & M.R. NEUTRA. 2003. Cholera toxin induces migration of dendritic cells from the subepithelial dome region to T- and B-cell areas of Peyer's patches. Infect. Immun. **71:** 504–509.
46. RESCIGNO, M. et al. 2001. Dendritic cells express tight junction proteins and penetrate gut epithelial monolayers to sample bacteria. Nat. Immunol. **2:** 361–367.
47. STEINMAN, R.M. et al. 2000. The induction of tolerance by dendritic cells that have captured apoptotic cells [comment]. J. Exp. Med. **191:** 411–416.
48. VINEY, J.L. et al. 1998. Expanding dendritic cells in vivo enhances the induction of oral tolerance. J. Immunol. **160:** 5815–5825.
49. WILLIAMSON, E., G.M. WESTRICH & J.L. VINEY. 1999. Modulating dendritic cells to optimize mucosal immunization protocols. J. Immunol. **163:** 3668–3675.
50. ITANO, A.A. et al. 2003. Distinct dendritic cell populations sequentially present antigen to CD4 T cells and stimulate different aspects of cell-mediated immunity. Immunity **19:** 47–57.
51. PULENDRAN, B. et al. 2001. Modulating the immune response with dendritic cells and their growth factors. Trends Immunol. **22:** 41–47.
52. FINKELMAN, F.D. et al. 1996. Dendritic cells can present antigen in vivo in a tolerogenic or immunogenic fashion. J. Immunol. **157:** 1406–1414.
53. HAWIGER, D. et al. 2001. Dendritic cells induce peripheral T cell unresponsiveness under steady state conditions in vivo. J. Exp. Med. **194:** 769–779.
54. LAVELLE, E.C. et al. 2003. Cholera toxin promotes the induction of regulatory T cells specific for bystander antigens by modulating dendritic cell activation. J. Immunol. **171:** 2384–2392.
55. BROMANDER, A., J. HOLMGREN & N. LYCKE. 1991. Cholera toxin stimulates IL-1 production and enhances antigen presentation by macrophages in vitro. J. Immunol. **146:** 2908–2914.
56. GAGLIARDI, M.C. et al. 2000. Cholera toxin induces maturation of human dendritic cells and licences them for Th2 priming. Eur. J. Immunol. **30:** 2394–2403.
57. ERIKSSON, K. et al. 2003. Cholera toxin and its B subunit promote dendritic cell vaccination with different influences on Th1 and Th2 development. Infect. Immun. **71:** 1740–1747.
58. BRAUN, M.C. et al. 1999. Cholera toxin suppresses interleukin (IL)-12 production and IL-12 receptor beta1 and beta2 chain expression. J. Exp. Med. **189:** 541–552.
59. VAJDY, M. et al. 1995. Impaired mucosal immune responses in interleukin 4-targeted mice. J. Exp. Med. **181:** 41–53.
60. XU-AMANO, J. et al. 1993. Helper T cell subsets for immunoglobulin A responses: oral immunization with tetanus toxoid and cholera toxin as adjuvant selectively induces Th2 cells in mucosa associated tissues. J. Exp. Med. **178:** 1309–1320.
61. HORNQUIST, E. & N. LYCKE. 1993. Cholera toxin adjuvant greatly promotes antigen priming of T cells. Eur. J. Immunol. **23:** 2136–2143.
62. SUN, J.B., J. HOLMGREN & C. CZERKINSKY. 1994. Cholera toxin B subunit: an efficient transmucosal carrier-delivery system for induction of peripheral immunological tolerance. Proc. Natl. Acad. Sci. USA **91:** 10795–10799.
63. CZERKINSKY, C. et al. 1991. Detection of human cytokine-secreting cells in distinct anatomical compartments. Immunol. Rev. **119:** 5–22.

64. AGREN, L. et al. 2000. The ADP-ribosylating CTA1-DD adjuvant enhances T cell-dependent and independent responses by direct action on B cells involving anti-apoptotic Bcl-2- and germinal center-promoting effects. J. Immunol, **164:** 6276–6286.
65. AGREN, L.C. et al. 1999. Adjuvanticity of the cholera toxin A1-based gene fusion protein, CTA1-DD, is critically dependent on the ADP-ribosyltransferase and Ig- binding activity. J. Immunol. **162:** 2432–2440.
66. SIMMONS, C.P. et al. 1999. MHC class I-restricted cytotoxic lymphocyte responses induced by enterotoxin-based mucosal adjuvants. J. Immunol. **163:** 6502–6510.
67. CHOI, A.H. et al. 2002. The level of protection against rotavirus shedding in mice following immunization with a chimeric VP6 protein is dependent on the route and the coadministered adjuvant. Vaccine **20:** 1733–1740.
68. MOWAT, A.M. & J.L. VINEY. 1997. The anatomical basis of intestinal immunity. Immunol. Rev. **156:** 145–166.
69. LYCKE, N. 1997. The mechanism of cholera toxin adjuvanticity. Res. Immunol. **148:** 504–520.
70. JANG, M.H. et al. 2003. Induction of cytotoxic T lymphocyte responses by cholera toxin-treated bone marrow-derived dendritic cells. Vaccine **21:** 1613–1619.
71. GRDIC, D. et al. 1999. The mucosal adjuvant effects of cholera toxin and immune-stimulating complexes differ in their requirement for IL-12, indicating different pathways of action. Eur. J. Immunol. **29:** 1774–1784.
72. MOWAT, A.M. et al. 2001. CTA1-DD-immune stimulating complexes: a novel, rationally designed combined mucosal vaccine adjuvant effective with nanogram doses of antigen. J. Immunol. **167:** 3398–405.

In Vivo Effectors
Summary of Part IV

MITCHELL KRONENBERG

La Jolla Institute for Allergy and Immunology, San Diego, California 92121, USA

Five speakers in session IV focused on emerging data, illustrating the diverse mechanisms of immune regulation that govern the balance between suppression and stimulation of immune responses. Emphasis was placed on the factors leading to the suppression of immune responses when antigen is given orally or following inhalation, to the means by which protective immune responses can be stimulated by adjuvants following mucosal immunization, and also to the factors leading to uncontrolled mucosal inflammation.

Caroline Whitacre reported that dendritic cells (DCs) are the cell type critical for the induction of oral tolerance. Expansion of immature DCs in mice, by treatment with the Fms-like tyrosine kinase-3 ligand (Flt3L), led to an increased efficacy of oral tolerance following feeding of myelin basic protein (MBP). This feeding regimen was effective at reversing established disease in an animal model of multiple sclerosis, and transfer of expanded DCs from the fed mice was shown to be protective. The DC susbset(s) responsible for protection remain to be identified. Thymectomy was shown to prevent oral tolerance from working in the same experimental system, and the data suggested that the rapid export of $CD4^+$ $CD25^+$ regulatory T cells from the thymus after high-dose MBP feeding might be required for protection.

For oral tolerance to be effective, bystander suppression must be induced. This means that feeding of one antigen from the target organ, for example MBP in the experimental models of nervous tissue damage in multiple sclerosis, must prevent immune responses to other antigens in the target organ. David Wraith reported that intranasal administration of peptides can be effective at inducing bystander suppression, but the choice of peptide is critical, with the precursor frequency of peptide-reactive T cells being one variable that must be taken into consideration. Repeated nasal administration of MBP peptide could induce resistance to autoimmune disease, and this was dependent upon the generation of an IL-10–producing regulatory $CD4^+$ T cell population. Peptide-induced regulatory T cells that produce IL-10 were not $CD25^+$, and cells with a similar phenotype were found to be present in the peripheral blood lymphocytes from humans. These data illustrate the complexity in both the phenotype and function of regulatory T cells, with at least some of the classical $CD4^+$ $CD25^+$ T cells generated centrally in the thymus, and perhaps the CD25 negative regulatory T cells generated in the periphery by chronic antigen exposure.

Address for correspondence: Mitchell Kronenberg, 10355 Science Center Drive, San Diego, California 92121. Voice: 858-678-4540; fax: 858-678-4595.
  mitch@liai.org

Arlene Sharpe reported on the increasing complexity in the family of immunoglobulin (Ig) superfamily costimulatory molecules. B7-1 and B7-2 bind to CD28, which is constitutively expressed by T cells, thereby providing T cell costimulation. The CTLA-4 homologue of CD28 interacts with these same two receptors to provide negative signals. Previous studies have emphasized the role of CD28 interaction with B7 molecules during primary responses, but the data presented indicate that CD28-B7 interactions are important for the survival of pathogenic T cells in the central nervous system as well. PD-1 is distantly related to CD28 and CTLA-4, and activated T cells express it. While the two B7 molecules are expressed primarily by B cells and DCs, the two PD-1 ligands, PD-L1 and PD-L2, are expressed in a variety of tissues, with PD-L1 being found in the brain. While the functional significance of this expression pattern remains to be determined, PD-L1 negatively regulates naive and effector $CD4^+$ T cell responses, and therefore its expression could be important for the induction of tolerance both within and outside lymphoid tissues.

Michael Briskin reported on progress in studies in an animal model of inflammatory bowel disease, which is induced by the transfer of naive, $CD4^+$ T cells to immune-deficient recipients. His studies focused on two molecules thought to be important for the homing of circulating T lymphocytes to intestinal tissue. The integrin $\alpha_4\beta_7$ mediates mucosal trafficking by binding to the addressin molecule MAdCAM-1. The chemokine receptor CCR9 mediates chemotaxis in response to the chemokine TECK, which is produced by intestinal epithelial cells. Peripheral T cells that express the integrin are also likely to express the chemokine receptor, providing a set of markers for circulating T cells likely to locate to the intestine. The importance of these molecules could be demonstrated in the transfer model of colitis, because CCR9-deficient T cells are less able to cause disease, and pathogenesis was inhibited with antibodies to $\alpha_4\beta_7$. These blocking strategies may be particularly effective because functions in addition to homing to the colon were affected.

There is a clear need for adjuvants that can be administered nasally with vaccines. Cholera toxin binds to ganglioside GM1 and can serve as a mucosal adjuvant, but toxicity, with accumulation in nervous tissue, is a significant problem. Nils Lycke reported on CTA1-DD, which contains the enzymatically active ADP-ribosyl transferase of the A subunit, but which is targeted to B cells because of fusion of the A subunit to the Ig-binding element from *Staphylococcus aureus* protein A. CTA1-DD did not accumulate in nervous tissue, and it is an effective adjuvant for a balanced Th1/Th2 cytokine response and the promotion of primary and secondary responses. The full effects of this molecule require an enzymatically active A subunit. The mechanism for the effectiveness of CTA1-DD remains to be determined, but it clearly does not require signaling by Toll-like receptors. Furthermore, it acts on B lymphocytes, which was expected because of their surface Ig expression, but also on dendritic cells.

These newly defined molecular interactions, important for the regulation of systemic and mucosal immunity, may provide new targets for modulating tolerance and immune responses following mucosal antigen administration.

Current Issues in the Treatment of Human Diseases by Mucosal Tolerance

HOWARD L. WEINER

Center for Neurologic Diseases, Brigham and Women's Hospital, Harvard Medical School, Boston, Massachusetts 02115-5817, USA

ABSTRACT: Tolerance has been defined as a lack of response to self but a more appropriate definition of tolerance is "any mechanism by which a potentially injurious immune response is prevented, suppressed, or shifted to a noninjurious class of immune response." Thus, tolerance is related to productive self-recognition, rather than blindness of the immune system to its autocomponents. Oral tolerance, in this sense, is of unique immunologic importance, as it is a continuous natural immunologic event driven by exogenous antigen. Because of their privileged access to the internal milieu, antigens that are continuously in contact with the mucosa are a frontier between foreign and self-components. Thus, oral tolerance is an immunological mechanism that evolved to treat external agents that gain access to the body via a natural route as internal components that then become part of self. Given this, it would seem logical that autoimmune diseases caused by an inappropriate response to self-antigens might ultimately be treated by presenting such autoantigens to the mucosal surface where they can be dealt with in a noninjurous (noninflammatory) immunologic environment. Furthermore, mucosal tolerance as a treatment for autoimmune diseases is an attractive concept, as antigen-specific therapy is the most physiologic means to manipulate immune responses, and mucosal antigen is nontoxic and can be given on a chronic basis. The efficacy of mucosal tolerance has been clearly demonstrated in several animal models.

KEYWORDS: mucosal tolerance; dendritic cells; oral antigen; atherosclerosis; Alzheimer disease; stroke; nerve injury

MECHANISMS OF ORAL TOLERANCE

It is now clear that oral tolerance is an active immunologic process and is mediated by more than one mechanism. Low doses of antigen favor the induction of active cellular regulation, whereas higher doses favor the induction of anergy or deletion. Among the active mechanisms induced by low doses of antigen, induction of regulatory T cells that secrete IL-4, IL-10, or TGF-β (Th3-type regulatory cells) is the most important one described so far.[1,2] The mucosal milieu generates tolerogenic dendritic cells that are crucial for the induction of regulatory T cells after mucosal

Address for correspondence: Howard L. Weiner, M.D., Brigham and Women's Hospital, 77 Avenue Louis Pasteur, HIM 730, Boston, Massachusetts 02115-5817. Voice: 617-525-5300; fax: 617-525-5252.
hweiner@rics.bwh.harvard.edu

exposure to antigen.[3] We have recently found that oral administration of antigen induces $CD4^+CD25^+$ regulatory T cells expressing CTLA-4. $CD4^+CD25^+$ cells fed from mice are able to transfer tolerance, proliferate poorly, and secrete high levels of IL-10 and TGF-β.[4,78] Intragraft $CD8^+$ T cells with regulatory function have also been described in a kidney allotransplantion model in rats. These cells exhibited high levels of IL-4 mRNA, and they could transfer tolerance to naive recipients.[5] In nasal tolerance and experimental models of colitis, IL-10–producing T cells (Tr1 type regulatory cells) have been shown to play an important modulatory role.[6,7]

Virtually all manifestations of specific immune responsiveness tested can be suppressed by oral antigen administration. This includes *in vivo* responses such as formation of immunoglobulin of different isotypes, including IgE responses,[8] delayed hypersensitivity reactions,[9] lymphocyte proliferation,[10] and cytokine production, including IFN-γ, IL-4, IL-5, and IL-10.[11,12] Nonetheless, these immunological parameters are differentially affected by oral antigen. Th1-type responses are easier to suppress by oral administration of antigen than Th2-type responses. Suppression of Th1 responses requires lower doses of antigen and lasts longer than the inhibition of Th2 immune responses.[1] Of note, the suppression of the TGF-β response by oral antigen has not been reported for any dose or regimen of orally administered antigen.

BYSTANDER SUPPRESSION AND MUCOSAL TOLERANCE IN DISEASE MODELS

Oral antigen–specific therapy can be effective in autoimmune diseases, even if the autoantigens are unknown or if there is reactivity to multiple autoantigens (epitope spreading) because of cytokine-mediated bystander suppression. During the course of chronic inflammatory autoimmune processes in animals, there is intra- and interantigenic spread of autoreactivity at the target organ.[13] Similarly, in human autoimmune diseases there are reactivities to multiple autoantigens in the target tissue.[14] In bystander suppression, regulatory cells induced by a fed antigen can suppress immune responses stimulated by different antigen as long as the fed antigen is present in the anatomic vicinity.[15] Bystander suppression has been demonstrated in several experimental models, such as adjuvant/antigen-induced arthritis that is inhibited by feeding collagen,[16,17] proteolipid protein (PLP)–induced experimental autoimmune encephalitis (EAE) that can be prevented by oral administration of myelin basic protein (MBP),[18] and lymphocytic choriomeningitis virus (LCMV)–induced diabetes that is inhibited by feeding insulin.[19]

Since the 1980s, oral tolerance has been shown to be an effective means of inhibiting immune responses to antigens of immunopathological importance in animals. Several autoantigens and experimental models of immunologically mediated diseases have been sucessfully used for oral tolerance studies. Examples include oral administration of MBP, PLP, myelin oligodendrocytic glycoprotein (MOG), and myelin in EAE models;[20–22] collagen II, HSP65, and streptococcal cell wall in arthritis;[23–25] insulin and glutamic acid decarboxylase (GAD) in diabetes;[26,27] S-antigen, interphotoreceptor binding protein (IRBP), and HLA-peptide in uveitis;[28–30] acetylcholine receptor (AchR) and its peptides in myasthenia gravis;[31] Derp1, mite protein, and pollen in allergy;[32–34] and allogeneic cells and allopeptides in transplantation.[35] Other experimental models of disease that have also been prevented by either oral or nasal administration of pathogenic antigens are colitis, thyroiditis, nickel sensitization, tracheal eosinophilia, antiphospholipid syndrome, immune complex disease, and experimental neuritis.[1] The potential clinical application of oral or mucosal tolerance has spread also to diseases not classically considered to be immune mediated but in which immune mechanisms play a role, such as atherosclerosis, stroke, nerve injury, and Alzheimer disease.

ATHEROSCLEROSIS

Although many factors may contribute to atherosclerosis, including lipid disorders and hypertension, the pathogenesis of atherosclerosis ultimately includes a major inflammatory component. Heat-shock proteins, known to be upregulated in inflammatory situations, are also a suitable target for bystander suppression strategies in inflammatory conditions such as this one. Recently, we examined the effect of nasal and oral administration of mycobacterial hsp65 on atherosclerotic lesion formation in mice lacking the receptor for LDL that were maintained on a high-cholesterol diet. Nasal administration of hsp65 induced a significant decrease in the size of atherosclerotic plaques, a reduction in macrophage-positive area in the aortic arch, downmodulation of IL-2 and IFN-γ production by spleen cells, increased IL-10 but not TGF-β expression, and reduced numbers of T cells in the arch. A similar trend was observed in orally treated mice, but not as significant as that in nasally treated.[36] Another study showed that oral treatment with hsp65 also reduced plaque size in *Mycobacterium tuberculosis*–induced atherosclerosis.[37]

NERVE INJURY

Axonal injury in the central nervous system (CNS) results in the degeneration of directly damaged fibers and the secondary degeneration of fibers that escaped the primary insult. Studies have shown that a protective T cell–mediated autoimmunity directed against myelin-related self-antigens is a physiological response to CNS injury, spontaneously elicited in strains that are constitutionally resistant to EAE but not in susceptible strains. Bystander suppression achieved by oral antigen in nonimmune pathological conditions may mimic this physiological protective reaction to self-antigens in response to inflammatory insult. Oral administration of low-dose MBP over a five-day period is beneficial for posttraumatic survival of retinal ganglion cells in Lewis rats following optic nerve injury. Protection was accompanied by increased expression of the costimulatory molecule B7.2 in the traumatized nerves, similar to that seen after passive transfer of MBP-specific T cells. These results support the contention that properly controlled autoimmunity is the body's defense mechanism against noninfective insults.[38]

STROKE

Ischemic stroke results from transient or permanent reduction in cerebral blood flow. It is one of the main causes of morbidity and mortality worldwide. Inflammation is also initiated by ischemia at the blood–microvascular endothelial cell interface and contributes significantly to CNS damage. Because inflammation plays an important role in ischemic stroke, strategies aiming at inducing immunological tolerance to the inflammatory event have already been reported using common CNS antigens. Oral administration of MBP decreased stroke size in a rat stroke model, presumably by decreasing inflammation associated with ischemic injury.[39] We used oral and nasal administration of MOG 35–55 peptide to C57BL/6 mice before middle cerebral artery occlusion (MCAO) to induce an anti-inflammatory T cell response directed at CNS myelin. Nasal MOG was most efficacious and reduced infarct size by 70% following stroke and also improved behavior score. Immunohistochemistry demonstrated increased IL-10 and reduced IFN-γ in the area surrounding the ischemic infarct in nasally tolerant mice. Nasal MOG did not reduce infarct size in IL-10–deficient mice. In addition, adoptive transfer of CD4$^+$ T cells from nasally treated wild-type but not IL-10–deficient mice was able to transfer tolerance.[40]

ALZHEIMER DISEASE

Alzheimer disease is a major cause of dementia in the adult population and is associated with the deposition of beta-amyloid (A-beta) in the brain, leading to neuronal degeneration and inflammatory responses. PDAPP transgenic mice serve as an animal model for the study of Alzheimer disease because these animals spontaneously accumulate A-beta in the CNS beginning at four to five months of age.

It has been shown that immunization with A-beta attenuates Alzheimer disease–like pathology in the PDAPP mouse. Antibodies play an important role, and their passive transfer seems to clear A-beta from the CNS. However, the use of this protocol in humans has shown detrimental inflammatory effects. Patients who were immunized with A-beta in adjuvant developed meningoencephalitis.[41]

Recently, we have developed a protocol for mucosal tolerance induction in PDAPP mice using oral and nasal administration of A-beta peptide before and during the course of the disease. Nasal but not oral administration of A-beta peptide significantly decreases cerebral amyloid burden. This reduced deposition is associated with circulating A-beta antibodies of the IgG1 and IgG2b isotypes, both of which are characteristic of a Th2-type immune response, and with the presence of mononuclear cells expressing IL-4, IL-10, and TGF-β in the brain. Our findings provide the basis for testing the effect of nasal A-beta administration for the prevention and/or treatment of Alzheimer disease in humans.[42]

HUMAN TRIALS OF MUCOSAL TOLERANCE

Trials of oral tolerance in human diseases have produced mixed results, and large-scale phase III trials in multiple sclerosis, rheumatoid arthritis, and type 1 diabetes have been unsuccessful in bringing oral tolerance immunotherapy to market.[43] Although clinical efficacy resulting in an approved drug has yet to be demonstrated, these initial trials suggest that there has been no systemic toxicity or exacerbation of disease. Results in humans have paralleled several aspects of what has been observed in animals, and there are several small studies demonstrating positive effects. Oral tolerance to keyhole limpet hemocyanin (KLH) was initially tested in volunteer human subjects who were experimentally immunized with the antigen. KLH administered orally and nasally decreased subsequent cell-mediated immune responses, although antibody responses were not affected,[44,45] and also decreased KLH-precursor frequency.[46] Mucosal tolerance has been reported as a means to help prevent rejection in maternal-donor renal allografts. It is known that a large number of maternal lymphocytes are present in breast milk, and there was a report in 1984 suggesting that breast-fed recipients may have done better after a maternal donor–related renal transplant procedure than non–breast-fed recipients.[47] Moreover, mucosal tolerance has been reported as successful in the treatment of contact sensitivity, allergic rhinitis, thyroditis, and uveitis. Oral desensitization to nickel in humans induces a decrease in nickel-specific T cells and affects cutaneous nickel-induced eczema.[48] In a double-blind placebo-controlled crossover trial for the treatment of perennial rhinitis due to house dust mite, low-dose sublingual therapy with house dust mite was reported to be effective in relieving symptoms in 72% of patients.[49] Mucosal tolerance has been used for the treatment of some allergic conditions in humans. Oral tolerance has also been shown to be effective in decreasing eye symptoms and allergy scores in conjunctival and respiratory allergy to birch pollen and ragweed.[50,51] Oral administration of porcine thyroid to patients with autoimmune thyroiditis previously receiving thyroid hormone replacement with synthetic thyroxin decreased cellular immunity to thyroid peptides when compared with the control patients who remained on synthetic T4.[52] In uveitis, a pilot trial of S-antigen and a retinal antigen mixture conducted at the National Eye Institute showed positive trends with oral bovine S-antigen but not the retinal mixture.[53] Feeding of peptide derived from a patient's own HLA antigen appeared to have an effect on uveitis, in that patients could discontinue their steroids because of reduced intraocular inflammation mediated by oral tolerance.[54]

Human trials involving multiple research centers and large numbers of patients have been performed in the past several years to test the efficacy of mucosal tolerance in the treatment of autoimmune diseases. Three diseases in particular have been studied: multiple sclerosis, rheumatoid arthritis, and diabetes.

MULTIPLE SCLEROSIS

A 515-patient, placebo-controlled, double-blind phase III trial of single-dose bovine myelin in relapsing-remitting multiple sclerosis (MS) did not show differences between placebo and treated groups in the number of relapses; a large placebo effect was observed (Autoimmune Inc., Lexington, MA, USA). The dose of myelin was 300 mg, given in capsule form, and contained 8 mg MBP and 15 mg PLP. Preliminary analysis of magnetic resonance imaging data showed significant changes favoring oral myelin in certain patient subgroups.

MBP- and PLP-specific TGF-β–secreting Th3-type cells were observed in the peripheral blood of MS patients treated with an oral bovine myelin preparation, but not in patients who were untreated.[55] This study suggests that it is possible to immunize for autoantigen-specific TGF-β–secreting cells in a human autoimmune disease by oral administration of the autoantigen.

Trials of oral tolerance in MS were carried out with the MBP analogue, glatiramer acetate, which is currently given by injection to MS patients, and which has been shown to be effective orally in animals and to induce regulatory cells that mediate bystander suppression.[56,57] A trial of glatiramer acetate in relapsing-remitting MS at a dose of 5 mg or 50 mg daily did not show immunologic or clinical effects. Trials of larger doses of oral glatiramer acetate are in progress.

RHEUMATOID ARTHRITIS

In rheumatoid arthritis (RA), a 280-patient double-blind phase II dosing trial of type II collagen in liquid doses ranging from 20 mg to 2500 mg per day for six months demonstrated statistically significant positive effects in the group treated with the lowest dose.[58] Oral administration of larger doses of bovine type II collagen (1 to 10 mg) did not show a significant difference between test and placebo groups, although a higher prevalence of responders was reported for the groups treated with type II collagen. An open-label pilot study of oral collagen in juvenile RA gave positive results with no toxicity.[59]

Five phase II randomized studies of oral type II collagen have been performed. On the basis of the results obtained, a multicenter double-blind phase III trial study of oral type II collagen (Colloral) was performed, but showed negative results (AutoImmune Inc.). In the five double-blind phase II studies, a total of 805 patients were treated with oral type II collagen and 296 were treated with placebo. Two of the studies have been published;[58,60] the other three studies were included in an integrated analysis that led to the decision to carry out a phase III trial. A dose refinement study tested doses of 5, 20, and 60 micrograms. Compared with the other doses, Colloral at 60 μg was found to be the most significant dose. Weighted averages for the Paulus 20 and Paulus 50 responses were calculated for the 60 μg dose and placebo. A significant effect favoring 60 μg was observed for both the Paulus 20 and the Paulus 50 response. Integrated efficacy analysis of predictors of response, including HLA, phenotype, rheumatoid factor, CII antibodies, duration of disease, and tender and swollen joint count, was performed, but no statistically significant predictors were identified. Use of NSAIDs did not appear to affect the clinical response of an RA patient to oral type II collagen. Safety analysis demonstrated that Colloral was safe with no side effects. The magnitude of the clinical responses with Colloral appear to be on the same level as with NSAIDs for the majority of patients. However, there is a subgroup of patients that appear to have a more significant response to the medication. On the basis of these data, a 760-patient phase III trial was performed comparing 60 μg of Colloral to placebo. However, no differences were observed. A large placebo effect (>50%) was observed in the control group. Subsequently, a placebo-controlled trial of bovine collagen showed significant effects in those receiving 0.5 mg, but not in those receiving 0.05 mg or 5 mg.[61] Oral collagen II in juvenile RA was associated with clinical improvement, decreased collagen II–specific IFN-γ, and increased TGF-β.[62] Clinical trials are underway to determine whether withholding NSAIDs and prednisone will allow oral tolerance to be induced and whether oral collagen II has meaningful clinical efficacy in RA.[63]

DIABETES

Six different trials are currently underway or completed in testing mucosally administered recombinant human insulin as a tolerizing agent in type 1 diabetes: (1) A multicenter double-blind study in the United States evaluating oral insulin therapy versus placebo in adults and children with new-onset disease. Preliminary analysis suggests preserved beta cell function as measured by endogenous C-peptide insulin responses in patients diagnosed after age 20 years and fed 1 mg versus placebo.[64] (2) A double-blind study in France to compare oral insulin therapy and parenteral insulin therapy versus placebo in patients during the remission phase. Evaluation criteria include duration of remission, measures of insulin secretion/sensitivity, and immunological parameters; no effect of treatment was observed with 2.5 or 7.5 mg oral insulin.[65] (3) A multicenter double-blind study in Italy to evaluate whether the addition of oral insulin is able to improve the integrated parameters of metabolic control and modify immunological findings compared with placebo in patients with recent onset disease treated with intensive insulin therapy (IMDIAB VI). (4) A multicenter double-blind study in the United States to determine whether diabetes can be prevented by subcutaneous insulin therapy or oral insulin therapy in subjects at risk for diabetes (DPT-1). (5) A double-blind study in Australia evaluating aerosolized insulin versus placebo in patients with new-onset disease. (6) A double-blind study in Finland evaluating nasally administered insulin versus placebo in patients with new-onset disease.

The recent randomized double-blind Intranasal Insulin Trial I (INIT I) was performed to test nasal tolerance in 38 first-degree relatives (median age = 10.8 years) who are positive for islet antibodies. The aim of this study was to determine whether administration of insulin to the nasal mucosa is safe and is able to induce changes in immunity that are consistent with mucosal tolerance induction. Two 10 U (400 mg) doses per nostril were administered daily for 10 consecutive days, and then on weekends. Antibody and T cell responses were monitored as well as insulin response to intravenous administration of glucose. Results of this trial showed no side effects of intranasal insulin administration and a first phase insulin response that was stable for more than four years. Moreover, a suppression in cellular but not in antibody responses was observed in treated individuals. These immunological changes were similar to those observed in NOD mice given nasorespiratory insulin or to those of human volunteers given oral or intranasal KLH. Results from the DPT-1 trial suggest positive effects of 7.5 mg of oral insulin in a subgroup of patients, and further trials of 7.5 mg oral insulin in these patients is being planned.

WORSENING OF AUTOIMMUNE DISEASES

Although mucosally administered antigens have been used successfully to treat a wide variety of autoimmune and inflammatory conditions, under certain experimental conditions worsening of autoimmune diseases in animals by oral antigen has been reported.

We have observed that neonatal administration of guinea pig MBP in the Lewis rat does not induce oral tolerance and in fact makes animals more susceptible to EAE induction as adults.[66] This raises the possibility that neonatal exposure to antigen may be a factor in the development of autoimmune disease in adulthood. This indeed has been postulated for diabetes in terms of exposure to cow's milk as a risk factor for development of diabetes. Interestingly, we fed insulin to neonatal NOD mice and did not find an enhancement of diabetes, but better protection against the development of diabetes.[67] We did not observe protection with oral MOG given to neonates, but it did not exacerbate EAE. Thus, worsening of autoimmunity by neonatal exposure may depend on strain of animal and antigen fed.

Meyer *et al.* reported that a single feeding of a small dose of guinea pig MBP exacerbated the clinical course of disease[68] in the B10.PL model of chronic relapsing EAE. Larger single doses suppressed the disease. These investigators also found that multiple oral doses of MBP were required to suppress clinical disease once it was established. We and others have found that there may be initial sensitization of Th1 responses when small doses of antigen are fed, followed by suppression as additional doses are given.[69,70] Thus, in animal models where immunization immediately follows feeding, exacerbation may be observed if only one feeding of a small dose is given. Nasal MBP has been associated with a trend of disease worsening in a protracted relapsing EAE model in DA rats.[71]

In diabetes models, Blanas *et al.* were able to induce diabetes by orally administering large doses of ovalbumin (OVA, 30 mg) to OVA double transgenic mice.[72] The animals expressed OVA on the islets under the rat insulin promoter and were made chimeric to enrich for OVA-specific transgenic TCR CTL. Although diabetes was induced, it is not clear the degree to which this transgenic model applies to conventional animals. It has been demonstrated that insulin given with an adjuvant may exacerbate diabetes in the BB rat model.[73] It has been difficult to protect the BB rat from diabetes by oral insulin, which may relate to defects the animals have in regulatory cell populations and could account for the ability to enhance diabetes by coadministered adjuvant. In results reported to date from human trials in which new-onset diabetics were fed 1 or 10 mg of insulin, there was no evidence of disease worsening.[74] Nonetheless, these studies demonstrate that orally administered antigen is active immunologically when it encounters the gut-associated lymphoid tissue (GALT), and under special circumstances the immune response generated can have a harmful effect.

FUTURE DIRECTIONS

In spite of the negative results of phase III human trials of mucosal tolerance, many lessons have been learned from them as well as from the successful experiments with animal models. On the basis of the results of oral tolerance in uveitis in humans,[53] and in animal models of myasthenia[31] and EAE,[75] it appears that protein mixtures may not be as effective oral tolerogens as purified proteins.

Data on animal models also show that a number of factors appear to modulate oral tolerance.[1] As oral tolerance has usually been defined in terms of Th1 responses, anything that suppresses Th1 and/or enhances Th2 or Th3 cell development would enhance oral tolerance. Th3 cells appear to use IL-4 and TGF-β itself as growth/differentiation factors. Thus, intraperitoneal IL-4 administration, oral IL-10, and IL-4 can also enhance oral tolerance when coadministered with antigen, and cytokines have also been administered by the nasal route.[77–81] Oral but not subcutaneous lipopolysaccharide (LPS) enhances oral tolerance to MBP and is associated with increased expression of IL-4 in the brain.[82] In the uveitis model, intraperitoneal IL-2 potentiates oral tolerance and is associated with increased production of TGF-β, IL-10, and IL-4.[83] Oral antigen delivery using a multiple emulsion system also enhances oral tolerance. In the arthritis model, intraperitoneal administration of TGF-β or dimaprid (a histamine type 2 receptor agonist), both of which are believed to promote the development of immunoregulatory cells, enhances the induction of oral tolerance to collagen II even after the onset of arthritis.[84] Coupling antigens to recombinant cholera toxin B subunit (CTB) enhances their ability to induce peripheral immune tolerance.[85] On the other hand, cholera toxin (CT) is one of the most potent mucosal adjuvants, and feeding CT abrogates oral tolerance when fed with an unrelated protein antigen. Large doses of IFN-γ given intraperitoneally abrogate oral tolerance, anti–IL-12 enhances oral tolerance and is associated both with increased TGF-β production and T cell apotosis, and subcutaneous administration of IL-12 reverses mucosal tolerance.[86] Oral IFN-β synergizes with the induction of oral tolerance in SJL/PLJ mice fed low doses of MBP. Antibody to chemokine monocyte chemotactic protein 1 (MCP-1) abrogates oral tolerance.[87] Gamma/delta T cells may have an important role in oral tolerance induction, as it seems more difficult to induce oral tolerance in animals depleted of such cells or in delta-chain–deficient animals. The steroid hormone dehydroepiandrosterone (DHEA) breaks intranasally induced tolerance.[88] We also have found recently that certain regimens of feeding may affect oral tolerance induction. Continuous feeding of antigen enhances oral tolerance by upregulating IL-10 and TGF-β.[76]

Although it is clear that oral antigen can suppress autoimmunity and inflammatory diseases in animals, it is also clear from all these studies that several factors need to be considered carefully to improve the therapeutic effectiveness of mucosal tolerance in human disease: (1) the dose of antigen, a crucial factor; (2) the route of administration, as it is now known that the nasal route is sometimes more effective than the oral route; (3) mucosal adjuvants, which can enhance induction of mucosal tolerance and may be required; (4) purified proteins, which are more effective oral tolerogens than protein mixtures; (5) combination therapy using conventional anti-inflammatory and immunosuppressive drugs, which may yield a better result; (6) early therapy, as mucosal tolerance is mostly effective before or shortly after disease onset; (7) a clear immunological marker or immunological effect that must be established as a parameter for the follow-up of each disease.

Many aspects of the mechanisms involved in mucosal tolerance induction also need to be investigated further. Cell surface molecules and cytokines associated with inductive events in the gut that generate and modulate oral tolerance are not completely understood. Important areas of investigation include cytokine milieu, antigen presentation and costimulation requirements, routes of antigen processing, form of the antigen, role of the liver, effect of oral antigens on antibody and IgE responses and on CTLs, and the role of γδ T cells. As the molecular events associated with the generation and modulation of oral tolerance are better understood, the ability to apply mucosal tolerance successfully for the treatment of human autoimmune and other diseases will be further enhanced.

REFERENCES

1. FARIA, A.M. & H.L. WEINER. 1999. Oral tolerance: mechanisms and therapeutic applications. Adv. Immunol. **73:** 153–264.
2. WEINER, H.L. 2000. Oral tolerance, an active immunologic process mediated by multiple mechanisms. J. Clin. Invest. **106:** 935–937.
3. WEINER, H.L. 2001. The mucosal milieu creates tolerogenic dendritic cells and T(R)1 and T(H)3 regulatory cells. Nat. Immunol. **2:** 671–672.
4. MAYER, L. & L. SHAO. 2004. Therapeutic potential of oral tolerance. Nat. Rev. Immunol. **4:** 407–419.
5. ZHOU, J., R.I. CARR, R.S. LIWSKI, et al. 2001. Oral exposure to alloantigen generates intragraft CD8+ regulatory cells. J. Immunol. **167:** 107–113.
6. AKBARI, O., R.H. DEKRUYFF & D.T. UMETSU. 2001. Pulmonary dendritic cells producing IL-10 mediate tolerance induced by respiratory exposure to antigen. Nat. Immunol. **2:** 725–731.
7. GROUX, H., A. O'GARRA, M. BIGLER, et al. 1997. A CD4+ T-cell subset inhibits antigen-specific T-cell responses and prevents colitis. Nature **389:** 737–742.
8. VAZ, N.M., L.C.S. MAIA, D.G. HANSON, et al. 1977. Inhibition of homocytotropic antibody responses in adult inbred mice by previous feeding of the specific antigen. J. Allergy Clin. Immunol. **60:** 110–115.
9. MILLER, S. & D. HANSON. 1979. Inhibition of specific immune responses by feeding protein antigens. IV. Evidence for tolerance and specific active suppression of cell-mediated immune responses to ovalbumin. J. Immunol. **123:** 2344–2350.
10. MOWAT, A.M. 1987. The regulation of immune responses to dietary protein antigens. Immunology Today **8:** 93–95.
11. MOWAT, A.M., M. STEEL, E.A. WORTHY, et al. 1996. Inactivation of Th1 and Th2 cells by feeding ovalbumin. Ann. N. Y. Acad. Sci. **778:** 122–132.
12. MELAMED, D., J. FISHMAN-LOVELL, Z. UNI, et al. 1996. Peripheral tolerance of Th2 lymphocytes induced by continuous feeding of ovalbumin. Int. Immunol. **8:** 717–724.
13. LEHMANN, P., T. FORSTHUBER, A. MILLER & E. SERCARZ. 1992. Spreading of T-cell autoimmunity to cryptic determinants of an autoantigen. Nature **358:** 155–157.
14. KERLERO DE ROSBO, N., R. MILO, M.B. LEES, et al. 1993. Reactivity to myelin antigens in multiple sclerosis: peripheral blood lymphocytes respond predominantly to myelin oligodendrocyte glycoprotein. J. Clin. Invest. **92:** 2602–2608.
15. MILLER, A., O. LIDER & H.L. WEINER. 1991. Antigen-driven bystander suppression following oral administration of antigens. J. Exp. Med. **174:** 791–798.
16. YOSHINO, S. 1995. Antigen-induced arthritis in rats is suppressed by the inducing antigen administered orally before, but not after immunization. Cell. Immunol. **163:** 55–58.
17. ZHANG, J.Z., C.S.Y. LEE, O. LIDER, et al. 1990. Suppression of adjuvant arthritis in Lewis rats by oral administration of type II collagen. J. Immunol. **145:** 2489–2493.
18. MILLER, A., A. AL-SABBAGH, L. SANTOS, et al. 1993. Epitopes of myelin basic protein that trigger TGF-β release following oral tolerization are distinct from encephalitogenic epitopes and mediate epitope driven bystander suppression. J. Immunol. **151:** 7307–7315.
19. VON HERRATH, M.G., T. DYRBERG & M.B. OLDSTONE. 1996. Oral insulin treatment suppresses virus-induced antigen-specific destruction of beta cells and prevents autoimmune diabetes in transgenic mice. J. Clin. Invest. **98:** 1324–1331.
20. BITAR, D.M. & C.C. WHITACRE. 1988. Suppression of experimental autoimmune encephalomyelitis by the oral administration of myelin basic protein. Cell. Immunol. **112:** 364–370.
21. HIGGINS, P. & H.L. WEINER. 1988. Suppression of experimental autoimmune encephalomyelitis by oral administration of myelin basic protein and its fragments. J. Immunol. **140:** 440–445.
22. AL-SABBAGH, A., A. MILLER, L.M. SANTOS, et al. 1994. Antigen-driven tissue-specific suppression following oral tolerance: orally administered myelin basic protein suppresses proteolipid induced experimental autoimmune encephalomyelitis in the SJL mouse. Eur. J. Immunol. **24:** 2104–2109.

23. NAGLER-ANDERSON, C., L.A. BOBER, M.E. ROBINSON, et al. 1986. Suppression of type II collagen-induced arthritis by intragastric administration of soluble type II collagen. Proc. Natl. Acad. Sci. USA **83:** 7443–7446.
24. HAQUE, M.A., S. YOSHINO, S. INADA, et al. 1996. Suppression of adjuvant arthritis in rats by induction of oral tolerance to mycobacterial 65-kDa heat shock protein. Eur. J. Immunol. **26:** 2650–2656.
25. CHEN, W., W. JIN, M. COOK, et al. 1998. Oral delivery of group A streptococcal cell walls augments circulating TGF-beta and suppresses streptococcal cell wall arthritis. J. Immunol. **161:** 6297–6304.
26. MA, S.W., D.L. ZHAO, Z.Q. YIN, et al. 1997. Transgenic plants expressing autoantigens fed to mice to induce oral immune tolerance. Nature Med. **3:** 793–796.
27. MA, S., Y. HUANG, Z. YIN, et al. 2004. Induction of oral tolerance to prevent diabetes with transgenic plants requires glutamic acid decarboxylase (GAD) and IL-4. Proc. Natl. Acad. Sci. USA **101:** 5680–5685.
28. NUSSENBLATT, R.B., R.R. CASPI, R. MAHDI, et al. 1990. Inhibition of S-antigen induced experimental autoimmune uveoretinitis by oral induction of tolerance with S-antigen. J. Immunol. **144:** 1689–1695.
29. RIZZO, L.V., N.E. MILLER-RIVERO, C.C. CHAN, et al. 1994. Interleukin-2 treatment potentiates induction of oral tolerance in a murine model of autoimmunity. J. Clin. Invest. **94:** 1668–1672.
30. WILDNER, G. & S.R. THURAU. 1994. Cross-reactivity between an HLA-B27-derived peptide and a retinal autoantigen peptide: a clue to major histocompatibility complex association with autoimmune disease. Eur. J. Immunol. **24:** 2579–2585.
31. OKUMURA, S. & K. MCINTOSH & D.B. DRACHMAN. 1994. Oral administration of acetylcholine receptor: effects on experimental myasthenia gravis. Ann. Neurol. **36:** 704–713.
32. HOYNE, G.F., B.A. ASKINAS, C. HETZEL, et al. 1996. Regulation of house dust mite responses by intranasally administered peptide: transient activation of CD4+ T-cells precedes the development of tolerance in vivo. Int. Immunol. **8:** 335–342.
33. ARAMAKI, Y., Y. FUJII, H. SUDA, et al. 1994. Induction of oral tolerance after feeding of ragweed pollen extract in mice. Immunol. Lett. **40:** 21–25.
34. SATO, M.N., A.F. CARVALHO, A.O. SILVA, et al. 1998. Oral tolerance induced to house dust mite extract in naive and sensitized mice: evaluation of immunoglobulin G anti-immunoglobulin G anti-immunoglobulin E autoantibodies and IgC-IgE complexes. Immunology **95:** 193–199.
35. SAYEGH, M.H., Z.J. ZHANG, W.W. HANCOCK, et al. 1992. Down-regulation of the immune response to histocompatibility antigen and prevention of sensitization by skin allografts by orally administered alloantigen. Transplantion **53:** 163–166.
36. MARON, R., G. SUKHOVA, A.M. FARIA, et al. 2002. Mucosal administration of heat shock protein-65 decreases atherosclerosis and inflammation in aortic arch of low-density lipoprotein receptor-deficient mice. Circulation **106:** 1708–1715.
37. HARATS, D., N. YACOV, B. GILBURD, et al. 2002. Oral tolerance with heat shock protein 65 attenuates *Mycobacterium* tuberculosis-induced and high-fat-diet-driven atherosclerotic lesions. J. Am. Coll. Cardiol. **40:** 133–138.
38. MONSONEGO, A., Z.P. BESERMAN, J. KIPNIS, et al. 2003. Beneficial effect of orally administered myelin basic protein in EAE-susceptible Lewis rats in a model of acute CNS degeneration. J. Autoimmun. **21:** 131–138.
39. BECKER, K.J., R.M. MCCARRON, C. RUETZLER et al. 1997. Immunological tolerance to myelin basic protein decreases stroke size after transient focal cerebral ischemia. Proc. Natl. Acad. Sci. USA **94:** 10873–10878.
40. FRENKEL, D., Z. HUANG, R. MARON, et al. 2003. Nasal vaccination with myelin oligodendrocyte glycoprotein redces stroke size by inducing Il-10 producing CD4$^+$ T cells. J. Immunol. **171:** 6549–6555.
41. NICOLL, J.A., D. WILKINSON, C. HOLMES, et al. 2003. Neuropathology of human Alzheimer disease after immunization with amyloid-beta peptide: a case report. Nat. Med. **9:** 448–452.
42. WEINER, H.L., C.A. LEMERE, R. MARON, et al. 2000. Nasal administration of amyloid-beta peptide decreases cerebral amyloid burden in a mouse model of Alzheimer's disease. Ann. Neurol. **48:** 567–579.

43. QUINN, S. 2001. Human Trials: Scientists, Investors, and Patients in the Quest for a Cure. Perseus Publishing. Cambridge, MA.
44. HUSBY, S., J. MESTECKY, Z. MOLDOVEANU, et al. 1994. Oral tolerance in humans. T cell but not B cell tolerance after antigen feeding. J. Immunol. **152:** 4663–4670.
45. WALDO, F.B, A.W. VAN DEN WALL BAKE, J. MESTECKY & S. HUSBY. 1994. Suppression of the immune response by nasal immunization. Clin. Immunol. Immunopathol. **72:** 30–34.
46. MATSUI, M., D.A. HAFLER & H.L. WEINER. 1996. Pilot study of oral tolerance to keyhole limpet hemocyanin in humans: down-regulation of KLH-reactive precursor-cell frequency. Ann. N. Y. Acad. Sci. **778:** 398–404.
47. CAMPBELL, D.A., JR., M.I. LORBER, J.C. SWEETON, et al. 1984. Breast feeding and maternal-donor renal allografts. Possibly the original donor-specific transfusion. Transplantion **37:** 340–344.
48. BAGOT, M., D. CHARUE, M.L. FLECHET, et al. 1995. Oral desensitization in nickel allergy induces a decrease in nickel-specific T-cells. Eur. J. Dermatol. **5:** 614–617.
49. SCADDING, G.K. & J. BROSTOFF. 1986. Low dose sublingual therapy in patients with allergic rhinitis due to house dust mite. Clin. Allergy **16:** 483–491.
50. TAUDORF, E., L.C. LAURSEN, A. LANNER, et al. 1987. Oral immunotherapy in birch pollen hay fever. J. Allergy Clin. Immunol. **80:** 153–161.
51. LITWIN, A., M. FLANAGAN, G. ENTIS, et al. 1997. Oral immunotherapy with short ragweed extract in a novel encapsulated preparation: a double-blind study. J. Allergy Clin. Immunol. **100:** 30–38.
52. LEE, S., N. SCHERBERG & L.J. DE GROOT. 1998. Induction of oral tolerance in human autoimmune thyroid disease. Thyroid **8:** 229–234.
53. NUSSENBLATT, R.B., I. GERY, H.L. WEINER, et al. 1997. Treatment of uveitis by oral administration of retinal antigens: results of a phase I/II randomized masked trial. Am. J. Ophthalmol. **123:** 583–592.
54. THURAU, S.R., M. DIEDRICHS-MOHRING, H. FRICKE, et al. 1997. Molecular mimicry as a therapeutic approach for an autoimmune disease: oral treatment of uveitis-patients with an MHC-peptide crossreactive with autoantigen—first results. Immunol. Lett. **57:** 193–201.
55. FUKAURA, H., S.C. KENT, M.J. PIETRUSEWICZ, et al. 1996. Induction of circulating myelin basic protein and proteolipid protein-specific transforming growth factor-beta1-secreting Th3 T-cells by oral administration of myelin in multiple sclerosis patients. J. Clin. Invest. **98:** 70–77.
56. TEITELBAUM, D., R. ARNON & M. SELA. 1999. Immunomodulation of experimental autoimmune encephalomyelitis by oral administration of copolymer 1. Proc. Natl. Acad. Sci. USA **96:** 3842–3847.
57. WEINER, H.L. 1999. Oral tolerance with copolymer 1 for the treatment of multiple sclerosis. Proc. Natl. Acad. Sci. USA **96:** 3333–3335.
58. BARNETT, M.L., J.M. KREMER, E.W. ST. CLAIR, et al. 1998. Treatment of rheumatoid arthritis with oral type II collagen: results of a multicenter, double-blind, placebo-controlled trial. Arthritis Rheum. **41:** 290–297.
59. BARNETT, M.L., D. COMBITCHI & D.E. TRENTHAM. 1996. A pilot trial of oral type II collagen in the treatment of juvenile rheumatoid arthritis. Arthritis Rheum. **39:** 623–628.
60. TRENTHAM, D., R. DYNESIUS-TRENTHAM, E. ORAV, et al. 1993. Effects of oral administration of type II collagen on rheumatoid arthritis. Science **261:** 1727–1730.
61. CHOY, E., D. SCOTT, G. KINGSLEY, et al. 2001. Control of rheumatoid arthritis by oral tolerance. Arthritis Rheum. **44:** 1993–1997.
62. MYERS, L.K., G.C. HIGGINS, T.H. FINKEL, et al. 2001. Juvenile arthritis and autoimmunity to type II collagen. Arthritis Rheum. **44:** 1775–1781.
63. POSTLETHWAITE, A.E. 2001. Can we induce tolerance in rheumatoid arthritis? Curr. Rheumatol. Rep. **3:** 64–69.
64. KRISCHER, J., S. TEN, J. MARKER, et al. 2001. Endogenous insulin retention by oral insulin in newly diagnosed antibody positive type-1 diabetes [abstract]. Diabetes **50:** A44.
65. CHAILLOUS, L., H. LEFEVRE, C. THIVOLET, et al. 2000. Oral insulin administration and residual beta-cell function in recent-onset type 1 diabetes: a multicentre randomised controlled trial. Diabete Insuline Orale group. Lancet **356:** 545–549.

66. MILLER, A., O. LIDER, O. ABRAMSKY, et al. 1994. Orally administered myelin basic protein in neonates primes for immune responses and enhances experimental autoimmune encephalomyelitis in adult animals. Eur. J. Immunol. **24:** 1026–1032.
67. MARON, R., M. GUERAU-DE-ARELLANO, X. ZHANG, et al. 2001. Oral administration of insulin to neonates suppresses spontaneous and cyclophosphamide induced diabetes in the NOD mouse. J. Autoimmun. **16:** 21–28.
68. MEYER, A.L., J.M. BENSON, I.E. GIENAPP, et al. Suppression of murine chronic relapsing experimental autoimmune encephalomyelitis by the oral administration of myelin basic protein. J. Immunol. **157:** 4230–4238.
69. GAUTAM, S.C., N.F. CHIKKALA & J.R. BATTISTO. 1990. Oral administration of the contact sensitizer trinitrochlorobenzene: initial sensitization and subsequent appearance of a suppressor population. Cell. Immunol. **125:** 437–448.
70. CHEN, Y., J. INOBE & H.L. WEINER. 1997. Inductive events in oral tolerance in the TCR transgenic adoptive transfer model. Cell. Immunol. **178:** 62–68.
71. BAI, X.F., H.L. LI, F.D. SHI, et al. 1998. Complexities of applying nasal tolerance induction as a therapy for ongoing relapsing experimental autoimmune encephalomyelitis (EAE) in DA rats. Clin. Exp. Immunol. **111:** 205–210.
72. BLANAS, E., F.R. CARBONE, J. ALLISON, et al. 1996. Induction of autoimmune diabetes by oral administration of autoantigen. Science **274:** 1707–1709.
73. BELLMAN, K., H. KOLB, S. RASTEGAR, et al. 1998. Potential risk of oral insulin with adjuvant for the prevention of Type I diabetes: a protocol effective in NOD mice may exacerbate disease in BB rats. Diabetology **41:** 844–847.
74. COUTANT, R., A. ZEIDLER, R. RAPPAPORT, et al. 1998. Oral insulin therapy in newly-diagnosed immune mediated (type I) diabetes. Preliminary analysis of a randomized double blind placebo controlled study [abstract]. Diabetes **47**(Suppl. 1): A97.
75. BENSON, J.M., S.S. STUCKMANN, K.L. COX, et al. 1999. Oral administration of myelin basic protein is superior to myelin in suppressing relapsing experimental autoimmune encephalomyelitis. J. Immunol. **162:** 6247–6254.
76. FARIA, A.M., R. MARON, S.M. FICKER, et al. 2003. Oral tolerance induced by continuous feeding: enhanced up-regulation of transforming growth factor-beta/interleukin-10 and suppression of experimental autoimmune encephalomyelitis. J. Autoimmun. **20:** 135–145.
77. INOBE, J., A.J. SLAVIN, Y. KOMAGAT, et al. 1998. Il-4 is a differentiation factor for transforming growth factor-beta secreting Th3 cells and oral administration of IL-4 enhances oral tolerance in experimental allergic encephalomyelitis. Eur. J. Immunol. **28:** 2780–2790.
78. ZHANG, X., L. IZIKSON, L. LIU, et al. 2001. Activation of CD25(+)CD4(+) regulatory T cells by oral antigen administration. J. Immunol. **167:** 4245–4253.
79. XIAO, B.G., X.F. BAI, G.X. ZHANG & H. LINK. 1998. Suppression of acute and protracted-relapsing experimental allergic encephalomyelitis by nasal administration of low-dose IL-10 in rats. J. Neuroimmunol. **84:** 230–237.
80. XIAO, B.G., X.F. BAI, G.X. ZHANG, et al. 1998. Decrease of LFA-1 is associated with upregulation of TGF-β in CD4(+) T-cells clones derived from rats nasally tolerized against experimental autoimmune myasthenia gravis. Clin. Immunol. Immunopathol. **89:** 196–204.
81. SLAVIN, A.J., R. MARON & H.L. WEINER. 2001. Mucosal administration of IL-10 enhances oral tolerance in autoimmune encephalomyelitis and diabetes. Int. Immunol. **6:** 825–833.
82. KHOURY, S.J., O. LIDER, A. AL-SABBAGH & H.L. WEINER. 1990. Suppression of experimental autoimmune encephalomyelitis by oral administration of myelin basic protein. III. Synergistic effect of lipopolysaccharide. Cell Immunol. **131:** 302–310.
83. RIZZO, L.V., R.A. MORAWETZ, N.E. MILLER-RIVERO, et al. 1999. IL-4 and IL-10 are both required for the induction of oral tolerance. J. Immunol. **162:** 2613–2622.
84. THORBECKE, G.J., R. SCHWARCZ, J. LEU, et al. 1999. Modulation by cytokines of induction of oral tolerance to type II collagen. Arthritis Rheum. **42:** 110–118.
85. SUN, J.-B., C. HOLMGREN & C. CZERKINSKY. 1994. Cholera toxin B subunit: an efficient transmucosal carrier-delivery system for induction of peripheral immunological tolerance. Proc. Natl. Acad. Sci. USA **91:** 10795–10799.

86. CLAESSEN, A.M., B.M. VON BLOMBERG, J. DEGROOT, *et al.* 1996. Reversal of mucosal tolerance by subcutaneous administration of interleukin-12 at the site of attempted sensitization. Immunology **88:** 363–367.
87. Karpus, W.J., K.J.Kennedy, S.L. Kunkel & N.W. Lukacs. 1998. Monocyte chemotactic protein 1 regulates oral tolerance induction by inhibition of T-helper cell-related cytokines. J. Exp. Med. **187:** 733–741.
88. WOLVERS, D.A., J.M. BAKKER, W.M. BAGCHUS & G. KRAAL. 1998. The steroid hormone dehydroepiandrosterone (DHEA) breaks intranasally induced tolerance, when administered at time of systemic immunization. J. Immunol. **89:** 19–25.

Failure to Induce Oral Tolerance in Crohn's and Ulcerative Colitis Patients: Possible Genetic Risk

THOMAS A. KRAUS, LISA TOY, LISA CHAN, JOSEPH CHILDS, ADAM CHEIFETZ, AND LLOYD MAYER

The Mount Sinai School of Medicine, Immunobiology Center, New York, New York 10029, USA

ABSTRACT: It has been proposed that defective activation of suppressor or regulatory T cells is one mechanism involved in the uncontrolled inflammatory process seen in inflammatory bowel disease (IBD). Because suppressor/regulatory T cells are thought to play a role in the promotion of oral tolerance, we attempted to induce oral tolerance in normal controls ($n = 21$) and patients with either Crohn's disease (CD; $n = 12$) or ulcerative colitis (UC; $n = 13$). In the first study, subjects were fed the neoantigen keyhole limpet hemocyanin (KLH) on days 1 to 5 and 11 to 15. Subcutaneous immunization with KLH was performed on day 26, with a booster immunization on day 35. Blood for KLH-induced T cell proliferation and serum for anti-KLH antibody production was obtained at baseline, on day 26 preimmunization (postfed), on day 35 after the first immunization, and again on day 42 after the second immunization. In normal individuals, KLH feeding prior to immunization and booster resulted in reduced KLH-specific T cell proliferation compared with the group that was not fed KLH. However, although on the same KLH-feeding protocol, both CD and UC patients demonstrated significantly enhanced proliferation without oral tolerance induction when compared with baseline values. These data suggest that oral tolerance induction is defective in patients with IBD. This may reflect an *in vivo* functional defect in mucosal suppression of immune responses in IBD. Both UC and CD appear to be multigenic disorders with evidence of familial segregation. We analyzed four multiplex Crohn's and two UC families to determine whether the defect in tolerance induction was genetically regulated. In three of the four CD families at least one unaffected family member also failed to tolerize (total 5 of 14 unaffected family members). In the UC families, the defect in tolerance segregated with disease. These data suggest a genetic defect in tolerance induction in Crohn's disease.

KEYWORDS: oral tolerance; inflammatory bowel disease; Crohn's disease; ulcerative colitis

Address for correspondence: Lloyd Mayer, M.D., Immunobiology Center, East Building Room 11-20, 1425 Madison Ave., New York, NY 10029. Voice: 212-659-9266; fax: 212-987-5593.
 lloyd.mayer@mssm.edu

INTRODUCTION

Noninvasive intestinal luminal antigens, both dietary and from commensal bacteria, are presented to T cells in the suppressive context of the gastrointestinal tract, which leads to an active inhibition or regulation of the immune response against these antigens. In animal models, genetic mutations that result in either barrier dysfunction or regulatory cell defects result in a dysregulation in the mucosal immune response to luminal antigens that leads to a spontaneous colitis reminiscent of the human inflammatory bowel diseases (IBD), ulcerative colitis (UC) and Crohn's disease (CD).[1,2] These results, as well as studies in IBD patients, suggest that IBD is caused by an imbalance or dysregulation in mucosal tolerance.

Oral tolerance is the active nonresponse to antigens given to the host via the oral route. In the murine system, it appears that the mechanism of tolerance is dependent upon the dose of antigen.[3] Repeated administration of low doses of antigen result in the activation of regulatory T cells that secrete inhibitory cytokines such as IL-10 and TGF-β.[4,5] High doses of antigen can lead to deletion or anergy of antigen-specific T cells.[6] Both types of tolerance lead to decreased T cell responses following subsequent immunizations, as well as decreased B cell responses as determined by specific antibody titer.

Less is known about the mechanisms of oral tolerance in humans. Early studies suggest that T cell responses to the fed antigen are diminished, but B cell responses are not.[7] The mechanisms involved in the generation of tolerance in humans are still undefined.

It appears that IBD patients have a defect in mucosal regulatory pathways. Studies have shown that IBD patients can mount immune responses against normal enteric bacteria.[8,9] Furthermore, IBD patients have elevated serum antibody titers against dietary antigens.[10]

We were interested in examining the ability of IBD patients to become orally tolerized. We adapted the oral tolerance protocol reported by Husby *et al.*[7] and attempted to induce oral tolerance, first in normal controls, and then in CD and UC patients, using different doses of KLH. We found that although we could induce a very strong inhibition of T cell responses in the normal controls, both CD and UC patients failed to develop oral tolerance. Furthermore, the immune responses seen in IBD patients suggested that oral feeding alone might have primed both a T cell and B cell response.

We further assessed the ability of unaffected family members from multiplex IBD families to orally tolerize. The data suggest that a subset of unaffected Crohn's disease family members also appear to have a defect in oral tolerance. Taken together, these results suggest that the genetic predisposition known to play a role in IBD might coincide with a genetic defect in oral tolerance induction. These findings could help elucidate the mechanism of disease as well as provide information for the diagnosis and treatment of IBD.

METHODS

Induction of Oral Tolerance

We followed the protocol established by Husby *et al.*, with some modifications, to induce oral tolerance to the neoantigen KLH.[7] Patients and normal controls were fed

KLH (Calbiochem, La Jolla, CA) at a dose of 5, 50, or 250 mg in 5 cc PBS on days 0 to 5 and 10 to 15. On day 26, subjects were given 100 g of KLH (in sterile PBS) subcutaneously (SC) and this was repeated on day 35. Blood for serum antibody and T cell proliferation studies was taken at baseline on day 0, postfed (day 26), postsystemic immunization (day 35), and postbooster immunization (day 42). Twenty-one normal controls, 13 UC and 12 CD patients, were studied in the oral tolerance protocol. All subjects signed informed consent according to Institutional Review Board guidelines. No untoward effects were seen as a result of the systemic immunization. Additionally, 8 normal controls and 13 IBD patients (6 UC, 7 CD) served as nontolerized controls who were immunized subcutaneously without prior feeding. In these individuals, blood was obtained prior to immunization on day 0 (baseline) and after immunization (day 10) and booster (day 17). This time frame was comparable to that used in the immunization and blood drawing following oral antigen administration.

Isolation and Culture of Peripheral Blood Mononuclear Cells

Heparinized venous blood was obtained, diluted in PBS, and layered over a Ficoll-Hypaque (Pharmacia Biotech, Uppsala, Sweden) density gradient. After centrifugation at 1800 r.p.m. for 30 min, peripheral blood mononuclear cells (PBMNC) were isolated from the interface, washed three times in PBS, and cultured in either RPMI 1640 (Gibco BRL, Gaithersberg, MD), 1% penicillin/streptomycin (Gibco BRL), 2 mM glutamine (Gibco BRL) with 20% autologous heated inactivated ($56°C \times 1$ h) serum, or in serum-free medium (AIM V, Gibco BRL) in the presence or absence of varying concentrations of KLH (10 and 100 g/mL) in triplicate microwell cultures at 1×10^5 cells/well (100 μL of medium). Purified endotoxin-free KLH (Pacific Biomarine, Venice, CA) was used *in vitro* to reduce background proliferation to contaminants within the Calbiochem-derived KLH. After 5 d of culture, 1 μCi ^{3}H-thymidine was added to each well and after an additional 18 h culture, cells were harvested by a TomTec harvester and counted in a Wallac MicroBeta Counter (Wallac, Gaithersberg, MD). The average c.p.m. of triplicate cultures was determined and compared with proliferation by T cells cultured in medium alone as well as with a positive control (PHA 1 g/mL added at day 2 of culture.) In all cases, baseline proliferation was low (< 1000 c.p.m.) and the response to PHA was greater than 25,000 c.p.m. Values for individual wells in triplicate cultures did not vary by greater than 20 percent. The data are presented as stimulation index (SI), to normalize for the variability inherent in using human samples (different background c.p.m.), and was defined by the following equation:

$$SI = (c.p.m. \ T + KLH)/(c.p.m. \ T + medium).$$

Statistical analysis was performed using the Student's *t* test. Comparisons were made within a specific patient group (denoted as "compared with baseline") as well as to appropriate values in the control group.

On the basis of control studies, an SI < 3 after booster immunization (day 42) was defined as a tolerized state.

Measurement of Anti-KLH Serum Antibody

KLH 10 and 100 g/mL in carbonate buffer was used to coat NUNC ELISA plates (Nalge NUNC, Naperville, IL) overnight at 4°C. After washing in ELISA wash buffer, serum collected at the varying time points was added to the plates for 4 h at room temperature. After washing, alkaline phosphatase–conjugated goat anti–human immunoglobulin (Biosource, Camarillo, CA) was added for an additional 1 hour. After washing again, 1 mg/mL of substrate 104 (Sigma, St. Louis, MO) was added to the wells and the reaction was read at 405 nm by an ELISA microplate reader. Serum from a systemically immunized normal individual served as a positive control for the assay. Serum antibody levels were depicted as absorbance values because an anti-KLH human antibody is not available. There was minimal variability in the duplicate samples (<5%). Serum was drawn and stored frozen until all time points were collected. All samples were run simultaneously to limit the variability inherent in the assay.

Patient Information

All patients chosen for study were in clinical remission as judged by a Crohn's disease activity index (CDAI) less than 150 (CD) or a Mayo Clinic activity index of less than 3 (UC). This was an important prerequisite for entry into the study to rule out any effects of increased permeability due to an ulcerated or edematous mucosa. One patient was receiving steroids, six patients were on 6-mercaptopurine (four CD, two UC), two were not on any 5-amino salicylic acid (ASA) product, and two were only using cortisone enemas nightly. The CD patients had either ileitis, ileocolitis (right colon), or segmental colitis. The UC patients had either left-sided colitis or pancolitis. One patient was status post total proctocolectomy and ileoanal pull-through. Three of the CD patients had had surgical intervention. The normal controls were age- and sex-matched and included four individuals with irritable bowel syndrome. No patients had any non-IBD inflammatory disease.

RESULTS

Oral Tolerance Responses in Normal Control Patients

The mechanism of oral tolerance in mice appears to be determined by antigen dose. Repeated low doses of oral antigen results in activation of regulatory T cells that can be transferred to a naive host, whereas a single high dose of oral antigen can lead to T cell deletion or anergy. In humans, the mechanism of oral tolerance is unknown. We were interested in the activation of regulatory T cells; therefore, we attempted to induce oral tolerance using a wide range of antigen doses.

We first measured T cell responses to KLH immunization in the absence of prior oral feeding in control patients (no IBD). Ten days after the first immunization, KLH-specific T cell proliferation ranged from a stimulation index of 2 to 22 ($P < .007$ compared with preimmunization), and further rose to between 4 and 48 after the second or booster immunization ($P < .002$; FIG. 1A). Following a 50 or 250 mg feeding regimen prior to immunization resulted in an SI of less than 3, even after the second immunization (FIG. 1C, D). Although KLH-specific T cell proliferation was low, the cells were viable and able to proliferate to mitogenic stimuli such as PHA (data not shown). Control patients that followed the 5 mg feeding regimen (FIG. 1B) generally exhibited baseline T cell proliferation until after the second

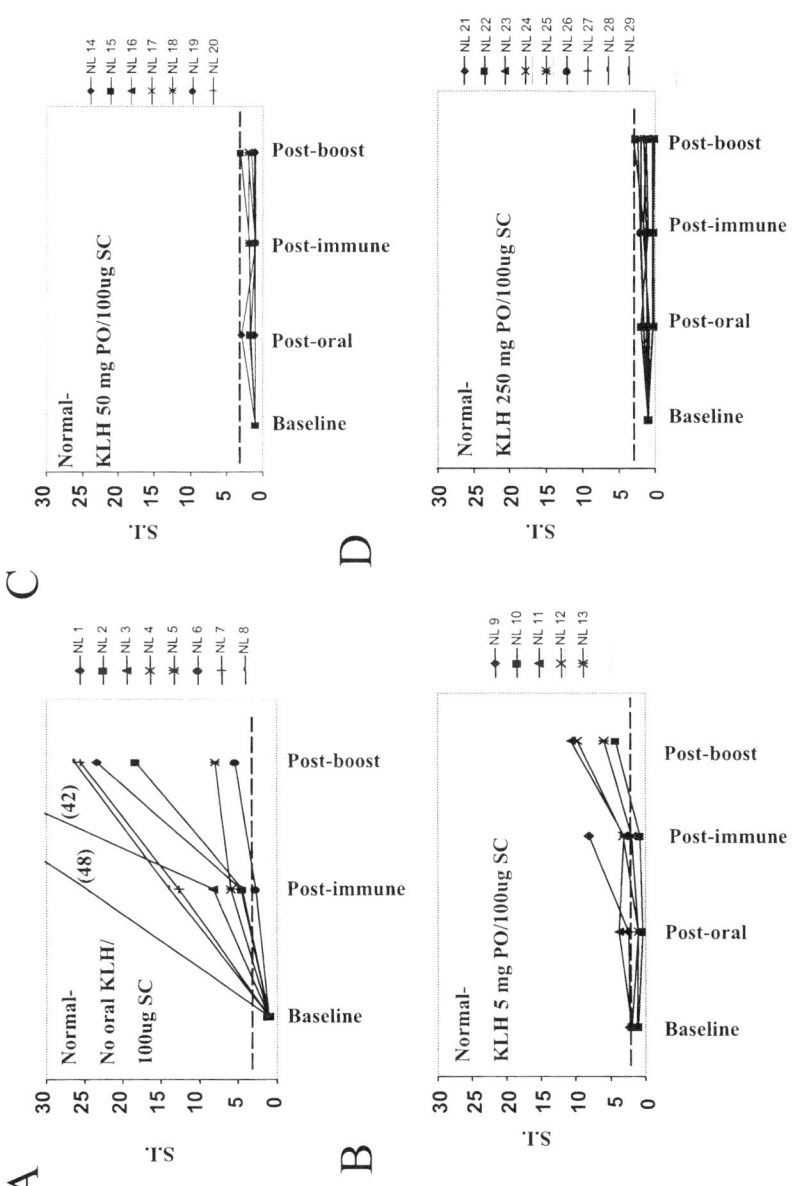

FIGURE 1. *See following page for legend.*

immunization. SI after the booster immunization ranged from 4 to 10, significantly lower than in patients without prior oral feeding ($P < .014$), but higher than the individuals fed 50 to 250 mg KLH. Therefore, we adopted the 50 mg protocol as our tolerizing dose, and the 5 mg protocol as our partially, or subtolerizing, dose. To help score the induction of tolerance in IBD patients, we adopted an SI < 3 to signify oral tolerance induction in patients following the 50 mg tolerizing protocol.

IBD Patients Cannot Orally Tolerize

We next attempted to assess T cell responses in IBD patients in response to KLH immunization in the absence of prior oral feeding. As in the control population, the responses of both the UC and Crohn's patients varied widely, but were in the range of normal controls (FIG. 2). However, unlike the normal controls, IBD patients following the 50 mg tolerizing dose protocol with KLH had significant T cell proliferative responses (SI ranging from 3 to 75) after the second immunization. Seven out of eight UC patients failed to meet our criterion for tolerance induction (FIG. 3B), whereas all eight Crohn's patients failed to tolerize (FIG. 3C). Furthermore, the stimulation indices were significantly higher than their respective baselines ($P < .035$ for UC and $P < .02$ for CD) as well as significantly higher than the SIs in the control group after the second immunization ($P < .03$ for UC and $P < .015$ for CD). Interestingly, the profile of responses was different in UC versus CD. Whereas in CD the majority of the T cell response occurred after the second immunization, KLH-specific T cell proliferation occurred after the first immunization in three UC patients and after oral feeding in two UC patients, suggesting that the luminal antigen was priming or possibly activating T cells *in vivo*.

We also tested the 5 mg partially tolerizing dose protocol with IBD patients. Although there were no significant differences in T cell responses after the second immunization in IBD versus control patients, SI increases after either feeding or after the first immunization in IBD patients were noted. SIs greater than 3 were generally seen only after the second immunization in the control patients, again suggesting that IBD patients were responding differently to the fed antigen (FIG. 4).

B Cell Responses

A fundamental difference between mouse and human oral tolerance is that the feeding protocols that inhibit T cell responses in mice also inhibit antibody production, whereas in the one published study of oral tolerance in humans this does not

---

FIGURE 1. Normal laboratory volunteers were given (**A**) no oral KLH, (**B**) 5 mg KLH, (**C**) 50 mg KLH, (**D**) or 250 mg KLH orally on days 0 to 5 and 10 to 15, followed by two subcutaneous immunizations of KLH (100 mg) on days 26 and 35 (day 0 and 10 for **A**). Heparinized venous blood and serum were obtained on days 0 (baseline), 26 (postoral, preimmunization with subcutaneous KLH), 35 (postimmune, after first immunization), and 42 (postboost, after booster). For **A**, blood was drawn on days 0, 10, and 17. T cell proliferation in response to KLH was measured as described in Materials and Methods. The response, fold increase in [^{3}H]thymidine incorporation (stimulation index = SI), represents the c.p.m. of the KLH-stimulated cultures divided by the c.p.m. of unstimulated cultures (range of c.p.m. in the unstimulated cultures was from 100 to 1000). Tolerance was defined as an SI < 3 following booster immunization (*dashed line*).

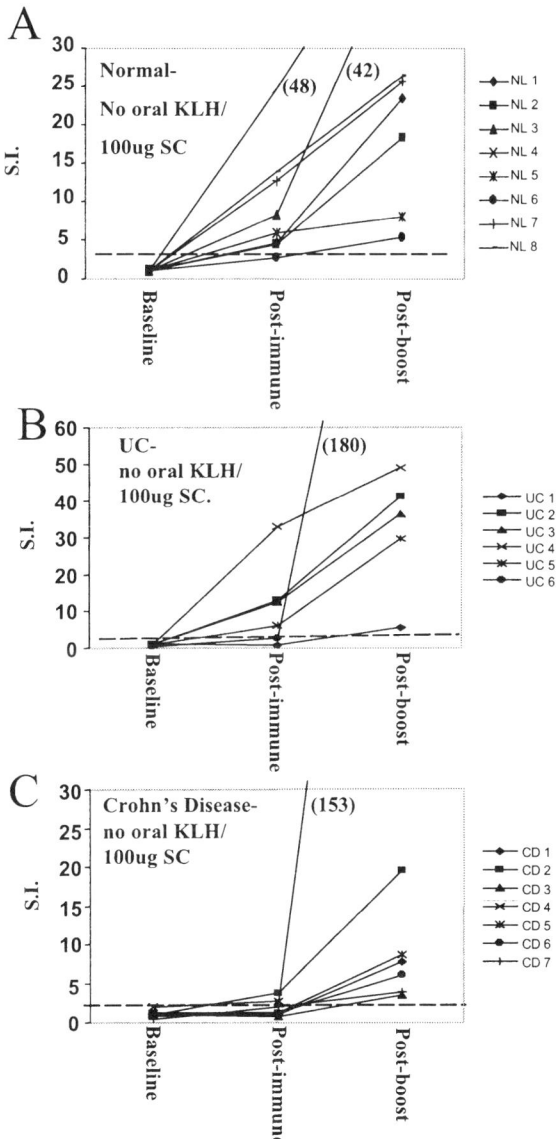

FIGURE 2. (**A**) Eight normal controls, (**B**) six UC patients, and (**C**) seven CD patients were immunized with 100 μg KLII on days 0 and 10 in the absence of prior oral feeding. Blood was drawn on days 10 and 17, and KLH-specific T cell proliferation was determined as described in FIGURE 1.

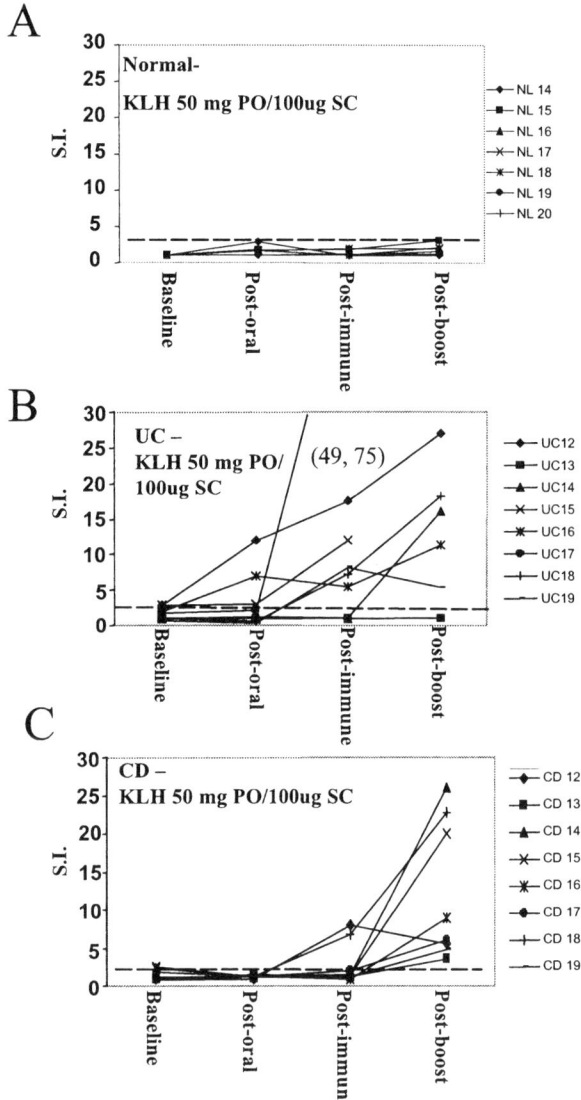

FIGURE 3. (**A**) Seven normal controls, (**B**) eight UC patients, and (**C**) eight Crohn's disease patients were given 50 mg KLH orally on days 0 to 5 and 10 to 15, followed by two subcutaneous immunizations of KLH (100 µg) on days 26 and 35. Blood was drawn and KLH-specific T cell proliferation was determined as described in FIGURE 1. Tolerance was defined as an SI < 3 following booster immunization (*dashed line*).

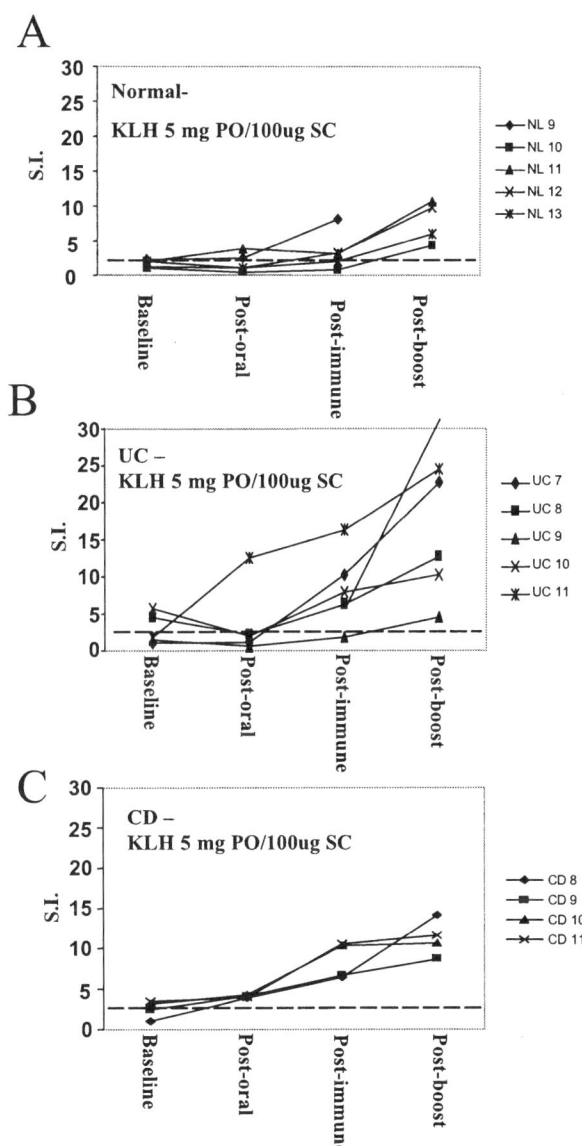

FIGURE 4. (**A**) Five normal controls, (**B**) five UC patients, and (**C**) four Crohn's disease patients were given 5 mg KLH orally on days 0 to 5 and 10 to 15, followed by two subcutaneous immunizations of KLH (100 µg) on days 26 and 35. Blood was drawn, and KLH-specific T cell proliferation was determined as described in FIGURE 1. Tolerance was defined as an SI < 3 following booster immunization (*dashed line*).

appear to hold true. We measured anti-KLH serum antibody concentrations in the control group and found that KLH-specific antibody concentrations increase after immunization, regardless of prior oral feeding (FIG. 5A–C). This is consistent with the published data. We also measured the antibody production from the IBD groups and found similar results (data not shown). Interestingly, there was increased anti-KLH antibody production in the IBD groups after oral feeding alone (FIG. 5D), again suggesting that feeding might be priming an immune response rather than inducing

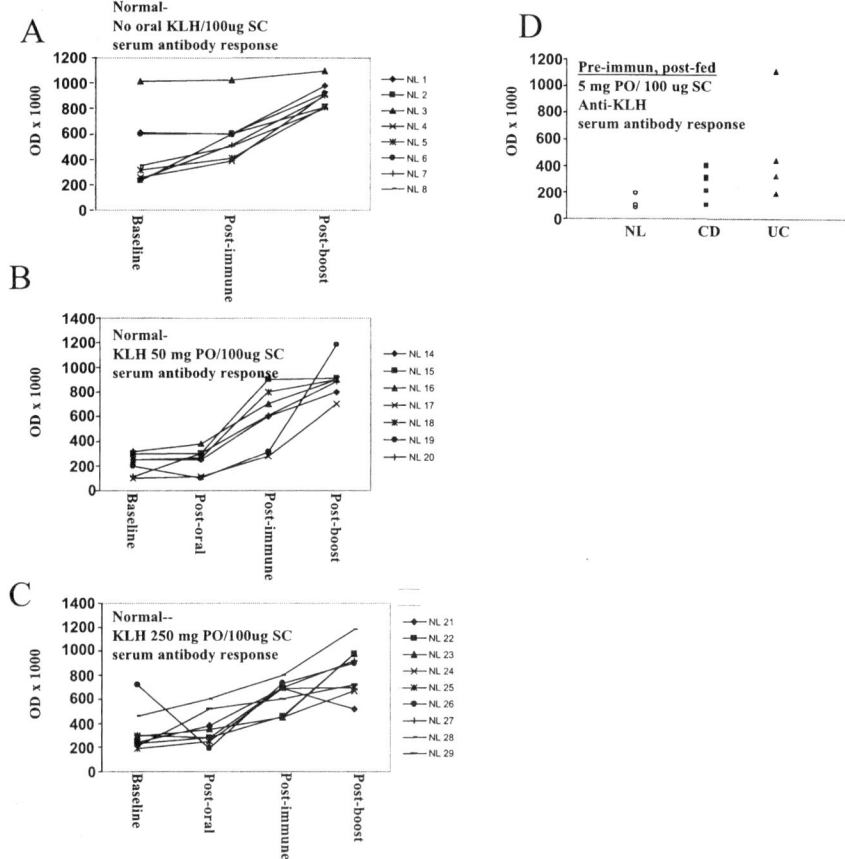

FIGURE 5. Sera were obtained from (**A**) normal volunteers, either not fed (KLH 0 mg), (**B**) fed KLH 50 mg, (**C**) or fed KLH 250 mg per the oral tolerance protocol and immunized with KLH, 100 μg SC, on days 26 and 35 (days 0 and 10 for nonfed controls). Anti-KLH antibody was determined by ELISA using KLH 10 μg/mL as a capture antigen and developed with a goat anti–human immunoglobulin–alkaline phosphatase–conjugated antibody (IgG and IgM). The results are depicted as OD units, as no specific anti-KLH control antibody is available. Similar data were obtained using KLH 100 μg as the capture antigen. (**D**) Sera were obtained from 5 mg KLH-fed normal controls, UC patients, and Crohn's patients. Anti-KLH antibody was determined by ELISA on day 26 (postoral feeding/preimmunization with KLH). All sera were assayed on the same day to control for variability. All sera were stored frozen (−20° C) until the time of assay.

tolerance. Taken together, these results further support a failure of oral tolerance induction in IBD patients. The immune responses seen after oral feeding alone suggest a possible defect in mucosal immunoregulation.

Evidence for Genetic Linkage

It has long been appreciated that there is an increased incidence of IBD in first-degree relatives of patients with either CD or UC. The concordance rate for CD in monozygotic twins is over 40%, whereas the rate is lower in UC.[11] Although these data speak to the importance of environmental factors, they are powerful lines of evidence for a true genetic linkage. We reasoned that because IBD is a genetic disorder, the failure to orally tolerize might also be a genetically regulated trait and, therefore, shared between family members of a multiplex IBD family. We attempted to induce oral tolerance in all first-degree family members of six multiplex IBD families. The four Crohn's disease and two UC families we studied had two affected family members each. We performed the oral tolerance protocol using the 50 mg tolerizing dose of KLH.

In each Crohn's family, the diseased family member failed to tolerize, consistent with the data described above. However, in three of the four CD families, at least one, and in two families, two, unaffected members also failed to tolerize (FIG. 6). In total, 5 out of 14 unaffected family members of the four multiplex CD families failed to orally tolerize to KLH, a significant difference ($P < .01$) compared with the control population without a family history of IBD.

In the two UC families, tolerance segregated with disease (FIG. 6). Three of four UC patients failed to tolerize (the fourth was the only patient who tolerized, as noted above), whereas all four unaffected family members tolerized normally. Although the sample size is too small for more definitive conclusions, these results suggest that oral tolerance might be genetically regulated and that first-degree relatives of IBD patients might share the genetic defect without exhibiting the clinical symptoms of inflammatory bowel diseases.

DISCUSSION

We have documented a failure to induce oral tolerance in IBD patients and in a subset of unaffected family members in multiplex IBD families.

The mechanism of oral tolerance induction in humans is unknown. As reported in mouse models, one possibility includes the generation of regulatory T cells that produce suppressive cytokines such as IL-10 (Tr1 cells) and TGF-β (Th3 cells). We have not been able to detect either IL-10 or TGF-β secreting T cells in *in vitro* T cell cultures stimulated with KLH from tolerized individuals (data not shown). An alternative mechanism of oral tolerance could be deletion of or the induction of anergy in antigen-specific T cells, as seen in high-dose oral tolerance in mice. Studies to address this mechanism are difficult to perform in humans.

Another possibility includes the generation of CD8$^+$ suppressor T cells. Early studies had identified these cells in the spleen following oral antigen administration.[12–14] These studies showed that transferring CD8$^+$ T cells, but not CD4$^+$ cells, transferred the tolerized state to a naive animal.

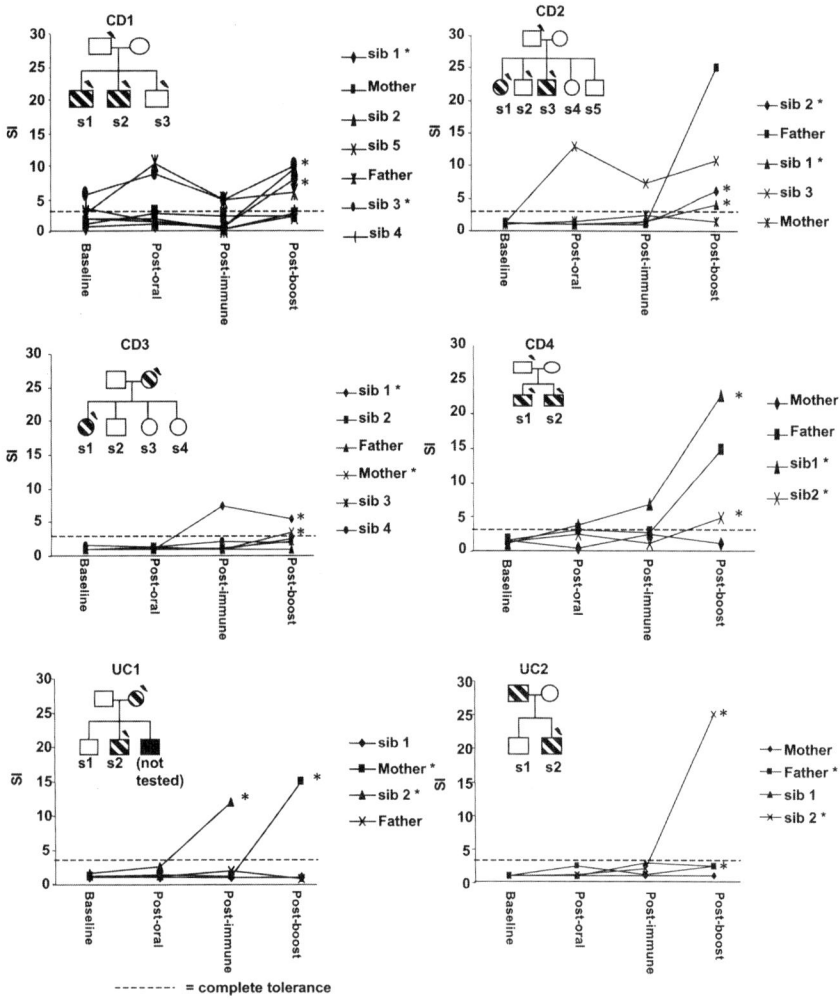

FIGURE 6. Four CD families and two UC families were tested for the ability to become orally tolerized. Each family member followed the 50 mg KLH feeding protocol, as outlined above, and T cell responses to KLH are shown in SI, as above. Each graph represents one multiplex family. Affected family members are denoted by an *asterisk*. Each inset describes the pedigree of the family, where *hatched bars* indicate affected patients. The presence of a *lightening bolt* indicates the failure of the individual to suppress KLH-induced T cell proliferation with prior oral feeding. Tolerance was defined as an SI < 3 following booster immunization (*dashed line*).

In studies that support a role for $CD8^+$ T cells in mucosal immunoregulation, we have published correlative data showing that normal intestinal epithelial cells can function as antigen-presenting cells *in vitro* and preferentially expand $CD8^+$ suppressor T cells. This is mediated by a complex of a CD8 ligand, gp180, and a class Ib molecule, CD1d, expressed by normal intestinal epithelial cells (IECs).[15] IECs from IBD patients fail to express the IEC glycoprotein gp180. Interestingly, in cocultures of IECs from IBD patients with peripheral blood T cells, $CD4^+$ T cells, and not $CD8^+$ T cells, preferentially expand.[16,17] In the presence of neutralizing antibodies to gp180, normal IEC:T cell cocultures replicate the disease state by preferentially expanding $CD4^+$ cells, suggesting that a defect in the CD8:gp180 interaction might contribute to the abnormal T cell response. Whether these *in vitro* defects correlate with our current *in vivo* findings has not been addressed.

Previous studies have documented immune responses against luminal antigens in IBD patients. One could imagine that this chronic immune stimulation in the gut could contribute to the pathology of disease. However, because intestinal permeability has been shown to be increased during active inflammation, luminal antigen might have transversed the mucosal barrier through transcellular pathways after the onset of active disease (resulting in priming of an immune response). In addition, medications that are used to treat IBD (e.g., 5-ASAs) have been shown to alter intestinal permeability. Therefore, immune responses to luminal antigens might be the result of active disease and/or treatment of IBD, and not a contributory factor in disease pathogenesis.

We attempted to induce oral tolerance to the neoantigen KLH to limit the risk of prior antigen exposure. The IBD patients were carefully selected to reduce the likelihood of increased intestinal permeability. All patients selected had to be in clinical remission for over six months. In addition, most were not taking any medications that are known to alter intestinal permeability, and six patients were off all medications throughout the study. Furthermore, a subset of these patients were tested for intestinal permeability using the lactose-mannitol test and were found to be within the normal range (Kraus *et al.*, manuscript in preparation). Therefore, it does not appear that increased permeability is the explanation for the failure to induce oral tolerance.

Moreover, the failure of oral tolerance induction in the unaffected family members, with no clinical symptoms of IBD, further suggests that permeability is not an issue. Although there are studies that suggest that unaffected family members can have increased intestinal permeability,[18,19] we tested a subset of these individuals using the lactose-mannitol test and found them also to be within the normal range.

The significant differences in tolerance induction in IBD patients and their first-degree relatives suggest that this approach might be valuable as a diagnostic aid. Furthermore, the defect represents a phenotype that can be used in the current study of genotype:phenotype correlations emanating from genome-wide screens in IBD patients and their families.

REFERENCES

1. BLUMBERG R.S., L.J. SAUBERMANN & W. STROBER. 1999. Animal models of mucosal inflammation and their relation to human inflammatory bowel disease. Curr. Opin. Immunol. **11:** 648–656.

2. BOUMA. G & W. STROBER. 2000. The immunological and genetic basis of inflammatory bowel disease. Nat. Rev. Immunol. **3:** 521–533.
3. FRIEDMAN, A. & H. WEINER. 1994. Induction of anergy or active suppression following oral tolerance is determined by antigen dose. Proc. Natl. Acad. Sci. USA **91:** 6688–6692.
4. FUKAURA, H., S.C. KENT, M.J. PIETRUSEWICZ, et al. 1996. Induction of circulating myelin basic protein and proteolipid protein-specific transforming growth factor beta-1 secreting Th3 T cells by oral administration of myelin in multiple sclerosis patients. J. Clin. Invest. **98:** 70–77.
5. GROUX H., A. O'GARRA, M. BIGLER, et al. 1997. A CD4+ T cell subset inhibits antigen-specific T-cell responses and prevents colitis. Nature **389:** 737–742.
6. MELAMED, D. & A. FRIEDMAN. 1993. Direct evidence for anergy in T lymphocytes tolerized by oral administration of ovalbumin. Eur. J. Immunol. **23:** 935–942.
7. HUSBY S., J. MESTECKY, Z. MOLDOVEANU, et al. 1994. Oral tolerance in humans. T cell but not B cell tolerance after antigen feeding. J. Immunol. **152:** 4663–4670.
8. DUCHMANN R., E. MAY, M. HEIKE, et al. 1999. T cell specificity and cross reactivity towards enterobacteria, bacteroides, bifidobacterium, and antigens from resident intestinal flora in humans. Gut **44:** 812–818.
9. DUCHMANN, R., M.F. NEURATH & K.H. MEYER ZUM BUSCHENFELDE. 1997. Responses to self and non-self intestinal microflora in health and inflammatory bowel disease. Res. Immunol. **148:** 589–594.
10. KNOFLACH P., B.H. PARK, R. CUNNINGHAM, et al. 1987. Serum antibodies to cow's milk proteins in ulcerative colitis and Crohn's disease. Gastroenterology **92:** 479–485.
11. TYSK C., E. LINBERG, G. JANEROT & B. FLODERUS-MYRNED. 1988. Ulcerative colitis and Crohn's disease in an unselected population of monozygotic and dizygotic twins. A study of heritability and the influence of smoking. Gut **29:** 990–996.
12. CHALLACOMBE, S.J. & T.B. TOMASI. 1980. Systemic tolerance and secretory immunity after oral immunization. J. Exp. Med. **152:** 1459–1472.
13. MOWAT, A.M. 1985. The role of antigen recognition and suppressor cells in mice with oral tolerance to ovalabumin. Immunology **56:** 253–260.
14. MATTINGLY, J.A. & B.H. WAKSMAN. 1978. Immunologic suppression after oral administration of antigen. I. Specific suppressor cells formed in rat Peyer's patches after oral administration of sheep erythrocytes and their systemic migration. J. Immunol. **121:** 1878–1883.
15. CAMPBELL N.A., M.S. PARK, L.S. TOY, et al. 2002. A non-class I MHC intestinal epithelial surface glycoprotein, gp180, binds to CD8. Clin. Immunol. **102:** 267–274.
16. MAYER, L. & D. EISENHARDT. 1990. Lack of induction of suppressor T cells by intestinal epithelial cells from patients with inflammatory bowel disease. J. Clin. Invest. **86:** 1255–1260.
17. TOY, L.S., X.Y. YIO, A. LIN, et al. 1997. Defective expression of gp180, a novel CD8 ligand on intestinal epithelial cells, in inflammatory bowel disease. J. Clin. Invest. **100:** 2062–2071.
18. HOLLANDER D., C.M. VADHEIM, E. BRETTHOLZ, et al. 1986. Increased intestinal permeability in patients with Crohn's disease and their relatives. Ann. Intern. Med. **105:** 883–885.
19. KATZ, K.D., D. HOLLANDER, C.M. VADHEIM, et al. 1989. Intestinal permeability in patients with Crohn's disease and their healthy relatives. Gastroenterology **97:** 927–931.

Oral Glatiramer Acetate in Experimental Autoimmune Encephalomyelitis

Clinical and Immunological Studies

DVORA TEITELBAUM,[a] RINA AHARONI,[a] ETY KLINGER,[b] RIVKA KREITMAN,[b] EMANUEL RAYMOND,[b] ARTHUR MALLEY,[c] RONA SHOFTI,[d] MICHAEL SELA,[a] AND RUTH ARNON[a]

[a]*Department of Immunology, The Weizmann Institute of Science, Rehovot 76100, Israel*

[b]*Innovative R & D Division, Teva Pharmaceutical Industries, Ltd, Petach Tikva, Israel*

[c]*Oregon Primate Center, Portland, Oregon, USA*

[d]*Faculty of Medicine, Technion Institute of Technology, Haifa, Israel*

> ABSTRACT: Glatiramer acetate (GA, Copaxone, copolymer 1) for injection is an approved drug for relapsing-remitting multiple sclerosis. The clinical and immunological effects of GA were extensively studied in experimental autoimmune encephalomyelitis (EAE), the experimental animal model for MS. The effect of oral administration of GA was tested in both rodents and primates in acute as well as in chronic relapsing (CR) models of EAE. Oral GA was found to suppress acute EAE induced in rats, mice, and rhesus monkeys. The effect of GA was also tested in several models of CR-EAE: proteolipid protein and myelin oligodendrocyte glycoprotein induced CR-EAE in mice, CR-EAE in Biozzi mice, and CR-EAE in cynomolgus monkeys. In all the murine models, oral treatment with GA initiated at the peak of first relapse reduced the severity of disease and suppressed further relapses. Suppression of EAE with oral GA was associated with marked inhibition of spleen cell proliferation and Th1 cytokine (IL-2 and IFN-γ) response to the respective autoantigens. GA-specific T cell lines of the Th2/3 type that inhibit EAE induction *in vivo*, similarly to those induced by injection of GA, could be isolated from spleens of GA-fed mice and rats. Furthermore, as demonstrated previously for GA-specific cells induced by the parenteral route, the orally induced GA-specific cells accumulate in the CNS and secrete *in situ* Th2 cytokines in response to both GA and MBP as well as brain-derived neurotrophic factor (BDNF). Although a clinical trial in MS with two doses of oral GA in enteric-coated tablets did not show a significant effect either at the clinical or immunological level, the results presented here suggest that oral GA may still be developed into a therapeutic modality in MS.
>
> KEYWORDS: glatiramer acetate; Copaxone; copolymer 1; multiple sclerosis; experimental autoimmune encephalomyelitis; oral tolerance immunomodulation; Th2/3 cells

Address for correspondence: Dr. Dvora Teitelbaum, Department of Immunology, The Weizmann Institute of Science, P.O. Box 26, Rehovot 76100, Israel. Voice: +972-8-9342537; fax: +972-8-9344141.

dvora.teitelbaum@weizmann.ac.il

INTRODUCTION

Experimental autoimmune encephalomyelitis (EAE) is a T cell–mediated autoimmune disease of the central nervous system (CNS) that serves as an experimental model for human multiple sclerosis (MS).[1] EAE can be induced in rodents and primates by several myelin autoantigens, such as myelin basic protein (MBP), proteolipid protein (PLP), myelin oligodendrocyte glycoprotein (MOG), and other minor myelin proteins. The clinical course of EAE may be acute or chronic relapsing; the latter resembles more closely the clinical and pathological manifestations of MS.[2]

Glatiramer acetate (GA), previously known as copolymer 1 (Cop 1), is a synthetic amino acid copolymer composed of L-alanine, L-lysine, L-glutamic acid, and L-tyrosine that was shown to suppress EAE in several animal species. Clinical trials in MS established the clinical efficacy of GA, and since 1996 GA for injection (brand name Copaxone) has been an approved drug for the treatment of relapsing-remitting MS.[2]

GA can affect EAE and MS at various levels of the immune response, and binding to MHC Class II molecules is a prerequisite for its effects. Studies from the experimental model and, recently, in MS indicate that the major important mechanism is the activation of GA-specific T regulatory/suppressor cells to secrete Th2 suppressive cytokines by suppressive determinants shared between MBP and GA. These GA-specific cells cross the blood-brain barrier, accumulate in the CNS, and release anti-inflammatory cytokines *in situ*.[2–4]

In the past decade, a large number of investigators have successfully applied oral tolerance to the treatment of experimental autoimmune diseases, including EAE, by feeding with the relevant autoantigens.[5] In view of the advantages of the oral route of administration over the parenteral one, it was of interest to test the effect of oral GA on the development of EAE.

In the following, we describe the suppression of both acute and chronic relapsing EAE by oral GA, and the immunological mechanisms involved.

SUPPRESSION OF ACUTE EXPERIMENTAL AUTOIMMUNE ENCEPHALOMYELITIS BY ORAL GLATIRAMER ACETATE

The ability of orally administered GA to prevent clinical manifestations of EAE was assayed in both rats and mice under conditions previously reported to induce oral suppression of EAE by MBP.[6,7] Oral GA was found to effectively suppress EAE in both species with an optimum dose-response activity.[8] Maximum effect was achieved with a dose of 1 mg GA in rats (57% reduction of disease incidence and 69% inhibition of disease severity) and 100 µg to 250 µg in mice (43% suppression of disease severity). Lower and higher doses were less effective.

The efficacy of oral GA was also reported by Maron *et al.*,[9] who showed that feeding GA markedly inhibits several EAE models in mice, including the disease induced in MBP TCR transgenic mice, but does not affect collagen-induced arthritis, another autoimmune disease, demonstrating the specificity of GA-induced tolerance.

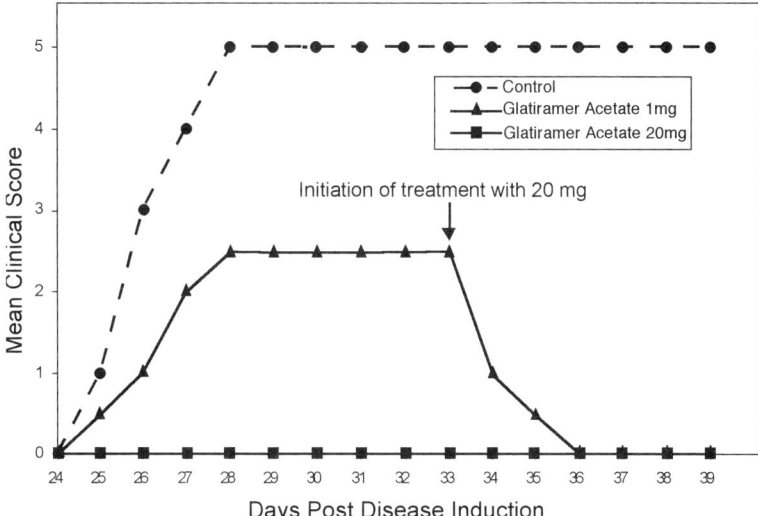

FIGURE 1. Prevention of EAE in Rhesus monkeys fed with GA. EAE was induced in Rhesus monkeys by injection of MBP emulsion in complete Freund's adjuvant (CFA). Monkeys were orally treated on alternate days starting 10 d prior to disease induction (5 treatments) and daily following disease induction. Various doses of GA were administered in enteric-coated capsules ($n = 1$ monkey per treatment group).

The efficacy of suppression induced by GA was found by both us and Maron et al.[9] to be more effective than MBP in modulating EAE.

The effect of oral GA was also tested in Rhesus monkeys. Experimental effects in primates are of particular importance because of the close phylogenetic relationship to humans and the similar pH in the gastrointestinal tract. The results obtained using enteric-coated (EC) GA capsules (the clinical formulation) are shown in FIGURE 1. Whereas an untreated monkey developed an acute fatal disease, a monkey that was fed 1 mg GA before disease induction developed mild disease. On day 33, when the disease was in a chronic steady stage, the monkey was fed 20 mg GA. This resulted in immediate improvement, and the monkey recovered completely within three days. Pretreatment with 20 mg GA resulted in complete suppression of EAE clinical symptoms.

INHIBITION AND THERAPY OF CHRONIC RELAPSING-EXPERIMENTAL AUTOIMMUNE ENCEPHALOMYELITIS BY ORAL GLATIRAMER ACETATE

Chronic relapsing EAE can be induced in various species using different encephalitogens and disease induction protocols. This disease more closely resembles the clinical and pathological manifestations of MS than does acute EAE. The ability of

TABLE 1. Suppression by glatiramer acetate of CR-EAE induced by several encephalitogens in different strains of mice

Strain	Inducing Antigen	Inhibition of First Attack (%)[a]	Inhibition of Relapses (%)[b]
(PL/J×SJL/J)F_1	MBP	46	57
(SJL/J×BALB/C)F_1	PLP139–151	68	50
	PLP178–191	69	No relapses
C57BL/6	MOG35–55	48	30

[a]Inhibition of first attack was calculated according to the mean maximal score.
[b]Inhibition of relapses was calculated according to the mean relapse rate.

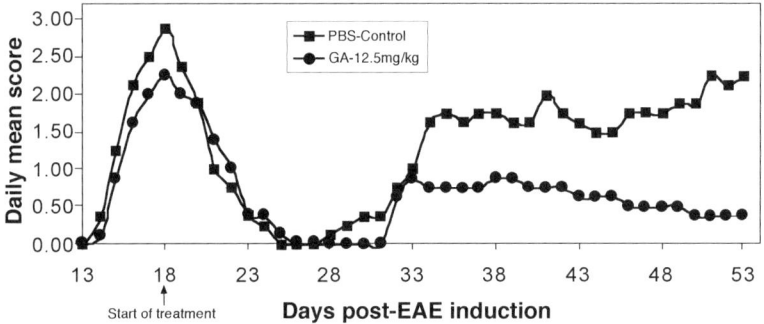

FIGURE 2. Treatment of CR-EAE in Biozzi mice by oral GA. EAE was induced by two injections of mouse spinal cord homogenate emulsified in CFA given one week apart. Treatment with daily feeding of PBS (control) or 250 µg GA was initiated 18 d following disease induction.

oral GA to inhibit and treat CR-EAE was, therefore, tested in several models of the disease induced in mice and primates.

The results obtained in several mouse strains in which CR-EAE was induced using different encephalitogens and that were fed daily with GA (250 µg) following disease induction are summarized in TABLE 1. As can be seen, oral GA was effective in suppressing both the first attack of the disease, as well as further relapses, regardless of the antigen used for induction: MBP, PLP peptides (p139–151 and p178–191), or MOG 35–55 peptide.

We also tested whether oral GA may possess not only a suppressive effect but also a therapeutic effect on the course of CR-EAE. FIGURE 2 illustrates such an effect on CR-EAE induced in Biozzi mice by injection of mouse spinal cord homogenate. Treatment was started at the peak of the first attack (day 18) and consisted of daily feedings with 250 µg GA. This treatment led to a marked reduction in the severity of further relapses. Therapeutic effect of oral GA could also be demonstrated in CR-EAE induced by PLP 139–151 and MOG 35–55.

CR-EAE can also be induced in cynomolgus monkeys by injection of MBP. The course of the disease in this experimental model was variable: in some of the animals

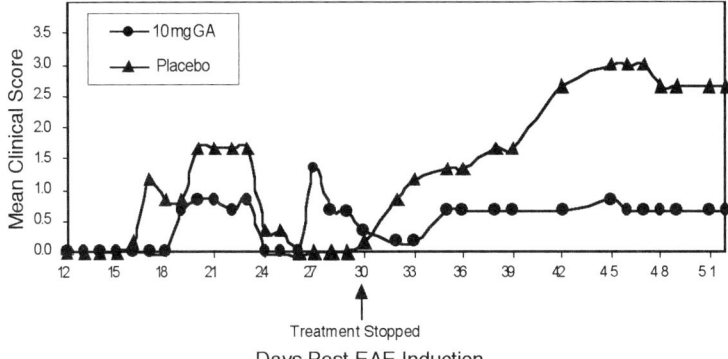

FIGURE 3. Prevention of CR-EAE in cynomolgus monkeys by oral GA. EAE was induced by immunization with MBP in CFA. Monkeys were orally treated on alternate days starting 10 d prior to disease induction (5 feedings), and daily following disease induction. GA (10 mg per feeding) was administered in enteric-coated tablets. Treatment was stopped 30 d following disease induction ($n = 3$ monkeys per group).

the course of the disease was chronic relapsing, whereas in others the course of disease was acute. The effect of feeding with the clinical formulation of enteric-coated GA tablets was tested in this disease model. Treatment was initiated 10 d prior to disease induction and stopped 30 d following disease induction. The results obtained are illustrated in FIGURE 3. Feeding with 10 mg GA in EC tablets delayed the onset and reduced the severity and duration of the disease. The beneficial effect of oral GA was sustained even after cessation of feeding. Treatment with a lower (5 mg per feeding) was not effective, and treatment with a higher dose (20 mg per feeding) was only partially effective.

THE IMMUNOLOGICAL MECHANISMS INVOLVED IN GA-INDUCED ORAL SUPPRESSION

The effect of oral administration of GA on the immune response to the disease-inducing antigen was evaluated in both rats and mice.[8] Feeding with various doses of oral GA inhibited both the proliferation of spleen cells and their secretion of the anti-inflammatory cytokines IL-2 and IFN-γ in response to the disease-inducing antigens. The inhibition of the immunologic response to the encephalitogen followed a dose-dependent bell-shaped curve consistent with the dose-response inhibition of clinical manifestations of EAE. The downregulation of the immune response to the encephalitogen was antigen specific, as no inhibition was observed in the response to the control antigen PPD. Similar results were also reported by Maron *et al.*,[9] demonstrating that oral GA differentially affected IFN-γ versus IL-10/TGF-β immune responses in MBP but not OVA TCR transgenic mice.

The nonresponsiveness induced by oral GA could be adoptively transferred by spleen cells of GA-fed donors or by GA-specific T cell lines established from such splenocytes. The ability of GA-specific lines established from spleen cells of GA-

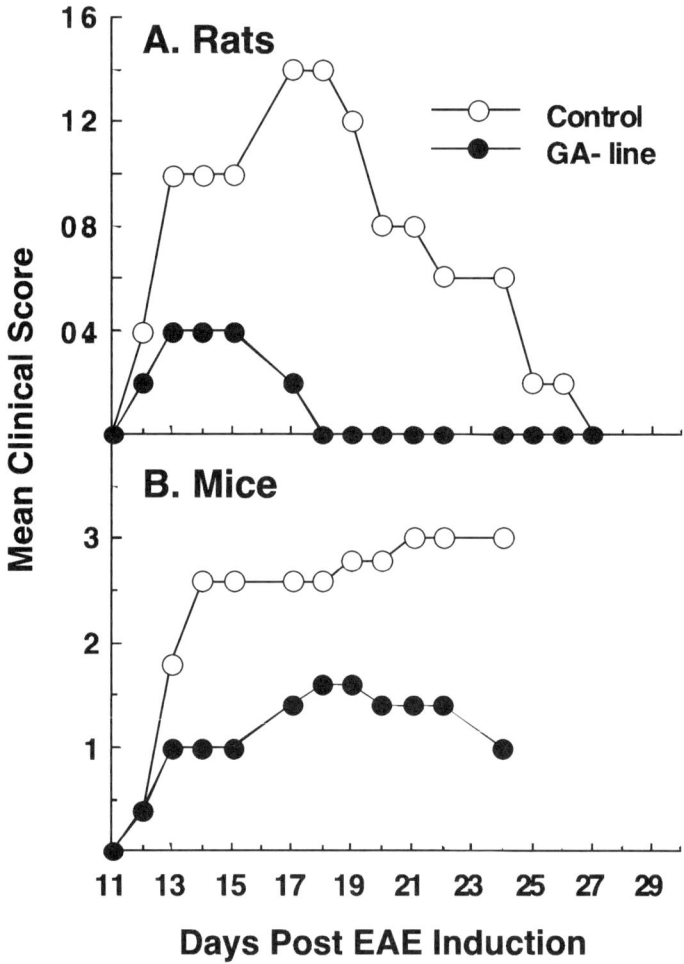

FIGURE 4. Inhibition of EAE by T cell lines derived from GA-fed donors. Activated Ts cell lines derived from spleens of GA-fed donors were injected 3 d after stimulation with GA into (**A**) naive rats (20×10^6 cells/rat, intraperitoneally) and (**B**) naive mice (15×10^6 cells/mouse, intravenously). Recipient animals were then challenged for EAE induction.

fed rats and mice to prevent EAE *in vivo* is illustrated in FIGURE 4. Both lines inhibited the disease considerably in the recipient animals, such that 44% inhibition was seen in mice and 88% inhibition in rats. Thus, both lines are T suppressor (Ts) lines capable of transferring the orally induced nonresponsiveness to EAE. To characterize the Ts-GA lines, we studied their proliferation response and the pattern of cytokine secretion in response to GA and the autoantigen MBP. The lines proliferated in response to GA, but not to MBP, and demonstrated a Th2/3 cytokine secretion profile (secretion of IL-10 and TGF-β) in response to GA. MBP did not induce proliferation or secretion of Th1 cytokines. On the other hand, MBP triggered the secretion of

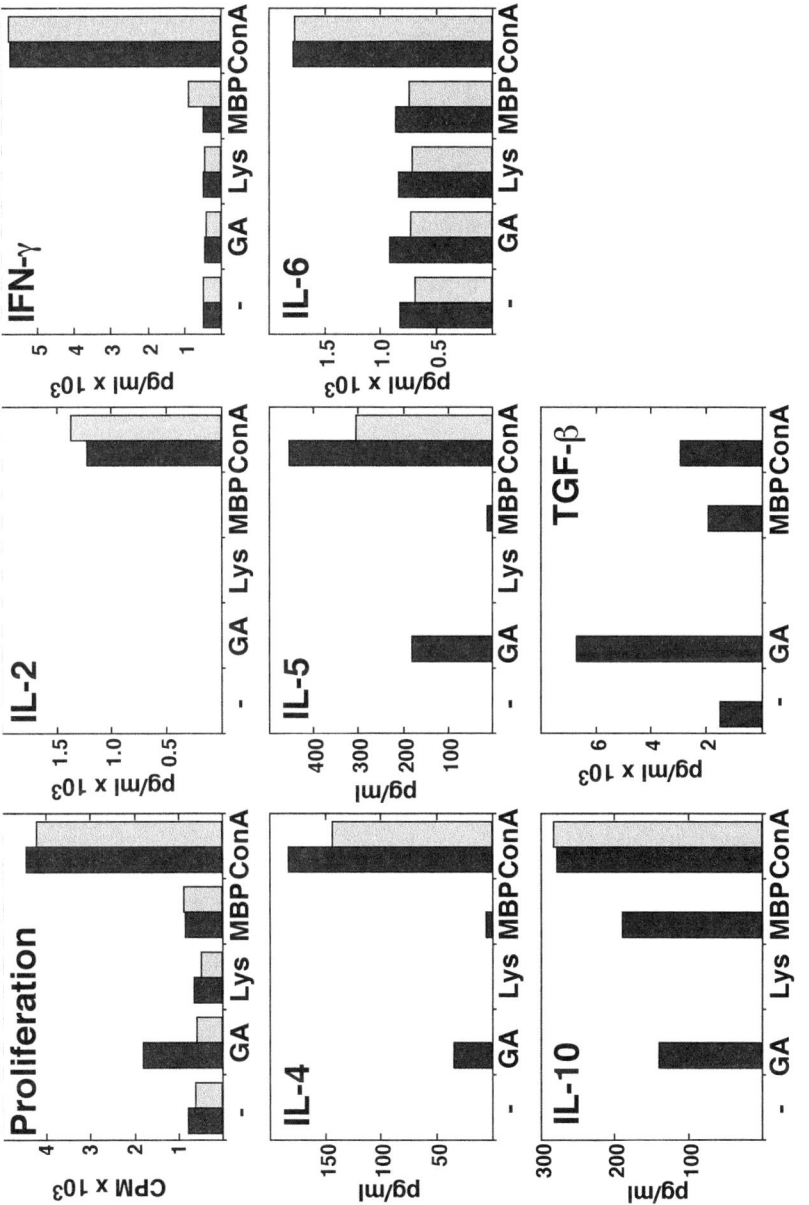

FIGURE 5. See following page for legend.

IL-10 and TGF-β. Thus, the cytokine secretion profile of these lines and the cross-reaction with MBP at the level of Th2 cytokines is similar to that previously demonstrated for GA-specific Ts lines obtained following injection of GA.[3]

We have previously demonstrated that GA-specific Th2 cells induced in the periphery by injection of GA cross the blood–brain barrier and accumulate in the target organ, the CNS.[4] We tested, therefore, whether the GA-specific Th2/3 cells induced by oral GA could also be demonstrated in the brain. Indeed, the presence of GA-specific cells induced by the oral route was established by using two different approaches: (1) by isolating GA-specific cells from the CNS of GA-fed mice, and (2) by following the appearance in the CNS of labeled adoptively transferred GA-specific cells.[10] FIGURE 5 demonstrates the proliferation and cytokine secretion patterns of whole lymphocyte populations isolated from brains of EAE-induced mice treated orally with GA or lysozyme. In all isolation experiments, the yield of CNS lymphocytes was very low ($\sim 1 \times 10^5$ cells/brain); still, proliferation and cytokine secretion could be detected in cultures of brain lymphocytes. Cells isolated from brains of mice treated orally with GA proliferated in response to GA and secreted IL-4, IL-5, IL-10, and TGF-β, but not IL-2 or IFN-γ. In contrast to the response to GA, no specific response to lysozyme could be observed in brains of control mice fed with lysozyme, although such response was observed in the periphery using spleen cells. Of particular interest is the response to MBP by the brain lymphocytes. Cells from brains of EAE-induced mice that had been fed with lysozyme responded to MBP by secretion of IFN-γ (928 pg/mL) but not IL-10. On the other hand, cells originating from brains of GA-treated mice secreted significant amounts of IL-10 and lower amounts of IFN-γ (471 pg/mL), indicating a Th1 to Th2 shift in the CNS in response to the autoantigen.

The cells isolated from CNS were cultured *in vitro* with the immunizing antigens to establish T cell lines. Three highly reactive T cell lines were generated from brains of mice treated orally with GA. They secreted high amounts of the Th2 cytokines IL-4, IL-5, IL-6, IL-10, and TGF-β in response to GA, and cross-reacted with MBP by Th2 secretion similarly to T cell lines established from peripheral splenocytes.

In contrast, no GA- or lysozyme-specific lines could be obtained from brains of mice fed with lysozyme, even after five *in vitro* stimulations.

The homing of orally induced GA-specific T cells to the CNS was followed by adoptive transfer of GA-specific T cell lines labeled with the fluorescent dye Hoechst that binds to the cell nucleus. Brains were removed seven days after cell injection, sectioned, and examined for the presence of fluorescent cells. In most of the sections (92%) accumulation of labeled cells was observed and penetration to the brain tissue was definitely visualized (FIG. 6). Recently, using a two-stage double-

---

FIGURE 5. Proliferation and cytokine secretion by lymphocytes isolated from the CNS of mice treated orally with GA or lysozyme. Mice were rendered resistant to EAE by feeding with GA (0.1 mg per mouse × 7 feedings); control mice were similarly fed with lysozyme. Ten days after disease induction, the mice were perfused and the whole lymphocyte population was isolated from the brains. Proliferation and cytokine secretion in response to medium alone (–), GA (50 µg/mL), lysozyme (Lys, 100 µg/mL), MBP (100 µg/mL), and ConA (5 µg mL) were tested. *Dark gray bars*=mice fed with GA; *light gray bars*=mice fed with lysozyme.

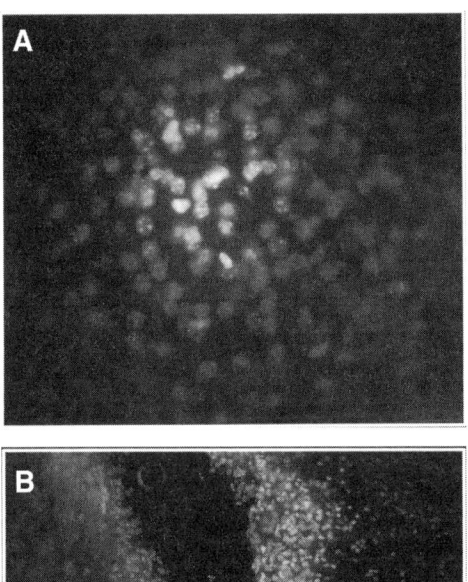
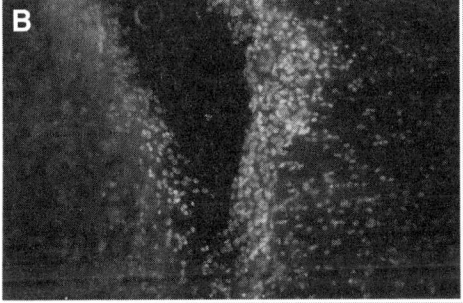

FIGURE 6. Brain sections of mice adoptively transferred with orally induced GA-specific T cell line. Activated T cells were labeled with Hoechst dye and injected intraperitoneally into normal mice (30×10^6 cells/mouse). After 7 d, brains were removed, fixed in paraformaldehyde, and sectioned. (**A**) Section showing perivascular infiltration (40 μ section, magnification ×400). (**B**) Section with periventricular infiltration (40 μ section, magnification ×100). Labeled cells were found in 101 out of 110 (92%) slides examined.

labeling system of fluorescent cell labeling and immunohistological staining, we demonstrated that the GA-specific T cells in the CNS exhibit intense expression of IL-10 and TGF-β, as well as of the brain-derived neurotrophic factor (BDNF). No expression of the inflammatory cytokine IFN-γ was observed.[11]

These results clearly indicate that T cells induced by GA by either parenteral or oral administration penetrate the CNS and function *in situ* as regulatory cells producing Th2/3 cytokines and neurotrophic factor.

THE IMMUNE RESPONSE TO GA IN MS PATIENTS TREATED WITH ORAL-GA

In view of the demonstrated efficacy of oral GA in the various EAE models, a double-blind and placebo-controlled study was initiated in relapsing-remitting MS patients. In this trial, given the code name "Coral," two active doses of oral GA, 5 mg and 50 mg, and placebo were given daily for 14 months. MS patients from 158 sites in 18 different countries were enrolled in this trial. The results of this trial were disappointing, as no significant effect on the clinical and MRI outcomes was observed.

In parallel to the clinical follow-up, the T cell–mediated immune response to GA was evaluated in an ancillary study in a few centers. It had previously been demonstrated[12] that GA-reactive T cells are present in peripheral blood mononuclear cells (PBMC) of both untreated MS patients and normal individuals. Following daily injections of GA, there is an initial slight increase followed by gradual reduction in T cell proliferation response to GA as a function of treatment time. When the cytokine secretion response was analyzed, it was demonstrated that a shift from Th1 to Th2 was also induced in response to GA.[2,13] The aim of the ancillary study was, therefore, to assess whether orally administered GA has systemic effects on the immune response to GA in MS patients, similar to those demonstrated following daily injections of GA. The results obtained in the ancillary study demonstrated no significant differences between the placebo group and the two treatment groups, either in the proliferation assay or in IFN-γ and IL-10 cytokine secretion. No decrease in the proliferation response to GA or shift from Th1 to Th2 was observed as a result of treatment with oral GA. These results, which correlated with the absence of clinical effects, may indicate that orally given GA either was not bioavailable to the systemic immune system or did not reach an effective bioactive dosage and, therefore, was not effective clinically. The latter may well be the case, in view of the bell-shaped dose-response curve of oral GA.

CONCLUSIONS

Oral GA was found to be effective in suppressing and treating different models of acute and chronic relapsing EAE induced by various encephalitogens in both rodents and primates. The beneficial effect of oral GA is associated with downregulation of the immune response to the disease-inducing antigens. The suppression of EAE by oral GA, similarly to injected GA, is mediated by GA-specific T cells that are of the Th2/3 type and secrete anti-inflammatory cytokines in response to GA and MBP. GA-specific T cells induced by both oral and subcutaneous administration accumulate in the brain and secrete anti-inflammatory cytokines and brain-derived neurotrophic factor (BDNF) *in situ*. Although the Coral clinical trial did not show significant effects, the experimental results suggest that oral GA may still be developed into a therapeutic modality in multiple sclerosis.

REFERENCES

1. MARTIN, R. & H.F. MCFARLAND. 1995. Immunological aspects of experimental allergic encephalomyelitis and multiple sclerosis. Crit. Rev. Clin. Lab. Sci. **32:** 121–128.
2. SELA, M. & D. TEITELBAUM. 2001. Glatiramer acetate in the treatment of multiple sclerosis. Expert Opin. Pharmacother. **2:** 1149–1165.
3. AHARONI, R. *et al.* 1997. Copolymer 1 induces T cells of T helper type 2 that cross react with myelin basic protein and suppress experimental autoimmune encephalomyelitis. Proc. Natl. Acad. Sci. USA **94:** 10821–10826.

4. AHARONI, R. *et al.* 2000. Specific Th2 cells accumulate in the central nervous system of mice protected against experimental autoimmune encephalomyelitis by copolymer 1. Proc. Natl. Acad. Sci. USA **97:** 11472–11477.
5. FARIA, A.M. & H.L. WEINER. 1999. Oral tolerance: mechanisms and therapeutic applications. Adv. Immunol. **73:** 153–264.
6. HIGGINS, P.H. & H.L. WEINER. 1998. Suppression of experimental autoimmune encephalomyelitis by oral administration of myelin basic protein and its fragments. J. Immunol. **140:** 440–445.
7. AL-SABBAGH, A. *et al.* 1994. Antigen-driven tissue-specific suppression following oral tolerance: orally administered myelin basic protein suppresses proteolipid protein-induced experimental autoimmune encephalomyelitis in SJL mouse. Eur. J. Immunol. **24:** 2104–2109.
8. TEITELBAUM, D., R. ARNON & M. SELA. 1999. Immunomodulation of experimental autoimmune encephalomyelitis by oral administration of copolymer 1. Proc. Natl. Acad. Sci. USA **96:** 3842–3847.
9. MARON, R. *et al.* 2002. Oral tolerance to copolymer 1 in myelin basic protein (MBP) TCR transgenic mice: cross reactivity with MBP-specific TCR and differential induction of anti-inflammatory cytokines. Int. Immunol. **14:** 131–138.
10. AHARONI, R. *et al.* 2002. Oral treatment of mice with copolymer 1 (glatiramer acetate) results in the accumulation of specific Th2 cells in the central nervous system. J. Neuroimmunol. **126:** 58–68.
11. AHARONI, R., B. KAYHAN, R. EILAM, *et al.* 2003. Glatiramer acetate-specific T cells in the brain express T helper 2/3 cytokines and brain-derived neurotrophic factor in situ. Proc. Natl. Acad. Sci. USA **100:** 14157-14162.
12. BRENNER, T. *et al.* 2001. Humoral and cellular immune responses to copolymer 1 in multiple sclerosis patients treated with Copaxone. J. Neuroimmunol. **115:** 152–160.
13. NEUHAUS, O. *et al.* 2001. Mechanisms of action of glatiramer acetate in multiple sclerosis. Neurology **56:** 702–708.

Constraints on the Efficacy of Mucosal Tolerance in Treatment of Human and Animal Arthritic Diseases

NORMAN A. STAINES, CATHERINE J. DERRY,
LILIA MARINOVA-MUTAFCHIEVA, NADIRA ALI,
D. HUW DAVIES, AND JOHN J. MURPHY

Infection and Immunity Research Group, King's College London, London, United Kingdom

ABSTRACT: Mucosal administration of an autoantigen has been shown to be a powerful way of inducing tolerance in both animal and human arthritis clinical trials. Bovine or chicken type II collagen has been administered orally to rheumatoid arthritis patients, resulting in some, although in many cases rather limited, clinical improvement. Animal studies have revealed that the mechanisms that underlie induction of mucosal tolerance include clonal deletion, suppression of the proinflammatory Th1 cells, and the induction of regulatory T cells. These cells, defined as a persistently CD25-expressing subset of CD4$^+$ cells, are frequently anergic, may produce anti-inflammatory cytokines such as IL-10 and TGF-β, and are likely to be agents of bystander suppression. A key feature that may affect the induction of these cells and other suppressive mechanisms is the dose of antigen administered. The results from human clinical trials suggest a daily dose of significantly less than 1 mg is optimal. Similarly data from collagen-induced arthritis studies reveal an optimal dose above and below which there is little or no immune suppression. Indeed, the incorrect dose can prime the immune response and aggravate disease. The timing and frequency of administration is also vital to the level of immune tolerance induced and the control of the pathological process. This and other findings derived from animal studies are discussed here in relation to the results from human clinical trials.

KEYWORDS: mucosal tolerance; arthritis; human clinical trials; dose

INTRODUCTION

Since the initial studies demonstrating the ameliorating effects of mucosal administration of antigen on arthritic diseases,[1,2] this method of suppressing disease pathology has attracted considerable interest. Similarly, oral tolerance induction is being investigated as a means of suppressing other autoimmune diseases, such as diabetes, multiple sclerosis, and uveitis.[3,4] Results of a number of clinical trials in rheumatoid arthritis (RA) patients published in the last 10 years have demonstrated that this interest was justified. However, the limited success of several of these trials also betrays the complexity of the mechanisms involved in both induction of mucosal tolerance and the pathological process in the arthritic joint. Animal studies have helped to focus future work and are discussed here in relation to clinical findings in humans.

HUMAN CLINICAL TRIALS

Type II collagen (CII) has been the antigen of choice in arthritis oral clinical trials, principally because it is the main structural component of cartilage against which both T and B cell responses can be demonstrated. Also, there is an animal model that makes use of this cardinal autoantigen. An early study of 60 severely arthritic patients demonstrated a decrease in the number of clinically affected joints in those who were fed chicken CII for three months, compared with those receiving placebo.[5] This encouraging finding was followed by a report of the effect of two doses of bovine CII in patients with less severe disease (duration of less than or equal to three years). Bovine CII was chosen as this has a higher peptide sequence homology to human CII than does chicken CII. Although the improvement in disease was not significant, there were small clinical benefits in patients receiving the higher dose of 10 mg/day.[6] In a separate trial, where the 10 mg daily dose was also shown to be more effective than 1 mg/day, this was associated with a reduction in anti-CII antibody titers, highlighting the need to understand the effect of oral administration of antigen on the immunology of RA.[7]

The effect of dose was investigated in a larger trial involving 274 patients administered with four oral doses of chicken CII (20, 100, 500 or 2,500 µg/d) over 24 weeks. Although the clinical benefit was small, the lowest dose (20 µg daily) evoked the most positive effects, with a baseline anti-CII antibody detection providing a predictive indicator of those patients that were likely to respond.[8] Choy *et al.*[9] have also shown that the middle dose administered in their study (0.05, 0.5, and 5 mg of bovine CII daily) produced small, but statistically significant, clinical improvements.

Interestingly, juvenile rheumatoid arthritis also appears to be susceptible to oral administration of CII, with clinical effects showing a correlation with a decrease in proinflammatory interferon (IFN)-γ and an increase in anti-inflammatory transforming growth factor (TGF)-β production.[10,11]

The studies are not strictly comparable, as different dose ranges of either bovine or chicken CII are used, and the type of patients included in trials varied (e.g., in terms of disease progression, and prior or ongoing treatment) from study to study. However, the clinical trials findings do share several features. Effects, where observed, are small and there does appear to be a relationship between dose of antigen administered and clinical effect, although this varies from study to study. Although not definitive, these studies suggest a daily dose significantly less than 1 mg is optimal. Regardless of the dose and level of efficacy, oral administration of CII does not appear to be toxic or have any side effects, although the durability of any effect has not been fully addressed.[12] Despite the clinical improvements reported in human disease, we have an incomplete understanding of their underlying mechanisms, although animal studies strongly suggest several key mechanisms at the heart of mucosal tolerance induction and expression.

ANIMAL ARTHROPATHIES

Five animal diseases have been used to study the mechanisms involved in mucosal tolerance induction in arthritis: rat and mouse collagen-induced arthritis (CIA), pristane-induced arthritis, adjuvant arthritis, and antigen-induced arthritis.[13] These all mimic aspects of the immunological and pathological processes of rheumatoid arthritis. For example, CIA in mice, induced by immunization with heterologous collagen, is mediated by Th1 cells that make proinflammatory cytokines, and B cells, and is restricted by the H-2A^q and H-2A^r alleles, which are homologous to human DR4. This has been the main model in which to investigate the induction of mucosal tolerance.[1]

The results of animal studies, however, urge caution in treatment of human disease. In many studies oral tolerance has been induced, but in others disease has been induced by oral or nasal administration of antigen.[14–16] Why this happens in some cases is unknown, but absorption in the gut may have been disturbed: there is a delicate balance between the gut microenvironment and induction of mucosal tolerance.[16]

However, and as in human studies, a key feature that has emerged from animal studies is the importance of the dose of orally administered antigen.

ANTIGEN DOSE

The outcome of each clinical trial has implied an optimum dose, compared with which higher or lower doses are ineffective. In animal studies on disease prevention, a U-shaped response curve has been seen in some situations, with low and high doses being ineffective or aggravating disease, and medium doses showing a beneficial effect.[13,17–19] We have observed similar dose-dependent effects when induction of nasal tolerance to CII has been used for the treatment of CIA (TABLE 1). In comparing three doses of CII (5 µg, 20 µg, and 80 µg), the highest dose of 80 µg gave the best protection against disease. For example, at day 40 after immunization only 12 percent of tolerant mice had the first signs of disease, whereas in the control group 92 percent of mice had arthritis. The mechanisms involved may depend upon dose: low doses may favor active suppression, whereas higher doses may lead to clonal deletion or anergy of activated cells.[3] This type of effect has also been seen in other autoimmune diseases, such as experimental autoimmune encephalomyelitis (EAE).[20]

Priming of T cells at low and high doses has been observed in other studies, and this suggests that there is a delicate balance between antigen uptake and processing and the threshold of activation required to activate a particular subset of regulatory or suppressive T cell.[13,21]

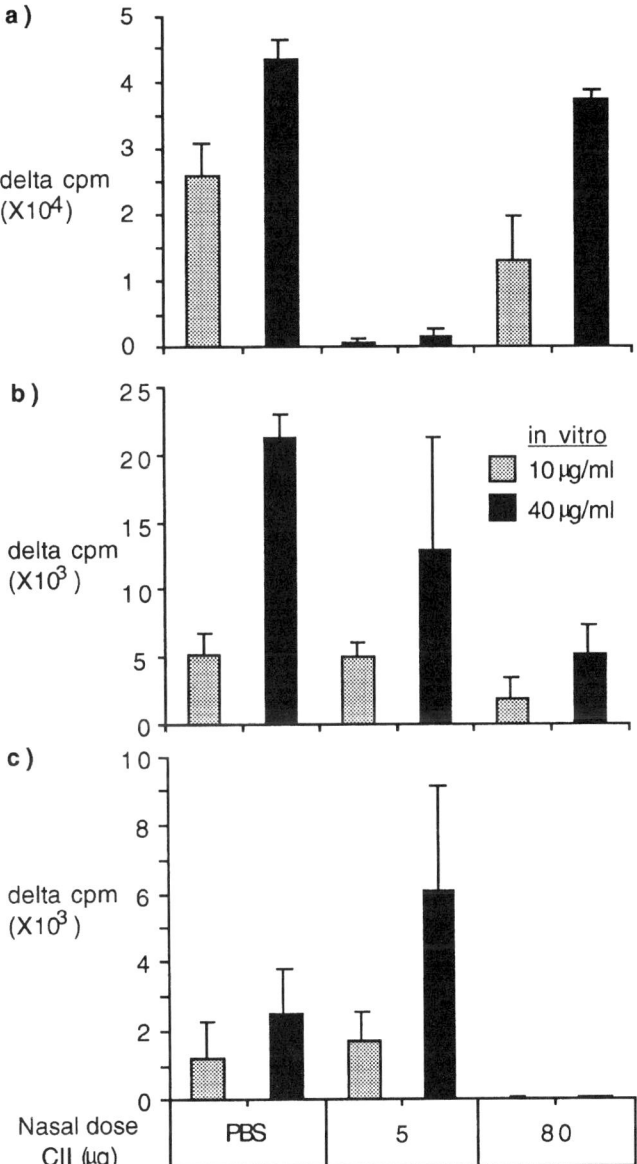

FIGURE 1. The same dose of bovine type II collagen (CII) administered nasally over different time frames may not suppress the T cell response to CII. Mice received PBS or CII over (**a**) 1 d, (**b**) 2 d, or (**c**) 4 d (to give the cumulative nasal doses indicated) on the days immediately preceding intradermal immunization with 100 µg CII in CFA. After 7 to 10 d, peripheral lymph nodes were removed, and proliferative responses to 10 and 40 µg/mL of CII were measured. Results are mean values from triplicate cultures corrected for mean background and representative of at least two experiments with a similar outcome.

TABLE 1. Efficiency of different doses of bovine type II collagen (CII) treatment on collagen-induced arthritis

Nasal Treatment	Arthritis Incidence (%) on Day 40
PBS	74
5 µg BSA	71
5 µg CII	77
80 µg BSA	92
80 µg CII	12

NOTE: DBA/1 mice were nasally dosed with either bovine type II collagen (CII) or BSA, as a control protein, after immunization with 100 µg CII in CFA. Three cumulative doses were studied (5 µg, 20 µg, and 80 µg CII), and treatment was started on day 14 (i.e., in the induction phase of arthritis, but before the onset of clinical disease). There were 8 to 10 animals in each treatment group. The experiment was repeated three times with similar results. The effect of treatment with 20 µg was similar to that observed with 5 µg (data not shown).

TIMING AND FREQUENCY OF DOSE

Although dose-response relationships in oral and nasal administration of antigen have been observed in both human and animal studies, it has become apparent that these may shift according to the timing and frequency of administration. In CIA, a single nasal administration of 5 µg CII will suppress subsequent T cell proliferation *in vitro* to CII (FIG. 1a). However, if this dose is split over two days (FIG. 1b) the level of suppression is minimal, and over four days (FIG. 1c) this dose will actually prime the T cells. Conversely, the 80 µg dose of CII is at its most suppressive when administered over four days (FIG. 1c), with a minimal level of suppression of T cell proliferation after a single administration (FIG. 1a). The reasons for this are unclear, although the issue of the frequency of feeding has been shown previously,[22] and highlights the importance of an appropriate dose administered over the correct time frame to dampen down the immune response.

Differential antigen uptake may also be a factor in the range of dose effects seen in both human and animal studies and, therefore, the nature and formulation of the antigen may be very important.

ANTIGEN TYPE AND FORM

Enhancing the tolerogenicity of an antigen may be an effective way of aiding tolerance induction, with some forms of an antigen being more tolerogenic than others.[23] The mode of delivery may also be influential, with entrapment of CII in nanoparticles prolonging the effect of a single oral dose, resulting in concomittant reduction of TNF-α and increase of TGF-β in Peyer's patches.[24]

An obvious criticism of all antigen-induced models is that type II collagen is unlikely to be the sole antigenic target in human disease. However, bystander suppression may be a key mechanism in initiating and maintaining mucosal tolerance, suggesting it is not crucial to know the predominant autoantigen. Studies with oral or nasal administration of peptides containing immunodominant T cell epitopes have

TABLE 2. Expression of TNF-α, IL-4, and TGF-β after nasal induction of tolerance followed by induction of arthritis

Cell Source	In Vivo Treatment	TNF–α	IL-4	TGF-β
CLN	PBS	16.3 ± 5.7	2.0 + 0.5	16.4 ± 2.1
ILN	PBS	18.4 ± 5.5	4.0 + 1.2	15.7 ± 5.5
CLN	80 µg CII	22.0 ± 4.1	6.8 + 2.3	38.0 ± 9.8
ILN	80 µg CII	4.3 ± 3.5	8.9 + 2.6	43.0 ± 21.0

NOTE: DBA/1 mice were nasally treated with a cumulative dose of 80 µg bovine collagen type II (CII), or PBS, on each of the 4 d before the induction of collagen-induced arthritis (CIA) by intradermal immunization with 100 µg CII in CFA. Five animals per group were used. Consecutive sections of the cervical and inguinal lymph nodes (CLN and ILN, respectively) were taken on day 7 after immunization and stained for the expression of TNF-α, IL-4, and TGF-β. Numbers represent the mean value ± SD of positive cells per high-power field.

reported successful tolerance induction.[25,26] It is possible that the heterogeneity of T and B cell epitopes, and determinant spreading, may frustrate tolerance induction using synthetic peptides.[27,28]

NASAL VERSUS ORAL TOLERANCE INDUCTION

Most studies on mucosal tolerance have used the oral route, but the nasal route provides a good alternative to induce suppression.[19,25,29] There is probably less degradation of antigens than in the gut, and the doses necessary to induce tolerance via the nasal mucosa may be smaller.[30] The mechanisms involved are likely to be similar to the oral route, but it is notable that nasal-associated lymphoid tissues have unique characteristics.[31,32] Recently, we have found that lymph nodes draining nasal mucosa in tolerized mice exhibited different cytokine expression patterns compared with other lymph nodes (TABLE 2), and this microenvironment might be favorable for tolerance induction. A key feature is that after nasally induced tolerance, more cells in the cervical and inguinal lymph nodes expressed anti-inflammatory cytokines (TGF-β and IL-4) and fewer cells in the inguinal lymph nodes expressed proinflammatory TNF-α.

MECHANISMS

Many mechanisms have been proposed for the induction of mucosal tolerance: a switch from a disease-causing Th1 to a protective Th2 phenotype; bystander suppression; anergy; apoptosis; deletion; and, more recently, regulatory cells.[3,4] Clearly the role of antigen presenting cells will be vital in these processes, with dendritic cells likely to play a key role here. Recent evidence suggests that the mucosal milieu creates tolerogenic dendritic cells that produce IL-10 and induce CD4$^+$ T regulatory cells.[33]

Different mechanisms may be associated with different doses of mucosally administered antigen,[3] but it has also been shown that there could be a dose-

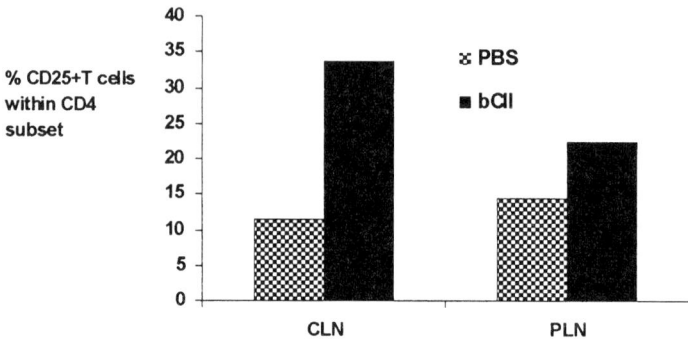

FIGURE 2. Nasal administration of bovine type II collagen (CII) expands CD25$^+$CD4$^+$ T cells. DBA/1 mice were nasally dosed with either 80 μg bovine type II collagen (CII) or PBS on days 14 to 18 after immunization with 100 μg CII in CFA. Expression of CD25 by CD4$^+$ T cells in lymph node cells was measured by flow cytometry 26 d after immunization. CLN, cervical lymph nodes draining nasal mucosa; PLN, peripheral lymph nodes (brachial, axillary, and inguinal) draining the site of intradermal immunization.

dependent induction of anergic phenotypes: hyporesponsiveness occurring at low doses and high doses resulting in induction of an anergic immunoregulatory cell.[34] Many phenomena observed in mucosal tolerance studies may be accounted for by the properties of regulatory cells: lack of T cell proliferation, reversal of an anergic state by addition of IL-2, and low levels of production of both pro- and anti-inflammatory cytokines.[19]

The regulatory cell pool is likely to include several types of cell. For example, adjuvant-induced arthritis can be inhibited by IL-10–producing regulatory cells induced by nasal administration of a peptide analogue of a heat shock protein 60 T cell epitope.[35] Similarly, Th3 cells producing TGF-β may play a role,[3] and latterly the CD4$^+$CD25$^+$ subset of regulatory cells has attracted much interest. CD25$^+$ regulatory cells are either "natural" or "induced." [36] Regulatory cells have certainly been shown to play a part in the downregulation of CIA, as depletion of a CD25$^+$ subset of CD4$^+$ T cells speeds up the onset of severe disease in this model.[37] In our hands, the protective effect of nasal tolerance on CIA is associated with elevated numbers of CD4$^+$ cells that are CD25$^+$. The proportion of these cells is significantly higher in lymph nodes draining nasal mucosae than in peripheral lymph nodes of tolerized mice (FIG. 2).

The induction of bystander suppression that plays a role in the generation of regulatory cells appears to be antigen specific, whereas its effect can be nonspecific. This feature could be exploited in the course of immunotherapy of autoimmune diseases, where there is likely to be more than one autoantigen involved. Understanding the relationship between the induced regulators and the "naturally" occurring populations of regulatory cells could have a significant practical implication for optimizing efficacy of mucosal tolerance.

CLINICAL POTENTIATORS OF MUCOSAL TOLERANCE

Clearly, in a human clinical situation, active established disease may be harder to control in the face of ongoing drug treatment, because induced tolerance is itself an immune response. Indeed, McKown et al.[38] reported that oral bovine CII added to existing arthritis medication may be ineffective. However, there are animal studies that suggest there could be ways to enhance mucosal tolerance induction. For example, administration of TGF-β or the histamine type II receptor agonist dimaprit (both of which will augment the action of immunoregulatory cells) enhances the induction of oral tolerance, even after the onset of arthritis.[39] Similarly, coupling of the cholera toxin B subunit, a potent enhancer of mucosal tolerance, increased the efficacy of low doses of nasally administered type II collagen in preventing disease and lowering the production of proinflammatory cytokines.[40]

FUTURE CONSIDERATIONS

Despite constraints, oral tolerance induction remains a safe, potentially nontoxic and antigen-specific means of controlling the immune mechanisms that underlie the arthritic process. Attention needs to be focused on those factors that influence its efficacy in any one individual, namely, stage of disease, prior exposure to infectious agents, the activation status of the immune system, and genetic background. In addition, use of drugs such as prednisolone and nonsteroidal anti-inflammatory drugs may have to be closely monitored in clinical trials. These inhibit generation of prostaglandins and thereby suppress oral tolerance induction.[41]

The challenge is twofold: to identify the optimum dose for each individual, and to augment a significant but as yet not impressive enough clinical benefit.

REFERENCES

1. THOMPSON, H.S. & N.A. STAINES. 1986. Gastric administration of type II collagen delays the onset and severity of collagen-induced arthritis in rats. Clin. Exp. Immunol. **64:** 581–586.
2. NAGLER-ANDERSON, C. et al. 1986. Suppression of type-II collagen-induced arthritis by intragastric administration of soluble type II collagen. Proc. Natl. Acad. Sci. USA **83:** 7443–7446.
3. WEINER, H.L. 1997. Oral tolerance for the treatment of autoimmune diseases. Annu. Rev. Med. **48:** 341–351.
4. KRAUSE, I. et al. 2000. Immunomodulation of experimental autoimmune diseases via oral tolerance. Crit. Rev. Immunol. **20:** 1–16.
5. TRENTHAM, D.E. et al. 1993. Effects of oral administration of type II collagen on rheumatoid arthritis. Science **261:** 1727–1730.
6. SIEPER, J. et al. 1996. Oral type II collagen treatment in early rheumatoid arthritis. Arthritis Rheum. **39:** 41–51.
7. GIMSA, U. et al. 1997. Type II collagen serology: a guide to clinical responsiveness to oral tolerance? Rheumatol. Int. **16:** 237–240.
8. BARNETT, M.L. et al. 1998. Treatment of rheumatoid arthritis with oral type II collagen. Results of a multicenter, double-blind, placebo-controlled trial. Arthritis Rheum. **41:** 290–297.
9. CHOY, E.H. et al. 2001. Control of rheumatoid arthritis by oral tolerance. Arthritis Rheum. **44:** 1993–1997.

10. BARNETT, M.L. *et al.* 1996. A pilot trial of oral type II collagen in the treatment of juvenile rheumatoid arthritis. Arthritis Rheum. **39:** 623–628.
11. MYERS, L.K. *et al.* 2001. Juvenile arthritis and autoimmunity to type II collagen. Arthritis Rheum. **44:** 1775–1781.
12. TRENTHAM, D.E. 1996. Evidence that type II collagen feeding can induce a durable therapeutic response in some patients with rheumatoid arthritis. Ann. N.Y. Acad. Sci. **778:** 306–314.
13. STAINES, N.A. *et al.* 1996. Arthritis: animal models of oral tolerance. Ann. N.Y. Acad. Sci. **778:** 297–305.
14. MELO, M.E. *et al.* 1996. Immune deviation during the induction of tolerance by way of nasal instillation: nasal instillation itself can induce Th-2 responses and exacerbation of disease. Ann. N.Y. Acad. Sci. **778:** 408–411.
15. FRANCIS, J.N. *et al.* 2000. The route of administration of an immunodominant peptide derived from heat-shock protein 65 dramatically affects disease outcome in pristane-induced arthritis. Immunology **99:** 338–344.
16. TERATO, K. *et al.* 1996. Induction of chronic autoimmune arthritis in DBA/1 mice by oral administration of type II collagen and *Escherichia coli* lipopolysaccharide. Br. J. Rheumatol. **35:** 828–838.
17. ZHANG, Z.Y. *et al.* 1990. Suppression of adjuvant arthritis in Lewis rats by oral administration of type II collagen. J. Immunol. **145:** 2489–2493.
18. YOSHINO, S. *et al.* 1995. Suppression of antigen-induced arthritis in Lewis rats by oral administration of type II collagen. Arthritis Rheum. **38:** 1092–1096.
19. DERRY, C.J. *et al.* 2001. Importance of dose of type II collagen in suppression of collagen-induced arthritis by nasal tolerance. Arthritis Rheum. **44:** 1917–1927.
20. WHITACRE, C.C. *et al.* 1996. Oral tolerance in experimental autoimmune encephalomyelitis. Ann. N.Y. Acad. Sci. **778:** 217–227.
21. HOYNE, G.F. *et al.* 1996. Regulation of house dust mite responses by intranasally administered peptide: transient activation of CD4+ T cells precedes the development of tolerance in vivo. Int. Immunol. **8:** 335–342.
22. FRIEDMANN, A. 1996. Induction of anergy in Th1 lymphocytes by oral tolerance. Importance of antigen dosage and frequency of feeding. Ann. N.Y. Acad. Sci. **778:** 103–110.
23. THOMPSON, H.S. *et al.* 1988. Tolerogenic activity of polymerized type II collagen in preventing collagen-induced arthritis in rats. Clin. Exp. Immunol. **72:** 20–25.
24. KIM, W.U. *et al.* 2002. Suppression of collagen-induced arthritis by single administration of poly(lactic-co-glycolic acid) nanoparticles entrapping type II collagen: a novel treatment strategy for induction of oral tolerance. Arthritis Rheum. **46:** 1109–1120.
25. STAINES, N.A. *et al.* 1996. Mucosal tolerance and suppression of collagen-induced arthritis (CIA) induced by nasal inhalation of synthetic peptide 184-198 of bovine type II collagen (CII) expressing a dominant T cell epitope. Clin. Exp. Immunol. **103:** 368–375.
26. BAYRAK, S & N.A. MITCHISON. 1998. Bystander suppression of murine collagen-induced arthritis by long-term administration of a self type II collagen peptide. Clin. Exp. Immunol. **113:** 92–95.
27. ZHANG, G.X. *et al.* 1998. Synthetic peptides fail to induce tolerance to experimental autoimmune myasthenia gravis. J. Neuroimmunol. **85:** 96–101.
28. CHU, C.Q. & M. LONDEI. 1999. Differential activities of immunogenic collagen type II peptides in the induction of nasal tolerance to collagen-induced arthritis. J. Autoimmun. **12:** 35–42.
29. MYERS, L.K. *et al.* 1997. Suppression of murine collagen-induced arthritis by nasal administration of collagen. Immunology **90:** 161–164.
30. HIGUCHI, K. *et al.* 2000. Comparison of nasal and oral tolerance for the prevention of collagen-induced murine arthritis. J. Rheumatol. **27:** 1038–1044.
31. WOLVERS, D.A. *et al.* 1999. Intranasally induced immunological tolerance is determined by characteristics of the draining lymph nodes: studies with OVA and human cartilage gp-39. J. Immunol. **162:** 1994–1998.
32. CSENCSITS, K.L. *et al.* 1999. Nasal-associated lymphoid tissue: phenotypic and functional evidence for the primary role of peripheral node address in naive lymphocyte adhesion to high endothelial venules in a mucosal site. J. Immunol. **163:** 1382–1389.

33. AKBARI, O. *et al.* 2001. Pulmonary dendritic cells producing IL-10 mediate tolerance induced by respiratory exposure to antigen. Nat. Immunol. **8:** 725–731.
34. TAAMS, L.S. *et al.* 1999. Dose-dependent induction of distinct anergic phenotypes: multiple levels of T cell anergy. J. Immunol. **162:** 1974–1981.
35. PRAKKEN, B.J. *et al.* 2002. Inhibition of adjuvant-induced arthritis by interleukin-10-driven regulatory cells induced via nasal administration of a peptide analog of an arthritis-related heat-shock protein 60 T cell epitope. Arthritis Rheum. **46:** 1937–1946.
36. VON HERRATH, M.G. & L.C. HARRISON. 2003. Antigen-induced regulatory T cells in autoimmunity. Nat. Rev. Immunol. **3:** 223–232.
37. MORGAN, M.E. *et al.* 2003. CD25+ cell depletion hastens the onset of severe disease in collagen-induced arthritis. Arthritis Rheum. **48:** 1452–1460.
38. MCKOWN, K.M. *et al.* 1999. Lack of efficacy of oral bovine type II collagen added to existing therapy in rheumatoid arthritis. Arthritis Rheum. **42:** 1204–1208.
39. THORBECKE, G.J. *et al.* 1999. Modulation by cytokines of induction of oral tolerance to type II collagen. Arthritis Rheum. **42:** 110–118.
40. TARKOWSKI, A. *et al.* 1999. Treatment of experimental arthritis by nasal administration of a type II collagen-cholera toxoid conjugate vaccine. Arthritis Rheum. **42:** 1628–1634.
41. POSTLEWAITE, A.E. 2001. Can we induce tolerance in rheumatoid arthritis? Curr. Rheumatol. Rep. **3:** 64–69.

Oral Insulin Therapy to Prevent Progression of Immune-Mediated (Type 1) Diabetes

BERRIN ERGUN-LONGMIRE,[a] JOHN MARKER,[b] ADINA ZEIDLER,[c] ROBERT RAPAPORT,[d] PHILIP RASKIN,[e] BRUCE BODE,[f] DESMOND SCHATZ,[g] ALFONSO VARGAS,[h] DOUGLAS ROGERS,[i] SHERWYN SCHWARTZ,[j] JOHN MALONE,[k] JEFFREY KRISCHER,[l] AND NOEL K. MACLAREN[m]

[a]*Division of Pediatric Endocrinology, New York-Presbyterian Hospital, Weill Medical College of Cornell University, New York, New York*

[b]*Tulane Medical School, New Orleans, Louisiana*

[c]*Department of Medicine, University of Southern California, Los Angeles, California*

[d]*Department of Pediatrics, Mount Sinai Medical Center, New York, New York*

[e]*University of Texas Southwestern Medical Center at Dallas, Dallas, Texas*

[f]*Endocrine Associates, Atlanta, Georgia*

[g]*Department of Pediatrics, University of Florida College of Medicine, Gainesville, Florida*

[h]*Department of Pediatrics, Louisiana State University Health Sciences Center, School of Medicine, New Orleans, Louisiana*

[i]*Cleveland Clinic, Cleveland, Ohio*

[j]*Diabetes and Glandular Disease Clinic, San Antonio, Texas*

[k]*University of South Florida Diabetes Center, St. Petersburg, Florida*

[l]*H. Lee Moffitt Cancer Center, University of South Florida, Tampa, Florida*

[m]*Bioseek Clinics, New York, New York 10022, USA*

ABSTRACT: Repeated ingestion of insulin has been suggested as an immune tolerization therapy to prevent immune-mediated (type 1) diabetes. We performed a placebo-controlled, two-dose, oral insulin tolerance trial in newly diagnosed (<2 years) diabetic patients who had required insulin replacement for less than 4 weeks and were found to have cytoplasmic islet cell autoantibodies (ICAs). No oral hypoglycemic agents were permitted during the trial. Endogenous insulin reserves were estimated at six-month intervals by plasma C-peptide responses to a mixed meal. Positive ICAs were found in 262 (31%) of the 846 patients screened. Of the 197 who agreed to participate, 187 could be followed for 6 to 36 months. Endogenous insulin retention was dependent upon initial stimulated C-peptide response, age at diabetes onset, and numbers of specific islet cell autoantibodies found. Oral insulin improved plasma C-peptide responses in patients diagnosed at ages greater than 20 years, best seen at the low (1 mg/day) over the high (10 mg/day) insulin dose ($P = .003$ and

Address for correspondence: Noel K. Maclaren, M.D., Bioseek Clinics, 5 East 57th Street, 16th Floor, New York, NY 10022. Voice: 212-371-0658; fax: 212-371-3744.
maclaren@endoclinics.com

Ann. N.Y. Acad. Sci. 1029: 260–277 (2004). © 2004 New York Academy of Sciences.
doi: 10.1196/annals.1309.057

$P = .01$, respectively). In patients diagnosed before age 20 years, the 1 mg dose was ineffective, whereas the 10 mg dose actually accelerated C-peptide loss ($P = .003$). There were no adverse effects. If confirmed, these findings suggest that diabetic patients over age 20 years with ICA evidence of late-onset immune-mediated diabetes should be considered for oral insulin at 1 mg/day to better retain endogenous insulin secretion.

KEYWORDS: type 1 diabetes; immune-mediated diabetes; oral insulin tolerance therapy; endogenous insulin reserve; mixed meal tolerance testing; islet cell autoantibodies (ICA); GAD_{65}; IA-2 autoantibodies; insulin autoantibodies; HLA-DR/DQ phenotypes

INTRODUCTION

The immune-mediated form of type 1 diabetes (IMD) is an incurable, life-long disease[1–3] replete with life-threatening complications. The Diabetes Control and Complication Trial clearly showed that better diabetes control lowers complication rates,[4] and good control is more likely when appreciable endogenous insulin secretion is preserved.[5] Such preserved secretion capacity of pancreatic β cells has been promoted by immunosuppressant agents.[6,7] The remissions achieved, however, were mostly transient, whereas the possible risks of lymphoma, renal damage, and/or infections likely outweighed the clinical benefits.[8] The evolution of autoimmunity and insulitis prior to the onset of clinical diabetes in nonobese diabetic (NOD) mice, as in human diabetes, has enabled investigators to use this animal model to design effective immunotherapies.[9] On the basis of such animal studies, autoreactivity of IMD can be manipulated by various islet cell autoantigen-based immunotherapies, including systemic or oral administration of antigen to induce either down regulatory processes (e.g., clonal anergy and deletion of autoreactive T cells) or a systemic deviation of autoimmune responses from destructive to nondestructive outcomes (e.g., Th2/3-dominated autoimmune responses with transferable suppression). It is now known that the frequency of diabetes can be lowered by repeated administrations of oral insulin in NOD mice without reducing insulitis.[9,10] However, this effect is dose dependent and the benefits seen at 1 mg doses disappear at higher doses (5 mg).[11,12] On the basis of encouraging results in NOD mice studies, the possible prevention or delay in the onset of type 1 diabetes in high-risk patients was tested by the administration of insulin in the Diabetes Prevention Trial–Type 1 diabetes (DPT-1) and by the administration of nicotinamide in the European Nicotinamide Diabetes Intervention Trial (ENDIT)[13,14] However, the results were disappointing, in that neither oral insulin at 7.5 mg/day nor low-dose insulin injections were able to prevent disease in either study.[14,15] In addition, smaller trials performed in Europe also did not show any benefit of oral insulin therapy in the prevention of diabetes.[16,17] However, these results highlight the need for better methods to detect disease onset, for delineating the critical time to begin intervention, and for determining the effective antigen dosage and time interval for administration. It was, therefore, the aim of this double-blind placebo-controlled study to learn whether oral insulin therapy taken daily from the time of clinical diagnosis of IMD could improve endogenous insulin retention and, if so, at what dose. We report herein that oral insulin delays progression of β cell failure in newly diagnosed patients, but only in those diagnosed after age 20 years who were given low (1 mg) doses.

MATERIALS AND METHODS

Study Subjects

A total of 846 patients were recruited by participating diabetes centers at the following: Children's Hospital of New Orleans and LSUHSC (Drs. Vargas, Chalew, and Maclaren); University of Florida, Gainesville (Drs. Schatz and Maclaren); University of Texas (Southwestern) at Dallas (Dr. Raskin); University of Southern California, Los Angeles (Dr. Zeidler); Joslin Center for Diabetes, Livingston, New Jersey (Dr. Rapaport); Cleveland Clinic (Dr. Rogers); Florida Hospital Diabetes Center, Orlando (Dr. Crockett); Atlanta Diabetes Associates (Drs. Davidson and Bode); Diabetes and Glandular Disease Clinic, San Antonio (Dr. Schwartz); University of Miami School of Medicine (Dr. Marks); Children's Clinic, Tallahassee, Florida (Dr. Deeb); and University of South Florida, Tampa (Dr. Malone and Shah).

Eligibility requirements for ICA screening were diagnosis according to the American Diabetes Association criteria[1] within the preceding two years, and less than four weeks insulin replacement therapy before entering the study. Some patients presented with a type 1 diabetes phenotype (especially children), whereas others did not (especially adults). Those found to have positive islet cell autoantibodies (ICAs) and who agreed to participate were asked to discontinue any oral hypoglycemic agents, and to have their diabetes managed exclusively by diet, exercise, and insulin injections to maintain optimal Hb_{A1C} levels.

Study Design

The study was conducted under an investigator IND No. 48,784 from the Food and Drug Administration, and under informed consent as approved by local institutional review boards. After an Hb_{A1C} test and a mixed-meal tolerance test (MMTT), patients were randomly assigned to placebo, 1 mg, or 10 mg insulin-containing capsules each day, balanced by the study center for age of onset (less than or greater than 20 years and treatment group. Repeat Hb_{A1C} levels were performed, weights recorded, and insulin doses calculated in units/kg/d every three months. At six-month intervals, MMTTs and multiple ICA levels were repeated. Patients were encouraged to remain in the trial for at least one year; for some patients, follow-up was extended up to three years. Patients with minimal plasma C-peptide responses (peak < 0.3 µU/mL) to the MMTT were considered to be treatment failures, and were removed from further study as identified.

Oral Insulin

The oral insulin used in the study was from a single batch of regular, recombinant human insulin, kindly donated by the Eli Lilly Co., Indianapolis, IN. The Belmar Pharmacy, Denver, CO, produced the insulin capsules under GMP conditions using methyl cellulose as excipient.

Mixed Meal Tolerance Tests

Patients were instructed to take a high-carbohydrate diet for at least three days and then to fast overnight before the test. Sustacal or Boost was given at 7 mL/kg up to a 13 oz. dose, and blood samples taken for glucose and plasma C-peptide levels at 0, 30, 60, 90, and 120 min thereafter.

Laboratory Analyses

Cytoplasmic islet cell autoantibodies (ICA) were determined using cryocut sections of freshly frozen human blood group O pancreas, as previously described.[18] Results equal to or greater than 20 JDFI units on two separate occasions were considered positive. Insulin autoantibodies (IAA) were assayed by a radio immunoassay binding method using human monospecific A-14A-14 ^{125}I-labeled insulin ligand, kindly provided by the Eli Lilly Co. as previously described.[19] A positive result was a displaceable insulin binding of >105 µU/mL or mean + 3 SDs of normal controls. Autoantibodies to Mr65Kda human glutamic acid ($GAD_{65}A$) and to the insulinoma-associated antigen-two (IA-2A) tyrosine phosphatase were performed as previously described by a double radioimmunoassay procedure using tritium and ^{35}S-labeled substrates produced recombinantly in a rabbit reticulocyte expression system.[20] Insulin and C-peptide analyses were performed by radioimmunoassay using kits purchased from Diagnostic Products, CA, and Linco, St. Louis MO. The Hb_{A1C} assay used a capillary electrophoretic method.[21] HLA phenotyping for DRB1 and DQB1 alleles was done by SSP as previously published.[20]

Statistical Analysis

The study was designed with approximately 60 subjects in each treatment group and had an 80% power to detect a 20% difference in the one-year failure-free survival rate overall and 80% power detect a 25% difference within each stratum. Kaplan-Meier life tables were constructed to describe the time from study enrollment until the peak plasma C-peptide response to MMTT fell below 0.3 µU/mL, a value that taken as evidence for near complete pancreatic β cell failure. The long-rank test was used to compare the life tables. Multivariate analysis of time until loss of peak C-peptide response to MMTT used the Cox proportional hazards general linear model. Covariates included age, peak C-peptide response, and antibody positivity at trial onset. The loss of C-peptide response over time was analyzed using the repeated measure analysis of variance, incorporating indicator variables for each subject that had serial results. Because the distribution of the C-peptide values were skewed, only log-transformed values were used in our analyses. When frequencies were sufficiently large, the Chi-square statistic was used to compare proportions. Otherwise, an exact test of proportions was used. The three-arm comparisons of variables at selected time points were made using either the Duncan or Tukey multiple-range tests. A two-tail P value of .05 was established for statistical significance. Values between .05 and .01 were considered to be marginally significant, to allow for the multiple comparisons made.

RESULTS

The numbers of patients who were screened for ICA, were found to be positive, and who participated in the oral insulin trial, together with their gender, ages, and initial Hb_{A1C} levels, are shown in TABLE 1. There were no statistical differences be-

TABLE 1. Baseline characteristics of the study subjects

	Screened for ICA	ICA+	Completed >6 Months of Trials
Number of Patients	846	262	187
Age Range in Years	5–78	5–72	5–60
Mean Age (years ± SD)	33.8 ± 16.1	22.4 ± 13.8	23.3 ± 13.7
Male/Female (%)	356/490 (73%)	114/147 (78%)	85/102 (83%)
Initial Hb_{A1C} (Mean % ± SD)	ND	ND	8.6% ± 2.4

TABLE 2. Metabolic outcomes and insulin requirements during follow-up

	Patient Treatment Group		
	1 mg Insulin Dose	10 mg Insulin Dose	Placebo
Basal Hb_{A1C} (mean % ± SD)	8.9 ± 2.8 (n=62)	8.6 ± 2.4 (n=62)	8.3 ± 2.4 (n=63)
6 months Hb_{A1C} (mean % ± SD)	8.0 ± 2.1* (n=34)	7.7 ± 1.6 (n=34)	6.8 ± 1.4 (n=35)
6 months insulin doses (U/kg/day)	0.46 ± 0.36 (n=55)	0.43 ± 0.29 (n=48)	0.43 ± 0.28 (n=54)
12 months Hb_{A1C} (mean % ± SD)	8.5 ± 2.4 (n=27)	7.8 ± 1.6 (n=20)	8.0 ± 2.6 (n=22)
12 months insulin doses (U/kg/day)	0.49 ± 0.33 (n=43)	0.46 ± 0.31 (n=34)	0.49 ± 0.31 (n=36)
24 months Hb_{A1C} (mean % ± SD)	8.5 ± 3.1 (n=9)	7.8 ± 0.48 (n=4)	7.3 ± 1.7 (n=9)
24 months insulin doses (U/kg/day)	0.63 ± 0.63 (n=14)	0.48 ± 0.36 (n=12)	0.50 ± 0.29 (n=15)

*Significantly different from placebo at $P=.03$.

tween the treatment groups for Hb_{A1c} levels or the insulin doses prescribed over the trial (TABLE 2). Subjects were studied for up to three years or until their peak C-peptide responses to a MMTT fell below 0.3 µU/mL. The median duration of follow-up was one year.

Of 191 randomized subjects, 153 (81%) maintained a C-peptide response greater than the 0.3 µU/mL threshold. The percentage of the subjects falling below this threshold did not differ significantly between the treatment arms. In a univariate analysis of time until peak C-peptide response failure, initial age and peak C-peptide were both statistically significant ($P = .03$ and $P = .0001$, respectively). Higher baseline C-peptide levels (a measure of endogenous insulin preservation) and older age were both associated with longer times until pancreatic β cell failure (FIG. 1A, B). However, after adjusting the results for the baseline peak C-peptide levels, age at study onset was no longer statistically significant; however, in 38% of subjects under

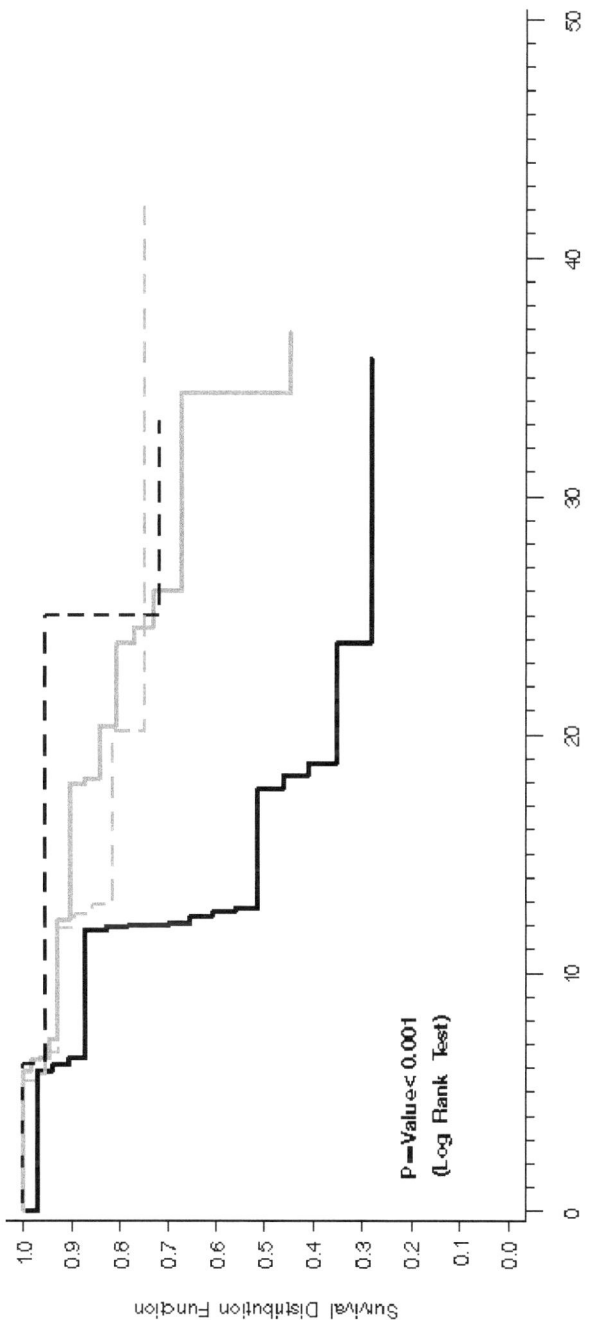

FIGURE 1A. Time until C-peptide loss by age at study onset. *Solid black line*, age <10; *dashed black line*, age ≥20 and <30; *solid gray line*, age ≥10 and <20; *dashed gray line*, age ≥30.

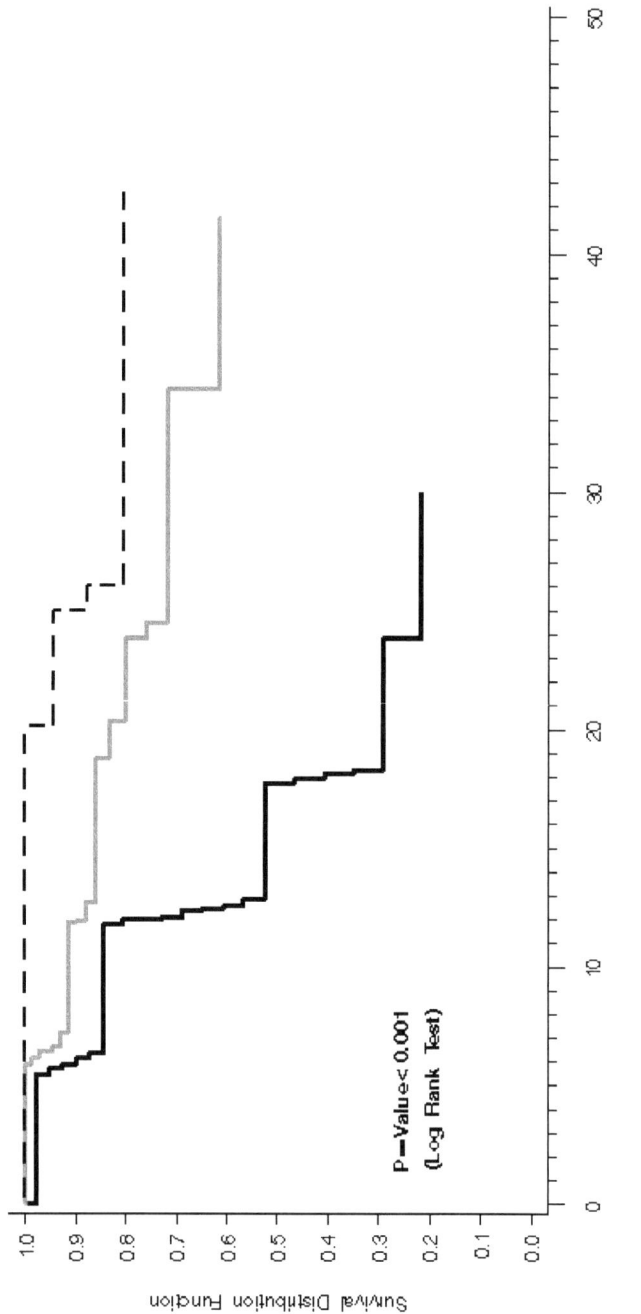

FIGURE 1B. Time until C-peptide loss by baseline C-peptide value. *Solid black line*, <1.98; *solid gray line*, 1.98–3.94; *dashed black line*, >3.94.

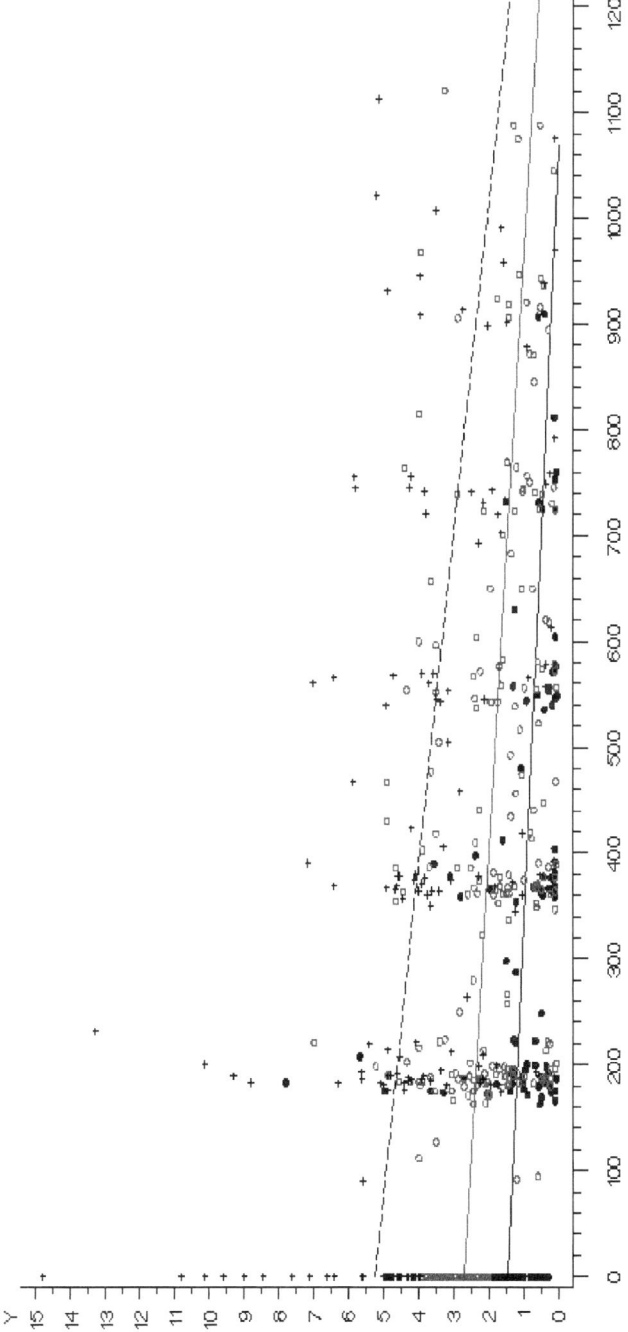

FIGURE 2A. C-peptide values (ng/mL) over time (days) by baseline C-peptide. *Solid circles*, <1.98; *open circles*, 1.98–3.94; *pluses*, >3.94.

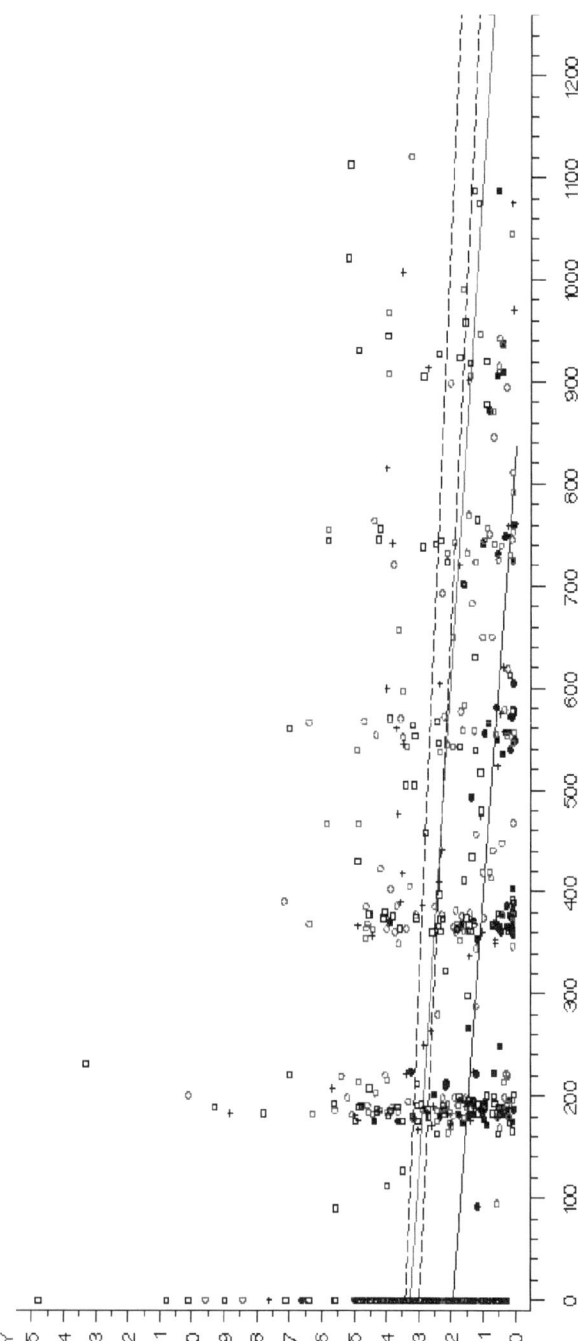

FIGURE 2B. C-peptide values (ng/mL) over time (days) by baseline age. *Solid circles*, age<10; *open circles*, age ≥10 and <20; *pluses*, age ≥20 and <30; *boxes*, age ≥30.

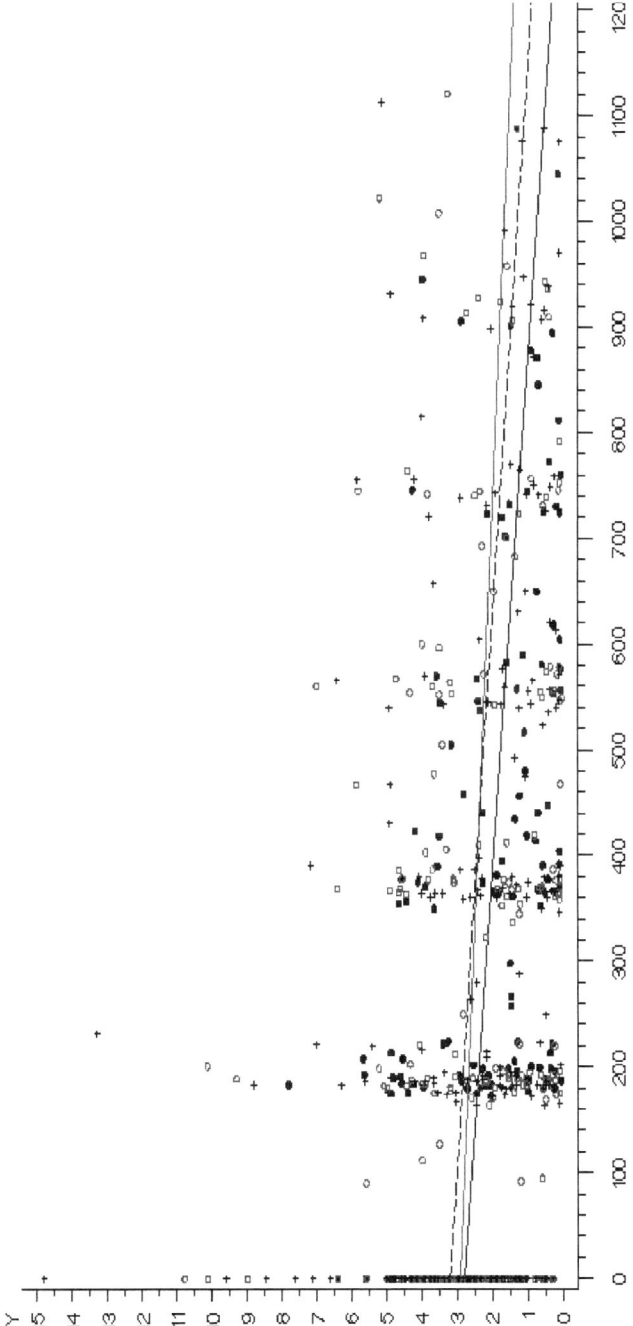

FIGURE 2C. C-peptide values (ng/mL) over time (days) by insulin dose. *Solid circles*, 10 mg; *open circles*, 1 mg; *pluses*, placebo.

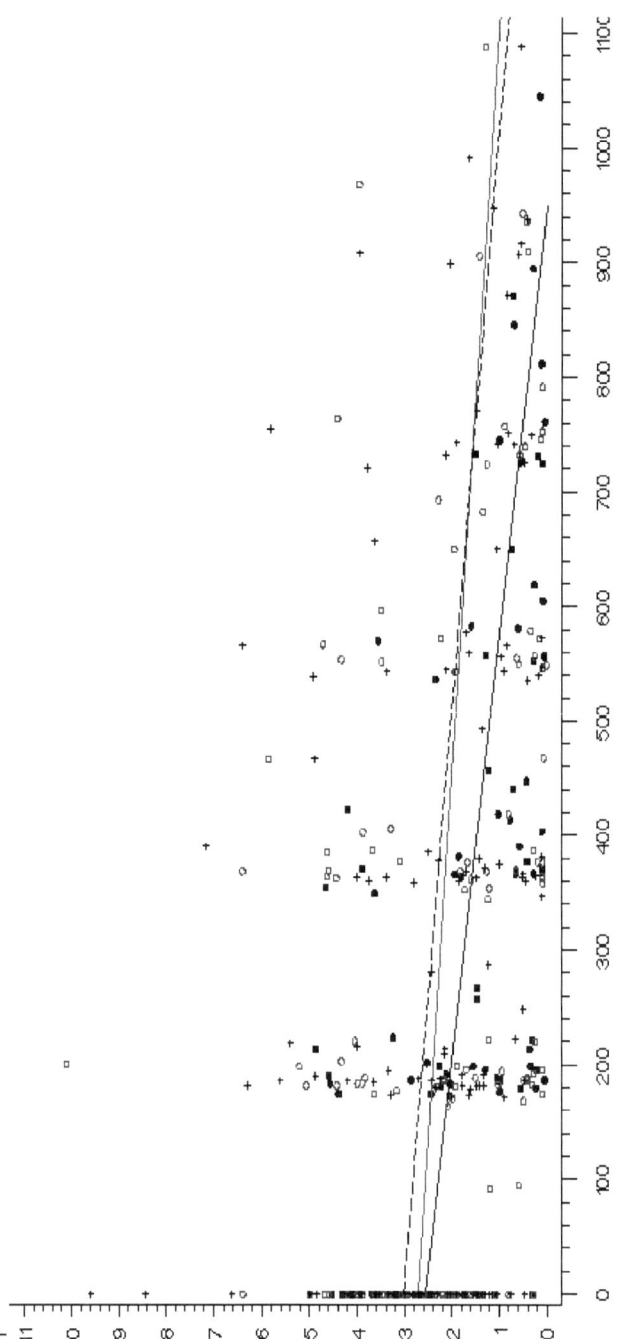

FIGURE 3A. C-peptide values (ng/mL) over time (days) by insulin dose (<20 years of age). *Solid circles*, 10 mg; *open circles*, 1 mg; *pluses*, placebo.

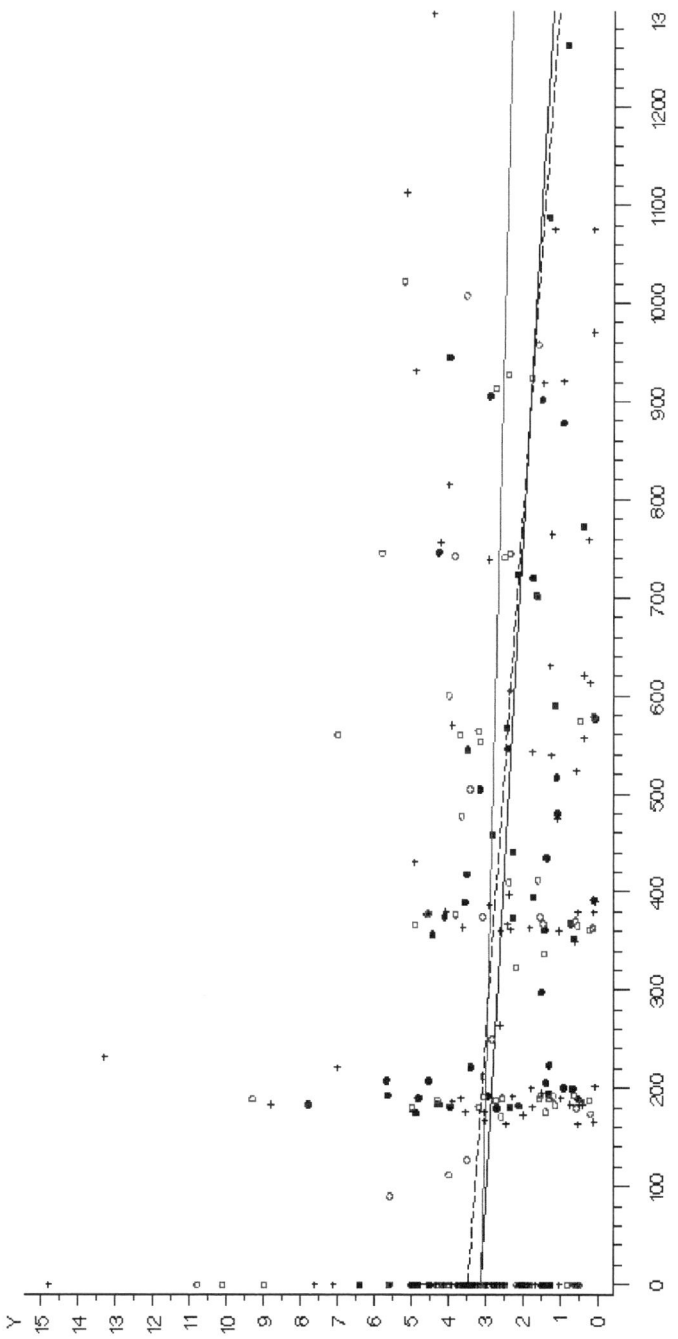

FIGURE 3B. C-peptide values (ng/mL) over time (days) by insulin dose (≥20 years of age). *Solid circles*, 10 mg; *open circles*, 1 mg; *pluses*, placebo.

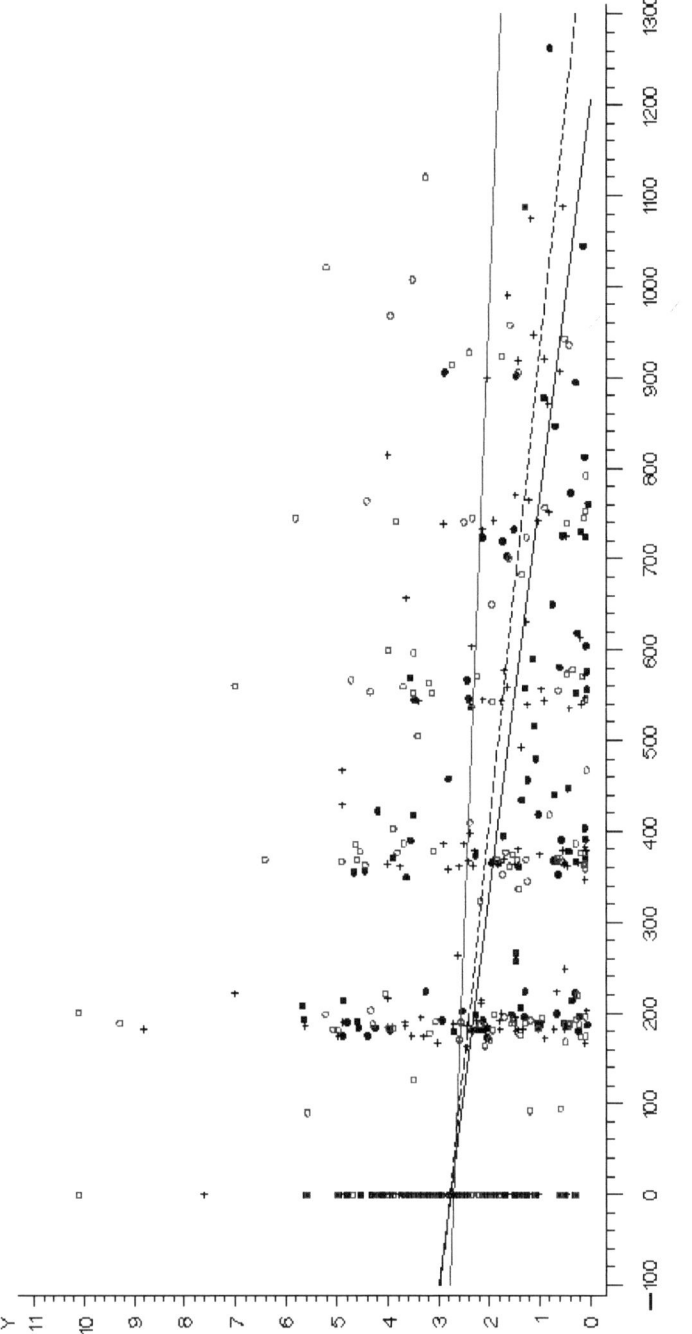

FIGURE 4. C-peptide values (ng/mL) over time (days) by insulin dose (2 or more positive antibodies at study onset). *Solid circles*, 10 mg; *open circles*, 1 mg; *pluses*, placebo.

10 years of age, age and baseline C-peptide levels were correlated with a mean baseline peak C-peptide ≤ 1.98, as compared with 18, 20, and 24% of subjects in the second, third, or higher decades of life, respectively ($P = .001$). When analyzed by age-at-treatment stratum, baseline peak C-peptide remained a statistically significant prognostic factor in each age group (data not shown).

There were no statistically significant differences in time until failure between the three experimental treatment groups ($P = .42$). The differences in time until C-peptide failure were not statistically significant in either age group (<20 or ≥ 20 years, $P = .08$ and $P = 0.21$, respectively). Although stratified by age, the study was not designed with sufficient power to adequately address this issue.

Changes in peak C-peptide values were also modeled over time to determine whether the rate of C-peptide loss was affected by oral insulin treatment. Whereas the peak C-peptide values generally declined over time, the rate of decline was marginally associated with baseline peak C-peptide levels, with the group with the lowest initial levels having a greater rate of loss after adjusting for repeated observations over time on each subject ($P = .05$; FIG. 2A). The rate of loss in C-peptide was statistically greatest for subjects under 10 years of age at study onset ($P = .0001$) as compared with other age groups (FIG. 2B). Subjects treated with 10 mg of oral insulin had greater declines in peak C-peptide than the others ($P = .02$; FIG. 2C). The greater rate of decline in C-peptide values over time in subjects treated with 10 mg of oral insulin was statistically significant in the group whose baseline C-peptide was between 1.98 and 3.94 ($P = .004$). Within the stratum of subjects under age 20 years at treatment onset, the association between treatment with 10 mg of oral insulin and a greater rate of C-peptide loss was statistically significant ($P = .003$; FIG. 3A). However, among subjects 20 years of age and older, there was a statistically significant benefit of treatment with 1 mg of oral insulin ($P = .002$), even after adjusting for baseline C-peptide values ($P = .003$; FIG. 3B). There was a smaller, yet statistically significant benefit ($P = .01$) from treatment with 10 mg of oral insulin as well in this group.

In a multivariate analysis that included number of specific autoantibodies (ICA, IAA, IA-2A, and GADA) and age at onset, a higher number of autoantibodies was associated with a greater rate of loss of C-peptide ($P = .05$); treatment with 1 mg of oral insulin was significantly associated with a lesser rate of loss of C-peptide in the ICA-only group ($P = .01$), but still statistically significant in those with multiple autoantibodies ($P = .03$; FIG. 4). After adjusting for baseline C-peptide value in the latter group, the lesser rate of C-peptide loss over time with the 1 mg oral insulin dose was still close to statistical significance ($P = .06$).

Patients with the youngest ages of onset had the highest frequencies of at-risk HLA haplotypes and the most numbers of autoantibodies, all of which were associated with the fastest loss of C-peptide response (data not shown).

Overall, we did not observe any side effects from either the low or high oral insulin doses when compared with placebo groups.

DISCUSSION

Oral insulin proved safe without adverse reactions of any kind. Although oral insulin administration did not reduce the overall endogenous insulin failure rate, the initial C-peptide response, number of specific autoantibodies, and age at onset were variables that were associated with a decreased failure rate. In our study, we demonstrated that in younger patients, more autoantibodies and/or a lower initial C-peptide level were associated with a more rapid loss of peak C-peptide (≤ 0.3 μU/mL). However, within the group of subjects with a moderate level of C-peptide at study entry, treatment with the 10 mg dosage was associated with greater rates of C-peptide loss, especially in the group under age 20. In patients over age 20, however, treatment with 1 or 10 mg oral insulin was associated with slower loss of C-peptide response, but not in those whose initial C-peptide responses were very low. Further, the linear dose-response relationship between oral insulin dose and maintenance of C-peptide suggests that there is a therapeutic dose window. Our study indicates that retention of endogenous insulin secretion after diagnosis of type 1 diabetes presenting after the pubertal years can be induced by the sustained, daily ingestion of oral insulin. These findings are in keeping with our preliminary report, which was performed as a blinded, interim safety analysis.[22] Further, there was a nonsignificant decline in the level of IAA in patients taking replacement insulin, but no declines in GAD65 or IA-2 autoantibodies. We previously reported that the prevalence of IMD as judged by islet cell autoantibodies and HLA markers of susceptibility for IMD varied among adult diabetic patients according to their ethnicity.[23] If insulin therapy could delay rapid progression to complete β cell destruction in this group, it would be beneficial to their long-term management. The Tokyo study demonstrated that small doses of insulin prevent β cell failure in slowly progressive of type 1 diabetes in adults with high GAD65 antibody levels.[24]

The lack of adverse effects make this an appealing way to intervene in the autoimmune process that continues beyond the time of clinical diagnosis. As in animal studies, the effect was strikingly dose related, being beneficial at moderate doses but non beneficial or perhaps even harmful at high doses.

The gut-associated lymphoid tissues (GALT) comprise the bulk of the body's immune system, as most foreign antigens are encountered as food. In general, antigen (peptide)-specific regulatory T cells generated by contact with cleaved peptides in the intraepithelial compartment are expanded in local nodes and Peyer's patches, so that subsequent contacts with that antigen will suppress possible T cell activation. Such T cells have a biased expression of cytokines, such as TGF-β, produced by T helper-3 (Th3) cells, or IL-4 and IL-10, produced by Th2 cells. Thus, it was hoped that repeated ingestion of an autoantigen targeted in an autoimmune disease could be used as tolerogenic therapy. Studies in NOD mice indicate that oral feedings of insulin generate insulin/insulin B chain–specific regulatory T cells, which, after clonal expansion, migrate to the pancreatic islets where (insulin/B chain) antigens are found. Once activated, these regulatory T (Tr) cells release their cytokines and thereby inhibit on going *in situ* autoimmune reactions to all antigens,[25] a process termed "bystander" immuno suppression. In this study, as in those reported in NOD mice, the protective effect was negated at increased antigen doses.[11] Relative to the doses of oral antigen used, the possible outcomes are immunization, active immunoregulation, or anergy.

Disappointingly, there were no clinical benefits discernible from our oral insulin tolerance therapy as reflected in improved diabetes control, lowered glycated hemoglobin levels, or reduced daily insulin dosages. Because the participating physicians were blinded as to the treatment groups, it is not unexpected that their care would have achieved similar levels of diabetes control, albeit lower replacement insulin requirements might have been anticipated with improved retention of endogenous insulin from oral insulin therapy, at least in the 20+ years at onset group. Nevertheless, these results are encouraging, and suggest that amendments to the 1 mg dose oral insulin protocol reported herein could lead to improved outcomes, which might be clinically valuable, at least in late-onset disease. Methods of enhancing the beneficial effects could include the addition of a second self-antigen to augment the affect of insulin. Our own group has, in fact, demonstrated augmented effects by the addition of GAD_{65} to oral insulin in NOD mice.[26] Other approaches include adding an adjuvant such as endotoxin[27] to promote Th2/3 responses, conjugating the antigen to a hapten such as cholera B chain, and/or adding cytokines therapies such as IL-4 of the Th2/3 types.

Before announcement of the DPT-1 trial,[15] two other trials of oral insulin therapy in newly diagnosed patients with type 1 diabetes were reported without significant improvements in residual β cell function.[16,17] All three studies used the same type and source of insulin, but the Italian group used a 5 mg dose, the French group 2.5 and 7.5 mg doses, and the DPT-1 trial a 7.5 mg dose. In our study, the 1 mg dose was superior to placebo, but only in patients diagnosed after age 20 years. The above the clinical trials were more limited studies than ours, with generally younger patients presenting clinically with a type 1 diabetic phenotype. The mean age for the Italian study was 14 years, with no patient over 35 years, whereas the mean age of the French study was 18 to 19 years, with no patient over 40 years. In the DPT-1 trial, the median age was 10 years, with a range of 3 to 45 years. This may have been significant, in that we documented worsening C-peptide responses in children, at least at the higher dose used. Further, our study was designed to include many ICA- positive adult diabetic patients in a relatively quiescent phase of their disease. In addition, endogenous insulin reserves in the other two studies were measured after a glucagon stimulus; however, it is unclear whether the mixed meal stimulus we used is the more powerful secretagogue.

Recently published data showed similar results with previous trials in attempt to prevent or delay the onset of IMD; however, preservation of C-peptide production in the prediabetic period appeared to indicate nonprogression to clinical disease.[28] This finding may serve as a new surrogate for determining response to preventative efforts.

In summary, ours is the first report to suggest a benefit from oral insulin tolerance therapy in newly diagnosed type 1 diabetic patients, albeit this benefit was chemical rather than clinical, and was confined to patients diagnosed after age 20 years and to low 1 mg daily doses of oral insulin. The result should encourage further trials, with multiple autoantigens (e.g., recombinant human GAD65 and insulin, which give additive protection in NOD mice), adjuvants (e.g., cholera B toxin), and suppressor cytokines (e.g., IL-4, TGF-β, IL-10) to amplify the benefits of oral insulin tolerance therapy, especially in adult-onset patients who have not yet progressed to a type 1 diabetic phenotype.

ACKNOWLEDGMENTS

We wish to thank all of the many patients who took part in this study, and the following physicians who assisted in the recruitment of their patients into the trial: Paul

Davidson, M.D. (Atlanta Diabetes Association), Stuart Chalew, M.D. (Lousiana State University Health Sciences Center, School of Medicine), Mary Luidens, M.D. (Albany Medical Center, NY), George Burghen, M.D. (University of Tennessee), Peterman Prosser, M.D. (Baton Rouge, LA), Mitchell Silverman, M.D. (Union, NJ), David Robbins, M.D. (Medlantic Research Center, Washington, DC), Peter Gottlieb, M.D. (Barbara Davis Center, CO), Jonathan Wise, M.D. (Institute for the Treatment of Diabetes & Metabolic Management, LA), Richard Kleinman, M.D. We also thank those who provided study coordination: Svetlana Ten (Maimoniades Medical Center, NY), Jihad Obeid, M.D. (Weill Medical College of Cornell University, NY), and Anjili Kureja, Ph.D. (Rockefeller University, NY). We thank the Eli Lilly Co. for the recombinant insulin used in the study and for their support through a grant-in-aid.

REFERENCES

1. Report of the Expert Committee on Diagnosis and Classification of Diabetes Mellitus. 1997. Diabetes Care **20**: 1183–1196.
2. Kukreja, A. & N.K. Maclaren. 1999. The autoimmunity of immune mediated diabetes. J. Clin. Endocrinol. Metab. **84**: 4371–4378.
3. Maclaren, N.K. & A. Kukreja. 2000. Type 1 diabetes. *In* The Metabolic and Molecular Bases of Inherited Disease. William S. Sly, Ed.: 1471–1478. McGraw-Hill. St. Louis.
4. Saudek, C. 1995. Non-ophthalmologic findings of the diabetes Control and Complications Trial. Surv. Ophthalmol. **40**: 157–162.
5. Diabetes Control and Complications Trial Research Group. 1998. Effect of intensive therapy on residual beta cell function in patients with Type-1 diabetes in the Diabetes Control and Complications Trial. Ann. Intern. Med. **128**: 517–523.
6. Silverstein, J., N. Maclaren, W. Riley, *et al.* 1988. Immunosuppression with azathioprine and prednisone in recent-onset insulin-dependent diabetes mellitus. N. Engl. J. Med. **319**: 599–604.
7. Stiller, C.R., J. Dupre, M. Gent, *et al.* 1984. Effects of cyclosporine immunosuppression in insulin-dependent diabetes mellitus of recent onset. Science **223**: 1362–1367.
8. Feutren, G., L. Papoz, R. Assan, *et al.* 1986. Cyclosporin increases the rate and length of remissions in insulin-dependent diabetes of recent onset. Results of multi-center double-blind trial. Lancet **2**: 119–124.
9. Kaufman, D.L., M. Clare-Salzler, J. Tian, *et al.* 1993. Spontaneous loss of T-cell tolerance to glutamic acid decarboxylase in murine insulin-dependent diabetes. Nature **366**: 69–72.
10. Muir, A., A. Peck, M. Clare-Salzler, *et al.* 1995. Insulin immunization of non-obese diabetic mice induces a protective insulitis characterized by diminished intra-islet interferon-gamma transcription. J. Clin. Invest. **95**: 628–634.
11. Zhang, Z.J., L. Davidson, G. Eisenbarth, *et al.* 1991. Suppression of diabetes in non-obese diabetic mice by oral administration of porcine insulin. Proc. Natl. Acad. Sci. USA **88**: 10252–10256.
12. Ramiya, V.K., M.S. Lan, C.H. Wasserfall, *et al.* 1997. Immunization therapies in the prevention of diabetes. J. Autoimmun. **10**: 287–292.
13. DPT-1 Study Group. 1995. The Diabetes Prevention Trial–Type 1 diabetes (DPT-1): implementation of screening and staging of relatives. Transplant Proc. **27**: 3377.
14. ENDIT Group. 2003. Intervening before the onset of type 1 diabetes: baseline data from the European Nicotinamide Diabetes Intervention Trial (ENDIT). Diabetologia **46**: 339–346.
15. Diabetes Prevention Trial–Type 1 Diabetes Study Group. 2002. Effects of insulin in relatives of patients with type 1 diabetes mellitus. Diabetes prevention trial–type 1 diabetes study group. N. Engl. J. Med. **346**: 1685–1691.

16. Chaillous, L., H. Lefevre, C. Thivolet, *et al.* 2000. Oral insulin administration and residual beta-cell function in recent-onset type 1 diabetes: a multicentre randomised controlled trial. Diabete Insuline Orale group. Lancet **356:** 545–549.
17. Pozzilli, P., D. Pitocco, N. Visalli, *et al.* 2000. No effect of oral insulin on residual beta-cell function in recent-onset type I diabetes (the IMDIAB VII). Diabetologia **43:** 1000–1004.
18. Riley, W.J., N.K. Maclaren, J. Krischer, *et al.* 1990. A prospective study of the development of diabetes in relatives of patients with insulin-dependent diabetes. N. Engl. J. Med. **323:** 1167–1172.
19. Vardi, P., L. Crisa & R.A. Jackson. 1991. Predictive value of intravenous glucose tolerance test insulin secretion less than or greater than the first percentile in islet cell antibody positive relatives of type 1 (insulin-dependent) diabetic patients. Diabetologia **34:** 93–102.
20. Maclaren, N., M. Lan, R. Coutant, *et al.* 1999. Only multiple auto-antibodies to islet cells (ICA), insulin, GAD65, IA-2 and IA-2β predict immune-mediated (Type 1) diabetes in relatives. J. Autoimmun. **12:** 279–287.
21. Hempe, J.M., J.N. Granger & R.D. Craver. 1997. Capillary iso-electric focusing of hemoglobin variants in the pediatric clinical laboratory. Electrophoresis **18:** 1785–1795.
22. Coutant, R., A. Zeidler, R. Rappaport, *et al.* 1998. Oral insulin therapy in newly diagnosed immune mediated (type-1) diabetes. Preliminary analysis of a randomized double blind placebo controlled study [abstract]. Diabetes **47**(Suppl. 1): A97.
23. Aviles-Santa, L., N. Maclaren & P. Raskin. 2004. The relationship between immune-mediated Type 1 diabetes mellitus and ethnicity. J. Diabetes Complications **18:** 1– 9.
24. Maruyama, T., A. Shimada, A. Kanatsuka, *et al.* 2003. Multicenter prevention trial of slowly progressive type 1 diabetes with small dose of insulin (the Tokyo study): preliminary report. Ann. N. Y. Acad. Sci. **1005:** 362–369.
25. Weiner, H.L. 1997. Oral tolerance: immune mechanisms and treatment of autoimmune diseases. Immunol. Today **18:** 335–343.
26. Ramiya, V.K., X.Z. Shang, P.G. Pharis, *et al.* 1996. Antigen based therapies to prevent diabetes in NOD mice. J. Autoimmun. **9:** 349–356.
27. Ramiya, V.K., X.Z. Shang, C.H. Wasserfall, *et al.* 1997. Effect of oral and intravenous insulin and glutamic acid decarboxylase in NOD mice. Autoimmunity **26:** 139–151.
28. Schatz, D., D. Cuthbertson, M. Atkinson, *et al.* 2004. Preservation of C-peptide secretion in subjects at high risk of developing type 1 diabetes mellitus—a new surrogate measure of non-progression? Pediatr. Diabetes **5:** 72–79.

Orally and Nasally Induced Tolerance Studies in Ocular Inflammatory Disease

Guidance for Future Interventions

ROBERT NUSSENBLATT

Laboratory of Immunology, National Eye Institute,
National Institutes of Health, Bethesda, Maryland 20892, USA

ABSTRACT: The induction of both oral and nasal tolerance has been used in both experimental models of ocular disease and clinically. Initial work centered around the abrogation of experimental autoimmune uveitis using either one or two whole uveitogenic antigens. Other models of ocular disease have included a corneal transplant model, demonstrating that feeding splenocytes from the donor strain of rats enhanced corneal engraftment. Fragments of pertinent antigens have been shown to alter the expression of experimental uveitis and possibly human disease. A randomized, masked study in uveitis provided valuable information for future studies, demonstrating that single antigen feeding provided far better protection than the feeding of multiple antigens. This review will deal with animal and human studies in the treatment of ocular inflammatory disease with the goal of extracting from past experience how to construct a future study in humans.

KEYWORDS: uveitis; oral tolerance; nasal tolerance; corneal engraftment

INTRODUCTION

Uveitis is a term that indicates any type of inflammation inside the eye. It is an old term that at one time suggested that the center of the inflammatory response in the eye is located in the uveal tract. We know that this is not the case for many types of inflammatory conditions. Further, the term indicates neither the anatomic location of the inflammatory response nor what the underlying cause of the disease might be. An inflammatory ocular response in the front of the eye is termed an anterior uveitis, while one involving the retina is a posterior uveitis. If the focus of the immune response appears to be in the vitreous of the eye then it is an intermediate uveitis, and if all coats of the eye are involved it is termed a panuveitis. As well, the inflammatory process may be due to an infectious process, such as toxoplasmosis or cytomegalovirus retinitis. Much of the disease seen in the developed world is believed not to be infectious in nature. Indeed, many of the disorders are conjectured to be driven by autoimmune mechanisms.

Address for correspondence: Robert Nussenblatt, M.D., Laboratory of Immunology, National Eye Institute, National Institutes of Health, Bldg. 10, Room 10S219, 10 Center Drive, Bethesda, MD 20892. Voice: 301-496-3123; fax: 301-402-0485.

    DrBob@nei.nih.gov

The therapy of intraocular inflammatory disease depends a great deal on whether the disease is believed to be infectious or noninfectious in origin. For uveitic conditions of noninfectious causes, there are essentially three approaches: intraocular, local, and systemic therapy. Topically applied medicines, such as corticosteroids, can effectively treat inflammations in the front of the eye but not in the back and so cannot be used to treat severe sight-threatening disease involving the retina. Periocular steroid injections can be used, and are effective, but have a relatively short half-life and have side effects. The use of intraocular anti-inflammatory therapy, usually steroid, is being employed more and more either by injection or by surgically placing an intraocular slow-release device. Though potentially effective, one can only treat one eye at a time and there are significant side effects, including cataract and glaucoma. As of this writing, the most commonly used therapy is systemic therapy. If it has become clear that long-term (i.e., greater than three months) therapy is needed, a second steroid-sparing agent will be added. The choices can include methotrexate, mycophenolate mofetil, or cyclosporine. More and more frequently, therapy has turned to the use of systemically administered biologic agents, directed against either the tumor necrosis factor or the interleukin-2 circuitry. It is clear that all of these approaches have potential benefits, but have substantial negatives as well. Therefore, the development of better, more effective therapies with fewer adverse events is an ongoing goal.

The study of immune-mediated ocular disease has been helped enormously by the animal models of disease currently available. One in particular, experimental autoimmune uveitis (EAU), has been especially helpful in delineating mechanisms of disease, with many of the observations seen in the animals corroborated in humans.[1,2] The induced disease is a bilateral inflammatory condition that affects the back of the eye. Th1 $CD4^+$, IL-2R bearing cells can transfer the disease. Uveitis patients demonstrate cell-mediated responses to retinal S-antigen[3]; these findings are similar to what is seen in the animal model. Further, *in vitro* cell culture of circulating cells from uveitis patients has not shown a dominant response to a specific fragment but rather to several.[4] This model has been used to test various therapeutic approaches.

Peripheral immune tolerance induced by either nasal or oral administration of antigen is an approach that has been studied with some degree of intensity in the past for both inflammatory ocular conditions and corneal transplantation.[5,6]

The goal of this paper is to examine the information that is available concerning the use of oral and nasal administration of ocular antigens in attempting to induce peripheral immune tolerance for uveitis but not other ocular conditions. It will deal with both animal data and the human trials that have been carried out to date in trying to maximize success in future human studies for uveitis.

EXPERIMENTAL UVEITIS STUDIES

Orally Administered Antigen

On the basis of our collaboration with Howard Weiner, we were able to reproduce the protective effect of orally administered antigens that has been seen in experimental autoimmune encephalomyelitis. In the original experiment,[5] female Lewis rats weighing 180–200 g were used. Animals were fed on day −7, −5, and −2 with either 200 μg or 1 mg of bovine retinal S-antigen or with 200 μg of one of two S-antigen fragments reported to induce uveitis, fragments N or M. Feeding with the whole antigen effectively diminished the expression of clinical disease, whether the immunizing antigen was the whole molecule or one of the fragments. Feeding with either of the fragments did not protect from immunization with the whole molecule, while M was better at downregulating clinical disease than was N. Of interest as well was that in a series of experiments not in this initial report, feeding animals with S-antigen beginning on day 7 after immunization still resulted in diminution of disease. However, although disease severity was markedly decreased, most eyes had a small amount of inflammatory disease. Other experiments performed by the group also gave hints as to what may occur in humans. The need for an intact spleen was noted in a series of experiments.[7] In addition, initial experiments suggested that the presence of cyclosporine may interfere with optimizing oral tolerization. Further, in a series of experiments using multiple antigens, tolerization appeared difficult to induce as well (Igal Gery, personal correspondence).

Reports have also looked at the use of fragments in the abrogation of experimentally induced uveitis. Some of the initial studies centered around peptide 35, a 20-amino acid peptide at position 341–360 of bovine S-antigen (GELTSSEVATEVPFR-LMHPQ) initially reported by Gregorson,[8] as well as another peptide, 36. Thurau and colleagues[9] fed animals either 1 mg of the full S-antigen molecule or 200 μg of one of these peptides at days −7, −5, and −2 before immunization with retinal S-antigen. The results suggested that orally administered peptide was not as effective as whole molecule. Animals fed KLH had a mean inflammatory index of 2.10, those fed the S-antigen molecule a mean inflammatory index of 0.38, and those fed peptide 35 an index of 1.00. Peptide 36 was even less effective than peptide 35.

Wildner and Thurau have reported a series of experiments using a common peptide sequence found in HLA B antigens. This peptide, designated B27PD and found in position 125–134 (ALNEDLSSWTAADT), mimics positions 341–354 of S-antigen, (FLGELTSSEVATEV).[10,11] Comparing the results of feeding this peptide with orally administered S-antigen, the peptide resulted in a diminution of uveitis and was felt to also have an effect on interphotoreceptor retinoid-binding protein (IRBP)-induced uveitis. The effect seen was not thought to be a bystander effect, but rather an effect of shared sequence homologies between IRBP and B27PD. In another series of experiments, Hu and colleagues,[12] using a heat shock peptide (336–351), were able to induce uveitis in a large percentage of animals tested. Of interest is the claim that immune responses to this particular peptide are specifically found in patients with Behçet's disease. However, giving this peptide nasally (see below) and/ or orally, the inflammatory disease induced with immunization was not abrogated.

Nasal Administration of Antigen

The second approach to therapy reviewed here is the nasal administration of antigen in attempting to elicit peripheral immune tolerance. Dick and colleagues have reported a series of studies in animals that suggest that this approach may be useful in inducing a positive immune effect with less antigen. In an early study, Dick and colleagues[13] gave either a retinal extract or retinal S-antigen nasally for 10 d before induction of disease. It would appear that a total of 12 μg of retinal S-antigen given over this period was effective in decreasing the severity of disease in immunized rats. A higher dose of a retinal extract was needed to effect a change, but still at much lower doses than needed when given orally. An interesting finding was that S-antigen nasally administered failed to suppress experimental uveitis induced with a retinal extract.

A later report[14] suggested that peripheral tolerance could still be induced with a nasal tolerant even if cyclosporine was used. However, the nasal administration of antigen could not reliably suppress active disease. Furthermore, peripheral tolerance using nasally applied antigens could not be induced if mycophenolate mofetil was used to pretreat the animals.[15]

HUMAN STUDIES

To date, two studies treating uveitis patients orally with ocularly derived antigens have been published.

Retinal S-Antigen

In a Phase I/II masked, randomized study, we tested the use of orally administered retinal antigens in the treatment of intermediate and posterior uveitis of noninfectious origin.[16] A total of 45 patients participated in the study. Patients were eligible if they required therapy for at least three months with immunosuppressive agents; if taking oral prednisone alone they must have received a daily dose of at least 20 mg. All patients were found to have minimal ocular inflammatory disease clinically. In addition, the patients' lymphocytes were screened *in vitro* for evidence of a positive

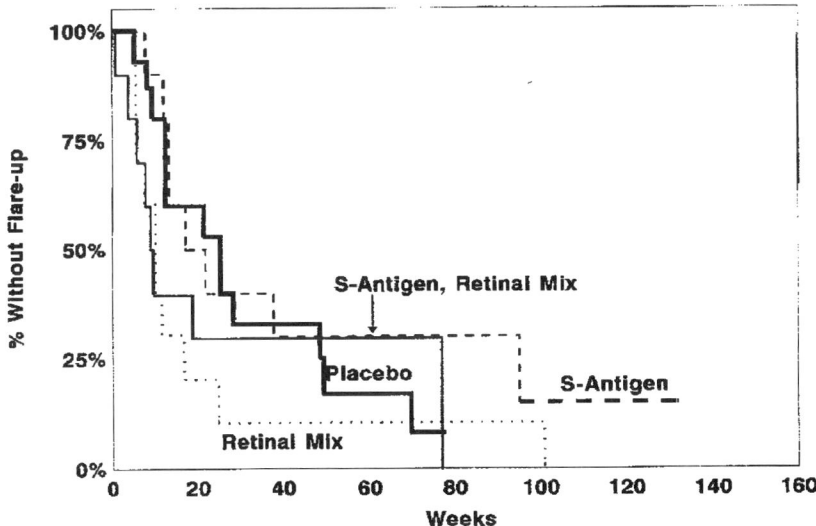

FIGURE 1. Life table analyses showing time to flare-up for all groups. From Nussenblatt *et al.*[16] Reproduced with permission.

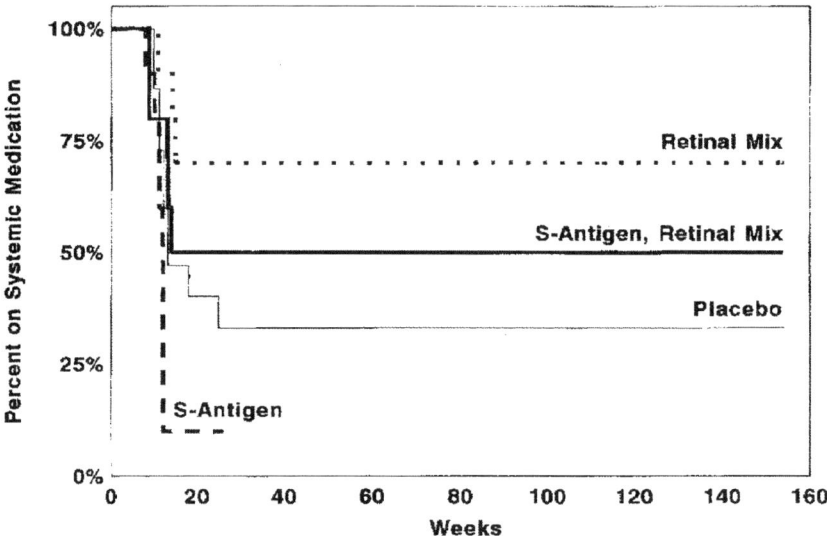

FIGURE 2. Life table analyses for all groups showing time to stopping medications. From Nussenblatt et al.[16] Reproduced with permission.

proliferative response to retinal S-antigen. A total of 230,000 bovine retinas were needed to prepare the antigens used in this study. Patients were randomized to four possible treatment arms: retinal S-antigen alone ($n = 10$), retinal mixture alone ($n = 10$), combination S-antigen and retinal mixture ($n = 10$), or placebo ($n = 15$). S-antigen was given in a 30-mg capsule, while the retinal mixture was given in a 50-mg capsule. For the first eight weeks of the study, patients received their regimen three times a week, and then were given the treatment once a week. Patients were tapered off their standard immunosuppressive therapy during that eight-week period. This was done by physicians who were masked as to the medications being given and the taper was done only if it was clinically indicated. The life tables from this study can be seen in FIGURES 1 and 2. Patients receiving retinal S-antigen could be tapered off their standard medication more readily and the recurrence of their disease occurred later than in the other groups. An interesting and unexpected finding was that patients receiving the retinal mixture did worse than the placebo group. It was initially assumed that patients receiving multiple antigens would, in fact, do as well or even better than the patients receiving soluble retinal S-antigen. A Cox proportional hazards model was used to assess the effect of various baseline characteristics on the ability of patients to stop their medication. Duration of disease and age of the patient were not found to be important variables. However, taking cyclosporine was found to be a variable that showed a trend toward making it more difficult to be tapered off medication, as compared with taking prednisone ($P = .07$).

Thurau and coworkers[17,18] have also published their results using B27PD, an HLA Class I fragment similar to a fragment in S-antigen, in the treatment of uveitis. In this open label, nonrandomized pilot study, nine patients were enrolled (three female, six male). The majority of these patients carried a diagnosis of iridocyclitis or iritis. Patients were treated for a 12-week period. They received a total of 4 mg of the fragment orally three times a week. Eight of the patients completed the study. In six of the patients, the steroid dosage was decreased (one patient stopped therapy just before going onto B27PD therapy) and had either stable or improved vision during this period. After finishing oral therapy, the inflammatory disease stayed quiescent for 18 weeks on average before relapses occurred.

CONCLUSIONS

What are the lessons learned from the animal and human studies that have been published to date? How might one ideally develop a human study in uveitis to assure as best one can a therapeutic success? Clearly, there are observations that do help, but several questions, of course, still remain.

On the basis of information that we have at present, it would be ideal to treat patients with a single full molecule, with S-antigen being the most favorable choice. An alternative would be a long segment of the molecule that contains several of the epitopes to which uveitis patients' lymphocytes responded.[4] IRBP is an excellent antigen for mouse studies, but we have not reliably seen *in vitro* cell-mediated proliferative responses to it from uveitis patients' lymphocytes. While administering a fragment of the molecule would be much easier and cheaper, we have seen in the animal studies that fragments of uveitogenic molecules do not protect against disease induced by the whole molecule. One antigen, not several, should be given. This is based on the striking results that we observed in our human study using a retinal extract. While this method worked in animal studies, patients receiving this retinal antigen combination did worse than placebo, perhaps reflecting negative results in other therapeutic trials when an antigen mix was used. One can argue that our batches may have contained material that prevented the oral administration of antigen from inducing a positive therapeutic effect; the mode of administration may also be important.

What of the route of administration, dosage, and frequency? On the basis of available information, it would seem that nasal administration of antigen is preferable to oral administration. Information from rat experiments would suggest that 1.2 µg of retinal S-antigen could be administered for daily therapy. A dosage of 200 µg to 1 mg of S-antigen was given to rats orally in order to see similar effects. Patients received 30 mg of S-antigen orally, or some 30 times the dose in rats. If this extrapolation held true for the nasal administration of antigen, one could foresee treating with 36 µg per day. One concern is that most of the nasal tolerance studies were performed by pretreating before immunization and treating after immunization has occurred. Therefore, it is very possible that higher doses would be needed. The use of an adjuvant would not be considered at this time, unless further studies showed it to be beneficial in this system. The use of cholera toxin components to enhance orally induced tolerance may have a downside, in that systemic immunization may occur, as these antigens have been used to induce a better immunizing effect when vaccines have been administered orally. One should consider daily therapy initially until a stable clinical state has been reached.

What type of patients would one consider treating? It would seem reasonable to again treat patients with noninfectious intermediate and posterior uveitis. *In vitro* proliferative responses to retinal S-antigen would be ideal, but practical issues may intervene with that strategy. It would seem reasonable to treat patients with disease that is being controlled by immunosuppressive therapy. It would be problematic at this stage treating patients with active disease because we are not sure of the effectiveness of the approach, and severe visual consequences could result in not treating patients effectively in a prompt fashion. Which other medications should the patients be taking? Could some inhibit the effectiveness of this therapy? On the basis of our human study, there was a trend for patients taking cyclosporine not doing as well as others. We know that cyclosporine may interfere with the induction of peripheral tolerance in other systems. It is interesting to note that animals receiving mycophenolate mofetil did not have beneficial results when ocular antigens were administered nasally. It may be that a completely different approach could be considered, such as not starting nasal administration until disease is rendered quiet by an antibody directed against lymphokine circuitry, that is, an anti–IL-2 receptor antibody.

It is clear that animal studies and the limited human studies performed suggest strongly that the administration of antigen, whether through the oral route or the nasal mucosa, has an effect on the expression of disease. Whether we will be able to standardize the response and maximize its effect so that it will be clinically relevant still remains the big challenge.

REFERENCES

1. CASPI, R.R. 2002. Th1 and Th2 responses in pathogenesis and regulation of experimental autoimmune uveoretinitis. Int. Rev. Immunol. **21:** 197–208.
2. NUSSENBLATT, R.B. 2002. Bench to bedside: new approaches to the immunotherapy of uveitis disease. Int. Rev. Immunol. **21:** 273–289.
3. NUSSENBLATT, R.B. *et al.* 1980. Cellular immune responsiveness of uveitis patients to retinal S-antigen. Am. J. Ophthalmol. **89:** 173–179.
4. DE SMET, M.D. *et al.* 2001. Human S-antigen determinant recognition in uveitis. Invest. Ophthalmol. Vis. Sci. **42:** 3233–3238.
5. NUSSENBLATT, R.B. *et al.* 1990. Inhibition of S-antigen induced experimental autoimmune uveoretinitis by oral induction of tolerance with S-antigen. J. Immunol. **144:** 1669–1695.
6. HE, Y.G., J. MELLON & J.Y. NIEDERKORN. 1996. The effect of oral immunization on corneal allograft survival. Transplantation **61:** 920–926.
7. SUH, E. *et al.* 1993. Splenectomy abrogates the induction of oral tolerance in experimental autoimmune uveoretinitis. Curr. Eye Res. **12:** 833–839.
8. GREGORSON, D.S. *et al.* 1990. Identification of a potent new pathogenic side in human retinal S-antigen which induces experimental autoimmune uveoretinitis in LEW rats. Cell Immunol. **128:** 209–219.
9. THURAU, S.R. *et al.* 1991. Induction of oral tolerance to S-antigen induced experimental autoimmune uveitis by a uveitogenic 20mer peptide. J. Autoimmun. **4:** 507–516.
10. WILDNER, G. & S.R. THURAU. 1994. Cross-reactivity between an HLA-B27 derived peptide and a retinal autoantigen peptide: a clue to major histocompatibility complex association with autoimmune disease. Eur. J. Immunol. **24:** 2579–2585.
11. THURAU, S.R. & G. WILDNER. 2003. An HLA-peptide mimics organ-specific antigen in autoimmune uveitis: its role in pathogenesis and therapeutic induction of oral tolerance. Autoimmun. Rev. **2:** 171–176.
12. HU, W. *et al.* 1998. Experimental mucosal induction of uveitis with the 60-kDa heat shock protein-derived peptide 336-351. Eur. J. Immunol. **28:** 2444–2455.

13. DICK, A.D. et al. 1993. Nasal administration of retinal antigens suppresses the inflammatory response in experimental allergic uveoretinitis. Br. J. Ophthalmol. **77:** 171–175.
14. KREUTZER, B. et al. 1977. Nasal administration of retinal antigens maintains immunosuppression of uveoretinitis in cyclosporin-A-treated Lewis rats: future treatment of endogenous posterior uveoretinitis. Eye **11:** 445–452.
15. DICK, A.D. et al. 1998. Effects of mycophenolate mofetil on nasal mucosal tolerance induction. Invest. Ophthalmol. Vis. Sci. **39:** 835–840.
16. NUSSENBLATT, R.B. et al. 1997. Treatment of uveitis by oral administration of retinal antigens: results of a Phase I/II randomized masked trial. Am. J. Ophthalmol. **123:** 583–592.
17. THURAU, S.R. et al. 1997. Molecular mimicry as a therapeutic approach for an autoimmune disease: oral treatment of uveitis-patients with an MHC-peptide crossreactive with autoantigen-first results. Immunol. Lett. **57:** 193–201.
18. THURAU, S.R. et al. 1999. Oral tolerance with an HLA-peptide mimicking retinal autoantigen as a treatment of autoimmune uveitis. Immunol. Lett. **68:** 205–212.

Oral Immune Regulation toward Disease-Associated Antigens

Results of Phase I Clinical Trials in Crohn's Disease and Chronic Hepatitis

YARON ILAN

Liver and Gastroenterology Units, Department of Medicine, Hebrew University Hadassah Medical Center, Jerusalem, Israel

ABSTRACT: Oral immune regulation is an immune response toward orally administered antigens, and is a balance between several types of responses. Recent studies in animal models have shown that antiviral immunity and the immune response toward colonic proteins can be modulated by oral feeding of these antigens. The effect of oral immune regulation on the outcome of various immune-mediated processes, including infectious, inflammatory, and neoplastic entities, has been the subject of much research and debate in recent years. Two phase I clinical trials have evaluated the effect of oral immune regulation in patients with chronic hepatitis B virus infection and Crohn's disease. Mechanisms and possible future clinical applications of this immune modulatory method are discussed.

KEYWORDS: Crohn's disease; hepatitis B virus; oral tolerance; immune response; treatment; antiviral immunity

ORAL IMMUNE REGULATION

The immunological outcome following oral antigen administration is in reality a balance between several different types of signals that may be mediated via different subtypes of lymphocytes (FIG. 1). Factors affecting this balance may be antigen related (i.e., nature and dose of an antigen) or host related (i.e., genetic background, immunological status, mucosal adjuvants).[1–4] Oral antigen administration may result in tolerance or in enhancement of epitope-specific immunity.[2] This effect may be mediated by a different subpopulation of antigen-specific or nonspecific cells that induces a Th1-type immune response in addition to the usually dominant Th2- and Th3-type immunity.[2,3] Immune enhancement can result from direct augmentation of the activity of these cells, or from inhibition of elements that suppress their function.

Address for correspondence: Yaron Ilan, M.D., Director, Department of Medicine, Hadassah-Hebrew University Medical Center, P.O.Box 12000, Jerusalem, Israel IL-91120. Voice: +972-2-6777816; fax: +972-2-6431021.

ilan@hadassah.org.il

Ann. N.Y. Acad. Sci. 1029: 286–298 (2004). © 2004 New York Academy of Sciences.
doi: 10.1196/annals.1309.059

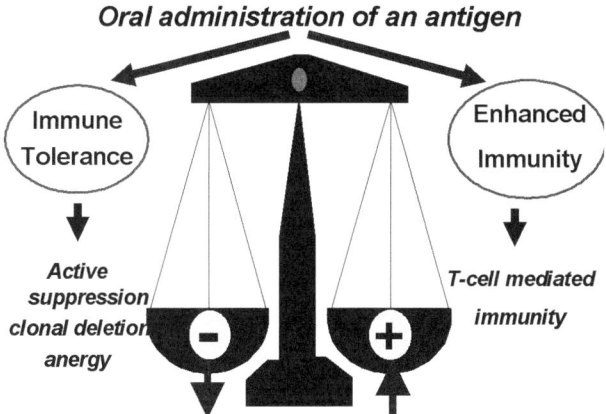

FIGURE 1. Oral immune regulation: the balance between immunity and tolerance.

ORAL IMMUNE REGULATION IN EXPERIMENTAL COLITIS

The current understanding of the pathogenesis of inflamatory bowel disease (IBD) is that in a genetically predisposed host, a pathogen or a nonpathogenic stimulus activates an abnormal mucosal response that cannot be regulated.[5] The defect can be at two levels: an inability to control an initial response to normal luminal contents, and/or subsequent failure of downregulatory mechanisms to become activated.[5,6] Both defects in host immune response and in host nonimmune defense mechanisms, such as abnormalities in mucin production, have been noted in patients with IBD.[6] IBD can be envisioned as a dysbalance between proinflammatory and anti-inflammatory cytokines. Secretion of proinflammatory cytokines, such as IFN-γ, contributes to an increase in mucosal permeability. Administration of anti–IL-12, anti-TNF-α, or anti-IFN-γ antibodies can prevent experimental colitis.[7–9] Immunosuppressive regimens lead to clinical and histological improvement in IBD patients. However, these drugs are associated with short-term and long-term complications. The advancing knowledge regarding the biology of chronic inflammation has led to development of specific biological therapies that target individual inflammatory pathways.[9] These treatments are non–antigen specific, and may have unwanted effects in the immune response in the bowel, as well as systemically. Induction of oral immune regulation for treatment of IBD can be viewed as an attempt to correct a defect in regulatory T cells or other defects in a regulatory process in the gut-associated and/or systemic immune system. This method could potentially allow for long-term alleviation of the disease, thereby leaving the general immunological defense of the recipient intact.

Oral Immune Regulation in Experimental Colitis

In animal models of experimental colitis, rectal administration of low doses of 2,4,6-trinitrobenzene sulfonic acid (TNBS) results in chronic transmural colitis with severe diarrhea, weight loss, and rectal prolapse, and mimics some of the characteristics of Crohn's disease in humans.[10,11] Lamina propria $CD4^+$ T cells exhibit a Th1

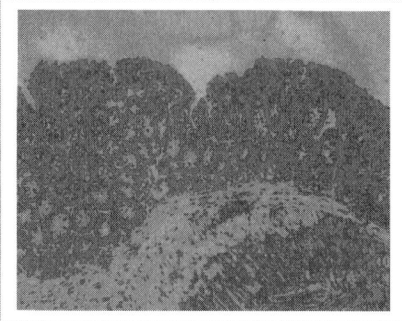 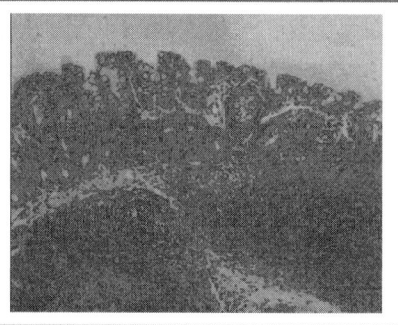

A: TREATED   **B: CONTROL**

FIGURE 2. Effect of oral immune regulation toward colitis-extracted proteins on experimental colitis in (**A**) orally immune–regulated and (**B**) control animals. A marked reduction in mucosal inflammation is noted in treated animals.

pattern of cytokine secretion, with an increase in IFN-γ and IL-2 and a decrease in IL-4 secretion. Induction of oral immune regulation toward colitis-extracted proteins (CEP) alleviated experimental colitis, manifested by a decrease in diarrhea, percentage of affected colonic area, degree of colonic ulceration, intestinal and peritoneal adhesions, and wall thickness.[12–14] Histologic evaluation of bowel tissue showed marked reduction in inflammatory response and mucosal ulceration (FIG. 2). Serum IFN-γ levels decreased in treated compared with control mice.[12,15–17]

Mechanisms of Oral Immune Regulation in Experimental Colitis

The mechanisms underlying induction of tolerance following feeding of soluble exogenous antigens, including proteins and haptens, are still unclear. Splenic lymphocytes from orally immune–regulated animals were capable of adoptively transferring immune tolerance upon transplantation into naive animals.[12] Surrogate antigens derived from normal mouse colonic wall induced a beneficial effect similar to that achieved by feeding of autologous-derived CEP.[15,16] When suppressor T cells activated by antigen-presenting cell (APC) presentation of these proteins encounter similar epitopes in the colon, they secrete anti-inflammatory cytokines.[17] A recent study demonstrates that cellular proteins from human colon epithelial cells, but not from human fibroblasts, can induce oral tolerance in experimental colitis.[13,14] It was recently suggested that haptenization of the colonic antigens is nonessential because oral feeding of nonhaptenized colonic antigens also protects rats from TNBS-induced colitis.[14]

The Role of the Liver and NKT Lymphocytes in Oral Immune Regulation

The liver plays a critical role in oral tolerance induction. A first pass of portal blood through portocaval shunt, or blockage of Kupffer cell function via injection of Gadolinium chloride, has been shown to prevent oral tolerance induction.[18,19] The adult liver is a meeting site for two subpopulations of lymphocytes: mainstream lymphocytes and alternative lymphocytes.[18] The latter include cells that are partially positive for NK markers (NKT lymphocytes). Upon primary activation NKT lymphocytes release a large variety of cytokines of both Th1 and Th2 origin.[20] NKT cells increase in the liver in response to IL-12 and TNF-α, and may be actively involved in administering a lethal hit to mainstream T cells during peripheral deletion. Depletion of NKT cells prevented oral tolerance induction in an animal model of experimental colitis.[21] NKT cytotoxicity function was associated with peripheral tolerance.[22] Adoptive transfer of NKT cells harvested from orally immune–regulated mice ameliorated colitis in recipient mice.[23,24] NKT cells may be involved in keeping a balance between anti-inflammatory and proinflammatory lymphocytes via cytokine secretion, or via killing of specific subsets of lymphocytes. They were suggested to play a dual role in regulating the immune-mediated damage in this model. In a "tolerized" environment they support immune hyporesponsiveness. In a "nontolerized" environment they support a proinflammatory immune response.

PATIENT-CUSTOMIZED MEDICINE: RESULTS OF PHASE I CLINICAL TRIAL OF INDUCTION OF ORAL IMMUNE REGULATION IN CROHN'S DISEASE

The aims of a recent study were to determine the safety and tolerability of oral administration of autologous colonic mucosal cells from Crohn's disease (CD) patients, and to determine the efficacy of this mode of treatment in patients with CD.[25]

Patients and Methods

One group of 10 patients, 6 males and 4 females, with a mean age of 37 years (19 to 59), was followed in an open-label, nonrandomized, single-center prospective trial. The diagnosis of Crohn's disease with clinical evidence of active (symptomatic) disease was based on clinical history, blood tests and/or histology, X-ray, or endoscopy, with a CDAI score between 200 and 350. Mean duration of disease was 11 years (range 2 to 37). Disease site was ileum (6 patients), ileocolon (2 patients), and colon (2 patients). Subjects who fulfilled the inclusion/exclusion criteria for participation in the study were scheduled for a colonoscopy, during which time colon biopsies were taken. The containing extract was prepared according to Enzo Therapeutics, Inc., Specification Number L0060-00-0109, "Preparation of Autologous Colon-Specific Antigen for Oral Immune Regulation for IBD: Crohn's Disease." All subjects were fed with antigen extracted from their own intestinal mucosa. Each subject ingested 3 doses per week for 16 weeks. Study individuals were monitored with a variety of safety, biological, and efficacy parameters.

Results

Administration of the study drug significantly ameliorated disease activity. During the course of treatment, all 10 subjects had a clinical response (CDAI decrease of at least 70 points), and 7 of 10 subjects achieved clinical remission (CDAI = 150). Median time to response was 5 weeks (FIG. 3). The median decrease of CDAI was 102 points at 6 weeks (264 to 162 points, $P = .003$), and 129 points at

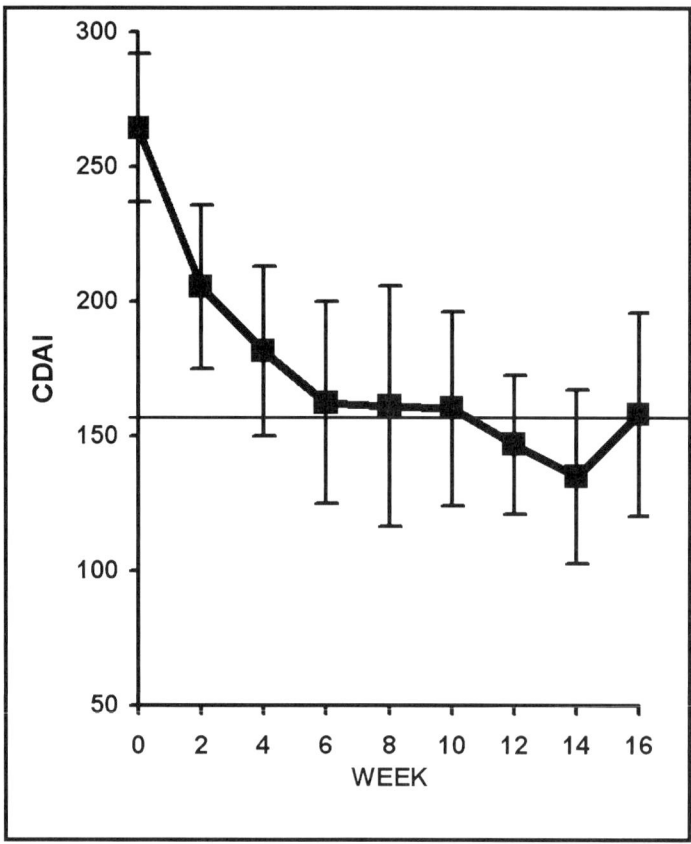

FIGURE 3. Effect of the study drug on CDAI score. Median (± SEM) CDAI scores over time during the treatment period.

14 weeks (95–158 points, $P = .0001$). At the end of the 16-week nontreatment follow-up period, CDAI score increased to 206 points. A significant increase in mean IBDQ score was noted on week 16 as compared with baseline (164 ± 12 vs. 134 ± 9, $P < .05$). Steroid treatment was discontinued in two patients and significantly reduced in one patient throughout the study period.

The antigen-specific effect of oral immune regulation on IFN-γ spot-forming cells (SFC) was determined using a CEP-specific ELISPOT assay. In five patients, positive T cell clones were detected prior to oral protein administration. In all five, a significant decrease in the number of IFN-positive SFC was noted. Administration of the study drug induced a significant increase in the $CD4^+/CD8^+$ lymphocyte ratio in 7 of 10 subjects. The peripheral NKT cell number increased significantly in 5 of 10 subjects (FIG. 4). An increase in IL-4 and IL-10 serum cytokine levels was observed in 7 of 10 subjects during the treatment period. Treatment was well tolerated by all patients and no major treatment-related adverse reactions were noted.

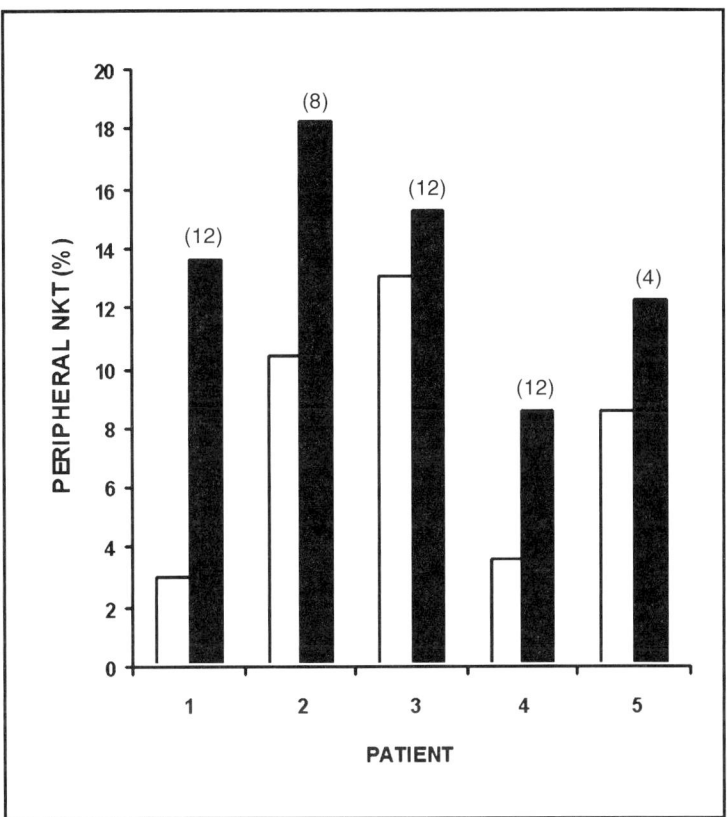

FIGURE 4. Peripheral NKT lymphocyte percent in 5 of 10 patients in whom a significant increase was observed during treatment. Baseline percent (*open bars*) as compared with maximal percent (*black bars*). Number of weeks of treatment shown in parenthesis above each bar.

The results of this preliminary study suggest that induction of oral immune regulation via oral administration of an autologous colon-specific protein-containing extract is a safe and possibly effective treatment for subjects with CD.[25] This mode of treatment could potentially enable long-term disease alleviation, while leaving the general immunological defense of the recipient intact. Antigen-specific oral immune regulation is unlikely to have unwanted long-term effects in other systems. Two explanations may elucidate these results, the first being the principle of induction of immune tolerization. Oral immune regulation may have altered the immune deviation, thereby removing a deleterious T cell population (such as those that secrete IFN-γ), thus uncovering a more efficacious subdominant response (secreting anti-inflammatory cytokines such as IL-4 and IL-10). The second possible explanation is induction of immunity. Oral immune regulation may have enhanced the effect of a beneficial subset of T cells toward the fed antigens in these patients, or of a regulatory subtype of T lymphocytes that reintroduce the required immunological balance in this setting. Correction of an immunological dysbalance can lead to an enhanced effect on the part of T cell subtypes, rather than a clearance or irreversible suppression of "unwanted" T cells. It is possible that simultaneous downregulation of one subset of T cells and augmentation of another occurs. During the follow-up period, 5 of 10 patients experienced a relapse of their symptoms. This loss of effect may suggest that long-term treatment involving continuous/constant exposure of the disease-associated antigens is required in these settings.

ORAL IMMUNE REGULATION TOWARD VIRAL PROTEINS

Employment of oral immune regulation to manipulate the host immune response to infectious agents in general—and viruses in particular—is a novel, exciting field of research. Both tolerance induction and enhancement of the immune response may be the object of such interventions. Induction of tolerance toward viruses may be desirable when the antiviral immune response entails substantial damage to the host. The basis for development of inadequate immunity, thus leading to chronic viral infections, is not known, and may be related to viral or host factors. These include mechanisms of evading the host's immune system, such as high mutation rate in HIV and hepatitis C virus (HCV), and establishment of latent infection in sites that are inaccessible to the immune system. In other cases, viral-related factors actively suppress the immune response. In view of the intricate involvement of immune mechanisms in several critical aspects of the pathogenesis and natural course of these infections—including viral persistence, destruction of infected cells, and control of viral replication—they present logical targets for active, specific immunotherapy.[4]

Tolerance Induction toward Adenoviruses

Recombinant adenoviruses are highly efficient vectors for gene therapy. However, host immune responses limit duration of viral expression and prevent transgene expression after reinjection of the virus.[26] Several strategies have been employed to induce immune hyporesponsiveness to adenoviral vectors, including injection into newborn Gunn rats, intrathymic inoculation of viral proteins, transient immunosuppression with FK-506, and expression of the adenoviral E3 gene.[27–30] Oral immune regulation toward viral proteins enabled induction of antiviral tolerance in a simpler and more effective way.[31,32] In Gunn rats fed with viral proteins, serum bilirubin levels were markedly reduced for a longer time following injection of an adenoviral vector containing the missing gene, and reinduction of the hypobilirubinemic effect was seen after rechallenge. Orally tolerized animals demonstrated markedly reduced antiadenoviral humoral and cellular immunity, and increased TGF-β1, IL-4, and IL-10, while decreasing IFN-γ production by lymphocytes upon exposure to adenoviral antigens. Tolerance induction was also feasible in the presence of preexisting antiviral immunity.[32]

Pathogenesis of Chronic Hepatitis B Virus Infection

Chronic hepatitis B virus (HBV) infection, affecting approximately five percent of the world's population, is a significant predisposing factor for the development of liver cirrhosis and hepatocellular carcinoma. Results of experimental infection in cultured hepatocytes, and the presence of asymptomatic carriers of the virus, indicate that the virus itself is noncytopathic, and suggest that the antiviral immune response may be accountable for both viral clearance and the severity of hepatitis.[33,34] Chronic HBV-associated liver inflammation is a result of a dysbalance between several types of immune responses. Both quantitative and qualitative differences may be held accountable for these differences among patients.[33] Following HBV infection, the majority of patients develop an effective antiviral response that leads to viral clearance and long-lasting antiviral immunity.[34,35] Upon recognition of viral peptides on MHC class I molecules of HBV-infected cells, $CD8^+$ T cells either cure HBV-infected cells via a noncytopathic cytokine-mediated inhibition of HBV replication, or destroy them via perforin-Fas ligand and TNF-α–mediated death pathways.[35] In contrast, the HBV-specific immune response is weak in chronically infected patients. In these patients, the immune response, being predominantly of Th2 type, fails to clear the virus and continues to be directed at the infected hepatocytes, thus leading to chronic liver disease.[35,36] High viral load, replication and mutation rates, infection of immunologically privileged sites, and viral immunosuppressive effects (including inhibition of antigen presentation) are some possible virus-associated mechanisms for chronic HBV infection. Host-related factors include induction of peripheral tolerance, exhaustion of the T cell response, immunosuppression of various causes, a variable baseline Th1/Th2 tone, ineffective antigen presentation, inefficient antigen processing, lack of costimulation, or defective cellular responsiveness to activating signals.[34]

Some HBV-infected patients who do not clear the virus may become "healthy" virus carriers. These patients are immunologically tolerant to the virus and may have normal liver histology despite chronic viremia.[33] In transgenic mice, several viral antigens have been shown to be potential tolerogens, leading to generation of antigen-specific suppressor T cell populations. In human neonates infected with HBV perinatally, tolerance is mediated by deletion of HBV-specific T cell clones.[37] In a recent study, we demonstrated that in a murine model oral administration of low doses of HBV antigens induces peripheral immune tolerance and downregulates preexisting anti-HBV immunity.[38] Oral immune regulation also led to downregulation of the anti-HBV cellular immune response, as demonstrated by decreased anti–HBV-specific IFN-γ spot-forming clones and HBV-specific T cell proliferation assays.

ORAL IMMUNE REGULATION TOWARD HBV ANTIGENS IN PATIENTS WITH CHRONIC HBV INFECTION

Various strategies have been employed in attempts to augment the anti-HBV response in humans, including administration of antiviral drugs such as interferon alpha and lamivudine, and immunization with therapeutic vaccines. These approaches have been only partially successful.[39] The aim of a recent study was to determine the safety and efficacy of oral administration of HBV envelope proteins to chronic HBV patients.[40]

Patients and Methods

One group of 42 patients, 27 males and 15 females, with a mean age of 56.5 years (range 22 to 72), was followed in an open-label, nonrandomized, single-center, prospective trial. Eligible participants were chronic HBV patients, positive for HBV DNA for at least three months, with a diagnosis of chronic active HBV infection based on liver biopsy. Both HbeAg- and anti-Hbe–positive patients were enrolled. Patients were fed with recombinant HBsAg+preS1+preS2 (BioHep B, BTG, Israel), every other day for 20 ($n = 20$) or 30 ($n = 22$) weeks. All patients were followed for clinical, biochemical, virological, and histological parameters.

Results

Normalization of liver enzymes occurred in 16 of 20 patients with elevated liver enzymes (80%). Two patterns of response were noted in responders: In 11 of 16 patients, a gradual decrease in enzymes beginning 2 to 4 weeks following the feeding was noted. In 5 of 16 additional patients, normalization of liver enzymes followed a transient increase in liver enzymes. In 13 of 16 of the responders (81.2%) enzymes

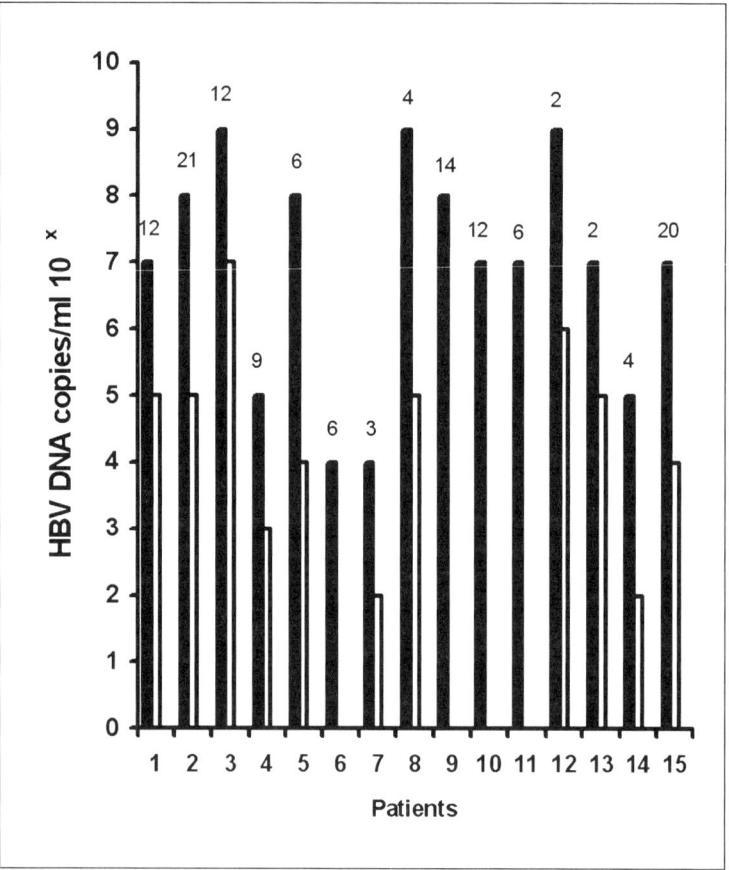

FIGURE 5. Effect of oral immune regulation toward HBV proteins on HBV DNA viral load before (*black bars*) and during (*white bars*) treatment in 15 of 42 patients. Numbers above bars represent week of maximal response.

remained normal throughout the follow-up period. Decrease in HBV DNA levels by two logs or more for two consecutive measurements occurred in 15 of 42 patients during the feeding period (35.7%, FIG. 5). In 9 of the responders, HBV DNA levels turned negative by hybridization (HBV DNA < 10^5 copies/mL). In 9 patients, a gradual decrease in HBV DNA levels was observed beginning from 2 to 8 weeks following feeding. In 8 of the responders, HBV DNA levels remained low throughout the follow-up period (53.3%). HBeAg was positive in 19 patients before the trial. Five HBeAg-positive patients turned HBeAg-negative (26%). Four of these developed anti-HBe antibodies. Improvement in the HAI histological score with a decrease of two or more points occurred in 12 of 40 patients (30%). Improvement in liver HBsAg score by more than one point was achieved in 16 of 39 (41.0%) patients, and improvement in liver HBcAg score by more than one point was achieved in 16 of 28 (57.1%) patients.

A favorable augmentation of the number of IFN-γ spot-forming colonies (SFC) was observed in 17 of 27 patients (62.9%). A decrease in the number of IL-10 SFC was observed in 13 of 27 patients (48.1%). An increase in HBV T cell stimulation index was observed in 21 of 27 (78.0%) of the treated patients. Peripheral NKT lymphocyte numbers increased twofold or more in all patients. The beneficial effect in some of the patients was dependent on continuous antigen administration. Following cessation of feeding, HBV DNA levels remained low in only half of the responders. The antiviral T cell response (IFN-γ ELISPOT and T cell proliferation studies) was lost in 30 to 70% of responders. Interestingly, IL-10 SPC number remained low throughout the follow-up period in all responders. Treatment was well tolerated by all patients. All patients completed the study, and no major adverse reactions in liver function or HBV measures were noted. No adverse effects were observed with regard to any other organs that were followed.[40]

The results of this preliminary uncontrolled study demonstrate that induction of oral immune regulation toward HBV antigens via oral administration of HBV envelope proteins alleviated immune-mediated liver damage, while enhancing effective antiviral immunity. The antiviral effect achieved in these patients was mediated via augmentation of an anti-HBV Th1 (IFN-γ)-mediated response along with a decrease in the Th2 (IL-10) response. These data support the concept that viral load is associated with a defective immune response, and that HBV replication is dependent on the antiviral immune status of the patient. Oral immune regulation may have altered the immune deviation, thus removing a deleterious T cell population (IL-10 producing) and, in so doing, uncovering a more efficacious response (IFN-γ producing). It is also possible that downregulation of viral growth occurred via both augmentation of an effective antiviral immunity and/or suppression of a proviral response. Similar approaches were recently described toward *Schistosoma mansoni* infection, in which the immune response to parasite eggs in the intestine and liver is responsible for the disease.[2]

FUTURE CLINICAL APPLICATION OF ORAL IMMUNE REGULATION

There is no obvious relationship between an immune response to antigens and what we see as "beneficial" or "protective" for the host. Inherent in this concept is the understanding that pathology is not essential for the development of a protective response. It is not always possible to separate pathology from protection, and to determine the role of different antigens and/or subsets of T cells in the induction of each type of response. It is critically important to have a thorough understanding of both pathogen-related and immune-mediated damage when immune modulation is considered. Oral immune regulation toward infectious pathogens is a promising tool for amelioration of immune-mediated injuries induced by infectious agents. It is a relatively simple antigen-directed mode of immune manipulation that allows for long-term alleviation of the disease, thus leaving the general immunological defense of the recipient intact. The potential of this novel method to simultaneously induce both tolerance and enhancement of antigen-specific immune responses that are beneficial to the host—as suggested by the preliminary results of the HBV trial—is beginning to be realized.

The following are the current limitations for use of this method in humans: (1) not knowing the disease target antigen, which may not necessarily be identical in all patients; (2) the possibility of inducing exacerbation of immune response in the bowel or of immune-mediated extraintestinal manifestation; (3) inability to predict which type of immune response (tolerance or augmentation) will develop; (4) defining attainable goals and issues of safety and applicability in humans; and (5) lack of success of prior human trials of oral tolerance.

The aims of ongoing trials using oral immune regulation are to test the role of different subsets of systemic and intrahepatic lymphocytes in oral immune modulation. Requirements for antigen presentation and costimulation, as well as cytokine milieu and roots of antigen processing, are being studied. The role of subsets of lymphocytes and their effects on antibody responses and on CTLs are being assessed. These trials hold promise for enabling use of this method in humans with immune-mediated disorders.

ACKNOWLEDGMENTS

This work was supported by grants from the Israel Academy of Sciences, the Roaman-Epstein Liver Research Foundation, and ENZO Biochem Inc. NY.

REFERENCES

1. WEINER, H.L. 2001. Oral tolerance: Immune mechanisms and generation of Th3-type TGF beta secreting regulatory cells. Microbes Infect. **3:** 947–954.
2. MCSORLEY, S.J. & P. GARSIDE. 1999. Vaccination by inducing oral tolerance. Immunol. Today **20:** 555–560.
3. STROBER, W., B. KELSALL, L. FUSS, *et al.* 1997. Reciprocal IFN-γ and TGF-β responses regulate the occurrence of mucosal inflammation. Immunol. Today **18:** 61–64.
4. ILAN, Y. 2002. Immune downregulation leads to upregulation of an anti-viral response: Lesson from the hepatitis B virus. Microbes Infect. **4:** 1317–1326.
5. PODOLSKY, D.K. 2002. Inflammatory bowel disease. N. Engl. J. Med. **347:** 417–429.
6. STROBER, W. & M.F. NOURISH. 1995. Immunological diseases of the gastrointestinal tract. *In* Clinical Immunology: Principles and Practice. R.R. Rich *et al.*, Eds.: 1401–1428. C.V. Mosby. St. Louis, MO.
7. MIZOGUCHI, A., E. MIZOGUCHI, C. CHIBA, *et al.* 1996. Cytokine imbalance and autoantibody production in T cell receptor-α mutant mice with inflammatory bowel disease. J. Exp. Med. **183:** 847–856.

8. NEURATH, M.F., I. FUSS, B.L. KELSALL, et al. 1995. Antibodies to IL12 abrogate established experimental colitis in mice. J. Exp. Med. **182:** 1281–1290.
9. SANDBORN, W.J. & S.R. TARGAN. 2002. Biologic therapy of inflammatory bowel disease Gastroenterology **122:** 1592–1608.
10. NEURATH, M., B.L. KELSALL, D.H. PRESKY, et al. 1996. Experimental granulomatous colitis in mice is abrogated by induction of TGF-β-mediated oral tolerance. J. Exp. Med. **183:** 2605–2616.
11. GALLIAERDE, V., C. DESVIGNES, E. PEYRON & D. KAISERLIAN. 1995. Oral tolerance to haptens: intestinal epithelial cells from 2,4-dinitrochlorobenzene-fed mice inhibit hapten-specific T-cell activation in vitro. Eur. J. Immunol. **25:** 1385–1390.
12. ILAN, Y., S. WEKSLER-ZANGEN, S. BEN-HORIN, et al. 2000. Treatment of experimental colitis by oral tolerance induction: A central role for suppressor lymphocytes. Am. J. Gastroenterol. **95:** 966–973.
13. DASGUPTA, A., K. RAMASWAMY, J. GIRALDO, et al. 2001. Colon epithelial cellular protein induces oral tolerance in the experimental model of colitis by trinitrobenzene sulfonic acid. J. Lab. Clin. Med. **138:** 257–269.
14. DASGUPTA, A., K.V. KESARI, K.K. RAMASWAMY, et al. 2001. Oral administration of unmodified colonic but not small intestinal antigens protects rats from hapten-induced colitis. Clin. Exp. Immunol. **125:** 41–47.
15. GOTSMAN, I., A. SHLOMAI, R. ALPER, et al. 2001. Amelioration of immune-mediated experimental colitis: Tolerance induction in the presence of pre-existing immunity and surrogate antigen bystander effect. J. Pharmacol. Exp. Ther. **297:** 926–932.
16. SHLOMAI, A., A. TROP, I. GOTSMAN, et al. 2001. Immunemodulation of experimental colitis: The role of NK1.1+ liver lymphocytes and surrogate antigen-bystander effect. J. Pathol. **195:** 498–507.
17. KOLKER, O., A. KLEIN, R. ALPER, et al. 2003. Early expression of interferon gamma following oral antigen administration is associated with peripheral tolerance induction. Microbes Infect. **5:** 807–813.
18. CRISPE, N. & W.Z. MEHAL. 1996. Strange brew: T cells in the liver. Immun. Today **11:** 236–245.
19. CALLERY, M.P., T. KAMEI & W. FLYE. 1989. The effect of portocaval shunt on delayed-hypersensitivity responses following antigen feeding. J. Surg. Res. **46:** 391–394.
20. GODFREY, D.J., K.J. HAMMOND, L.D. POULON, et al. 2000. NKT cells: facts, functions and fallacies. Immunol. Today **21:** 573–583.
21. TROP, S., D. SAMSONOV, I. GOTSMAN, et al. 1999. Liver-associated lymphocytes expressing NK1.1 are essential for oral tolerance induction in a murine model. Hepatology **29:** 746–755.
22. SAMSONOV, D., S. TROP, R. ALPER, et al. 2000. Enhancement of immune tolerance via induction of NK1.1 positive liver-associated-lymphocytes under immunosuppressive conditions in a murine model. J. Hepatol. **32:** 812–820.
23. TROP, S. & Y. ILAN. 2002. NK 1.1+ T cell: A two-faced lymphocyte in immune modulation of the IL4/IFNγ paradigm. J. Clin. Immunol. **22:** 270–280.
24. TROP, S., A. NAGLER & Y. ILAN. 2003. Role of NK1.1+ and AsGm-1+ cells in oral immune-regulation of experimental colitis. Inflamm. Bowel Dis. **9:** 75–86.
25. ISRAELI, E., E. GOLDIN, N. HEMED, et al. 2003. Oral immune rgulation using colitis extracted proteins—A new mode of treatment for Crohn's disease: Results of a phase I clinical trial. Gastroenterology **124:** 518A.
26. ILAN, Y., H. SAITO, N.R. THUMMALA & N.R. CHOWDHURY. 1999. Adenovirus-mediated gene therapy of liver diseases. Semin. Liver Dis. **19:** 49–59.
27. TAKAHASHI, M., Y. ILAN, K. SENGUPTA, et al. 1996. Induction of tolerance to recombinant adenoviruses by injection into newborn rats: Long-term amelioration of hyperbilirubinemia in Gunn rats. J. Biol. Chem. **271:** 26536–26542.
28. ILAN, Y., P. ATTAVAR, M. TAKAHASHI, et al. 1996. Induction of central tolerance by intrathymic inoculation of adenoviral antigens into the host thymus permits long-term gene therapy in Gunn rats. J. Clin. Invest. **98:** 2640–2647.
29. ILAN, Y., V.K. JONA, K. SENGUPTA, et al. 1997. Transient immunosuppression with FK506 permits long-term expression of therapeutic genes introduced into the liver using recombinant adenoviruses. Hepatology **26:** 949–956.

30. ILAN, Y., G. DROGUETT, N.R. CHOWDHURY, *et al.* 1997. Insertion of the adenoviral E3 region into a recombinant viral vector prevents anti-viral humoral and cellular immune responses and permits long-term gene expression. Proc. Nat. Acad. Sci. USA **94:** 2587–2592.
31. ILAN, Y., R. PRAKASH, A. DAVIDSON, *et al.* 1997. Oral tolerization to adenoviral antigens permits long-term gene expression using recombinant adenoviral vectors. J. Clin. Invest. **99:** 1098–1106.
32. ILAN, Y., B. SAUTER, N.R. CHOWDHURY, *et al.* 1998. Oral tolerization to adenoviral proteins permits repeated adenovirus-mediated gene therapy in rats with pre-existing immunity to adenovirus. Hepatology **27:** 1368–1376.
33. ILAN, Y. & J.R. CHOWDHURY. 1999. Induction of oral tolerance towards hepatitis B virus: can we eat the disease and live with the virus? Med. Hypotheses **52:** 505–509.
34. CHISARI, F.V. & C. FERRARI. 1995. Hepatitis B virus immunopathogenesis. Annu. Rev. Immunol. **13:** 29–45.
35. REHERMANN, B. 2000. Intrahepatic T cells in hepatitis B: viral controls versus liver cell injury. J. Exp. Med. **191:** 1263–1268.
36. GUIDOTTI, L.G. & F.V. CHISARI. 2000. Cytokine-mediated control of viral infections. Virology **273:** 221–227.
37. KUROSE, K., S.M. AKBAR, K. YAMAMOTO & M. ONJI. 1997. Production of antibody to hepatitis B surface antigen by murine hepatitis B virus carriers: neonatal tolerance versus antigen presentation by dendritic cells. Immunology **92:** 494–500.
38. GOTSMAN, I., R. BEINART, R. ALPER, *et al.* 2000. Induction of oral tolerance towards hepatitis B envelope antigens in a murine model. Antiviral Res. **48:** 17–26.
39. HOOFNAGLE, J.H. & A.M. DI BISCEGLIE. 1997. The treatment of chronic viral hepatitis. N. Eng. J. Med. **325:** 347–356.
40. SAFADI, R., E. ISRAELI, O. PAPO, *et al.* 2003 Treatment of chronic HBV infection via oral immune regulation towards hepatitis B virus proteins. Am. J. Gastroenterol. **98:** 2505–2515.

Oral Tolerance in Humans

Failure to Suppress an Existing Immune Response by Oral Antigen Administration

ZINA MOLDOVEANU, FRED OLIVER, JIRI MESTECKY, AND CHARLES O. ELSON

Departments of Medicine and Microbiology, University of Alabama at Birmingham, Birmingham, Alabama 35294, USA

ABSTRACT: Orally administered antigens can induce systemic tolerance. In animal models, oral tolerance can both prevent and treat experimental autoimmune diseases. The induction of oral tolerance to human autoantigens has been envisioned as a potential treatment for human autoimmune conditions. The results of previous human studies from our laboratory have provided evidence that oral administration of a model antigen, keyhole limpet hemocyanin (KLH), prior to systemic immunization, can decrease the magnitude of subsequent T cell proliferative and skin test responses to KLH. The present study was designed to test the hypothesis that orally administered KLH could attenuate a preexisting immune response to KLH. Thus, human subjects ($n = 8$) were primed subcutaneously with KLH without adjuvant prior to a 42-day feeding regimen of 100 mg of KLH per day. At the end of the feeding regimen, the subjects were boosted with KLH, again without adjuvant. Eight control subjects were immunized as above with KLH, but fed ovalbumin. The measurement of antigen-driven T cell proliferation, serum and salivary antibody, and dermal delayed hypersensitivity responses to KLH failed to reveal significant differences between subjects fed KLH and those fed ovalbumin. These results indicate that the KLH dose and feeding regimen used in this study failed to attenuate the primary response or to prevent the secondary response to KLH. Therefore, some form of immunomodulation greater than that provided by oral administration of antigen alone is required in humans for suppression of an existing immune response.

KEYWORDS: tolerance; antigen feeding; humans; T cell; antibody

INTRODUCTION

Mucosal tolerance is defined by a marked reduction in systemic immune responses to an antigen previously administered by the mucosal route. This phenomenon

Address for correspondence: Charles O. Elson, M.D., Division of Gastroenterology and Hepatology, The University of Alabama at Birmingham, 633 Ziegler Research Building, 703 S. 19th Street, Birmingham, AL 35294-0407. Voice: 205-934-6060; fax: 205-934-8493.
coelson@uab.edu

was demonstrated by Chase in animals fed a contact sensitizing agent and later challenged systemically with the same antigen.[1] Since this pioneering work, many subsequent studies have been performed in animals using a broad spectrum of soluble (e.g., ovalbumin, bovine gammaglobulin, human gammaglobulin) or particulate (e.g., sheep erythrocytes) antigens.[2] Furthermore, in animal models of autoimmune diseases such as allergic autoimmune encephalomyelitis, collagen type 2–induced arthritis, uveitis, and diabetes mellitus, initial feeding of the autoantigen has prevented disease otherwise induced by systemic immunization with the relevant antigen in adjuvant.[2] Compared with the large number of experiments performed in animals, basic studies in humans are quite limited. Evidence for the existence of mucosal tolerance in humans was provided in our previous study, in which we administered keyhole limpet hemocyanin (KLH) antigen for 10 days either orally[3] or intranasally.[4] Upon subsequent systemic challenge, cellular immune responses were inhibited, as manifested by decreased T cell proliferation and decreased delayed-type hypersensitivity skin test responses to KLH. In contrast, antibody responses were increased rather than inhibited, with increased levels of KLH-specific antibodies in serum and external secretions, and increased numbers of specific antibody-secreting cells in peripheral blood.

We next examined the immunologic effects of long-term feeding of antigen. For this we used dietary antigen as a surrogate for what might happen if one fed protein antigens long term. To this end, immune responses to the common dietary antigens bovine gammaglobulin (BGG), ovalbumin (OVA), and soybean protein were evaluated in 50 normal human volunteers. Humoral and T cell responses to these antigens were measurable but low, consistent with immune tolerance.[5] T cell proliferation to dietary antigens was increased significantly by addition of low doses of recombinant human interleukin-2. Peripheral blood mononuclear cells stimulated with BGG or OVA expressed IL-2 receptor α chain, but not IL-2 mRNA, consistent with T cell anergy. In some individuals, T cell proliferation to an unrelated vaccine antigen (tetanus toxoid or purified protein derivative) was suppressed by addition of BGG or OVA, but this inhibition could be reversed with low doses of rIL-2. The conclusion of these studies was that the major mechanism of tolerance to chronic antigen feeding in humans is anergy. We did not find evidence of regulatory T cells or active suppression mediated by inhibitory cytokines such as IL-10 or TGFβ.

A number of attempts have been made in humans to use mucosal tolerance in the treatment of human autoimmune disease, with little success to date, as is detailed elsewhere in this volume. Despite this, mucosal tolerance is attractive as a therapeutic modality if it can be translated to humans with autoimmune or chronic inflammatory diseases. However, it remains unknown whether antigen feeding can inhibit a preexisting immune response in humans, which is a requirement for an effective therapy in patients who are already sensitized at the time of diagnosis. It is known in animals that oral tolerance is most effective when the antigen is fed to naive animals prior to systemic immunization. In experimental models of autoimmune disease, antigen feeding in the setting of a preexisting immune response has been much less effective. In the studies reported here, we addressed this question by feeding either KLH or OVA as a control antigen for six weeks to human volunteers who had been primed with a small dose of KLH prior to the antigen feeding.

MATERIALS AND METHODS

Human Subjects and Study Protocol

Sixteen human volunteers (8 males and 8 females), ranging from 22 to 46 years of age, were recruited for this study. The study protocol was approved by the UAB Institutional Review Board, and informed consent form was obtained from all subjects. The volunteers were immunized intramuscularly (i.m.) with 100 µg of endotoxin-free KLH (Pacific Biomarine, Venice, CA) without adjuvant. The antigen-feeding protocol, which consisted of a daily ingestion of 100 mg of either KLH (Calbiochem, La Jolla, CA) or chicken ovalbumin (OVA; Sigma, St. Louis, MO) in gelatin capsules on an empty stomach, commenced on day 7 and ended on day 49. On day 56, all subjects were systemically boosted with 100 µg of endotoxin-free KLH. Delayed-type hypersensitivity (DTH) skin test reactions were measured after intradermal (i.d.) injection of 10 µg of KLH on days 49 and 63. Peripheral blood and saliva samples were collected at the beginning of the study, and on days 7, 28, 49, and 63 thereafter. Peripheral blood was collected by venipuncture with heparin for isolation of cells, or without anticoagulants to obtain serum. Unstimulated parotid saliva was collected with the use of plastic Schaefer cups placed over the opening of the duct of the parotid gland.[6] After collection, samples were centrifuged and the supernatants aliquoted and frozen at $-70\,°C$ until assay.

Measurement of Antigen-Specific T Cell Proliferation

T cells were isolated from peripheral blood mononuclear cell fraction (PBMC, obtained by Ficoll-Hypaque gradient centrifugation) by rosetting with 2-aminoethyl-isothiouronium bromide-treated sheep red blood cells.[7] The nonrosetting cells were irradiated (3000 R) and used as antigen-presenting cells (APC). A mixture of 2×10^5 T cells and 5×10^4 APC suspended in RPMI 1640 supplemented with 5% human AB serum were plated in each well of a 96-well flat bottom plate (Costar, Cambridge, MA). After the addition of 100 µg/mL of antigen (KLH or OVA), the cells were cultured for five days at 37°C, and 5% CO_2. On the fifth day, 0.1 µCi ^{3}H-thymidine was added to each well and the incubation was continued for an additional six hours. Cells were then harvested and T cell proliferation was measured by ^{3}H-thymidine incorporation with a liquid scintillation counter (Beckman, Fullerton, CA).

Measurement of Cytokine Secretion

Isolated T cells were cultured in the presence of irradiated APC at 37°C in a 5% CO_2 for 24 h in complete medium (RPMI 1640 supplemented with 10% fetal calf serum (FCS), 1.5 mM L-glutamine, 50 µM 2-mercaptoethanol, 100 U/mL penicillin, and 100 µg/mL streptomycin) in the presence or absence of 10 µg/mL KLH or OVA. The supernatants were collected after 24 or 72 h and assayed for levels of IFN-γ, IL-4, IL-10, and TGF-β by ELISA (R& D Systems, Minneapolis, MN).

Measurement of Skin Delayed-Type Hypersensitivity Responses

The diameter of induration and erythema was measured 24 h after the volunteers were challenged intradermally with 10 µg of KLH on days 7, 49, and 63.

Measurement of B Cell Responses by ELISPOT Assay

The number of KLH- and OVA-specific as well as total antibody-secreting cells (ASC) was determined by enzyme-linked immunospot assay (ELISPOT), as described by Czerkinsky[8] and previously used by our group for a similar study.[3] Because of the high degree of variability among the volunteers in the number of ASC per 10^6 PBMC, we expressed the KLH- or OVA-specific ASC as percentage of total isotype.

Measurement of Antibody Responses in Serum and Secretions

Antibodies were measured by ELISA as previously described.[5] Quantitation of specific and total levels of antibodies was accomplished by ELISA. Ninety-six-well polystyrene plates (Nalge Nunc International, Roskilde, Denmark) were coated with the same concentrations of antigens or antibodies as those used for ELISPOT assay. Serial dilutions of samples or standards (100 µL /well) were added to plates blocked with 5% heat-inactivated FCS in PBS-Tween 20 and then incubated overnight at 4°C. The standards consisted of a pool of human sera calibrated against WHO standards (Moni-Trol, Dade International, Miami, FL) and, for saliva, of purified colostral S-IgA prepared in our laboratory. The same biotin-labeled reagents as those used for the ELISPOT assay were added to the plates and incubated for three hours at 37°C. After another hour, incubation with ExtrAvidin peroxidase-conjugate (Sigma), the peroxidase substrate, O-phenylenediamine-H_2O_2 (Sigma), was added, and the color reaction was stopped with 1 M sulfuric acid. The absorbance was measured in an EL312 Bio-Kinetics microplate reader (Bio-Tek Instruments Inc., Winooski, VT) at 490 nm. The results were calculated by interpolation of optical densities on calibration curves constructed using the Delta Soft 3 computer program. Antigen-specific and total immunoglobulin levels were calculated by interpolating the optical densities on calibration curves, as previously described[9] using the DeltaSoft 3 program (BioMettalics, Inc., Princeton, NJ).

Statistical Analysis

Data are expressed using descriptive statistics such as mean and standard deviation. A nonparametric two-tailed test (Wilcoxon or Mann-Whitney) was employed to determine the significance between the two groups, and a paired t test was used to test the significance in the same group at different times.

RESULTS

Antigen-Specific T Cell Proliferation

The effect of prolonged KLH or OVA ingestion on the KLH-specific T cell responses of the intramuscularly KLH-primed individuals was tested by an *in vitro* proliferation assay. T cell proliferation of KLH-fed volunteers increased during the feeding and particularly 1 week after the systemic boost at day 56. Importantly, no significant differences were detected between the group of volunteers fed KLH or those fed OVA (FIG. 1). The OVA-specific T cell proliferation was modest, and even in the OVA-fed group, there was very little increase over the baseline values.

DTH Responses

Skin testing was used to determine whether the DTH mediated by KLH-sensitized CD4 T lymphocytes could be abolished or diminished by KLH feeding. As shown in TABLE 1, the prolonged ingestion of large amounts of KLH by KLH-primed

TABLE 1. Skin test responses to KLH

Volunteers Ingesting:	Day 8[a]	Day 50[a]	Day 64[a]
KLH	2.0 (0–5)	10 (0–40)	17 (0–60)
OVA	1.3 (0–3)	15 (10–30)	14.5 (1–30)

[a]None of the differences were statistically significant. Data represent mean and range (in parentheses) of induration diameter expressed in millimeters.

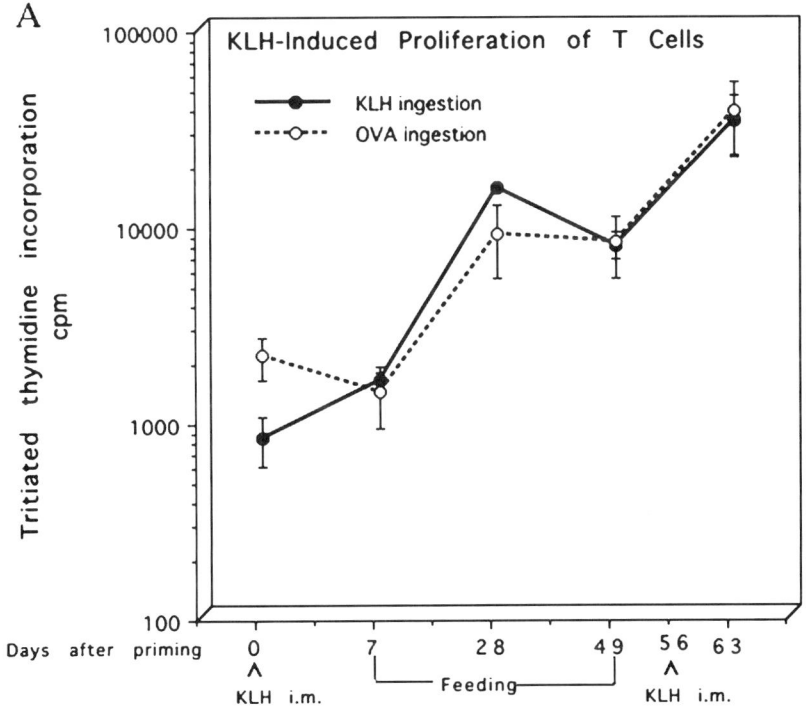

FIGURE 1. Antigen-induced proliferation of T cells isolated from peripheral blood of volunteers before and after systemic priming with KLH, after ingestion of either KLH ($n = 8$ individuals) or OVA ($n = 8$ subjects), and following intramuscular challenge with KLH. Proliferative responses to KLH (**A**) and OVA (**B**) were measured by ^{3}H-thymidine incorporation and expressed as mean Δ cpm (stimulated–unstimulated) ($\pm$ SD).

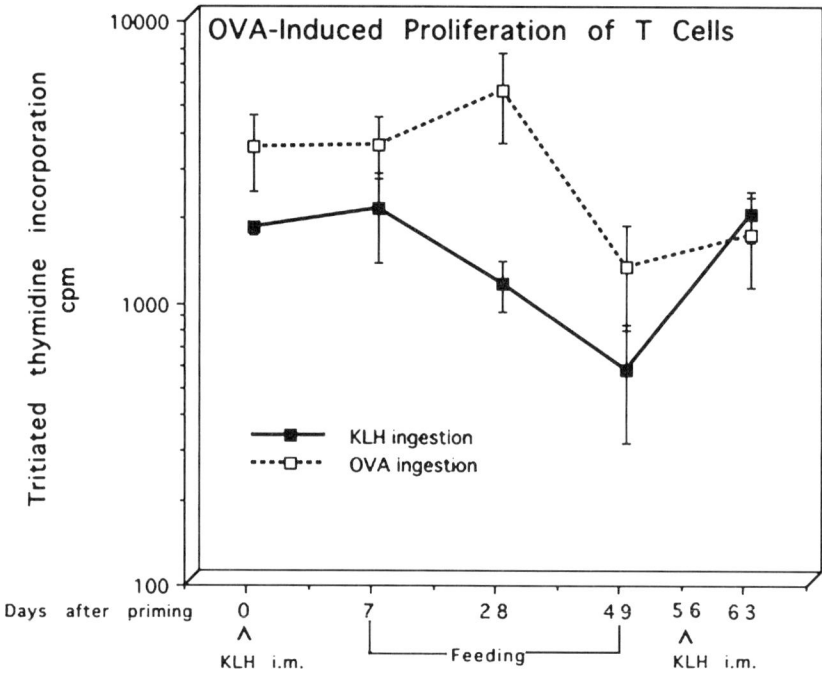

FIGURE 1 — *continued.*

individuals did not affect their DTH reactions. These data complement the antigen-stimulated T cell proliferation data, and demonstrate that oral tolerance, manifested as reduced T cell responsiveness, was not induced on the background of a preexisting systemic response.

Secretion of Cytokines by T Cells after in Vitro *Stimulation with Antigen*

Cells isolated from the peripheral blood of volunteers after the systemic challenge were cultured with KLH, OVA, or the mitogen ConA (as a control), and cytokines (see Methods) secreted in culture supernatants were measured. An increase in secreted IL-2 was detected after KLH stimulation of cells; however, the difference between the KLH- and OVA-fed volunteers was not statistically significant. Likewise, IFN-γ, TGF-β, and IL-4 secretion were not significantly different between the two groups. A small increase in secreted IL-10 was measured in KLH-stimulated cells isolated from KLH-fed volunteers, but it was not statistically significant (data not shown).

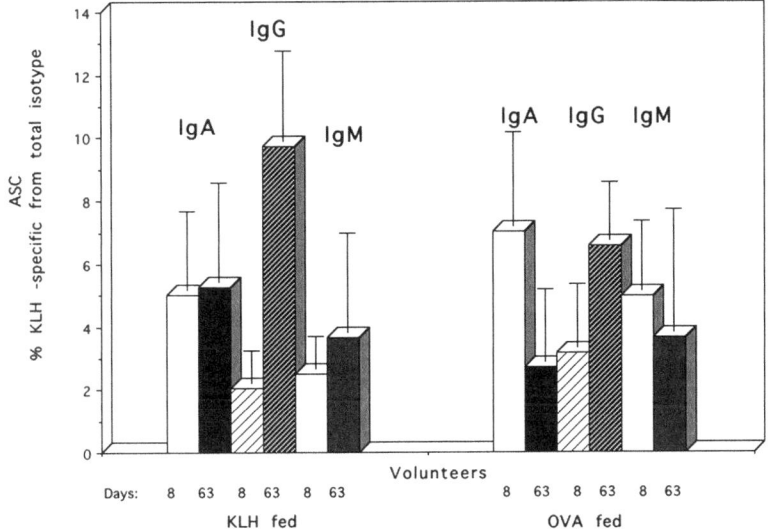

FIGURE 2. ELISPOT assay of IgA, IgG, or IgM isotypes from KLH-specific antibody-secreting cells (ASC) in peripheral blood of volunteers fed KLH or OVA, from samples taken one week after each intramuscular injection with KLH. The bars represent mean percentage of total IgA, IgG, or IgM ASC secreting anti-KLH antibodies (± SD).

Peripheral Blood ASC to KLH or OVA

The percentages of cells secreting KLH- or OVA-specific antibodies as a percentage of the total IgA, IgG, or IgM isotypes are presented in FIGURE 2. One week following the priming injection with KLH of the 16 volunteers, 1% or more of total isotype of ASC was KLH specific: IgA in 12 volunteers (more than 5% in 7 volunteers), IgM in 14 (more than 5% in 6), and IgG in 9. The response against OVA was low, not exceeding 0.14% of total IgA-, 0.23% of the IgG-, and 1.49% of IgM-secreting cells. The OVA feeding did not increase the number of peripheral blood lymphoblasts secreting anti-OVA antibodies, and the OVA-specific IgM-secreting cells were not detectable. One week after the booster challenge with KLH of volunteers fed with either KLH or OVA (day 63), the proportion of cells secreting KLH-specific antibodies was not statistically significantly different between the two groups, nor was the difference significant between the percentages measured after the booster compared with after the primary immunization (FIG. 2). After the systemic challenge, the percentage of cells secreting IgA antibodies against KLH was decreased in OVA-fed volunteers, consistent with a stimulatory effect on B cell responses, although this difference did not reach statistical significance.

Levels of KLH-Specific Antibodies in Sera and in Saliva

The measurement of antigen-specific and of total immunoglobulin isotypes indicated that systemic priming with KLH resulted in the induction of antigen-specific

A

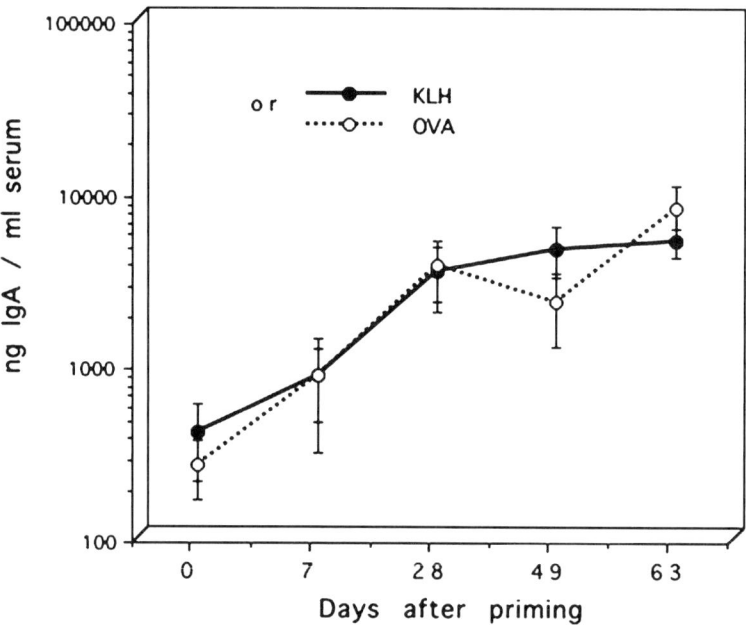

FIGURE 3. KLH-specific IgA (**A**) and IgG (**B**) antibodies in sera collected from volunteers enrolled into this study. At each time point, the values represent the mean (± SD) of the ELISA data generated from the eight volunteers in the experimental (fed KLH) or control (fed OVA) groups.

antibodies in sera of all 16 participants in this study. After feeding, KLH-specific IgA increased in sera of three out of the eight volunteers fed KLH, and decreased in the other five, as well as in all volunteers who ingested OVA capsules. The subcutaneous challenge with KLH increased the anti-KLH IgA titers in all individuals who ingested OVA and in four of the KLH-fed volunteers (FIG. 3a). IgG anti-KLH increased in all 16 volunteers (FIG. 3b). Little or no increase in IgM titers was observed in either KLH- or OVA-fed groups (data not shown). None of the changes were statistically significant. Neither feeding nor systemic injection with KLH induced statistically significant changes in salivary KLH-specific IgA.

B

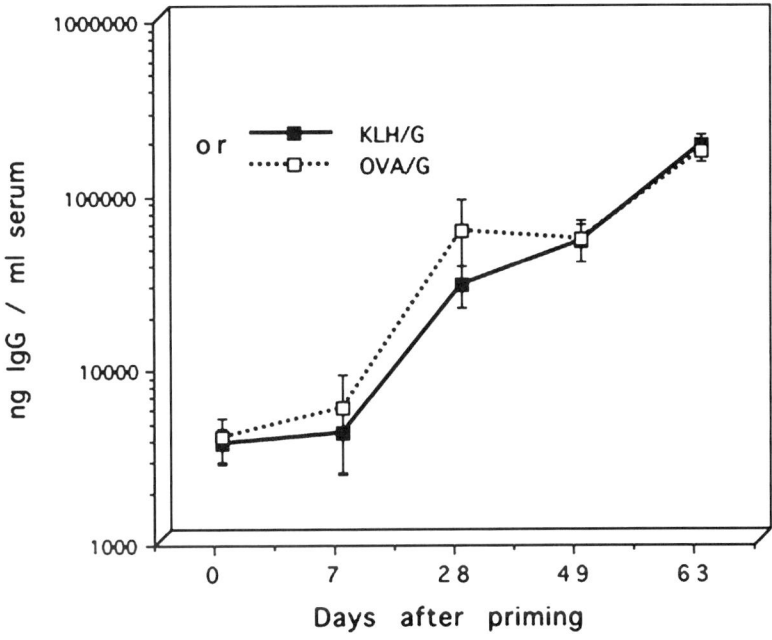

FIGURE 3 — *continued.*

DISCUSSION

These results demonstrate that extended oral administration of KLH to individuals with preexisting immunity to it failed to induce a state of tolerance, as manifested by diminished T cell proliferative responses or delayed hypersensitivity skin test responses. Both of the latter have previously been demonstrated in naive human volunteers fed KLH at similar doses. These results confirm and extend studies previously performed in animals and in humans. Chase,[1] using oral feeding, was unable to suppress cellular responses in animals previously sensitized to the antigen that was subsequently fed. Czerkinsky et al.[10] were unable to improve the clinical status or to arrest the development of collagen type 2 arthritis or autoimmune allergic encephalomyelitis by mucosal administration, either oral or nasal, to animals sensitized systemically two weeks before the mucosal antigen exposure. In humans, oral administration of extracts of poison ivy or poison oak failed to suppress cutaneous delayed-type hypersensitivity reactions in previously sensitized individuals and, for lack of efficacy, were abandoned.[11,12] As mentioned above, antigen feeding in experimental models of autoimmune disease is much more effective when antigen is given prior to systemic immunization rather than after. These results are consistent with the negative results of the multiple clinical trials, reported elsewhere in this volume, in which autoantigen feeding of patients with various diseases has failed to provide any clinical efficacy. These present data plus those of the negative clinical trials indicate that simple antigen feeding by itself is unlikely to be an effective therapeutic modality in patients.

From experiments in animals it is clear that oral tolerance is a complex phenomenon and that multiple factors influence its development, including the dose of antigen, frequency of feeding, the route of administration, the immunogenicity of the antigen, the age of the animals, and the genetic background of the individual.[2] These multiple variables make comparison of results difficult, even in rodents. There appears to be an early and a late phase of oral tolerance, and each probably has different mechanisms. Clearly, oral tolerance is not one entity, and multiple mechanisms exist, including deletion, anergy, and the induction of regulatory cells, all of which are probably operating simultaneously to varying degrees.

In contrast to the rich data in experimental animals, particularly in mice, there is a dearth of basic immunology studies on oral tolerance in humans. Most experiments performed in mice are carried out in inbred strains that are genetically uniform. These mice represent, in essence, monoclonal reagents, and results in a given strain would be equivalent to the reactivity that would be expected from a single person. Humans have very diverse responses to immunization and antigen feeding,[5] and overall their oral tolerance response appears to be less than that seen in inbred strains of mice. That may be more a reflection of the genetic diversity of humans relative to the inbred strains than anything else. It is clear that oral tolerance is an active form of immune response and not simply the absence of a response. Thus, the effective use of oral tolerance to treat human disease will require adjuvants and delivery systems, just as is required for oral immunization. Adjuvants and delivery systems that enhance oral tolerance have already been described in experimental systems.[10,13,14]

If mucosal tolerance as a therapeutic modality is to advance, where does it go from here? Clearly, the development of adjuvants and delivery systems to enhance tolerance are needed and should be a high priority. In humans, the induction of anergy to a single antigen is unlikely to be beneficial, and thus studies should target the induction of regulatory cells that are able to mediate bystander suppression. The latter has been demonstrated clearly in multiple experimental models,[15–19] although not yet demonstrated in humans. Systems are available to test for bystander suppression in humans[5] and could be applied after antigen feeding. Clearly, more studies on the mechanisms involved in humans, and, for that matter, in mice, are needed, particularly studies dissecting early versus late events. Dose is a critical variable in rodent models but has been chosen fairly arbitrarily in human trials. Dose-ranging studies on volunteers or individuals with a given disease are crucial and should be done prior to large clinical trials or antigen feeding. The notion of exploiting mucosal tolerance as a therapeutic approach to human disease remains attractive, and the initial trials attempting simple antigen feeding were worthwhile. However, the negative results are clearly telling us that the situation in humans with various diseases and preexisting immunity is quite complex, and new approaches are needed.

REFERENCES

1. CHASE, M.V. 1946. Inhibition of experimental drug allergy by prior feeding of the sensitizing agent. Proc. Soc. Exp. Biol. Med. **61:** 257–259.
2. MOWAT, A.M. & H.L. WEINER. 1999. Oral tolerance. Physiological basis and clinical applications. *In* Mucosal Immunology, 2nd edit. P.L. Ogra, J. Mestecky, M.E. Lamm, W. Strober, J. Bienenstock & J. R. McGhee, Eds.: 587–618. Academic Press. San Diego.
3. HUSBY, S., J. MESTECKY, Z. MOLDOVEANU, *et al.* 1994. Oral tolerance in humans. T cell but not B cell tolerance after antigen feeding. J. Immunol. **152:** 4663–4670.
4. WALDO, F.B., A.W.L. VAN DEN WALL BAKE, J. MESTECKY & S. HUSBY. 1994. Suppression of the immune response by nasal immunization. Clin. Immunol. Immunopathol. **72:** 30–34.
5. ZIVNY, J.H., Z. MOLDOVEANU, H.L. VU, *et al.* 2001. Mechanisms of immune tolerance to food antigens in humans. Clin. Immunol. **101:** 158–168.
6. SCHAEFER, M.E., M. RHODES, S.J. PRINCE, *et al.* 1977. A plastic intraoral device for the collection of human paratid saliva. J. Dent. Res. **56:** 728–733.
7. SAXON, A., J.FELDHAUS & R.A. ROBINS. 1976. Single step separation of human and B cells using AET treated SRBC rosettes. J. Immunol. Methods **12:** 285–288.
8. CZERKINSKY, C. 1986. Antibody secreting cells. *In* Methods of Enzymatic Analysis, Vol. 3. H.U. Bergmeyer, J. Bergmeyer & M. Grassl, Eds.: 23– 44. VCH. Weinheim.
9. RUSSELL, M.W., J. MESTECKY, B. JULIAN & J. GALLA. 1986. IgA-associated renal diseases: antibodies to environmental antigens in sera and deposition of immunoglobulins and antigens in glomeruli. J. Clin. Immunol. **6:** 74–86.
10. CZERKINSKY, C., F. ANJUERE, J.R. MCGHEE, *et al.* 1999. Mucosal immunity and tolerance: relevance to vaccine development. Immunol. Rev. **170:** 197–222.
11. STEVENS, F.A. 1945. Council on pharmacy and chemistry. Report of the council: Status of poison ivy extracts. J. Am. Med. Assoc. **127:** 912–921.
12. Klingman, A.M. 1958. Poison ivy (*Rhus*) dermatitis. Arch. Dermatol. **77:** 149–180.
13. TOMASI, M., M.T. DERTZBAUGH, T. HEARN, *et al.* 1997. Strong mucosal adjuvanticity of cholera toxin within lipid particles of a new multiple emulsion delivery system for oral immunization. Eur. J. Immunol. **127:** 2720–2725.
14. SUN, J.B., C. RASK, T. OLSSON, *et al.* 1996. Treatment of experimental autoimmune encephalomyelitis by feeding myelin basic protein conjugated to cholera toxin B subunit. Proc. Natl. Acad. Sci. USA **93:** 7196–7201.
15. AL-SABBAGH, A., A. MILLER, L.M. SANTOS & H.L. WEINER. 1994. Antigen-driven tissue-specific suppression following oral tolerance: orally administered myelin basic protein suppresses proteolipid protein-induced experimental autoimmune encephalomyelitis in the SJL mouse. Eur. J. Immunol. **24:** 2104–2109.
16. MILLER, A., O. LIDER & H.L. WEINER. 1991. Antigen-driven bystander suppression after oral administration of antigens. J. Exp. Med. **174:** 791–798.
17. THOMPSON, S.J., H.S.THOMPSON, N. HARPER, *et al.* 1993. Prevention of pristane-induced arthritis by the oral administration of type II collagen. Immunology **79:** 152–157.
18. YOSHINO S., E. QUATTROCCHI & H.L. WEINER. 1995. Suppression of antigen-induced arthritis in Lewis rats by oral administration of type II collagen. Arthritis Rheum. **38:** 1092–1096.
19. ZHANG, Z.Y., C.S. LEE, O. LIDER & H.L. WEINER. 1990. Suppression of adjuvant arthritis in Lewis rats by oral administration of type II collagen. J. Immunol. **145:** 2489–2493.

Oral Tolerance: Animal Disease Models and Human Trials

Summary of Part V

WARREN STROBER

The Mucosal Immunity Section, Laboratory of Host Defense, NIAID, National Institutes of Health, Bethesda, Maryland 20892, USA

In this segment of the conference the possible use of oral tolerance induction as a therapeutic modality in humans was the focus of discussion. While it is fair to say that the record of success of this treatment approach is, at best, mixed, there are nevertheless reasons to hope that oral administration of antigens can eventually be a useful way of controlling inflammatory diseases, and we are gradually learning how this goal can be accomplished. Weiner and his colleagues provide an in-depth review of oral tolerance and how it may be used in the therapy of patients, and our aim here is to highlight and discuss certain observations that relate to the immune mechanisms that underlie the clinical usage of this approach.

We can start our commentary with a discussion of a well-executed and provocative study by Moldoveanu and her associates that very clearly shows that oral antigen administration *after* initial immunization does not reduce a subsequent booster response to the same antigen; in other words, oral antigen administration does not influence (downregulate) an already established response and, by extension, would not influence the ongoing response to self-antigens in autoimmune disease. These authors point out that this "negative" result mimics prior studies of "after-the-fact" oral tolerance induction in experimental animals, and, indeed, it fits with the fact that the success of oral tolerance induction in the treatment of experimental inflammation in rodents usually involves administration of the oral antigen at the time of initiation of disease, not after the disease has developed. It should be added that this result obtained by Moldoveanu can conceivably be explained by the studies of Strober and his colleagues (this volume, pages 115–131) who show that an ongoing Th1 response inhibits either the expansion of regulatory cells or the negative signaling by these cells.

These results clearly bode ill for reversal of disease by oral tolerance induction, which necessarily involves treatment of an already established immune response. However, several facts may mitigate this poor prognosis for this form of treatment. First, the study was done with an exogenous antigen (KLH) and thus may not lead to the stimulation of natural $CD25^+$ regulatory cells that have been shown to be specific for self-antigens. Thus, if the antigen selected for the induction of oral tolerance results in the expansion of already existent regulatory cells, it may have a

Address for correspondence: W. Strober, The Mucosal Immunity Section, Laboratory of Host Defense, NIAID, NIH, Bethesda, MD 20892. Voice: 301-496-6810; fax: 301-402-2240.
wstrober@niaid.nih.gov

greatly improved chance of success. It is important to remember here that the antigenic specificity of the regulatory cell does not have to be directed to the autoantigens actually causing tissue damage, only to the self-antigens present in the inflammatory site that can stimulate the regulatory cells to quell the inflammation by their bystander effects. This requirement for oral tolerance induction by a self-antigen may explain the interesting finding of Nussenblatt and his colleagues that a purified antigen had a better therapeutic effect in the treatment of uveitis by oral tolerance than did the mixture of antigens. In this situation, the limited number of antigenic epitopes of a purified antigen may mimic self-antigens and thus may better target regulatory cells than a mixture of antigens that may actually target effector cells and enhance cell injury.

A second fact to be considered in this context is that, as shown by Powrie and her colleagues (this volume, pages 132–141), administration of $CD25^+$ regulatory cells seemed able to overcome an ongoing inflammation, even though the latter was the robust inflammation seen in cell-transfer colitis. One factor in this success was again the fact that the stimulating antigens for the regulatory cells were probably the abundant self-antigens in the mucosal milieu. Another factor, however, may have been that in this situation the regulatory cells were operative in an immunodeficient host and thus may have been better able to expand because they were unhindered by homeostatic controls of lymphocyte expansion existent in a more normal host. This leads to the possibility that oral tolerance induction may be enhanced in conditioned patients that more readily allow regulatory cell expansion. Such conditioning may involve controlled immunoablative procedures, such as the use of anticytokines that cause apoptosis of Th1 T cell effector cell populations prior to the institution of oral tolerance induction. In addition, as suggested by Staines and his colleagues, it may also involve the use of regulatory cell "adjuvants" that allow for expansion of the latter in the face of Th1 inflammatory responses.

The studies reported here highlight the wide spectrum of possible diseases subject to treatment by oral tolerance. In studies of experimental mice, new data from Weiner and colleagues indicate that the field of possible use for this therapeutic modality must now be widened to include treatment of atherosclerosis, stroke, and Alzheimer disease, diseases not normally included within the category of autoimmune states. Indeed, from these data it is fair to say that all inflammations, not only autoimmune inflammations, may be subject to control by oral tolerance induction. One disease addressed in this section that is of particular interest is Crohn's disease, a Th1-mediated inflammation of the small and/or large intestine that is thought to be due to excess reactivity to antigens in the mucosal microflora (i.e., antigens that are equivalent to self-antigens). As shown by Kraus and his colleagues, there is some reason to believe that this disease is, in fact, associated with a defect in oral tolerance induction, although it is far from clear whether this is a primary or secondary effect. Interestingly, this study was performed with the same exogenous antigen, KLH, as used in the Moldoveanu study and thus may not reflect oral tolerance mediated by self-antigen–reactive cells. In any case, Ilan and his colleagues report promising therapeutic results by feeding patients a colonic antigen preparation in an uncontrolled clinical trial. This brings us back to the point made above, that it is possible that this positive result was obtained because in this situation one is administering antigen that does address the self-antigens in the intestinal milieu that are widely thought to be the causative antigens in this disease.

A further point emphasized by several of the authors of clinical studies is that not only the choice of antigen, but also the dose and timing of the antigen may be critical to the success of oral tolerance induction as a treatment of disease. From the work of Teitelbaum and his colleagues, for instance, we learn that oral glatiramer acetate (copolymer I) administration was an effective means of preventing experimental autoimmune encephalomyelitis in two rodent species and in primates. In addition, these authors reported that in the rodent model this treatment was effective in chronic disease, that is, after the disease had been already established. In view of these positive results in experimental animals, it was disappointing that oral glatiramer acetate administration was not effective in treating patients with MS in a large multicentered trial. A possible reason for this failure was suggested by the fact that in the animal studies, oral glatiramer acetate induced a Th2 response as well as cells that produced suppressive cytokines, such as TGF-β, whereas in the study of humans this was not the case. In view of this qualitatively different response in humans, it is possible that either the dose or timing of the treatment did not quite match that used in the animal studies and that further manipulation of how this material was given would lead to more positive results.

Finally, it is important to mention an exquisitely well-designed study of treatment of patients at risk for the development of diabetes with oral insulin conducted by Ergun-Longmire and colleagues. While the overall results of this double-blind, placebo-controlled study was generally negative, oral insulin did delay beta cell failure in a subset of patients: those with newly diagnosed disease who were given a low dose of insulin. These results deserve follow-up and again point out the role of dose in the effectiveness of oral tolerance induction. However, another point to emerge clearly from this work is that the therapy seemed to work early in the course of disease, again emphasizing that suppressor cell response induced by oral antigen may only be effective before the effector cell response becomes too overwhelming.

Overall, it seems apparent that these early studies of the use of oral tolerance induction to treat inflammation have shown some successes tucked among the several failures of this treatment. On this basis, additional studies that take into consideration the nature of the oral agent that is used, its dose, and its time with respect to disease will yield more positive results. In addition, the whole question of how to "condition" the patient to respond to treatment by oral tolerance induction needs to be more fully explored.

Class II MHC–Expressing Myofibroblasts Play a Role in the Immunopathogenesis Associated with Staphylococcal Enterotoxins

C. A. BARRERA,[a] I. V. PINCHUK,[a,b] J. I. SAADA,[b] G. SUAREZ,[a] D. A. BLAND,[a] E. BESWICK,[a] P. A. ADEGBOYEGA,[c] R. C. MIFFLIN,[b] D. W. POWELL,[b] AND V. E. REYES[a]

[a]*Child Health Research Center, Department of Pediatrics,*
[b]*Division of Gastroenterology, Department of Internal Medicine,*
[c]*Department of Pathology, University of Texas Medical Branch, Galveston, Texas 77555, USA*

ABSTRACT: Food poisoning due to staphylococcal enterotoxins (SEs) affects hundreds of thousands of people each year. Little is known about how SEs initiate immune responses and cause pathogenesis. Here, we demonstrate that cultured human intestinal myofibroblasts (IMFs) bind SEs in an MHC class II–dependent fashion. IMFs respond to SE exposure with increased secretion of IL-6, IL-8, and TNF-α. A significant proliferative T cell response was observed when MHC class II–expressing IMFs were pulsed with SEA and co-cultured with human CD4$^+$ T cells. In conclusion, our findings support the hypothesis that IMFs may play an important role in pathology associated with staphlococcocal enterotoxigenic disease.

KEYWORDS: myofibroblast; staphylococcal enterotoxins; superantigen; cytokines; MHC class II molecule

INTRODUCTION

Food-borne diseases have a major public health impact in the world. Staphylococcal enterotoxins A and B (SEA and SEB, respectively) represent the most common enterotoxins associated with food poisoning outbreaks in the United States, where 10% of affected individuals visited or were admitted to hospitals.[1] Functionally, SEs act through two major mechanisms in the host: potent gastrointestinal toxins and superantigens. Superantigens are characterized by their ability to bypass normal MHC-restricted, intracellular antigen processing and presentation. SEs bind directly to the MHC class II molecule and trigger various cellular events. The MHC class II–SE complex interacts with the Vβ element of the T cell receptor, initiating polyclonal T cell proliferation and excessive production of cytokines. In this way,

---

Address for correspondence: V.E. Reyes, Child Health Research Center, Department of Pediatrics, Mail # Rt. 0366, University of Texas Medical Branch, Galveston, TX 77555-0366. Voice: 409-772-3897; fax: 409-772-1761.
vreyes@utmb.edu

SEs activate up to a vast segment of the T cell repertoire rather than the small (<1%) fraction stimulated by conventional antigens.[2,3] This massive T cell proliferation and cytokine production can lead to fever, hypotension, and toxic shock.[1-4] Although the mode of action of superantigens is well understood, little is known about how SEs trigger the initial T cell response in the gastrointestinal tract and cause their characteristic pathologic effects. Considering that class II MHC molecules are the receptors for SEs and are required as part of a complex to engage T cells, cells that express class II MHC molecules are candidates for a central role in the induction of SE-associated pathogenesis.

Intestinal myofibroblasts (IMFs), which are located directly subjacent to the epithelial basement membrane, express MHC class II molecules *in vitro* and *in vivo*. Given the unique location of IMFs with respect to mucosal lymphocytes and SEs that cross the epithelial barrier, we hypothesize that class II MHC–expressing myofibroblasts play an important role in the pathogenesis of SE disease. The present study was designed to explore the ability of myofibroblasts to respond to exposure to SEs through class II MHC cross-linking, with the secretion of cytokines involved in the toxic effect of SEs, and to determine the ability of IMFs to activate $CD4^+$ T cells.

MATERIALS AND METHODS

The human colonic myofibroblast cell isolate 18Co (CRL-1459), obtained from the American Type Culture Collection (ATCC), was used as a representative IMF. 18Co cells were stimulated for 7 to 9 d with IFN-γ, to restore expression of MHC class II molecules, and were used as indicated for each experiment. Human $CD4^+$ T cells were purified from the peripheral blood mononuclear cells (PBMC) of healthy donors by a magnetic bead negative selection method using a cocktail of anti-class II MHC antibodies (IVA-12, L243, 9.3F10 derived from the hybridomas HB145, HB55 and HB180, respectively, from ATCC) and anti-CD8 antibodies (B9.4, kindly provided by Dr. E. Brooks, UTMB, Galveston, TX) to eliminate the non–$CD4^+$ T cells.

A superantigen-binding assay was performed to determine whether SEs bind MHC class II molecules on IMFs. Briefly, 18Co cells were preincubated with SEs at 37°C for 48 h in the presence or absence of anti–HLA-DR monoclonal antibody (Becton Dickinson, CA), then washed and stained with unconjugated anti-SEA or anti-SEB rabbit antisera (Sigma, MO) for 45 min, followed by 45 min staining with PE-conjugated anti–rabbit IgG (H+L) antibodies (Caltag, CA). Then cells were analyzed using a FACScan flow cytometer (Becton Dickinson, CA).

Cytokine production (IL-1β, IL-6, IL-8, IL-10, and TNF-α, TGF-β) in supernatants of IMFs exposed to SEA or SEB (Sigma) was measured using ELISA and Cytometric Bead Array (CBA) kits (PharMingen and Becton Dickinson, respectively) according to the manufacturer's instructions.

T cell proliferation assay was used to determine whether IMFs activate T cells bearing the appropriate T cell receptors. Briefly, the assay was performed in 96-well plates, in which $1-5 \times 10^5$ MHC II–expressing, irradiated (8000 rad) 18Co cells were used in coculture with $1-5 \times 10^4$ of purified $CD4^+$ T cells in the presence or absence of SEs (5 μg/mL). The plates were incubated for 4 d at 37°C, 5% CO_2. The cells were pulsed with [^{3}H]thymidine (1 μCi, ICN Pharmaceuticals Inc., CA) 18 h

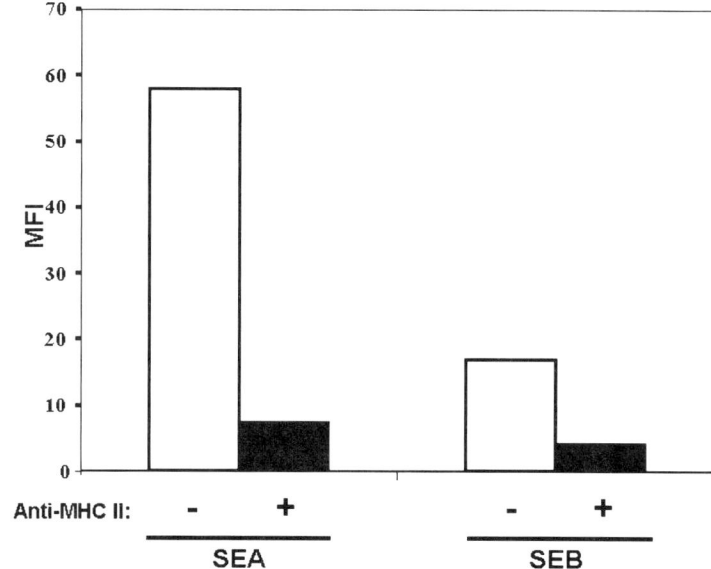

FIGURE 1. SEA and SEB superantigens bind to MHC class II molecules expressed by 18Co colonic myofibroblasts. 18Co cells were incubated for 7 d in the presence of IFN-γ (100 U/mL); 24 h after removal of IFN-γ, the cells were exposed to 5 μg/mL of SEA or SEB in the presence (*solid bars*) or absence (*open bars*) of anti-HLA-DR antibody. Binding of SEs to 18Co cells was measured 48 h later using immunostaining, followed by flow cytometric analysis. The results are expressed as a mean of fluorescence intensity (MFI).

prior to the end of coculture, and [^{3}H]thymidine incorporation was measured using a liquid scintillation counter (Beckman Instrument Inc.).

RESULTS AND DISCUSSION

Although we have studied various myofibroblast isolates derived from mucosal sections of human colon, a commercially available isolate (18Co) was used for the studies reported here. IMFs freshly isolated from surgical intestinal tissue express high levels of MHC II. However, after several passages *in vitro*, they lose MHC II expression.[5] Pretreatment of IMF with IFN-γ (100 U/mL) restores expression of MHC II in these cells. In the present study, we demonstrated that MHC II–expressing 18Co cells bind SEA and SEB in a dose-dependent manner. This SE binding was significantly decreased when anti-MHC class II antibodies were added to the IMF culture, proving the MHC II binding specificity of SEs (FIG. 1). Moreover, the specific binding of SEA to 18Co cells expressing MHC II was comparable to that observed for a B cell line used as a positive control. The observed difference in binding between SEA and SEB is probably owing to the fact that SEA binds both the a and b chains of HLA-DR and leads to cross-linking of MHC II molecules.[6] In contrast, SEB interacts exclusively with a chain of HLA-DR and does not effectively cross-link MHC class II molecules.[4,6]

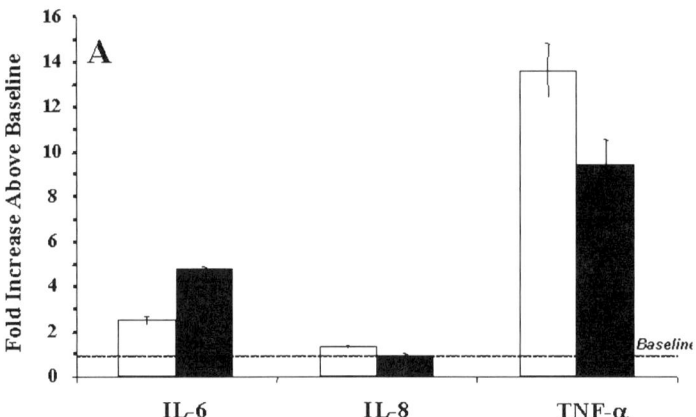

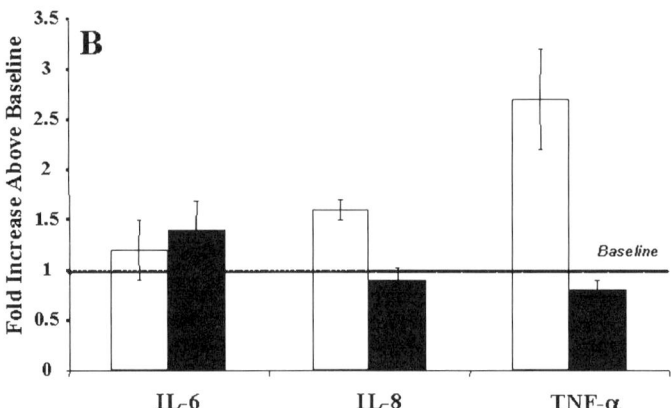

FIGURE 2. Exposure of 18 Co colonic myofibroblasts to SEs *in vitro* results in production of IL-6, IL-8, and TNF-α. 18Co cells were incubated for 7 d in the presence (*solid bars*) or absence (*open bars*) of IFN-γ (100 U/mL) and then exposed to 5 μg/mL of SEA (**A**) or SEB (**B**) 24 h after removal of IFN-γ. The cytokine level in the cell supernatant 72 h after SE exposure was measured using ELISA kits. Cytokine levels are expressed as the increase over baseline, which is defined as the level of the indicated cytokine in the supernatant of untreated 18Co cell cultures. All assays were performed in duplicate, and the data are expressed as means ± standard deviation.

Using a combination of RT-PCR and microarray analyses of IMF isolates (including 18Co), we have recently identified receptors for many of the cytokines on IMFs, including receptors for IL-1, IL-6, and TNF-α. These cytokines play a central role in SE-associated pathogenesis. The induction of IL-6 and TNF-α by SEs in human MHC class II–positive antigen–presenting cells in the absence of T cells has been described previously.[6] We, therefore, analyzed IMF 18Co cytokine production *in vitro* in response to SEA or SEB. Significant increases in IL-6, IL-8, and TNF-α production were observed when 18Co cells were exposed to SEA (FIG. 2A). Moreover, treatment of 18Co cells with IFN-γ to restore MHC II expression prior to SEA exposure led to higher production of IL-6. IFN-γ by itself had no significant effect on the expression of these cytokines (data not shown). This increased IL-6 production by MHC class II–expressing and SEA-exposed 18Co cells, compared with production by 18Co cells with low MHC class II expression, is probably due to the potent effect of MHC II cross-linking by SEA. Similar results have previously been described for human peripheral blood monocytes.[6]

In contrast to SEA, SEB exposure significantly increased the level of IL-8 and TNF-α, but not IL-6 (FIG. 2B). Interestingly, we observed a decrease in IL-8 and TNF-α production in 18Co cells treated with IFN-γ before SE exposure. This decrease in IL-8 and TNF-α production may be a result of downregulation of intracellular cAMP by IFN-γ.[7] It has previously been shown that decreases in intracellular cAMP, an important second messenger in the differential induction of proinflammatory mediators, may be implicated in the downregulation of IL-8 and TNF-α.[8] Using ELISA and CBA, no significant level of IL-1β, IL-12, and TGF-β was detected in the supernatants of SE-exposed 18Co cells (with or without IFN-γ pretreatment).

Finally, the ability of MHC class II–expressing 18Co cells to stimulate proliferation of purified human CD4$^+$ T cell in the presence or absence of SEA was determined. IMFs cocultured with SEA induced a robust T cell proliferative response (stimulation index: 29).

In conclusion, our results show that IMFs are able to bind SEs via surface class II MHC molecules and respond with the production of proinflammatory cytokines. Also, IMFs with associated SEs are able to stimulate CD4$^+$ T cell proliferation. These observations provide insights into the mechanisms by which superantigens may initiate and/or propagate inflammatory pathological processes associated with staphlococcal enterotoxigenic diarrheal disease.

ACKNOWLEDGMENTS

This work was supported by the NIH grants (DK50669, DK 55783), the UTMB's Gastrointestinal Research Interdisciplinary Program (GRIP), the Sealy Foundation, and the Texas Gulf Coast DDC (DK 56338).

REFERENCES

1. BALABAN, N. & A. RASOOLY. 2000. Staphylococcal enterotoxins. Int. J. Food Microbiol. **61:** 1–10.

2. MOURAD, W., R. AL-DACCAK, T. CHATILA & R.S. GEHA. 1993. Staphylococcal superantigens as inducers of signal transduction in MHC class II-positive cells. Semin. Immunol. **5:** 47–56.
3. ULRICH, R. 2000. Evolving superantigens of *Staphylococcus aureus*. FEMS Immun. Med. Microbiol. **27:** 1–7.
4. LLEWELYN, M. & J. COHEN. 2002. Superantigens: microbial agents that corrupt immunity. Lancet Inf. Dis. **2:** 156–162.
5. SAADA, J.I., C.A. BARRERA, V.E. REYES, *et al.* 2004. Intestinal myofibroblasts and immune tolerance. Ann. N.Y. Acad. Sci. **1029:** 379–381.
6. KRAKAUER, T. 1999. Immune response to staphylococcal superantigens. Immunol. Res. **20:** 163–173.
7. LEVI, G., L. MINGHETTI & F. ALOISI. 1998. Regulation of prostanoid synthesis in microglial cells and effects of prostaglandin E_2 on microglial function. Biochemie **80:** 899–904.
8. TAYLOR, C.T., N. FUEKI, A. AGAH, *et al.* 1999. Critical role of cAMP response element binding protein expression in hypoxia-elicited induction of epithelial tumor necrosis factor-alpha. J. Biol. Chem. **274:** 19447–19454.

Early Upregulation of T Cell IL-10 Production Plays an Important Role in Oral Tolerance Induction

Y. CONG, C. LIU, C. T. WEAVER, AND C. O. ELSON

Departments of Medicine and Pathology, University of Alabama, Birmingham, Alabama 35294, USA

ABSTRACT: Early in oral tolerance induction, IL-10–producing $CD4^+$ T cells were increased, and adoptive transfer of IL-10–deficient $CD4^+$ T cells failed induction of oral tolerance, suggesting a key role of IL-10 production in such a process.

KEYWORDS: IL-10 production; dendritic cells; transgenic mice

The induction of oral tolerance involves an initial phase of immune activation in which T cells proliferate and produce cytokines, such as interferon. This early stage of activation after antigen feeding provides a window in which the tolerogenic process or pathways can be altered. However, the cells, cytokines, and costimulatory molecules involved in this early phase of tolerance induction are still largely unknown. The purpose of this study was to determine whether T cell IL-10 production is required during oral tolerance induction. Oral tolerance was examined in BALB/c mice adoptively transferred with $CD4^+$ T cells from ovalbumin (OVA)-specific wild-type or IL-10–deficient DO11.10 TCR transgenic (Tg) mice. The mice were fed 1 mg OVA five times every other day in a multiple emulsion (ME) antigen delivery system. Control groups were fed KLH in ME or PBS in ME. Two days after the last feeding, T cell responses were determined by culture of $CD4^+$ T cells with OVA peptide in the presence of antigen-presenting cells (APCs), and cytokine production was measured. In the recipient mice given OVA in ME, but not in controls, Tg T cell number was decreased in spleen, mesenteric lymph nodes (MLN), and Peyer's patches (PP). Expression on dendritic cells (DCs) of CD40 and CD86 but not MHC class II was decreased. CD40L but not CD28 or CD69 on Tg $CD4^+$ T cells was decreased in PP but not in MLN or spleen and not in control mice. When cultured with OVA peptide, $CD4^+$ T cells from the mice receiving OVA in ME had significantly decreased proliferation and decreased IL-2 production in PP, MLN, and spleen. Interestingly, IL-10 production was increased, as was IFN production. IL-4 was not detected in any cultures. Feeding 1 mg OVA plus 100 ng IL-10 in ME moderately enhanced oral tolerance induction as compared with mice receiving only OVA in ME; that is, the CD4$^+$ T cell responses and IL-2 production were further decreased. Recipients of IL-10–deficient DO11 CD4$^+$ T cells failed to induce oral tolerance after feeding with OVA in ME, in that no decreases of T cell proliferation or of DC CD40 expression were observed. We conclude that in this system the induction of oral tolerance requires early CD4$^+$ T cell IL-10 production that inhibits costimulatory molecule expression on DCs and their ligands on T cells.

Study of Oral Tolerance and Its Indirect Effects in Adoptive Cell Transfer Experiments

ANDRÉ PIRES DA CUNHA,[a] NELSON MONTEIRO VAZ,[a] AND CLÁUDIA ROCHA CARVALHO[b]

[a]*Departmento de Bioquímica-Imunologia ICB-UFMG, Brazil*
[b]*Departmento de Morfologia, ICB-UFMG, Brazil*

ABSTRACT: Parenteral exposure to antigens to which oral tolerance had been previously induced results in the inhibition of immune responses to other unrelated antigens. Herein we tested whether indirect effects of oral tolerance could be adoptively transferred. Anti-Ova– and antihemoglobin-specific responsiveness as well as oral tolernace to Ova were transferred to irradiated, but not to normal, nonirradiated recepients. Irradiation, thus, facilitated adoptive transfer of oral tolerance. However, the inhibitory (indirect) effects upon the unrelated immunogen were not adoptively transferred, even to irradiated recepients. In addition, we studied adoptively transferred CFSE-labeled spleen cells by flow cytometry in recipient spleen, inguinal lymph nodes, and bone marrow, both in irradiated and nonirradiated recipients, 1, 3, or 5 days after cell transfer. Comparing the percent and absolute number of CFSE-labeled cells in each organ displayed significant differences in the dynamics of decay of adoptively transferred cells from tolerant or immune donors.

KEYWORDS: oral tolerance; syngeneic barrier; indirect effects; adoptive transference

INTRODUCTION

Oral tolerance was first described by Wells in 1911.[1] In recent years, there has been renewed interest in this phenomenon as a possible therapy for autoimmunity.[2] Although many aspects of oral tolerance have been resolved, its fundamental nature remains elusive.

Several results from our laboratories[3,4] and the laboratories of others[5] have shown that in addition to blocking immune responsiveness to the specific antigen, parenteral exposure to an antigen against which oral tolerance has been previously induced can induce blockage of the initiation of immune responses to unrelated antigens.

Many laboratories have used the adoptive transfer of cells between syngeneic animals as a tool for seeking a better understanding of the mechanisms involved in

Address for correspondence: Nelson Monteiro Vaz, Laboratório de Imunobiologia, Departamento de Bioquímica e Imunologia, ICB-UFMG, Av. Antônio Carlos, 6627, Pampulha, Belo Horizonte, MG, Brazil, CEP: 31270-901 Caixa Postal 486. Voice: +5531 3499-2662; fax: +5531 3499-2640.

   nvaz@icb.ufmg.br; nvaz@superig.com.br

immunological phenomena. A dominant consideration in these studies is based on the fact that the main determinant in cell transplantation is MHC dependent, such that histocompatibility determines whether transferred cells will be incorporated in the immunological activities of the recipient or not. However, a more fundamental role of the recipient's cells in the survival of transferred cells and the establishment of these immunological activities, which prevails even in syngeneic transplants, has also been demonstrated: the so-called "syngeneic barrier."[6] Some form of depletion of the recipient's lymphocytes is believed to be necessary to provide "space" for transferred cells to operate. Experimentally, this is usually achieved by whole-body irradiation of recipient animals,[6] or other immunosuppressive treatments. Notwithstanding, adoptive transference of oral tolerance has been demonstrated using syngeneic animals with an intact immune system.[7] The subject, however, is still a matter of debate, with most authors proposing that depletion of the recipient's cells is necessary for the persistence of isogeneic transferred cells and, beyond this, to promote homeostatic expansion of transferred cells.[8,9]

With these questions in mind, the present experiments were undertaken to assess the possibility of adoptively transferring oral tolerance and its indirect effects to normal or previously irradiated syngeneic animals, and to evaluate which factors interfere in these events and by what means.

MATERIALS AND METHODS

Young adult C57BL/6 mice (7 to 10 weeks of age) were made orally tolerant to ovalbumin (Ova) by drinking a solution of 4 mg/mL Ova (Ova, Sigma Grade III; Sigma Chemical Co., St Louis, MO, USA) for 3 days. Seven days later, they received intraperitoneally 2 µg of hemoglobin from Biomphalaria glabrata (Hb, kindly provided by Prof. Marcelo Santoro from our department) mixed with 10 µg of Ova plus 3 mg aluminum hydroxide ($Al(OH)_3$). Fourteen days thereafter, 5×10^7 spleen cells from these mice or from nontolerant controls were transferred intravenously into normal or previously irradiated mice (600 rad). All recipients were boosted intraperitoneally with a mixture of 2 µg Hb and 10 µg Ova without adjuvant immediately after cell transfer and 7 d later. Serum was collected 7 d thereafter and analyzed by ELISA; results are represented as Elisa* as previously described.[4] Results are expressed as means plus one standard deviation (1 SD). To test significance, Student's t test was performed. CFSE-labeled cells were adoptively transferred as previously described.[10] Pooled donor spleen cells were traced by flow cytometry in irradiated and nonirradiated recipient spleen, inguinal lymph nodes, and bone marrow 1, 3, or 5 d after cell transfer, using the same protocol described above.

RESULTS

We investigated the possibility of adoptively transferring the "indirect (inhibitory) effects" of parenteral exposures to a tolerated antigen. In mice that were orally exposed to Ova and then immunized with Ova+Hb mixtures, anti-Ova and anti-Hb titers were both significantly lower than in mice not orally exposed to Ova, as expected (FIG. 1). These mice were used as donors of spleen cells to normal or previ-

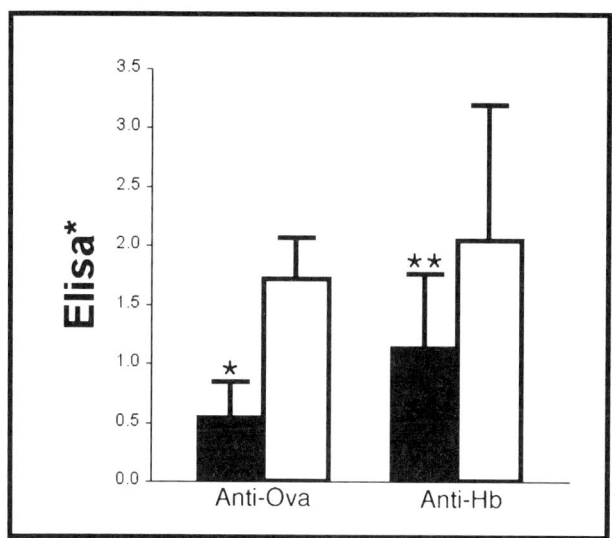

FIGURE 1. Anti-Ova and anti-Hb antibodies in C57BL/6J donor mice 14 d after primary immunization with Ova+Hb+Al(OH)$_3$. Figure indicates immune (*open bars*) and tolerant (*black bars*) donors. *$P<.0001$ and **$P<.05$.

ously irradiated syngeneic recipients. Subsequent bleedings of mice that received cells from nontolerant donors showed that antibody responses to Ova and Hb were present in irradiated, but not in nonirradiated syngeneic recipients (FIG. 2, B and D). Irradiated recipient mice that received cells from tolerant donors showed low responses to Ova but stronger responses to Hb. This showed that oral tolerance was adoptively transferred, but its indirect (inhibitory) effects were not (FIG. 2, A and C). In nonirradiated recipients, there was no evidence of adoptive transfer (FIG. 2) of immunization, tolerance, or its indirect effects, a phenomenon that may be ascribed to the so-called "syngeneic barrier."[6]

Further experiments were performed by adoptively transferring CFSE-labeled cells. Preliminary results indicate that more CFSE-labeled donor cells may be recovered from nonirradiated recipients (data not shown). However, owing to the lymphocyte depletion caused by irradiation, a larger percentage of CFSE cells may be recovered from irradiated recipients, independent of the origin of the transferred cells (tolerant or normal donors).

DISCUSSION

We were unable to transfer the indirect (inhibitory) effects of parenteral exposures to a tolerated antigen to either normal or irradiated recipients, whereas immune responsiveness (immunization) and tolerance could be successfully transferred to irradiated recipients. This suggests that the indirect (inhibitory) effects of the tolerated antigen are more demanding of a systemic architecture than oral tolerance.

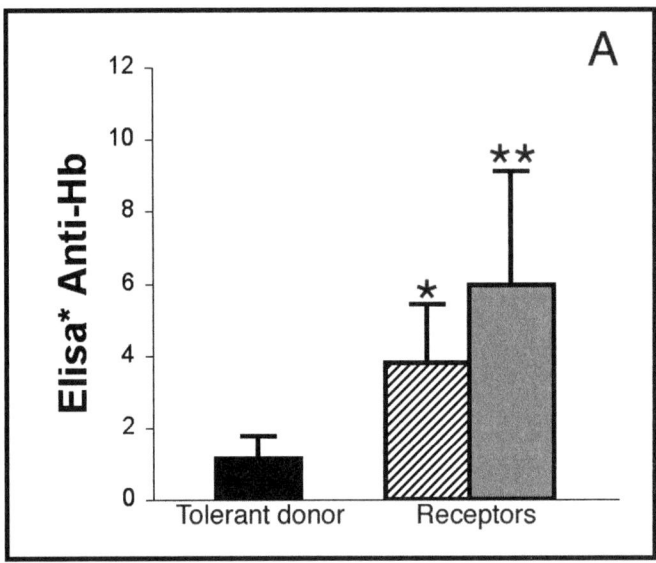

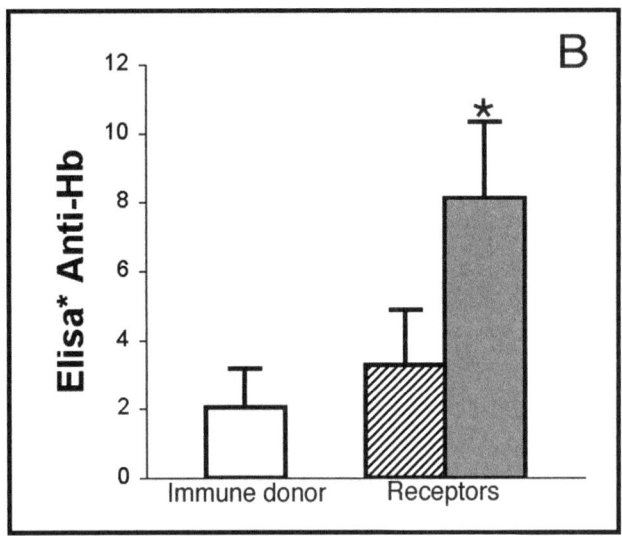

FIGURE 2. Anti-Ova and anti-Hb antibodies in C57BL/6J donor and recipient mice. Donors were immunized with Ova+Hb+Al(OH)$_3$; 14 days later, sera were collected for antibody testing, and 5×10^7 spleen cells from these mice were transferred intravenously to syngeneic irradiated (*dotted bars*) or normal (*hatched bars*) mice. These recipients were then immunized intraperitoneally with Ova+Hb immediately after transference and 7 d thereafter. The figure indicates immune (*open bars*) and tolerant (*black bars*) donors. (**A**) Anti-Hb Elisa∗ of tolerant donors × recipients (∗$P<.0001$ in relation to donors). (**B**) Anti-Hb Elisa∗ of immune donors × recipients (∗$P<.05$ and ∗∗$P<.001$ in relation to donors).

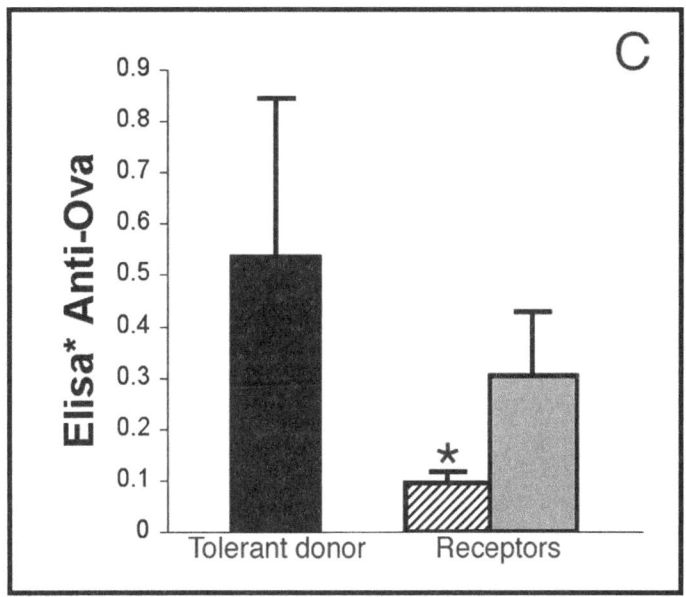

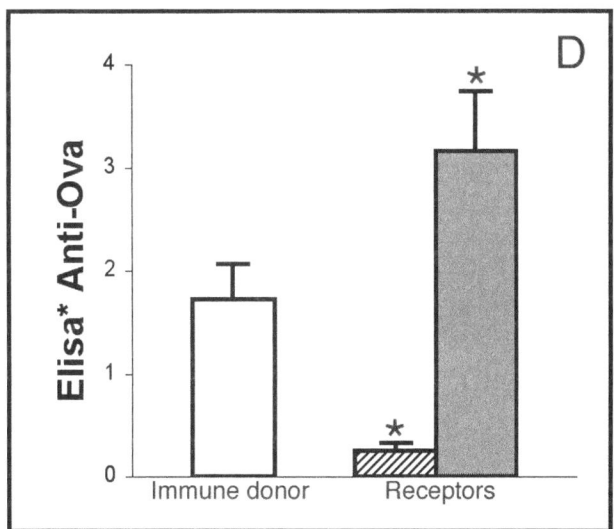

FIGURE 2 — *continued*. (**C**) Anti-Ova Elisa* of tolerant donors × recipients (*$P<.0001$ in relation to donors). (**D**) Anti-Hb Elisa* of immune donors × recipients (*$P<.01$ in relation to donors).

Cells transferred to nonirradiated syngeneic recipients have their specific activities strikingly blocked, such that neither immunization nor tolerance could be transferred to nonirradiated recipients. However, a few previous studies have demonstrated the possibility of transferring oral tolerance to intact recipients.[7,11] Nonetheless, the transference is made at different time points after oral tolerance induction and usually donor mice are fed but not challenged before donation. We are unaware whether this could be an explanation for this discrepancy.

Overall, these results imply that there are barriers other than MHC-mismatch to the functional implantation of the transferred lymphocytes. As classically demonstrated by Celada,[6] antibody-producing cells transferred to normal syngeneic recipients of different ages face a "syngeneic barrier" that significantly hinders their operation, even in newborn recipients, and grows steadily thereafter. In irradiated recipients, who had most of their cycling cells destroyed, transferred cells may be fully operant and may respond 50- to 100-fold better to subsequent exposures to the specific antigen than when transferred to normal recipients.

A further point is worth attention: We could only tell that oral tolerance was transferred to irradiated recipients because we compared this group with another that had also been irradiated and received cells from immune donors. However, we could not evaluate whether oral tolerance was transferred to nonirradiated recipients because immunization was not transferred to the immune control group.

We used CFSE cell-labeling to study the distribution of cells derived from tolerant or immune donors in irradiated or normal syngeneic recipients. Our preliminary results suggest that on the first day the pattern of distribution of cells derived from immune or tolerant donors did not differ in any of the analyzed organs (data not shown). By the third day, however, recipients of cells from immune but not tolerant donors showed a decrease in both the relative and absolute number of cells (data not shown). This suggests that there may be differences in the dynamics of decay of adoptively transferred cells from tolerant or immune donors.

An issue arising from these results is why oral tolerance is transferable only to irradiated recipients if, as mentioned above, nonirradiated recipients maintain a higher absolute number of donor cells. It may be that although animals with an intact immune system display a higher number of donor-derived cells, they represent a smaller proportion of total cells, and may be unable to establish the interactions necessary to maintain tolerance. An environment where transferred cells predominate may be necessary to form the connections involved in the production of activating or inhibitory cytokines.

ACKNOWLEDGMENTS

We thank Ms. Ilda Marçal and Frankcinéia Assis for their excellent technical assistance. CNPq and FAPEMIG, Brazil supported this work.

REFERENCES

1. WELLS, H.G. 1911. Studies on the chemistry of anaphylaxis. III. Experiments with isolated proteins, specially those of the hen's egg. J. Infect. Dis. **8:** 147–171.

2. FARIA, A.M. & H.L. WEINER. 1999. Oral tolerance: mechanisms and therapeutic applications. Adv. Immunol. **73:** 153–264.
3. VAZ, N.M., D.G. HANSON, L.C.S. MAIA, et al. 1981. Cross-suppression of specific immune responses after oral tolerance. Mem. Inst. Oswaldo Cruz. **76:** 83–91.
4. CARVALHO, C.R., B.A. VERDOLIN & N.M. VAZ. 1997. Indirect effects of oral tolerance cannot be ascribed to bystander suppression. Scand. J. Immunol. **45:** 276–281.
5. MILLER, A., O. LIDER & H.L. WEINER. 1991. Antigen driven bystander suppression after oral administration of antigen. J. Exp. Med. **174:** 791–798.
6. CELADA, F. 1966. Quantitative studies of the adoptive immunological memory in mice. I. An age-dependent barrier to syngeneic transplantation. J. Exp. Med. **124:** 1–14.
7. RICHMAN, L.K., J.M. CHILLER, W.R. BROWN, et al. 1978. Enterically induced immunologic tolerance. I. Induction of suppressor T lymphocytes by intragastric administration of soluble proteins. J. Immunol. **121:** 2429–2434.
8. MAINE, G.N. & J.J. MULÉ. 2002. Making room for T cells. J. Clin. Invest. **110:** 157–159.
9. TANCHOT, C., A. LE CAMPION, B. MARTIN, et al. 2002. Conversion of naive T cells to a memory-like phenotype in lymphopenic hosts is not related to a homeostatic mechanism that fills the peripheral naive T cell pool. J. Immunol. **168:** 5042–5046.
10. OEHEN, S., K. BRDUSCHA-RIEM, A. OXENIUS, et al. 1997. A simple method for evaluating the rejection of grafted spleen cells by flow cytometry and tracing adoptively transferred cells by light microscopy. J. Immunol. Methods. **207:** 33–42.
11. CHEN, Y., J. INOBE, H.L. WEINER. 1995. Induction of oral tolerance to myelin basic protein in CD-8 depleted mice: both CD4+ and CD8+ cells mediate active suppression. J. Immunol. **155:** 910– 916.

Differential Immune Induction with Subcutaneous versus Oral Administration of a Diabetogenic Insulin Peptide in the NOD Mouse

DEVASENAN DEVENDRA, JOHANNA PARONEN, EDWIN LIU,
HIROAKI MORIYAMA, DONGMEI MIAO, LIPING YU,
AND GEORGE S. EISENBARTH

Barbara Davis Center for Childhood Diabetes,
University of Colorado Health Sciences Center, Denver, Colorado 80862, USA

ABSTRACT: The B chain insulin peptide 9 to 23 (B:9–23) is a dominant T cell epitope of the NOD mouse. Given in oral form with multiple different vehicles, it did not alter expression of insulin autoantibodies in contrast to subcutaneous administration.

KEYWORDS: insulin; diabetes; NOD; insulin autoantibody; oral tolerance

INTRODUCTION

Subcutaneous insulin peptide B:9–23 in incomplete Freund's adjuvant (IFA) has been shown to be very effective in preventing diabetes and inducing insulin autoantibodies (IAAs) in NOD mice.[1] B:9–23 peptide given subcutaneously (SQ) in saline alone also induces IAA but is not as protective. Given the previously reported efficacy of an orally administered (PO, *per os*) insulin B chain peptide in inducing regulatory T cells,[2] we investigated the effects of PO B:9–23 peptide (given in different adjuvants) in NOD mice. Because of previous reports of the ability of lipid emulsions and lipopolysaccharide (LPS)[3] to modulate the immune response, combinations with B:9–23 peptide were given to mice as well.

RESEARCH DESIGN AND METHODS

Eight groups of NOD mice (6 to 8 in each group) each were given one of the following: (1) B:9–23 100 μg/dose in saline PO; (2) B:9–23 in soybean oil emulsion PO; (3) soybean oil emulsion alone PO; (4) B:9–23 peptide in LPS 0.5 mg/dose PO;

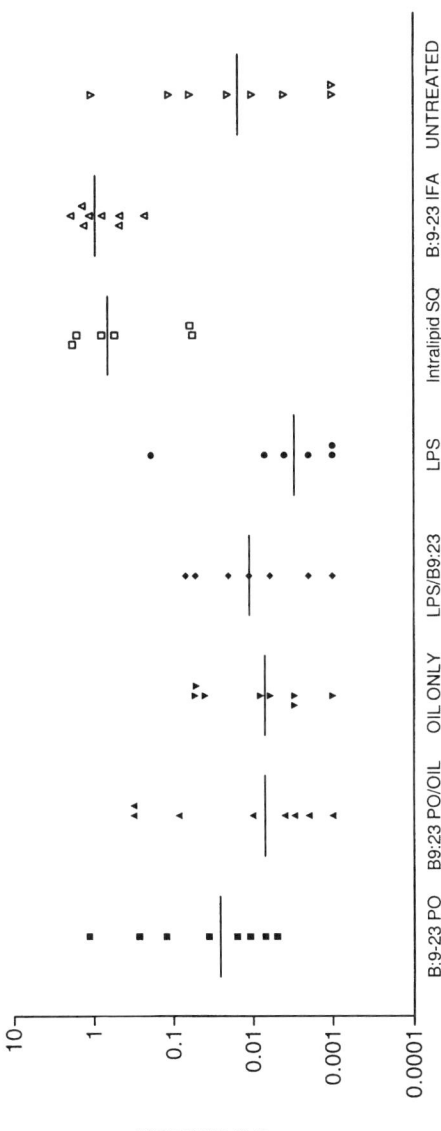

FIGURE 1. Insulin autoantibody (IAA) index and median value at 10 weeks of age in NOD mice given B:9–23 insulin peptide orally (PO) or subcutaneously (SQ), with or without adjuvant. IFA, incomplete Freund's adjuvants; LPS, lipolysaccharide.

(5) LPS alone PO; (6) B:9–23 peptide in intralipid SQ; (7) B:9–23 peptide in IFA; or (8) no treatment. Oral gavage was given weekly from 4 through 15 weeks of age. Subcutaneous injections were given once only at 4 weeks of age. Blood sugars were monitored weekly, starting at 12 weeks of age, until 40 weeks of age. Diabetes was defined as two consecutive blood sugars greater than 250 mg/dL. IAAs and anti–B:9–23 antibodies were measured regularly as well.

RESULTS

None of the oral regimens with or without B:9-23 peptide were able to induce higher IAAs or suppress spontaneous IAA production in NOD mice compared with unmanipulated controls. However, B:9–23 given in intralipid or in IFA SQ induced significantly higher levels of IAA compared with all other groups at all times tested. There were no differences in the levels of IAA among the groups receiving oral B:9–23 in saline, soybean oil emulsion, or LPS. The IAA index at 10 weeks of age for groups 1 to 8 is shown in FIGURE 1. In addition, there were no detectable IgG1 antibodies against B:9–23 peptide in those mice receiving oral therapy. Only B:9–23 in IFA was able to prevent diabetes (88% diabetes-free at 40 weeks of age) compared with controls.

DISCUSSION

Insulin peptide B:9–23 given orally alone or in combination with an oil emulsion or LPS was not able to prevent diabetes in NOD mice, nor was it able to alter the natural course of spontaneous IAA production. Furthermore, anti–B:9–23 antibodies (which are usually seen in mice receiving subcutaneous B:9–23 injections) were undetectable in mice receiving oral B:9–23. This lack of effect from oral B:9–23 peptide compared with subcutaneous peptide injections may be a result of the inability of the peptide to induce oral tolerance. Alternatively, lack of effect could be a result of peptide instability or lack of mucosal absorption when delivered intragastrically. Higher doses of peptide or other means of oral adjuvant delivery may be needed to induce an immunological effect.

REFERENCES

1. ABIRU, N., A.K. MANIATIS, L. YU, et al. 2001. Peptide and MHC specific breaking of humoral tolerance to native insulin with the B:9-23 peptide in diabetes prone and normal mice. Diabetes **50:** 1274–1281.
2. MARON, R., M. GUERAU-DE-ARELLANO, X. ZHANG & H.L. WEINER. 2001. Oral administration of insulin to neonates suppresses spontaneous and cyclophosphamide induced diabetes in the NOD mouse. J. Autoimmun. **16:** 21–28.
3. BELLMANN, K., H. KOLB, B. HARTMANN, et al. 1997. Intervention in autoimmune diabetes by targeting the gut immune system. Int. J. Immunopharmacol. **19:** 573–577.

Comparative Study of Oral versus Subcutaneous B:9–23 Insulin Peptide in Balb/c Mice as an Experimental Model for Autoimmune Diabetes

DEVASENAN DEVENDRA, JOHANNA PARONEN, EDWIN LIU,
HIROAKI MORIYAMA, ROBERT TAYLOR, DONGMEI MIAO, LIPING YU,
AND GEORGE EISENBARTH

Barbara Davis Center for Childhood Diabetes,University of Colorado Health Sciences Center, Denver, Colorado 80262, USA

ABSTRACT: Insulin peptide B:9–23 (amino acids 9 to 23 of the B chain) can induce immune targeting of insulin and islets in normal Balb/c mice. The insulin autoantibodies induced react with insulin and not the immunizing peptide. Oral administration of insulin as well as subcutaneous insulin can sensitize to insulin.

KEYWORDS: insulin; diabetes; Balb/c; autoantibody; poly IC

INTRODUCTION

Proinsulin/insulin and the insulin B-chain 9–23 peptide have been studied extensively as islet autoantigens, and insulin was an early subject of immune response gene-dependent recognition, with interest in the observation that the response to the B-chain of insulin was $H-2^d$ restricted.[1,2] The insulin peptide B:9–23 given subcutaneously (SQ) has been shown to be an effective antigen in inducing insulin autoantibodies (IAA); when given with poly-IC, a viral mimic, it induces insulitis in Balb/c mice.[3] In contrast, administration of the B:9–23 peptide to C57BL/6 mice did not induce IAA. These studies demonstrate that "normal" mice have autoreactive T lymphocytes able to rapidly target islets and that peripherally administered insulin peptide can enhance specific anti-islet autoimmunity. We were interested in investigating whether the administration of B:9–23 peptide orally, with or without poly-IC and/or SQ B:9–23, is able to induce IAA, insulitis, and possibly even diabetes.

Address for correspondence: George S. Eisenbarth, M.D., Ph.D., Barbara Davis Center for Childhood Diabetes, University of Colorado Health Sciences Center, 4200 East 9th Avenue, B-140, Denver, CO 80262. Voice: 303-315-4891; fax: 303-315-4892.
george.eisenbarth@uchsc.edu

TABLE 1. Induction of insulin autoantibodies (IAA), anti–B:9–23 antibodies, and insulitis in Balb/c mice using oral (PO) B:9–23 insulin peptide alone or in combination with poly-IC and/or subcutaneous (SQ) B:9–23 peptide

Group	Initial Treatment	Subsequent Treatment	IAA	Anti–B:9–23 Antibodies	Insulitis
1	B:9–23 PO	none	2/11	0/11	1/11
2	B:9–23 PO	B:9–23 SQ	3/3	3/3	2/3
3	Saline PO	B:9–23 SQ	3/3	3/3	2/3
4	B:9–23 PO + poly-IC	none	3/11	0/11	1/11
5	B:9–23 PO + poly-IC	B:9–23 SQ	6/6	6/6	6/6
6	Saline PO + poly-IC	B:9–23 SQ	3/3	3/3	3/3
7	B:9–23 SQ	B:9–23 SQ	6/6	6/6	6/6
8	Saline PO	none	0/11	0/11	0/11

RESEARCH DESIGN AND METHODS

Eight groups of Balb/c mice (3 to 11 in each group) were each given one the following: (1) oral B:9–23 in saline; (2) oral B:9–23 and subsequently SQ B:9–23; (3) oral saline and subsequently SQ B:9–23; (4) oral B:9–23 plus poly-IC; (5) oral B:9–23 plus poly-IC, followed by SQ B:9–23; (6) oral saline plus poly-IC, followed by SQ B:9–23 (7) SQ B9-23 insulin in saline; or (8) oral saline only. Oral gavages (500 μg B:9–23 insulin) were given weekly from ages 4 through 10 weeks. SQ doses were given weekly from ages 11 to 19 weeks, except in group 7, in which they were given weekly from ages 4 through 19 weeks. Poly-IC was given daily during weeks 4 and 5. Blood sugars were checked every 2 weeks through 30 to 32 weeks of age. The mice were sacrificed at 30 to 32 weeks of age and pancreatic histology was examined. Anti-B:9–23 antibodies (B:9–23 Ab) and IAA were checked regularly. The microfiltration radioimmunoassay was used to detect IAA, and an ELISA format was used for the detection of B:9–23 insulin antibodies.

RESULTS

The results are summarized in TABLE 1. Although marginal IAA was detected in two mice in group 1 (mice receiving oral B:9–23 only), there was a marked delay in IAA expression (first detected at 20 weeks age) compared with group 7 mice receiving B:9–23 SQ only (first detected at 8 weeks of age). The median levels of IAA were higher in all groups given B:9–23 SQ, regardless of the immunization protocol. Oral B:9–23 did not induce IAA in Balb/c mice, but also did not prevent subsequent formation of IAA in those mice later receiving B:9–23 SQ. Furthermore, oral B:9–23 did not induce anti–B:9-23 antibodies as compared with B:9-23 SQ. As expected, the presence of poly-IC induced insulitis; however when B:9–23 was given orally, this only promoted insulitis when given with subsequent SQ immunization.

DISCUSSION

Insulin B chain peptide B:9–23 administered subcutaneously can induce IAA in normal strain BALB/c mice. The current study indicates that oral B:9–23 may have a priming effect for later insulin-specific immune responses, although by itself it induces no clear insulin autoimmunity serologically or histologically. Oral administration of B:9-23 peptide may be involved in inducing normal mice to break both humoral and cellular tolerance, thus possibly underscoring the role of the mucosal immune system in the pathogenesis of type 1 diabetes.

REFERENCES

1. ZHANG, Z.J., L. DAVIDSON, G. EISENBARTH & H.L. WEINER. 1991. Suppression of diabetes in nonobese diabetic mice by oral administration of porcine insulin. Proc. Natl. Acad. Sci. USA **88:** 10252–10256.
2. WEGMANN, D.R., M. NORBURY-GLASER & D. DANIEL. 1994. Insulin-specific T cells are a predominant component of islet infiltrates in pre-diabetic NOD mice. Eur. J. Immunol. **24:** 1853–1857.
3. MORIYAMA, H., L. WEN, N. ABIRU, *et al.* 2002. Induction and acceleration of insulitis/diabetes in mice with a viral mimic (polyinosinic-polycytidylic acid) and an insulin self-peptide. Proc. Natl. Acad. Sci. USA **99:** 5539–5544.

CCL25 Enhances CD103-Mediated Lymphocyte Adhesion to E-Cadherin

ANNA ERICSSON,[a] ANU ARYA,[b] AND WILLIAM AGACE[a]

[a]*Immunology Section, Department of Cell and Molecular Biology, Lund University, Lund, Sweden*

[b]*Enanta Pharmaceuticals, Inc., Watertown, Massachusetts 02472, USA*

ABSTRACT: Our results demonstrate that (1) CD103 is upregulated on CD8$^+$ T cells subsequent to their entry into the small intestinal epithelium, and (2) that the chemokine CCL25 enhances CD103-mediated adhesion to E-cadherin. These results suggest a novel role for chemokines in modulating interactions between lymphocytes and epithelial cells at mucosal surfaces.

KEYWORDS: CCL25; CD103; CD8$^+$ T cells; E-cadherin

INTRODUCTION

The chemokine CCL25 is constitutively expressed in the murine and human small intestine,[1] and its receptor CCR9 is functionally expressed on human and murine small intestinal intraepithelial lymphocytes (IEL).[2,3] IEL adherence to intestinal epithelial cells is mediated through interactions between the integrin CD103 and its epithelial ligand E-cadherin.[4] This interaction appears important, since mice deficient in CD103 have reduced numbers of IEL;[5] however, it must be regulated, because the half-life of IEL is much greater than that of epithelial cells.[6] In the current study, we have examined the expression and regulation of CD103 on CD8$^+$ IEL and the ability of CCL25 to enhance CD103-mediated IEL adhesion to E-cadherin.

RESULTS

CD8$^+$ Lymphocytes Upregulate CD103 after Entry into the Small Intestinal Epithelium

To determine the expression and regulation of CD103 in lymphocytes entering the small intestinal epithelium, we used an ovalbumin (OVA)-specific TCR transgenic (OT-1) T cell adoptive transfer system. OT-1 T cells were transferred into

---

Address for correspondence: Anna Ericsson, Immunology Section, Department of Cell and Molecular Biology, Lund University, BMC I-13, SE-22184 Lund, Sweden. Voice: +46-46-222-0434; fax: +46-46-222-4218.
  Anna.Ericsson@immuno.lu.se

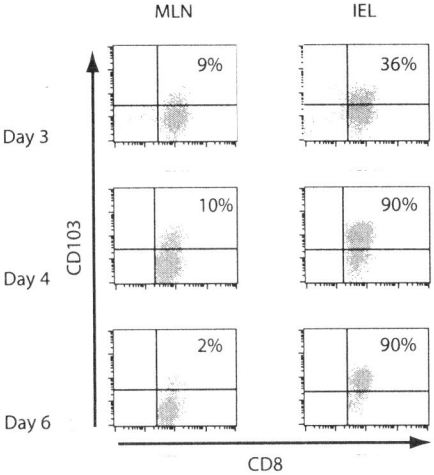

FIGURE 1. CD103 expression is induced on CD8$^+$ lymphocytes after their entry into the small intestinal epithelium. CD103 expression on CD8$^+$ OT-1 T cells in MLN and IEL 3, 4, and 6 days after an intraperitoneal injection of OVA (5 mg) and LPS (100 μg). Representative results from one of three experiments performed are shown.

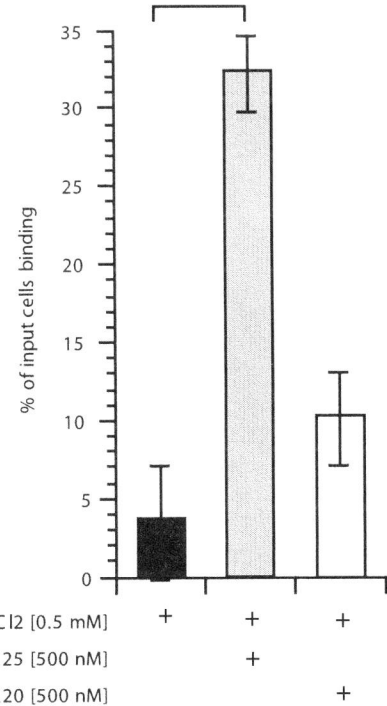

FIGURE 2. CCL25 promotes IEL adhesion to murine E-cadherin human-Fc fusion protein. CD8$^+$ IEL were incubated with CCL25 (*gray bar*) or CCL20 (*white bar*) at a suboptimal concentration of MgCl$_2$ (*black bar*). Results are mean (SEM) from triplicate wells and are representative from one of six experiments performed.

congenic recipient mice. One day after transfer, OVA-specific T cells were activated by intraperitoneal injection of OVA and lipopolysaccharide (LPS). In this model, OT-1 cells enter the intestinal epithelium following activation in gut-associated lymphoid tissue. As shown in FIGURE 1, CD103 was expressed by 9% to 10% of the OT-1 cells in mesenteric lymph nodes (MLN) 3 and 4 d after activation, and 2% of the OT-1 cells 6 d after activation. CD103 was expressed by 36% of the OT-1 cells that had entered the intestinal epithelium at day 3. However, by day 4, CD103 expression had increased to 90%, and levels remained high at day 6.

CCL25 Enhances CD103-Mediated Adhesion of IEL to E-Cadherin-Fc

Next, we examined the ability of CCL25 to regulate CD103-mediated adhesion to its epithelial ligand E-cadherin. For this purpose, we constructed a murine E-cadherin human Fc fusion protein (mE-Fc). Adhesion of IEL to mE-Fc was efficiently blocked by anti-CD103 antibody, but not by cell-binding control antibody (data not shown). Furthermore, CCL25, but not CCL20, whose receptor CCR6 is not expressed by IEL, enhanced IEL adhesion to E-cadherin (FIG. 2).

REFERENCES

1. WURBEL, M.A., J.M. PHILIPPE, C. NGUYEN, et al. 2000. The chemokine TECK is expressed by thymic and intestinal epithelial cells and attracts double- and single-positive thymocytes expressing the TECK receptor CCR9. Eur. J. Immunol. **30:** 262–271.
2. ZABEL, B.A., W.W. AGACE, J.J. CAMPBELL, et al. 1999. Human G protein-coupled receptor GPR-9-6/CC chemokine receptor 9 is selectively expressed on intestinal homing T lymphocytes, mucosal lymphocytes, and thymocytes and is required for thymus-expressed chemokine-mediated chemotaxis. J. Exp. Med. **190:** 1241–1256.
3. SVENSSON, M., J. MARSAL, A. ERICSSON, et al. 2002. CCL25 mediates the localization of recently activated CD8alphabeta(+) lymphocytes to the small-intestinal mucosa. J. Clin. Invest. **110:** 1113–1121.
4. CEPEK, K.L., C.M. PARKER, J.L. MADARA, et al. 1993. Integrin alpha E beta 7 mediates adhesion of T lymphocytes to epithelial cells. J. Immunol. **150:** 3459–3470.
5. SCHON, M.P., A. ARYA, E.A. MURPHY, et al. 1999. Mucosal T lymphocyte numbers are selectively reduced in integrin alpha E (CD103)-deficient mice. J. Immunol. **162:** 6641–6649.
6. PENNEY, L., P.J. KILSHAW & T.T. MACDONALD. 1995. Regional variation in the proliferative rate and lifespan of alpha beta TCR+ and gamma delta TCR+ intraepithelial lymphocytes in the murine small intestine. Immunology **86:** 212–218.

Bacterial Translocation in the Normal Human Appendix Parallels the Development of the Local Immune System

JAN-OLAF GEBBERS[a] AND JEAN-ALBERT LAISSUE[b]

[a]*Institute of Pathology, Kantonsspital, Luzern, Switzerland*
[b]*Institute of Pathology, University of Bern, Switzerland*

ABSTRACT: Experimental modes and pathological conditions may result in bacterial translocation (BT), that is, the passage of indigenous bacteria colonizing the intestine through the intestinal mucosa to mesenteric lymph nodes. Yet no data are available on BT in the normal human gut. We determined the occurrence of BT and its extent in histologically normal, incidentally removed human vermiform appendices (VA) from individuals of different ages and correlated the findings with the development with age of associated lymphatic tissue. BT appears to pertain to normal antigen-sampling processes of the GALT in the VA. It also parallels the development of the GALT and its maintenance during adulthood. In the first two weeks after birth, when bacterial colonization of the gut evolves and when the VA lacks the protection of secretory IgA, BT was not detected. Thereafter, BT occurs along with development of the local GALT, which is fully built up after the first year. A physiological uptake of, or invasion by, bacteria may be instrumental (1) for tolerance induction against the indigenous flora and (2) for the stimulation and normal development of the GALT.

KEYWORDS: bacterial translocation; human vermiform appendix; GALT; postnatal development

INTRODUCTION

Bacterial translocation (BT), defined as the passage of both viable and nonviable microbes and microbial products of the flora across the intestinal mucosal barrier,[1,2] may be instrumental in the induction of the development of the gut-associated lymphoid tissue (GALT) as well as in the induction of tolerance against indigenous flora, particularly in the newborn. However, it has not been established whether BT occurs in the normal human gut or not.

Few quantitative data are available on the postnatal development of the GALT[3] and its maintenance during life. Immunologic protection, primarily by secretory IgA, seems to be insufficient for a variable period after birth.[4,5] However, there is little clinical evidence concerning age-related alterations in mucosal immunity.[6]

Address for correspondence: Jan-Olaf Gebbers, M.D., Institute of Pathology, Kantonsspital, CH-6000 Luzern 16, Switzerland. Voice: +41-41-205-3470; fax: +41-41-205-3496.
janolaf.gebbers@ksl.ch

To understand the association between postnatal microbial colonization of the intestine and the development of the human GALT we tried to determine in normal vermiform appendices (VA) from individuals of different ages (1) the postnatal occurrence of BT; (2) the postnatal development of the lymphoid tissue and the time of appearance of plasma cells containing immunoglobulins (Ig); (3) the distribution of Ig classes in mucosal plasma cells; and (4) the size of the organ and the amount of lymphoid tissue during adult life.

MATERIALS AND METHODS

We studied postnatal human VA removed incidentally, without histologic signs of active inflammation or luminal obliteration. Newborn and infant VA were all from breast-fed children. We examined 33 VA from individuals of different ages (1 d to 54 years) by electron microscopy to detect bacteria. Mucosal samples of the proximal, middle, and distal part of the organ were processed. Bacterial structures were counted per electron microscopic field in at least 250 fields per sample. Further, in 203 uninflamed VA from individuals ages 1 d to 89 years, weight, volume, length, and diameter were determined. In histologic cross sections of the proximal, middle, and distal parts of the VA, number and size of the lymphatic follicles and germinal centers were assessed; the mucosal areas were measured. In serial histologic sections, plasma cells stained by the peroxidase-antiperoxidase (PAP) method for IgA, IgG, IgM, and IgE were counted in the mucosa.

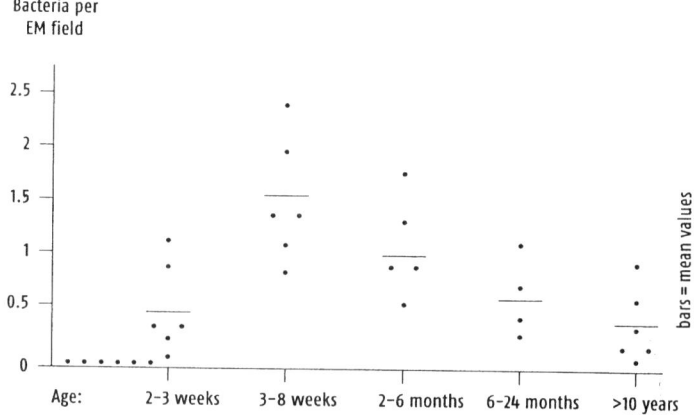

FIGURE 1. Semiquantitative evaluation by electron microscopy of the bacterial translocation in the human vermiform appendix versus age. Horizontal bars indicate mean numbers. Electron microscopy, $n=33$.

RESULTS

Free bacterial structures within the mucosa of VA were not detected in the first two weeks after birth (6 VA), but were constantly present in persons older than two weeks; increased in number between the third and eighth postnatal week; decreased after 2 to 24 months; and were seen almost constantly in low numbers in adults (FIG. 1). Bacteria were located beneath the follicle-associated epithelium, within follicles, in the epithelium, and in lymphatics (FIG. 2).

Median and mean values of the morphometric parameters were almost identical. In the first year after birth, the elongation rate of the VA exceeded the increase in

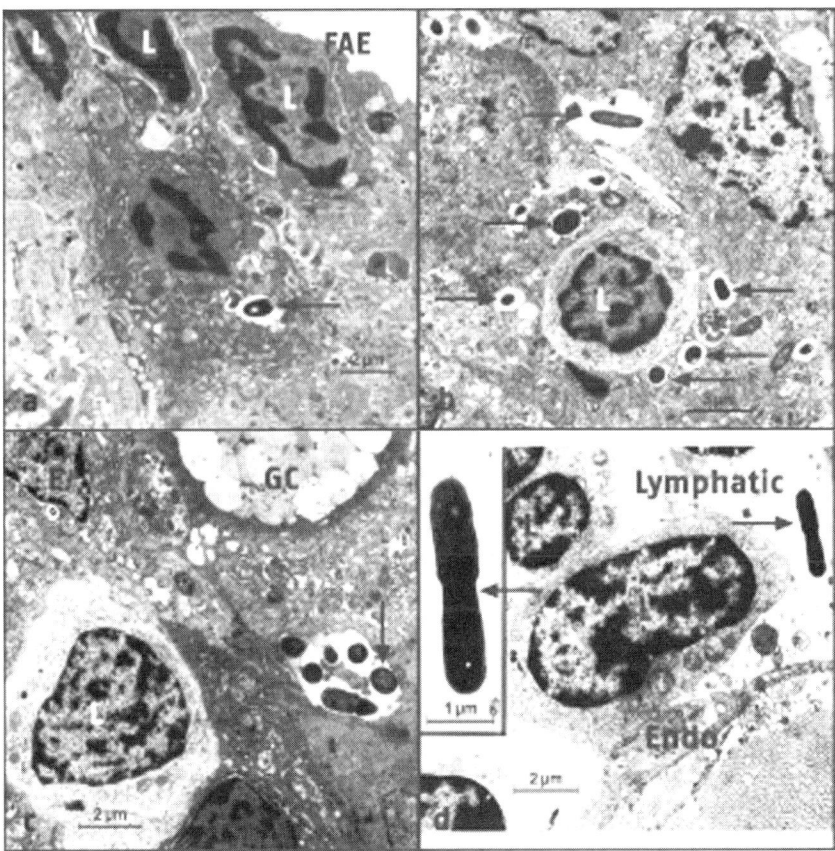

FIGURE 2. Electron micrographs of bacterial structures in the uninflamed human vermiform appendix. (**a**) Bacterium (*arrow*) beneath the follicle-associated epithelium (FAE); 14-day-old VA (L, lymphocyte). (**b**) Free bacteria (*arrows*) in a lymphatic follicle; 25-day-old VA (L, lymphocyte). (**c**) Intraepithelial bacteria (*arrow*); 36-year-old VA (E, enterocyte; GC, goblet cell; L, lymphocyte). (**d**) Bacterium (*arrows*) in a lymphatic, 6-month-old VA (L, lymphocyte; Endo; endothelium).

volume; length and volume reached maximum values in the first decade and remained constant during adult life; there was no decrease in volume in old age.

The mucosal area increased rapidly, reached a maximum during the first year, and remained constant thereafter, even in old persons.

Very few small lymphatic follicles were present in the VA of the newborn (FIGS. 3 and 4). Germinal centers did not appear until the fourth week after birth. Thereafter, number and size of both structures increased in parallel, reached a peak in the second decade, and decreased rapidly in the third decade and slowly after the fifth decade (FIGS. 3 and 4).

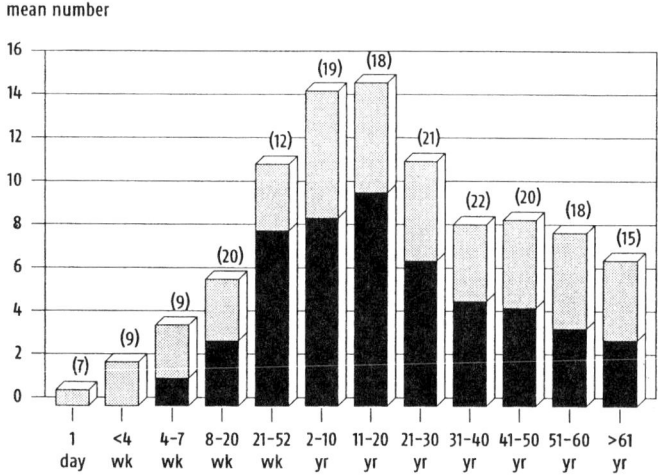

FIGURE 3. Number of germinal centers (*black box*) and lymphatic follicles (*gray box*) in vermiform appendix versus age. $n = 199$.

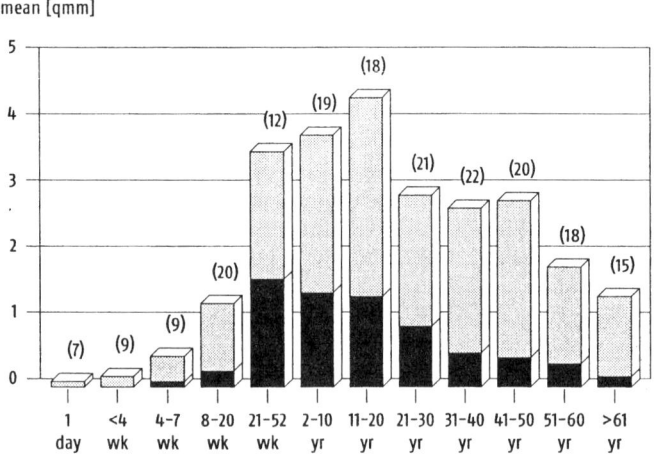

FIGURE 4. Areas of germinal centers (*black box*) and lymphatic follicles (*gray box*) in vermiform appendix versus age. $n = 190$.

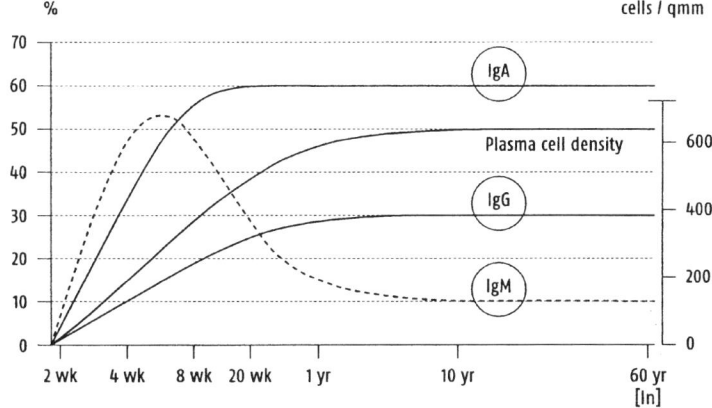

FIGURE 5. Mucosal plasma cell density and immunoglobulin classes of the vermiform appendix versus age. $n=82$.

Few plasma cells were present during the first months after birth (FIG. 5). The highest plasma cell numbers were measured in the first decade. After a decrease in the second decade, their number remained almost constant until old age. In the VA of the newborn, we did not observe cells containing Ig, but the secretory component of IgA was already detectable in the epithelium. The first plasma cells appeared two weeks after birth. After four weeks, there was a marked increase in IgA and IgM cells. Twenty weeks after birth, the number of IgA cells reached a maximum value that changed little until old age (FIG. 5). Two months after birth, IgM and IgG cell number showed an inverse relationship until old age: the IgM cell population decreased while the number of IgG cells increased (FIG. 5). The IgE cell number was low (1 to 2%) in all age groups with a small peak during the first two weeks after birth.

DISCUSSION

Some authors describe BT as a spontaneous event in humans,[1,2,7–9] whereas others attribute BT exclusively to pathological conditions.[10] In our study, BT appears to pertain to normal antigen-sampling processes of the appendiceal GALT throughout life. However, we could not demonstrate BT before the second week after birth, although bacterial colonization of the human newborn intestinal tract begins immediately after birth and lasts throughout the first year of life.[5,11] Particulate antigens are known to be absorbed through M cells of the follicle-associated epithelium[12,13] (FIG. 2a). As BT parallels the postnatal development of the appendiceal GALT, it can be assumed that bacterial uptake occurs only upon the development of the lymphatic follicles, two weeks after birth (FIGS. 3 and 4). BT in newborn rabbits depends on small bowel colonization[8] and peaks as early as six days after birth; maturity of the GALT results in a loss of BT.[9] The types of bacteria colonizing the intestine of newborns and the timing of colonization may determine the immunomodulation of the naive immune system.[5]

It is evident that for the first two weeks after birth, the VA lacks mature plasma cells and secretory IgA. Thereafter, there is a rapid numerical rise and a predominance of IgM-containing cells, complete by the age of one to two months. This finding is in keeping with observations that young infants respond to mucosal stimuli with IgM class antibodies that may compensate for the relative absence of IgA in early life.[5] The rise in IgA-containing cells is much slower and lasts up to five months. Thereafter, the IgA-cell population remains constant and predominant until old age (FIG. 5). In humans, the immune barrier in the intestine is provided by secretory immunoglobulins, mainly IgA, and IgM.[12] Our results show that the human intestine lacks this system in the first two weeks after birth. This deficiency in secretory immunoglobulins is probably the most important factor in the high permeability of the neonatal intestine.[5,14] The high proportion of IgG plasma cells (30 %) in the VA has also been found in Peyer's patches of rats, mice, and humans. The high local production of IgG differs markedly from the much lower values observed in the other gut mucosa. This difference can be ascribed to preferential accumulation of IgG immunocytes adjacent to the many lymphatic follicles in the VA. Presumably, these immunocytes represent follicle-derived B cells that have reached terminal maturation locally.[15]

There appears to be no decrease in size of the normal VA and only little involution of lymphoid tissue with age. Nor does the average number of solitary lymphatic follicles in the intestine of humans obviously decrease in old age.[16] Most experimental studies on gastrointestinal immunity failed to detect an age-related decline in immunoglobulin titers in the gut lumen.[17–20]

REFERENCES

1. WELLS, C.L., M.A. MADDAUS & R.L. SIMMONS. 1988. Proposed mechanisms for the translocation of intestinal bacteria. Rev. Infect. Dis. **10:** 958–979.
2. ALEXANDER, J.W., S.T. BOYCE, G.F. BABCOCK, et al. 1990. The process of microbial translocation. Ann. Surg. **212:** 496–512.
3. MACDONALD, T.T. (ed.) 1990. Ontogeny of the Immune System of the Gut. CRC Press, Inc. Boca Raton.
4. MACDONALD, T.T. 1994. Development of mucosal immune function in man: potential for GI disease states. Acta Paediatr. Jpn. **36:** 532–536.
5. GRÖNLUND, M.-M., H. ARVILOMMI, P. KERO, et al. 2000. Importance of intestinal colonisation in the maturation of humoral immunity in early infancy: a prospective follow up study of healthy infants aged 0-6 months. Arch. Dis. Child. Fetal Neonatal. Ed. **83:** F186–F192.
6. SCHMUCKER, D. & C. DANIELS. 1985. Aging, gastrointestinal infections and mucosal immunity. J. Am. Geriatr. Soc. **34:** 377–385.
7. SEDMAN, P.C., J. MACFIE, P. SAGAR, et al. 1994. The prevalence of gut translocation in humans. Gastroenterology **107:** 643–649.
8. URAO, M., J. MOY, J. VAN CAMP, et al. 1995. Determinant of bacterial translocation in the newborn: small bowel versus large bowel colonization. J. Pediatr. Surg. **30:** 831–836.
9. URAO, M., D.H. TEITELBAUM, R.A. DRONGOWSKI & A.G. CORAN. 1996. The association of gut-associated lymphoid tissue and bacterial translocation in the newborn rabbit. J. Pediatr. Surg. **31:** 1482–1487.
10. BERG, R.D. 2002. Promotion or inhibition of bacterial translocation from the GI tract by bacterial components. In Host-microflora interactions in the first years after birth. P. J. Heidt et al., Eds.: 73–85. Herborn Litterae. Herborn-Dill, Germany.

11. ROLFE, R.D. 2002. The development of the colonisation resistance in the infant. *In* Host-microflora interactions in the first years after birth. P.J. Heidt *et al.*, Eds.: 41–60. Herborn Litterae. Herborn-Dill, Germany.
12. BRANDTZAEG, P. 1996. History of oral tolerance and mucosal immunity. Ann. N.Y. Acad. Sci. **778:** 1–27.
13. NEUTRA, M.R., N.J. MANTIS & J.-P. KRÄHENBÜHL. 2001. Collaboration of epithelial cells with organized mucosal lymphoid tissues. Nat. Immunol. **2:** 1004–1009.
14. TAYLOR, B., A.P. NORMAN, H.A. ORGEL, *et al.* 1973. Transient IgA deficiency and pathogenesis of infant atopy. Lancet **2:** 111–113.
15. BJERKE, K., P. BRANDTZAEG & T.O. ROGNUM. 1986. Distribution of immunoglobulin producing cells is different in normal human appendix and colon mucosa. Gut **27:** 667–674.
16. DUKES, C. & H.J.R. BUSSEY. 1926. The number of lymphoid follicles of the human large intestine. J. Pathol. Bacteriol. **19:** 11–16.
17. EBERSOLE, J., D. SMITH & M. TAUBMAN. 1985. Secretory immune response in aging rats. I. Immunoglobulin levels. Immunology **56:** 345–351.
18. KAWANISHI, H. & J. KIELY. 1985. The effect of aging on murine gut-associated lymphoid tissue. Gastroenterology **88:** 1440 (abstract).
19. SENDA, S., E. CHENG & H. KAWANISHI. 1986. Aging-associated changes in murine intestinal immunoglobulin secretes. Gastroenterology **90:** 1626–1631.
20. LIM, T., N. MESSIHA & R. WATSON. 1981. Immune components of the intestinal mucosa of aging and protein deficient mice. Immunology **43:** 401–408.

Hyporesponsiveness of CD4 T Cells Induced in Oral Tolerance Is Maintained by Selective Impairment in the TCR-Induced Calcium/NFAT Signaling Pathway Resulting from Caspase Activation

SATOSHI HACHIMURA,[a] TOMOHIRO KAJI,[a] KAZUMI ASAI,[a] WATARU ISE,[a] TOSHINORI NAKAYAMA,[b] AND SHUICHI KAMINOGAWA[a,c]

[a]*Department of Applied Biological Chemistry, University of Tokyo, Tokyo, Japan*

[b]*Department of Medical Immunology and Molecular Immunology, Graduate School of Medicine, Chiba University, Chiba, Japan*

[c]*Department of Food Science and Technology, Nihon University, Kanagawa, Japan*

ABSTRACT: We examined intracellular signaling of hyporesponsive CD4 T cells induced by continuous feeding with high-dose antigen in a TCR transgenic mouse system. The results demonstrated a selective impairment in their TCR-induced calcium/NFAT-signaling pathway. Proteomic analysis revealed caspase activation in these cells, which resulted in cleavage of GADS. Further analysis of the TCR-signaling complex showed that GADS-LAT-SLP-76-associated PLC-γ1 was decreased in both phosphorylation and association. Thus, as a consequence of caspase activation, orally tolerant CD4 T cells could not form normal TCR signaling complexes associated with GADS and showed downregulated PLC-γ1 activation, which resulted in impairment of TCR-induced calcium signaling.

KEYWORDS: CD4 T cells; caspase activation; TCR-transgenic mice

The molecular mechanisms of oral tolerance have been poorly defined. We investigated the molecular basis underlying the hyporesponsiveness of orally tolerant CD4 T cells using a TCR transgenic mouse system in which oral tolerance was induced by long-term feeding with high-dose antigen.[1,2]

OVA-specific TCR-transgenic mice (OVA 23-3; Ref. 3) were fed a 20% egg-white diet for four weeks to obtain orally tolerant splenic CD4 T cells. These CD4 T cells exhibited reduced proliferation and reduced IL-2, IL-4, and IFN-γ cytokine production when stimulated with OVA + APC *in vitro*. We analyzed the TCR-mediated signaling pathway in these orally tolerant CD4 T cells.[1] We found (1) impaired phosphorylation of TCR-ζ, ZAP-70, LAT, and phospholipase C-γ1 (PLCγ-1); (2) impaired calcium responses and decreased NFAT nuclear translocation; and (3)

Address for correspondence: Satoshi Hachimura, Department of Applied Biological Chemistry, Graduate School of Agricultural and Life Sciences, The University of Tokyo, 1-1-1 Yayoi, Bunkyo-ku, Tokyo 113-8657, Japan. Voice: +81-3-5841-5137; f ax: +81-3-5841-8029.
  ahachi@mail.ecc.u-tokyo.ac.jp

normal activation of ERK and SAPK (MAPK pathway). These results suggest that the hyporesponsive state of the CD4 T cells was maintained by a selective impairment in the TCR-induced calcium/NFAT signaling pathway.

We further used two-dimensional electrophoresis to compare intracellular protein expression patterns of orally tolerant and unsensitized CD4 T cells.[2] Twenty-six increased and 16 decreased protein spots were detected, and 35 of these were identified by mass spectrometry. The results indicate that the expression of caspases was upregulated and that the protein levels of intact proteins susceptible to caspase cleavage, such as Grb2-related adaptor downstream of Shc (GADS),[4] were decreased in orally tolerant CD4 T cells. Western blotting confirmed that expression of the active form of caspase-3 was upregulated in orally tolerant CD4 T cells. Nevertheless, these CD4 T cells were found to be nonapoptotic as demonstrated by annexin V staining and DNA fragmentation analysis. Furthermore, these cells were found to express the antiapoptotic factor, X-linked inhibitor of apoptosis (XIAP), which may contribute to their survival.

We hypothesized that the degradation of GADS contributed to the impairment in TCR-induced signaling in the orally tolerant CD4 T cells. First, the formation of cleaved GADS was confirmed by Western blotting. Furthermore, GADS-associated molecules were analyzed by immunoprecipitation with anti-GADS antibody. It was demonstrated that GADS-associated SLP-76 and GADS-LAT-SLP-76-associated PLC-γ1 were decreased in both phosphorylation and association in orally tolerant CD4 T cells. The results demonstrate that orally tolerant CD4 T cells could not form normal TCR signaling complexes associated with GADS and showed downregulated PLC-γ1 activation, which are likely to contribute to the impairment of TCR-induced calcium signaling.

Taken together, our results indicate that orally tolerant CD4 T cells upregulate caspase activation with decreased levels of caspase-targeted proteins, including TCR signaling-associated molecules, while upregulating antiapoptotic factors, all of which appear to contribute to their unique tolerant characteristics. As a consequence of caspase activation, orally tolerant CD4 T cells could not form normal TCR signaling complexes associated with GADS and showed downregulated PLC-γ1 activation, which appears to result in impairment of TCR-induced calcium signaling. Our findings provide new insights concerning the molecular mechanisms of T cell hyporesponsiveness in oral tolerance.

REFERENCES

1. ASAI, K., S. HACHIMURA, M. KIMURA, et al. 2002. T cell hyporesponsiveness induced by oral administration of ovalbumin is associated with impaired NFAT nuclear translocation and p27^{kip1} degradation. J. Immunol. **169:** 4723–4731.
2. KAJI, T., S. HACHIMURA, W. ISE & S. KAMINOGAWA. 2003. Proteome analysis reveals caspase activation in hyporesponsive CD4 T lymphocytes induced *in vivo* by the oral administration of antigen. J. Biol. Chem. **278:** 27836–27843.
3. SATO, T., T. SASAHARA, Y. NAKAMURA, et al. 1994. Naive T cells can mediate delayed-type hypersensitivity response in T cell receptor transgenic mice. Eur. J. Immunol. **24:** 1512–1516.
4. BERRY, D.M., S.J. BENN, A.M. CHENG, & C.J. MCGLADE. 2001. Caspase-dependent cleavage of the hematopoietic specific adaptor protein Gads alters signaling from the T cell receptor. Oncogene **20:** 1203–1211.

The Presentation of Haptenated Proteins and Activation of T Cells in the Mesenteric Lymph Nodes by Dendritic Cells in the TNBS Colitis Rat

YOH ISHIGURO, HIROTAKE SAKURABA, KAZUFUMI YAMAGATA, AND AKIHIRO MUNAKATA

First Department of Internal Medicine, Hirosaki University School of Medicine, Hirosaki University School of Medicine, Hirosaki, Japan

ABSTRACT: We described the role of dendritic cells (DCs) in aspects of T cell activation at the mesenteric lymph nodes (MLN) in trinitrobenzene sulfonic acid (TNBS)–induced colitis. An antigenic-immune response is induced at the MLN, and dendritic cells are the affected cell type. Cross-linking and GRO/CINC-1 have synergistic effects for DC maturation.

KEYWORDS: cytokine; Th1; inflammatory bowel disease; antigen-presenting cell; function chemokine

INTRODUCTION

The dendritic cell (DC) is central to induction of the antigen (Ag)-driven immune response.[1] Recent reports have highlighted the importance of activated innate immunity that is required for induction of the Th1 response.[2] In this mechanism, polarization occurs in regional lymph nodes of various local induction sites, such as the stomach, lung, and skin.[3] It has been well established that interleukin (IL)-12/IL-23 induce polarization of Th1-type T cells,[4,5] and that in conjunction with this, DC maturation is also important for polarizing the T cell phenotype. It has been reported that DCs stimulated with interferon (IFN)-γ and LPS induce the Th1 response at the initial step, while with maturation of DCs, T cells polarize into TGF-β–producing cells.[6]

ANTIGEN-DRIVEN IMMUNE RESPONSE IN REGIONAL LYMPH NODES IN TNBS COLITIS

We have described the role of DCs in certain aspects of T cell activation in the mesenteric lymph nodes (MLN) in trinitrobenzene sulfonic acid (TNBS)–induced

---

Address for correspondence: Y. Ishiguro, First Department of Internal medicine, Hirosaki University School of Medicine, 5 zaifu-cho, Hirosaki, Japan. Voice: +81-172-39-5053; fax: +81-172-32-5529.
 yishi-hki@umin.ac.jp

colitis, and have also assessed the regulatory mechanism of DC maturation in the context of T cell polarization, as TNBS colitis is a well-characterized Th1-mediated model.

In the OX-62–positive DC fraction of MLN, IL-2 production was enhanced in a dose-dependent manner by bovine serum albumin (BSA) coupled with TNBS, whereas in the OX-62–depleted fraction this enhancement was not apparent. The same antigen (BSA-TNBS) also resulted in elevated IL-12 production, and IL-12 transcripts were present in purified OX-62 cells, whereas analysis of the negative fraction of OX-62 cells showed IL-2, IL-10, and IFN-γ transcripts. The presence of either the foreign haptenated antigen or the autologous haptenated antigen enhanced IL-2 production.

DENDRITIC CELL MATURATION

From our findings, it was suggested that an antigenic immune response is induced at the MLN in hapten-induced colitis and that dendritic cells are the cell type affected. Haptenated macromolecules are likely to induce cross-reactivity. However, the triggers that stimulate DC maturation in T cell polarization are still enigmatic. We assessed the effect of growth-related oncogene/cytokine-induced neutrophil chemoattractant (GRO/CINC-1) on MLN DC maturation, and found that in the presence of TNBS, GRO/CINC-1 enhanced the expression of costimulatory molecules on DC, suggesting that cross-linking and GRO/CINC-1 have a synergistic effect on DC maturation. Further study will be needed to elucidate the mechanism underlying DC maturation and the role of highly expressed costimulatory molecules on dendritic cells.

REFERENCES

1. LANZAVECCHIA, A. & F. SALLUSTO. 2001. Regulation of T cell immunity by dendritic cells. Cell **106:** 263–266.
2. ITO, T., R. AMAKAWA, T. KAISHO, *et al.* 2002. Interferon-alpha and interleukin-12 are induced differentially by Toll-like receptor 7 ligands in human blood dendritic cell subsets. J. Exp. Med. **195:** 1507–1512.
3. SALLUSTO, F. 2001. Origin and migratory properties of dendritic cells in the skin. Curr. Opin. Allergy Clin. Immunol. **1:** 441–448.
4. OPPMANN, B., R. LESLEY, B. BLOM, *et al.* 2000. Novel p19 protein engages IL-12p40 to form a cytokine, IL-23, with biological activities similar as well as distinct from IL-12. Immunity **13:** 715–725.
5. NEURATH, M.F., B. WEIGMANN, S. FINOTTO, *et al.* 2002. The transcription factor T-bet regulates mucosal T cell activation in experimental colitis and Crohn's disease. J. Exp. Med. **195:** 1129–1143.
6. LANGENKAMP, A., M. MESSI, A. LANZAVECCHIA, *et al.* 2000. Kinetics of dendritic cell activation: impact on priming of TH1, TH2 and nonpolarized T cells. Nat. Immunol. **1:** 311–316.

Macrophage Migration Inhibitory Factor and Activator Protein-1 in Ulcerative Colitis

YOH ISHIGURO,[a] KAZUFUMI YAMAGATA,[a] HIROTAKE SAKURABA,[a] AKIHIRO MUNAKATA,[a] AKIO NAKANE,[b] TAKAYUKI MORITA,[c] AND JUN NISHIHIRA[d]

[a]*First Department of Internal Medicine,* [b]*Department of Bacteriology,*
[c]*Second Department of Surgery, Hirosaki University School of Medicine, Hirosaki, Japan*

[d]*Department of Molecular Chemistry, Hokkaido University of Graduate School of Medicine, Sapporo, Japan*

ABSTRACT: Macrophage migration inhibitory factor (MIF) is a cytokine that has potent antisteroid effects. We determined that MIF is involved in the glucocorticoid-resistant inflammatory process of ulcerative colitis (UC), and the altered AP-1 signal is a potent therapeutic target for refractory UC.

KEYWORDS: glucocorticoids; inflammatory bowel disease; transcriptional factors

INTRODUCTION

There are several transcriptional factors that exacerbate steroid resistance in the inflammatory process, such as RelA, c-Jun of activator protein (AP)-1 transcriptional factor. Glucocorticoid receptor (GR) is reported to exert its activity through binding to the cytoplasmic GR, and the complex translocates into the nucleus. In the nucleus, this binds to a specific palindromic DNA sequence in the promoter region of several genes (glucocorticoid response elements (GREs) and negative GREs), thus regulating the respective transcriptional gene activity. More recently, it has been shown that GR can also modulate proinflammatory activity through another pathway without binding to GREs and negative GREs.[1,2] In these states, AP-1 is an established interference transcriptional factor of GR through direct protein–protein interaction.

MACROPHAGE MIGRATION INHIBITORY FACTOR IN THE PROINFLAMMATORY CASCADE

Macrophage migration inhibitory factor (MIF) is a cytokine that also has potent antisteroid effects in LPS-induced lung and hepatic injury models. Its pivotal role in human chronic inflammatory diseases such as rheumatoid arthritis[3] and Crohn's disease[4] has also been clarified. However, a recent report has highlighted its antagonistic effect on AP-1 activation[5] and this mechanism appeared to conflict with the activation pathway of matrix metalloproteinases in synovial fibroblasts.[3] In addition, Bucala[6] has advocated the hypothesis that MIF signaling is mediated through two distinct pathways: phagocytosis and receptor-dependent signaling.

Furthermore, the promoter region of human MIF has specific binding sites for AP-1, GRE, and NF-κB. The role of MIF in ulcerative colitis (UC), especially refractory cases, and its relationship to these transcriptional factors has not been well defined.

MIF AND TRANSCRIPTIONAL FACTORS IN UC

We determined the amount of MIF in tissue samples from glucocorticoid (GC)-unresponsive UC and simultaneously evaluated the DNA-binding of phospho-RelA.

MIF was reduced in the cytoplasmic fraction of lamina propria mononuclear cells (LPMCs) from UC compared with normal controls. AP-1 levels were also higher in the nuclear fraction of LPMCs from UC, whereas the levels of RelA were lower than in the controls. Anti-MIF antibody ameliorated GC-resistant interleukin-8 production in LPMCs from the UC patients.

These results suggest that MIF is involved in the GC-refractory inflammatory process of UC. MIF and the altered AP-1 signal are potent therapeutic targets for patients with refractory ulcerative colitis.

REFERENCES

1. BELVISI, M.G., S.L. WICKS, C.H. BATTRAM, et al. 2001. Therapeutic benefit of a dissociated glucocorticoid and the relevance of in vitro separation of transrepression from transactivation activity. J. Immunol. **166:** 1975–1982.
2. GONZALEZ, M.V., B. JIMENEZ, M.T. BERCIANO, et al. 2000. Glucocorticoids antagonize AP-1 by inhibiting the activation /phosphorylation of JNK without affecting its subcellular distribution. J. Cell Biology **150:** 1199–208. .
3. ONODERA, S., K. KANEDA, Y. MIZUE, et al. 2000. Macrophage migration inhibitory factor up-regulates expression of matrix metalloproteinases in synovial fibroblasts of rheumatoid arthritis. J. Biol. Chem. **275:** 444–450.
4. DE JONG, Y.P., A.C. ABADIA-MOLINA, A.R. SATOSKAR, et al. 2001. Development of chronic colitis is dependent on the cytokine MIF. Nat. Immunol. **2:** 1061–1066.
5. KLEEMANN, R., A. HAUSSER, G. GEIGER, et al. 2000. Intracellular action of the cytokine MIF to modulate AP-1 activity and the cell cycle through Jab1. Nature **408:** 211–216.
6. BUCALA, R. 2000. Signal transduction. A most interesting factor. Nature **408:** 146–147.

Genetic Selection for Resistance or Susceptibility to Oral Tolerance to Ovalbumin Affects General Mechanisms of Tolerance Induction in Mice

ALICE O. KAMPHORST,[a] MARIA F. S. DA SILVA,[b] ANTÔNIO C. DA SILVA,[b] CLAUDIA R. CARVALHO,[c] AND ANA MARIA C. FARIA[a]

[a]*Departamento de Bioquímica e Imunologia ICB-UFMG, Brazil*
[b]*Departamento de Biologia Celular e Genética, IB-UERJ, Brazil*
[c]*Departamento de Morfologia, ICB-UFMG, Brazil*

ABSTRACT: To study the genes involved in oral tolerance susceptibility, two strains of mice were genetically selected for susceptibility (TS) and resistance (TR) to oral tolerance to ovalbumin by bidirectional breeding. Herein we show that the genetic selection process is restricted neither to ovalbumin nor to oral tolerance. It affected oral tolerance to other proteins, such as casein, and tolerance induced the intravenous route.

KEYWORDS: genetic selection; oral tolerance; immunoregulation; continuous feeding; TS mice; TR mice

INTRODUCTION

Two strains of mice were genetically selected for susceptibility (TS) or resistance (TR) to oral tolerance by genetic bidirectional breeding.[1] The protocol used for induction and selection of oral tolerance consisted of one gavage of 5 mg ovalbumin (OVA) followed by intraperitoneal (i.p.) immunization with OVA plus aluminum hydroxide ($Al(OH)_3$) and subsequent analysis of anti-OVA antibodies. The two selected strains have extreme phenotypes for anti-OVA antibody production: TS OVA-fed mice have drastic suppression of their serum anti-OVA antibody production, whereas feeding OVA to TR mice has no suppressive effects on their specific antibody response.

It has previously been reported that TR mice can be rendered tolerant to OVA for cellular immune responses, such as delayed-type hypersensitivity (DTH), in spite of their resistance to induction of tolerance for antibody response.[2] Therefore, their resistance to oral tolerance induction is not absolute, as they can still be orally tolerized to cellular responses, which are known to be more easily suppressed.[3]

Address for correspondence: Ana Maria C. Faria, Laboratório de Imunobiologia, Departamento de Bioquímica e Imunologia, ICB-UFMG, Av. Antônio Carlos, 6627 Pampulha, Belo Horizonte–MG Brazil, CEP: 31270-901 Caixa Postal 486. Voice/fax: +55-31 3499-2640.
afaria@icb.ufmg.br

It is well established that the antigen dose and frequency of oral exposure interferes with induction of oral tolerance.[3] Continuous feeding of antigen is more effective in inducing oral tolerance, being able to tolerize otherwise refractory aged mice and to upregulate the production of TGF-/IL-10.[3–5]

Therefore, the aim of this study was to test oral induction of tolerance in TS and TR strains under different feeding protocols (continuous oral exposure and higher doses) and to learn whether the extreme phenotypes observed for OVA feeding were also detectable for other proteins.

MATERIALS AND METHODS

Mice

Two- to three-month-old mice of both sexes from an F_{18} generation of the susceptible (TS) and resistant (TR) strains were used. In some experiments, we also used B6D2F1 mice as a control strain that was not genetically selected for oral tolerance induction.

Antigens

Ovalbumin (OVA) and casein (Cas) were purchased from Sigma Chemical Co., St. Louis, MO, USA. The casein-containing diet was purchased from Rhoster Indústria e Comércio LTDA, SP, Brazil.

Oral Tolerance Induction

Mice received either 5 or 20 mg OVA by gavage or diluted in the drinking water (continuous feeding). To induce oral tolerance to casein, mice were fed a diet containing 15% casein for three days (1.5 g/mice).

Intravenous Tolerance Induction

Mice were injected intravenously with 2 mg soluble OVA in 0.2 mL saline seven days before immunization.

Immunization Protocol

Seven days after the tolerance induction protocols, mice were immunized with 10 μg OVA in 3 mg of intraperitoneal $Al(OH)_3$. After two weeks, they received a booster of 10 μg OVA i.p.; serum was collected seven days thereafter. In the experiments with casein, mice were immunized with 100 μg casein in alum and boosted with 100 μg casein.

Antibody Analysis

Serum antibody production was assessed by ELISA (FIGS. 1 and 2). ELISA scores are shown by bars that represent the mean value of the running sums of optical densities between 1/100 and 1/6,400 serum dilutions for each individual mouse.

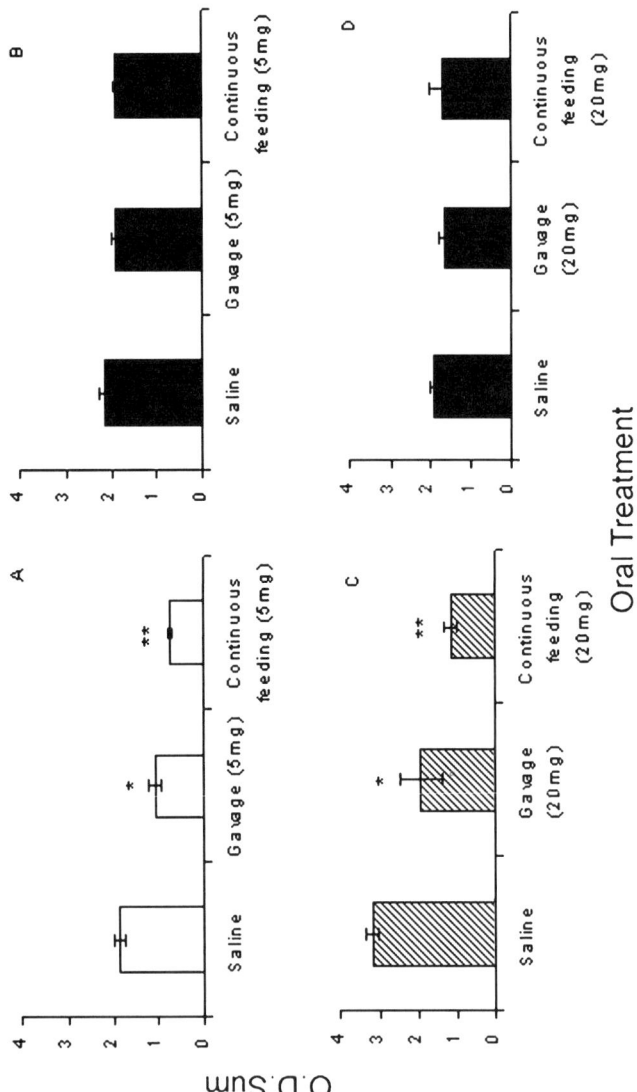

FIGURE 1. Anti-OVA antibody production in TS (*open bars*), TR (*filled bars*), and B6D2F1 (*hatched bars*) mice. Mice received an oral treatment consisting of saline or either 5 mg or 20 mg (**A**, **B**) or 20 mg (**C**, **D**) of OVA by gavage or continuous feeding. They were immunized with OVA and Al(OH)$_3$ seven days later and after two weeks received an i.p. booster. Seven days thereafter they were bled for antibody measurement. n = 5–7 mice; *P<.05; **P<.01.

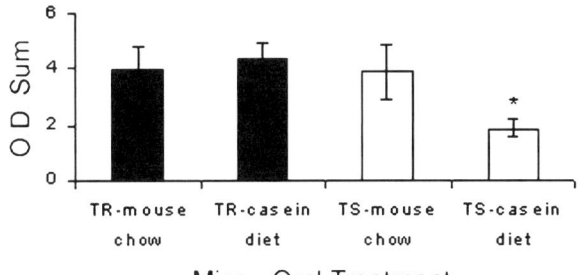

Mice - Oral Treatment

FIGURE 2. Anti-casein antibody production in TS (*open bars*) and TR (*filled bars*) mice. Mice were fed a casein-containing diet or regular mouse chow and were immunized with casein and $Al(OH)_3$ seven days after the last feeding regiment. They received an i.p. booster 2 weeks later and were bled seven days thereafter for antibody measurement. $n = 4$–6 mice; $*P < .05$.

Statistical Analysis

Differences in the ELISA scores among groups were determined by Kruskal Wallis and subsequently compared by Student's *t* test.

RESULTS AND DISCUSSION

Our results show that in TS mice continuous feeding is more effective than gavage in suppressing antibody production. However, this regimen is not able to render TR mice tolerant, not even when a dose of 20 mg OVA is administered (FIG. 1). These results indicate that the mouse strain TR generated by the genetic selection has a strong resistance to tolerance induction, not only for the conditions for which they were selected.

To confirm the robustness of their resistance to oral tolerance induction, we tested whether oral treatment with OVA would stabilize the production of anti-OVA antibodies in TR mice when given several i.p. boosters with OVA. Stabilization of specific antibody production is a phenomenon that was described by Verdolin *et al.*[6] as a usual consequence of feeding antigen even in conditions where tolerance cannot be detected. When OVA-fed TR mice received several OVA i.p. boosters, their anti-OVA antibody production increased to the same level as the control group that was fed only saline (data not shown). Therefore, feeding 5 mg OVA to TR mice is not even able to stabilize their antibody response. Conversely, TS mice maintained their low level of anti-OVA serum antibodies even after several boosters.

We also tested oral tolerance induction to casein and several other antigens in order to verify whether the genetic selection had affected oral tolerance to other antigens as well. Oral tolerance was induced to casein in TS but not in TR mice (FIG. 2). Similar results were also found with other tested antigens (data not shown).

To investigate whether the genetic selection had affected tolerance induced by other routes, we tested intravenous tolerance in TS and TR mice. Only TS mice became tolerant after intravenous injection of disaggregated OVA prior to immunization (TABLE 1).

TABLE 1. Anti-Ova IgG production in mice treated with OVA intravenously

Intravenous Administration	TR Mice (O.D. sum)	TS Mice (O.D. sum)
Saline	3.22 ± 1.23	3.09 ± 1.16
OVA	3.13 ± 1.17	1.37* ± 0.80

NOTE: Mice received an i.v. injection of either saline or soluble OVA and were i.p. immunized with OVA and Al(OH)$_3$ seven days later. After two weeks they received a booster. Serum was collected seven days thereafter and tested by ELISA for anti-OVA antibody production. Numbers represent the average of a running sum of serum dilutions SD. $n = 4–7$ mice; * $P < .05$.

These results suggest that the resistance features selected in TR mice are specific neither to OVA nor to oral administration, implying that the selection acted on general regulatory genes for tolerance induction. Experiments to determine the selected features in TR and TS mice that are responsible for their opposite phenotypes are ongoing. We are especially interested in studying OVA handling and presentation in the gut-associated lymphoid tissue. Preliminary experiments have shown that there are differences in intestinal absorption of orally administered OVA between the TR and TS mice. We believe that the information obtained with these two strains of mice will be very helpful in clarifying the mechanisms that operate in oral tolerance induction.

ACKNOWLEDGMENTS

The authors wish to thank Ms. Ilda Marsal and Frankcinéia Assis for their excellent technical assistance. CNPq and FAPEMIG, Brazil supported this work.

REFERENCES

1. DA SILVA, A.C., K.W. DE SOUZA, R.C. MACHADO, et al. 1998. Genetics of immunological tolerance: I. Bidirecional selective breeding of mice for oral tolerance. Res. Immunol. **149:** 151–161.
2. DA SILVA, M.F., S.C. DA COSTA, R.C. RIBEIRO, et al. 2001. Independent genetic control of B- and T-cell tolerance in strains of mouse selected for extreme phenotypes of oral tolerance. Scand. J Immunol. **53:** 148–154.
3. FARIA, A.M.C. & H.L. WEINER. 1999. Oral tolerance: mechanisms and therapeutic applications. Adv. Immunol. **73:** 153–264.
4. FARIA, A.M., S.M. FICKER, E. SPEZIALI, et al. 1998. Aging and immunoglobulin isotype patterns in oral tolerance. Braz. J. Med. Biol. Res. **31:** 35–48.
5. FARIA, A.M., R. MARON, S.M. FICKER, et al. 2003. Oral tolerance induced by continuous feeding: enhanced up-regulation of transforming growth factor-beta/interleukin-10 and suppression of experimental autoimmune encephalomyelitis. J. Autoimmun. **20:** 135–145.
6. VERDOLIN, B.A., S.M. FICKER, A.M. FARIA, et al. 2001. Stabilization of serum antibody responses triggered by initial mucosal contact with the antigen independently of oral tolerance induction. Braz. J. Med. Biol. Res. **34:** 211–209.

CD45 Knockout Mice, Diet, and Colitis

In the Absence of CD45, Colitis Follows Dietary Changes

MARÍA C. LÓPEZ[a] AND NICK HOLMES

Department of Pathology, University of Cambridge, Cambridge, CB2 1QP, United Kingdom

> ABSTRACT: Healthy CD45 KO mice show a Th2-type cytokine secretion profile in their small intestines. Dietary supplementation with human infant formula induced colitis and a shift toward a Th1-type profile, suggesting that diet can alter cytokine secretion.
>
> KEYWORDS: CD45KO mice; gut lymphocytes; intestinal intraepithelial lymphocyte cytokines

INTRODUCTION

CD45 is a transmembrane glycoprotein expressed by all cells of hemopoietic lineage. A CD45 knockout (KO) mouse was generated by targeting exon 9, which is common to all isoforms.[1] This mouse model has shown that CD45 expression is required for the full differentiation and maturation of both T cells and B cells. CD45 null mice are characterized by a diminished number of peripheral T cells.[1] Intestinal intraepithelial (IEL) T cells in the gut mucosa have a phenotypic and ontogenic origin different from peripheral T cells, as at least some subsets have an extrathymic origin.[2] Therefore, we studied whether gut T cells could develop in CD45 null mice. We observed a dramatic decrease in the percentage of $\alpha\beta TCR^+$ and $\gamma\delta TCR^+$ cells in the small intestine. In contrast, the percentage of natural killer (NK) cells was increased, but their phenotype was quite different from that in normal mice, as gut NK cells in CD45 KO mice had lost T cell markers.[3]

CD45 KO mice presented problems breeding; they had small litters with low weight. Taking into account that other mouse strains respond very well to supplementation with human infant formula, dietary changes were introduced to improve litter weight. After several weeks all mice with supplemented diets began to develop colitis. The presence of an infectious agent was ruled out. Supplementation was stopped and after one week on the previous unsupplemented diet, mice began to present less flatulent feces. We hypothesized that the combination of dietary changes and abnormal T- and NK-cell populations induced a different pattern of cytokine secretion.

Address for correspondence: María C. López, Ph.D., Center for Immunology and Microbial Disease, Albany Medical College, 47 New Scotland Ave. MC-151, Albany, NY 12208. Voice: 518-262-6263; fax: 518-262-6161.
  lopezma@mail.amc.edu

MATERIALS AND METHODS

To test our hypothesis, we sacrificed several mice, isolating small intestine IELs to study their cytokine secretion profile. The analysis was done using flow cytometry to estimate the percentage of cells producing specific cytokines[4] in normal and CD45 null IELs.

RESULTS

Data obtained in one experiment, one week after diet supplementation was stopped, indicated that there was an increase in the percentage of CD45 KO IELs producing IFN-γ, IL-2, and TNF-α when compared with normal mice (FIG. 1, top panel). In contrast, several experiments showed a consistent increase in the percentage of healthy CD45 KO IELs producing IL-4 (5 out of 5 experiments) and in the production of IFN-γ (3 out of 5 experiments) (FIG. 1, bottom panel).

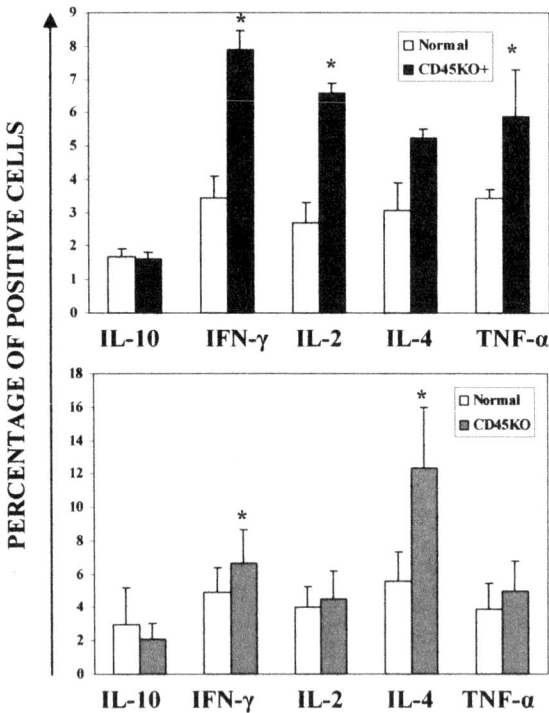

FIGURE 1. Small intestine IELs were isolated, cultured for 5 h in the presence of PMA/ionomycin and brefeldin A, fixed, permeabilized, stained with directly conjugated anti-mouse cytokine (IL-10, IFN-γ, IL-2, IL-4, and TNF-α) monoclonal antibodies, and analyzed in a FACScan to determine the percentage of cells producing each cytokine in normal, CD45 KO healthy, and CD45 KO[+] (postcolitis) mice.

CONCLUSION

Taking into account that in healthy CD45 KO mice it is mainly the percentage of IL-4 secreting cells that is increased, and that in CD45 KO mice recovering from colitis the percentage of IFNγ-, IL-2, and TNF-α–secreting cells was higher than in wild-type mice, we conclude that the introduction of dietary changes shifted the cytokine secretion profile toward an inflammatory profile. Therefore, we consider CD45 KO mice to be a suitable model for studying the relationship between abnormal T cell phenotype and induction of colitis resulting from dietary modifications.

REFERENCES

1. BYTH, K.F., L.A. CONROY, S. HOWLETT, et al. 1996. CD45-null transgenic mice reveal a positive regulatory role for CD45 in early thymocyte development, in the selection of $CD4^+CD8^+$ thymocytes, and in B-cell maturation. J. Exp. Med. **183:** 1707–1718.
2. GUY-GRAND, D. & P. VASSALLI. 2002. Gut intraepithelial lymphocyte development. Curr. Opin. Immunol. **14:** 255–259.
3. LOPEZ, M.C. & N. HOLMES. 2004. Phenotypical and functional alterations in the mucosal immune system of CD45 exon 9 KO mice. Int. Immunol. In press.
4. OPENSHAW, P.J.M., E.E. MURPHY, N.A. HOSKEN, et al. 1995. Heterogeneity of intracellular cytokine synthesis at the single-cell level in polarized T helper 1 and T helper 2 populations. J. Exp. Med. **182:** 1357–1367.

Noise and Microflora Behavior

MÁXIMO LORENZO,[a] PABLO SÁNCHEZ,[a] AND ENRIQUE REWALD[b]

[a]*Facultad de Ciencias Exactas y Naturales, Universidad Nacional de Mar del Plata, Mar del Plata, Argentina*

[b]*H. Yrigoyen 2184, 7600 Mar del Plata, Mar del Plata, Argentina*

ABSTRACT: Noise is ubiquitous, and in any discussion about regulation of immune diversity, oral tolerance, commensal microflora, and "health" homeostasis, stochastic resonance should not be omitted. It also may have a role in immune receptor regulation, transplant tolerance, and host reaction against intruders. It would be in line with nature's tendency to adapt to available network patterns.

KEYWORDS: noise; digestion; commensal flora; gene rearrangement; ambiguity

From the mixing of food during the process of digestion, an ample variety of antigens as well as microbes come in contact with or cross the mucosa of the gut, and may prime a systemic immune response and/or cause disease. Commensal flora are essential for our health and usually are not targeted by the host, although facultative pathogens are to be considered, and invaders in *sensu stricto* often are at hand. Their microscopic size may cause the cells' significant dependence on the dynamics of the digestive tract. Microbes perhaps experience these dynamics as Niagara Falls–like. In attempting to comprehend the riches of the variables, including the complexity of gene rearrangements, much of this highly complicated scenario understandably remains in the dark. Linking the events with oral tolerance, the involvement of noise may play some role. Intracellular and cellular noise patterns must be regarded in the environmental context to which background noise belongs. Also worthy of mention is the intestinal barrier that, like other delimiting functions in the body, is somewhat virtual, although, by keeping crowded microflora apart from microbe-free tissues, its efficacy is real. How does the host sense what happens in the luminal compartment? Oral tolerance is thought to depend heavily on cross-talk between gut-associated lymphoid tissue (GALT) and commensal flora. The epithelial lining dividing the two is by no means inert either. Though it is appealing to see the digestive tract as a whole, its setting suggests two main segments. The major segment typically is one of active flow. Resulting from ingesta/secretions/absorption, alongside the colon, it passes through its second "sedentary" counterpart. The latter encompasses GALT and intestinal flora; their multifaceted interplay is characteristic.

Address for correspondence: E. Rewald, M.D., Facultad de Ciencias Exactas y Naturales, Universidad Nacional de Mar del Plata, Hipolito Yrigoyen 2184, 7600 Mar del Plata, Argentina. Voice: +54-223-4948478; fax: +54-11-4756-2245.
 e.rewald@speedy.com.ar

From the general consideration of noise as a nuisance, we are coming to understand its functional properties. Inside the digestive tract, micro- as well as macroenvironments are "noisy," and noise may play a pivotal role in gene circuit functionality.[1] Ranging in relationships from symbiotic to hostile, stochastic effects (biochemical noise) in gene expression may participate in producing the cell variations observed in isogenic populations (phenotypic noise). Elowitz et al.[2] postulate a crucial biological role for stochastic resonance (SR) by establishing initial asymmetries that feedback mechanisms may amplify to determine cell fate, and they approach the question as to whether cell–cell variation is set by noise in expression of the gene itself or by fluctuations in the amounts of other cellular components. Any cellular component that suffers intrinsic fluctuation in its own concentration will act as extrinsic noise for other components with which it interacts. Reliable functioning of the cell may require that it suppresses, or is capable of a robust response to, fluctuations. Fedoroff and Fontana recognize the importance of stochastic genetic mechanisms that generate diversity in the immune system.[3] When coupled to suitable feedback mechanisms, such as the clonal amplification of cells expressing a particular antigen, this constitutes a powerful means of learning balanced reaction. On the other hand, phase variation in bacteria with genes randomly alternating between expression and silence is thought by Rao et al.[4] to be a form of cultivated noise. Noise-induced synchronization of oscillations is shared by a large number of cell types. As to whether molecular noise will, in effect, be found to be a factor in the process of modifying the dynamics of bacterial ties, either by weakening or by intensifying them, is another question (one that remains elusive).

Unlike lateral gene transfer or other major changes, we focus, rather, on common options by which a strain re-edits its classical core of genes, adapting its phenotype to the priorities of circumstance (though the outcome may be ambiguous). Thus far, much may depend on cognitive properties such as quorum sensing, and molecular noise is increasingly being considered as a component in the process to adjust intercellular ties. Furthermore, links between both "cognitive" cell resources may complicate the puzzle even more, theoretically for the better.[1]

CONCLUSION

SR may have a supporting role in the homeostasis of "health" in an individual. It also may emerge at the level of commensal microflora and relate to the development of immune diversity, including oral tolerance. It would be consistent with the Darwinian hypothesis concerning the need of living systems to adapt network patterns to whatever is available in nature. Noise is ubiquitous. It is now being targeted to regulate immune receptor function so as to improve transplant tolerance and defenses against dangerous intruders. By succeeding, it could perhaps avoid problematic drug effects in the treatment of severe disease conditions.

ACKNOWLEDGMENTS

We thank Dr. Lazar y Cía, S.A.Q.e I., Buenos Aires, Argentina, for sponsoring this paper.

REFERENCES

1. Cox, C.D., G.D. Peterson, M.S. Allen, *et al.* 2003. Analysis of noise in quorum sensing. OMICS **7:** 317–334.
2. Elowitz, M.B., A.J. Levine, E.D. Siggia & P.S. Swain. 2002. Stochastic gene expression in a single cell. Science **297:** 1183–1186.
3. Fedoroff, N. & W. Fontana. 2002. Small numbers of big molecules. Science **297:** 1129–1131.
4. Rao, C.V., D.M. Wolf & A.P. Arkin. 2002. Control, exploitation and tolerance of intracellular noise. Nature **420:** 831–837.

Decreased Nasal Tolerance to Allergic Asthma in Mice Fed an Amino Acid–Based Protein-Free Diet

DANIEL SOUSA MUCIDA,[a] DUNIA RODRÍGUEZ,[a] ALEXANDRE CASTRO KELLER,[a] ELIANE GOMES,[a] JUSCILENE SILVA MENEZES,[a] ANA MARIA CAETANO DE FARIA,[b] AND MOMCHILO RUSSO[a]

[a]*Departamento de Imunologia, Universidade de São Paulo-USP, São Paulo, Brasil*

[b]*Departamento de Bioquímica e Imunologia, Universidade Federal de Minas Gerais-UFMG, Belo Horizonte, Brasil*

ABSTRACT: Intranasal (i.n.) administration of soluble proteins induces a state of specific unresponsiveness to subsequent immunization, known as nasal tolerance. It is thought that newborns are less susceptible to nasal tolerance induction. Recently, we have shown that feeding adult animals with a protein-free diet (Aa) resulted in their arrest at an immature immunological profile. Here, we examined the effects of the Aa diet on the development of nasal tolerance to ovalbumin (OVA) in a murine model of allergic asthma. Nasal OVA administration suppressed almost totally the OVA-induced asthma-like responses (airway eosinophilia, type 2 cytokine production, and OVA-specific IgE antibodies) in chow- or casein-fed BALB/c mice. In contrast, in Aa-fed animals the suppression of asthma-like responses by nasal OVA was partial, being effective in suppressing airway eosinophilia, but not airway type 2 cytokine or OVA-specific IgE response. We conclude that animals fed the Aa diet are more resistant to the induction of nasal tolerance. Our animal model may mimic the features of the immune system of human infants.

KEYWORDS: diet; tolerance; asthma; eosinophils; IgE

INTRODUCTION

Allergic asthma results from an intrapulmonary allergen-driven Th2 response and is characterized by intermittent airway obstruction, airway hyperreactivity, and airway inflammation. Intranasal (i.n.) administration of soluble proteins (allergens) before immunization induces a state of specific unresponsiveness known as nasal tolerance.[1] However, in human infants airborne allergens may cause long-term allergic sensitization instead of inducing tolerance.[2] Indeed, mucosal tolerance to allergens is relatively slow to develop in newborns.[3,4]

Address for correspondence: Momchilo Russo, Departamento de Imunologia, Instituto de Ciências Biomédicas, Universidade de São Paulo, São Paulo 05508-900, SP, Brazil. Voice/fax: +55-11-3091-7377.

momrusso@icb.usp.br

We have previously shown that mice fed a diet in which intact dietary proteins were replaced by equivalent amounts of amino acids from weaning (day 21 of life), presented an immunological profile similar to neonates.[5] Adult animals reared in this balanced amino acid–based protein-free diet (Aa-fed mice) grew and looked like normal mice but showed local and systemic abnormalities in their immune system. Aa-fed mice had poorly developed gut-associated lymphoid tissue (GALT), and presented a predominant Th2 profile, resembling preweaned mice.[5] Most of the reports on the impairment in Th1 responses in neonates refers to the neonatal period as the early postnatal time in suckling animals.[4,6] In the present work, we examined whether animals fed an Aa diet are susceptible to the induction of nasal tolerance. We used ovalbumin (OVA) as allergen in an established murine model of allergic asthma.[7]

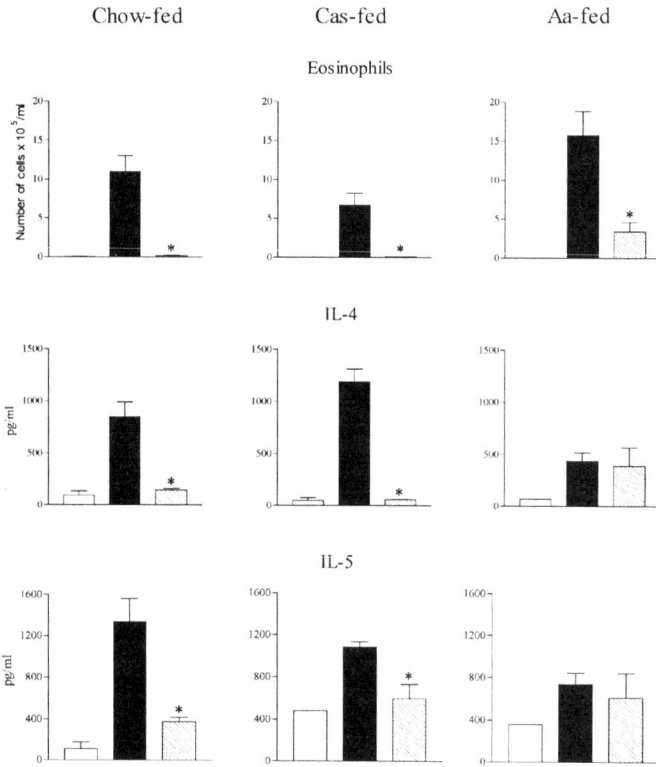

FIGURE 1. The effect of nasal OVA administration on antigen-induced airway eosinophilic inflammation and BAL fluid IL-4 and IL-5 levels in Chow-fed (*left*), Cas-fed (*middle*), or Aa-fed (*right*) BALB/c mice. Groups of five mice received OVA 100 µg i.n. (nasal) or PBS i.n. (immune) for three consecutive days, before OVA-alum immunization and challenge. The control group received only OVA intranasally. Experiments were performed 24 h after the last OVA challenge. Results are expressed as means ± standard error of the mean (SEM). *Significant difference ($P < .05$) between values of Immune versus Nasal groups. *Open bars*, control; *black bars,* immune; *striped bars,* nasal.

MATERIALS AND METHODS

BALB/c mice were fed normal chow (Chow), casein (Cas)-, or an amino acid–based protein-free diet (Aa) after weaning (21 days of life), as previously described.[5] At 7 weeks of age, groups of five animals received OVA 100 μg/50μL PBS i.n. delivered into the nostrils for 3 consecutive days to induce nasal tolerance. Control animals received only 50 μL PBS. Four days after, the animals were immunized, and boosted at weekly intervals, by a subcutaneous injection of OVA (Sigma grade V) 4 μg/1.6 mg alum, followed by two intranasal OVA challenges with 10 μg OVA/ 50 μL PBS. Twenty-four hours after the last intranasal challenge, lungs were lavaged (BAL). Total and differential cell counts and the levels of IL-4 and IL-5 in the BAL fluid were assessed by hemocytometer and cytospin preparation, and by ELISA, respectively, and OVA-specific IgE levels of serum samples were related to an internal standard that was set at 10,000 arbitrary units (A.U.) as previously described.[7]

RESULTS

Both normal Chow- and Cas-fed BALB/c mice that received OVA intranasally before OVA immunization and challenge showed almost complete inhibition (>99%) of airway eosinophilia when compared with OVA-immunized and challenged animals that received i.n. PBS (FIG. 1). The inhibitory effect of nasal OVA administration was less pronounced (~75% of inhibition) in Aa-fed animals (FIG. 1). Similar results were obtained when the total number of BAL cells was determined (data not shown).

Nasal tolerance in Chow- or Cas-fed animals also suppressed airway type 2 cytokine production (IL-4 and IL-5) (FIG. 1). In addition, intranasal OVA administration resulted in a significant suppression of OVA-specific IgE antibody production

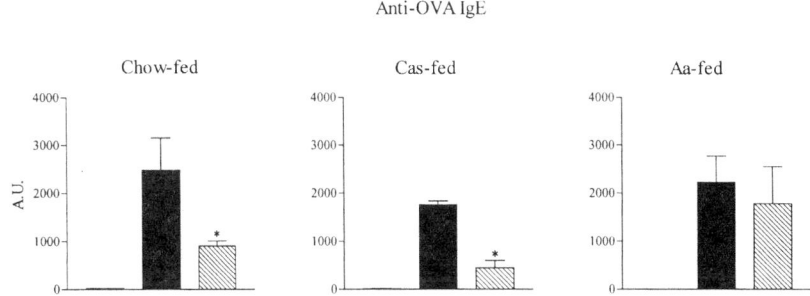

FIGURE 2. The effect of nasal OVA administration on antigen-induced anti-OVA IgE antibody production in Chow-fed (*left*), Cas-fed (*middle*), or Aa-fed (*right*) BALB/c mice. Groups of five mice received OVA 100 μg i.n. (nasal) or PBS i.n. (immune) for three consecutive days before OVA-alum immunization and challenge. The control group received only OVA intranasally. Experiments were performed 24 h after last OVA challenge. Results are expressed as arbitrary units of means ± standard error of the mean (SEM). *Significant difference ($P < .05$) between values of immune versus nasal groups. *Open bars*, control; *black bars*, immune; *striped bars*, nasal.

in Chow- or Cas-fed animals (FIG. 2). In contrast, nasal OVA administration did not suppress type 2 cytokine production or OVA-specific IgE response in Aa-fed animals (FIGS. 1 and 2).

DISCUSSION

The results presented here show that nasal tolerance is fully effective in suppressing asthma-like responses in Chow- or Cas-fed animals, but not in Aa-fed animals. The resistance of Aa-fed animals to nasal tolerance was clearly documented by the elevated production of IL-4 and IL-5 cytokines, as well as the high levels of OVA-specific IgE antibodies in the nasally treated group. Interestingly, airway eosinophilia was significantly suppressed (~75%) in these mice despite the high levels of IL-5 attained in their BAL fluid. It is known that IL-5 and eotaxin cooperate locally in pulmonary tissues to selectively and synergistically promote eosinophilia.[8] Thus, the inhibition of airway eosinophilia observed in Aa-fed animals could be attributed in part to inhibition of chemokines such as eotaxin, or RANTES and MIP-1α that are also involved in eosinophilic inflammation.[9,10] Conversely, the high production of IgE antibodies in these Aa-fed mice is consistent with the lack of suppression of IL-4 by intranasal OVA administration, inasmuch as IL-4 and IL-13 are key cytokines for IgE production.[11,12]

Our results are in consonance with a previous study showing that the nasal tolerance for IgE response does not function during the early postnatal period,[3] and we extend this finding to type 2 cytokine production and airway eosinophilia. The mechanism(s) responsible for the partial resistance to nasal tolerance in Aa-fed animals remains to be determined.

ACKNOWLEDGMENTS

This work was supported by grants from FAPESP (99/03778-3, 01/01748-1, 01/06212-2, 03/02070-4) and by a fellowship from CNPq to M.R.

REFERENCES

1. HOLT, P.G. 1997. Development of sensitization versus tolerance to inhalant allergens during early life. Pediatr. Pulmonol. Suppl. **16:** 6–7.
2. HOLT, P.G. 1994. Immunoprophylaxis of atopy: light at the end of the tunnel? Immunol. Today **15:** 484–489.
3. HOLT, P.G., J. VINES & D. BRITTEN. 1988. Suppression of IgE responses by antigen inhalation: failure of tolerance mechanism(s) in newborn rats. Immunology **63:** 591–593.
4. NELSON, D.J. & P.G. HOLT. 1995. Defective regional immunity in the respiratory tract of neonates is attributable to hyporesponsiveness of local dendritic cells to activation signals. J. Immunol. **155:** 3517–3524.
5. MENEZES, J.S. et al. 2003. Stimulation by food proteins plays a critical role in the maturation of the immune system. Int. Immunol. **15:** 447–455.
6. HUSBAND, A.J. & M. GLEESON. 1996. Ontogeny of mucosal immunity. Environmental and behavioral influences. Brain Behav. Immun. **10:** 188–204.

7. Russo, M. et al. 2001. Suppression of asthma-like responses in different mouse strains by oral tolerance. Am. J. Respir. Cell Mol. Biol. **24:** 518–526.
8. Foster, P.S. et al. 2001. Elemental signals regulating eosinophil accumulation in the lung. Immunol. Rev. **179:** 173–181.
9. Jia, G.Q. et al. 1999. Selective eosinophil transendothelial migration triggered by eotaxin via modulation of Mac-1/ICAM-1 and VLA-4/VCAM-1 interactions. Int. Immunol. **11:** 1–10.
10. Gonzalo, J.A. et al. 1996. Eosinophil recruitment to the lung in a murine model of allergic inflammation. The role of T cells, chemokines, and adhesion receptors. J. Clin. Invest. **98:** 2332–2345.
11. Finkelman, F.D. et al. 1988. IL-4 is required to generate and sustain in vivo IgE responses. J. Immunol. **141:** 2335–2341.
12. Wills-Karp, M. et al. 1998. Interleukin-13: central mediator of allergic asthma. Science **282:** 2258–2261.

Peyer's Patch Dendritic Cells Capturing Oral Antigen Interact with Antigen-Specific T Cells and Induce Gut-Homing CD4$^+$CD25$^+$ Regulatory T Cells in Peyer's Patches

KATSUYA NAGATANI, KAYO SAGAWA, YOSHINORI KOMAGATA, AND KAZUHIKO YAMAMOTO

Department of Allergy and Rheumatology, Graduate School of Medicine, University of Tokyo, Tokyo, Japan

> ABSTRACT: Antigen-specific naive T cells accumulated in Peyer's patches only after the feeding of antigen. DCs that captured oral antigen interacted with these T cells in the IFR of PP. Some of these T cells acquired a similar phenotype to CD4$^+$ CD25$^+$ regulatory T cells and CCR9$^+$ gut-homing T cells.
>
> KEYWORDS: Peyer's patch; dendritic cell; chemokine receptor; regulatory T cell

INTRODUCTION

It is thought that antigen-specific regulatory T cells are generated in the gut-associated lymphoid tissue (GALT), including Peyer's patches (PPs), after antigen is orally administered. However, the importance of dendritic cells (DCs) in the generation of regulatory T cells, and the kind of regulatory T cells generated in PPs are still unclear. Here, we show that PP DCs capturing oral antigen interacted with antigen-specific T cells and induced gut-homing CD4$^+$CD25$^+$ regulatory T cells in PPs.

MATERIALS AND METHODS

We transferred naive T cells of ovalbumin (OVA)-TCR transgenic mice (DO11.10) into BALB/c mice, which were then fed FITC-conjugated OVA (FITC-OVA) (30 mg/mouse) 24 h later. Kinetics of oral antigen–loaded cells and interaction between antigen-specific T cells and antigen-loaded DCs in PPs after the feeding of OVA (or FITC-OVA) were checked by immunofluorescence staining.

Address for correspondence: Yoshinori Komagata, Department of Allergy and Rheumatology, Graduate School of Medicine, University of Tokyo, 7-3-1 Hongo, Bunkyo-ku, Tokyo 113-8655, Japan. Voice: +81-3-3815-5411, ext. 37263; fax: +81-3-3815-5954.
 komagata-tky@umin.ac.jp

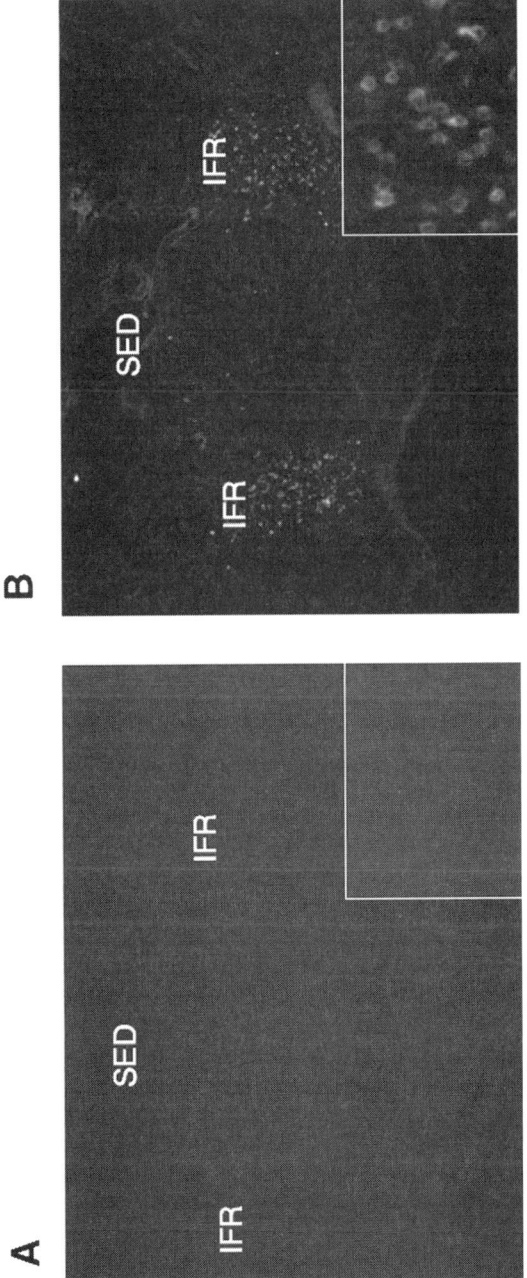

FIGURE 1. OVA-specific T cells accumulated in IFR of Peyer's patch by OVA feeding. We transferred OVA-specific T cells of DO11.10 mice into naive BALB/c mice, then fed 30 mg OVA to these mice. We collected Peyer's patches 24 h after the transfer and stained with FITC anti-KJ1.26 antibody. (A) Peyer's patch of nonfed mouse. OVA-specific T cells are not detected (inset magnified ×200). (B) Peyer's patch of OVA-fed mouse. OVA-specific T cells accumulated in IFR (inset magnified ×200).

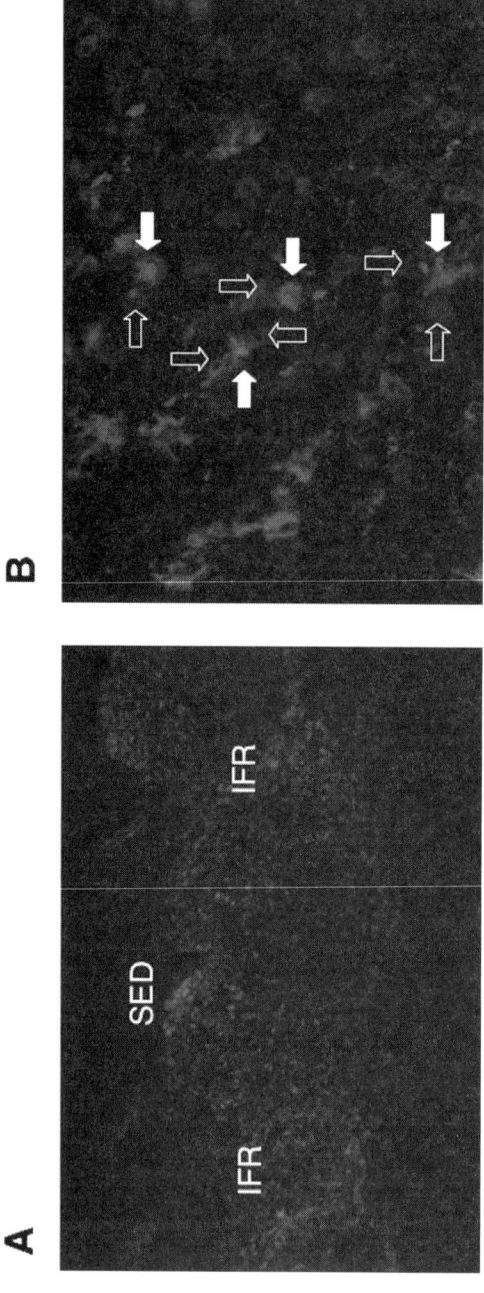

FIGURE 2. FITC-OVA–loaded DCs interact with OVA-specific T cells in IFR of Peyer's patches. (**A**) We transferred OVA-specific T cells of DO11.10 mice into naive BALB/c mice, then fed 30 mg of FITC-conjugated OVA (FITC-OVA) to these mice. We collected Peyer's patches 24 h after the transfer, and stained with FITC anti-KJ1.26 antibody and PE anti-CD11c antibody. (IFR, interfollicular region; SED, subepithelial dome; magnified ×40). (**B**) FITC-OVA–loaded DCs (*closed arrows*) contact OVA-specific T cells (*open arrows*) in IFR after FITC-OVA feeding (magnified ×400).

To examine the phenotype of OVA-specific T cells accumulated in PPs after OVA feeding, we purified KJ1.26 positive T cells from PPs by magnetic beads (MACS, Miltenyi Biotec, Bergisch Gladbach, Germany) and checked relative gene expression by real-time RT-PCR (iCycler iQ; Bio-Rad, CA).

RESULTS

FITC-positive cells appeared in the subepithelial dome (SED) of PPs as early as three hours after the feeding of FITC-OVA. Double staining with PE anti-CD11c antibody showed that FITC-positive cells in SEDs were CD11c-positive DCs (data not shown). Twenty-four hours after the feeding of FITC-OVA, DCs capturing FITC-OVA migrated from the SED to the interfollicular region (IFR) and interacted with OVA-specific T cells accumulated in the IFR of PPs (FIG. 1B and FIG. 2). In contrast, OVA-specific T cells were not detected in IFRs in nonfed mice (FIG. 1A).

We investigated the gene expression levels of chemokine receptors such as CCR4, CCR7, CCR8, CCR9, and CXCR3 in OVA-specific T cells by quantitative

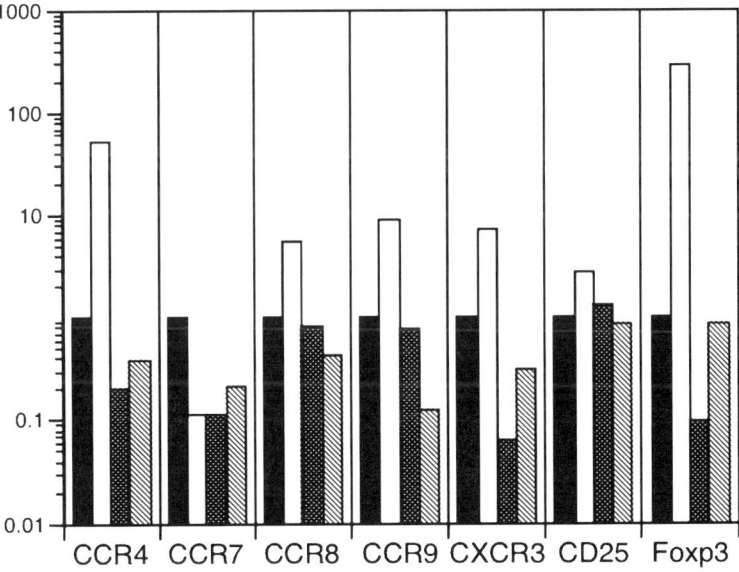

FIGURE 3. Gene expression in OVA-specific T cells accumulating in Peyer's patches after OVA feeding. We transferred OVA-specific T cells of DO11.10 mice into naive BALB/c mice, followed by feeding of 30 mg OVA. Twenty-four hours after the transfer, KJ1.26-positive OVA-specific T cells were purified from Peyer's patches, and total RNA was extracted. We checked relative gene expression of OVA-specific T cells accumulated in Peyer's patch by quantitative real time RT-PCR (*open box*). As controls, KJ1.26-positive T cells from spleens of OVA-fed (*black box with white dots*), nonfed mice (*striped box*), and KJ1.26-positive T cells before transfer (*black box*) were also checked.

real-time PCR. Gene expression of CCR4, CCR8, CCR9, and CXCR3 was substantially higher in OVA-specific T cells accumulated in PPs after OVA feeding (FIG. 3).

It has been reported that CCR4 and CCR8 are expressed on $CD4^+CD25^+$ regulatory T cells.[1] Therefore, we next checked the gene expression of Foxp3, which is a $CD4^+CD25^+$ regulatory T cell–specific transcription factor,[2] in OVA-specific T cells. Surprisingly, the Foxp3 gene level in OVA-specific T cells accumulated in PPs after OVA feeding was 294-fold more abundant than in OVA-specific T cells before the transfer. Expression of CCR7, which is regarded as a marker of naive T cells, in the OVA-specific T cells before the transfer, was relatively high (FIG. 3).

DISCUSSION

Recent studies have shown that CCR4, CCR8, and CXCR3 are expressed on $CD4^+CD25^+$ regulatory T cells and that Foxp3 is exclusively expressed in these T cells.[1,2] In addition, CCR9 has been reported to be expressed by gut-homing T cells.[3] These results suggest that DCs that capture oral antigens in the SED migrate into the IFR and interact with antigen-specific T cells, and that some antigen-specific T cells acquire a similar phenotype to $CCR9^+$ gut-homing T cells and $CD4^+CD25^+$ regulatory T cells.

REFERENCES

1. IELLEM, A., M. MARIANI, R. LANG, et al. 2001. Unique chemotactic response profile and specific expression of chemokine receptors CCR4 and CCR8 by $CD4^+CD25^+$ regulatory T cells. J. Exp. Med. **194:** 847–854.
2. HORI, S., T. NOMURA & S. SAKAGUCHI. 2003. Control of regulatory T cell development by the transcription factor Foxp3. Science **299:** 1057–1061.
3. ZABEL, B.A., W.W. AGACE, J.J. CAMPBELL, et al. 1999. Human G protein–coupled receptor GPR-9-6/CC chemokine receptor 9 is selectively expressed on intestinal homing T lymphocytes, mucosal lymphocytes, and thymocytes and is required for thymus-expressed chemokine–mediated chemotaxis. J. Exp. Med. **190:** 1241–1256.

The Role of Transforming Growth Factor–β in a Model of Oral Tolerance to the Diet Antigen Dextrin

SOFÍA OLMOS,[a] MARIA GABRIELA MARQUEZ, MARÍA C. LÓPEZ,[a] AND MARIA ESTELA ROUX

Department of Biological Sciences, University of Buenos Aires, Buenos Aires, Argentina

ABSTRACT: In a model of immunodeficiency provoked by protein deficiency, cytosol fractions from gut IELS isolated from immunodeficient rats presenting oral tolerance to dextrin showed increased expression of TGF-β to reduce the effect of higher levels of inflammatory cytokines.

KEYWORDS: oral tolerance; TGF-β; intestinal intraepithelial lymphocytes; immunodeficiency; CD8αα; γδTCR

INTRODUCTION

The specific immune response to fed antigens is characterized by antigen-specific systemic unresponsiveness called oral tolerance.[1] After oral administration of a protein antigen, CD8 T cells capable of transferring oral tolerance into naive recipients are induced.[2] Several mechanisms have been associated with different forms of tolerance, including the secretion of immunomodulatory cytokines such as IL-4, IL-10, and TGF-β.[3] TGF-β has been shown to be a key mediator of oral tolerance and is mainly produced by antigen-specific T cells (Th3 cells).[4]

In a model of secondary immunodeficiency due to malnutrition, we have shown that oral tolerance to a polysaccharide can be induced.[5] Studying intestinal intraepithelial lymphocytes (iIEL), we have demonstrated that there is a significant increase in the CD8αα population that expresses γδTCR, and that CD8αα cells, as well as CD8αβ cells, express CD25. Moreover, CD8α+-γδTCR+ cells inhibited the delayed-type hypersensitivity (DTH) response to dextrin after transfer into naive recipients, but not to another carbohydrate (levan), indicating the specificity of the response.[5,6] The aim of this study was to analyze the expression of TNF-α, IFN-γ, and TGF-β by iIELs of control (C) and malnourished (R21) animals in our model of oral tolerance to dextrin.

[a]Current address, and address for correspondence: Sofía Olmos, Ph.D., Center for Immunology and Microbial Disease, Albany Medical Center, 47 New Scotland Ave. MC-151, Albany, NY 12208. Voice: 518-262-6220; fax: 518-262-5061.
olmoss@mail.amc.edu

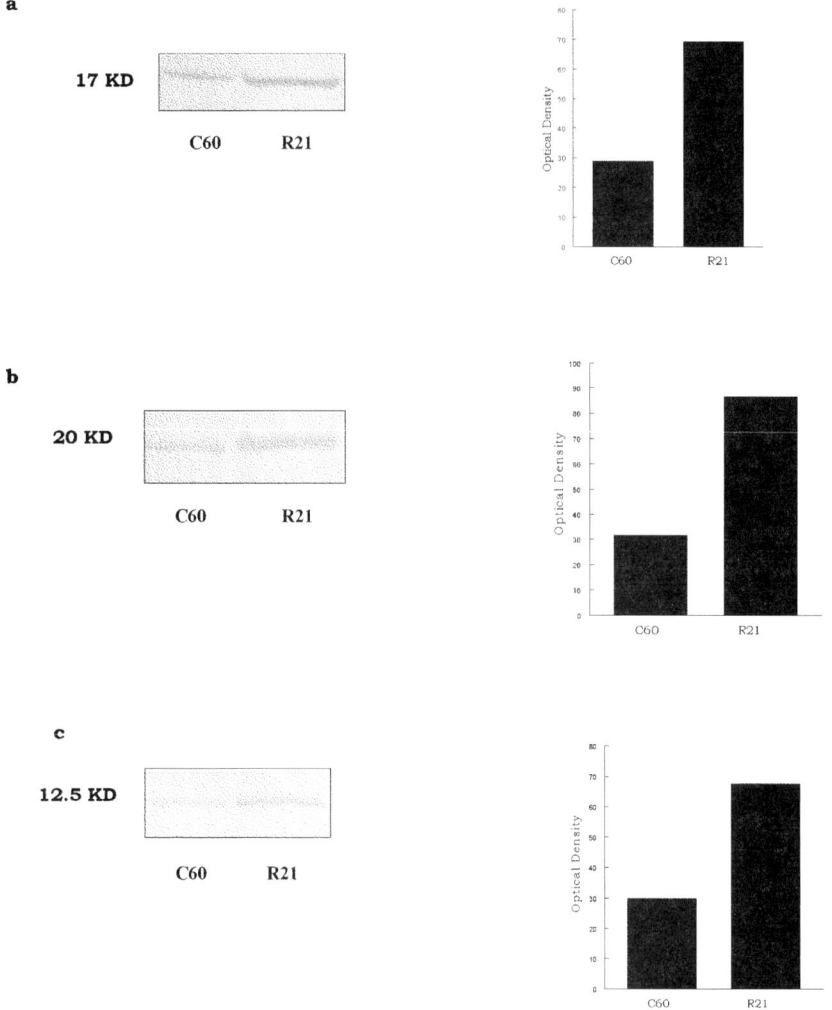

FIGURE 1. Representative immunoblot showing expression of (**a**) TNF-α; (**b**) IFN-γ, and (**c**) TGF-β in cytosol fractions from isolated iIELs. Similar results were obtained from a second independent repetition of the experiment.

MATERIALS AND METHODS

A model of secondary immunodeficiency due to protein malnutrition was used. Rats were fed a protein-free diet from the time of weaning until they had lost 25% of their initial body weight and were then fed for 21 days with a 20% casein diet (R21 group). Cytosol fractions from isolated iIELs were used to analyze the presence of TNF-α, IFN-γ, and TGF-β using Western blot analysis.

RESULTS

The expression of all cytokines studied was increased in R21 when compared with the control group, as shown in FIGURE 1.

DISCUSSION

Our results confirm the existence of an inflammatory process in the immunodeficient animals (R21), not detectable at the histological level, that is characterized by an increase in the proportion of activated cells (CD8$\alpha\alpha^+$CD25$^+$) and by an increase in the proinflammatory cytokines TNF-α and IFN-γ. We believe that the increase in TGF-β expression is antigen specific, and that it appears in order to downregulate the increased expression of inflammatory cytokines and maintain oral tolerance. This would be in agreement with the concept that TGF-β is produced by Th3 or T regulatory cells as part of the cascade of events required to establish oral tolerance. Therefore, we conclude that in our experimental model, the iIEL CD8$\alpha\alpha^+$/TCR$\gamma\delta^+$ population that increased in R21 and transferred hyporesponsiveness to dextrin is the T cell regulatory population responsible for the production of TGF-β.

REFERENCES

1. BRANDTZAEG, P. 1996. History of oral tolerance and mucosal immunity. Ann. N.Y. Acad. Sci. **778:** 1–27.
2. WEINER, H.L., A. FRIEDMAN, A. MILLER, et al. 1994. Oral tolerance: immunologic mechanisms and treatment of animal and human organ-specific autoimmune diseases by oral administration of autoantigens. Ann. Rev. Immunol. **12:** 809–837.
3. LETTERIO, J. & A. ROBERTS. 1998. Regulation of immune responses by TGF-β. Ann. Rev. Immunol. **16:** 137–161.
4. WEINER, H.L. 2001. Induction and mechanism of action of transforming growth factor-beta-secreting Th3 regulatory cells. Immunol. Rev. **182:** 207–214.
5. LOPEZ, M.C., M.G. MARQUEZ, N. SLOBODIANIK & M.E. ROUX. 2003. Oral tolerance to dextrin mediated by specific suppressor T-cells induced in the intestinal intraepithelium and their systemic migration. Lymphology **36:** 26–38.
6. MÁRQUEZ, M.G., A. GALEANO, S. OLMOS & M.E. ROUX. 2000. Flow cytometric analysis of intestinal intraepithelial lymphocytes in a model of immunodeficiency in Wistar rats. Cytometry **41:** 115–122.

Commonly Used Drugs Impair Oral Tolerance in Mice

SOPHIE PECQUET, GUÉNOLÉE PRIOULT, JOHN CAMPBELL, BRUCE GERMAN, AND MARCO TURINI

Nestlé Research Center, Lausanne, Switzerland

ABSTRACT: Ibuprofen and antibiotics are commonly prescribed during early childhood. When given to mice at the time at which oral tolerance is induced, both treatments affect either the induction or the maintenance of oral tolerance. These results suggest that the coadministration of these and similarly acting drugs should be considered cautiously for infants at risk of allergy.

KEYWORDS: oral tolerance; allergy; antibiotics; NSAIDs; weaning; food

INTRODUCTION

A food allergy arises when the natural processes of oral tolerance fail to occur in response to the ingestion of specific food proteins. In children, examples of failed oral tolerance include cow's milk allergy, when oral tolerance does not develop to β-lactoglobulin (BLG) or caseins, and peanut allergy when oral tolerance to peanut conglycinin fails. Exogenous factors separate from, and in addition to, the presence of the allergens themselves are now recognized to modulate the processes of oral tolerance.[1–3] The goal of this work was to determine in mice whether drugs commonly administered to children for the treatment of infections alter the signals and processes of oral tolerance. To address these questions, the induction of oral tolerance to BLG was evaluated in mice[4] that were treated concurrently at the time of induction either with antibiotics or with a nonsteroidal anti-inflammatory drug (NSAID); both types of medication are commonly used in pediatric practice during the first year of life.[5–7] This period coincides with the period of life during which oral tolerance is normally induced to a large range of food proteins, including cow's milk.

MATERIALS AND METHODS

Mice

Three-week-old conventional Balb/c mice were treated for seven days either with ibuprofen (intraperitoneal injection 50 mg/kg body weight/d) or with antibiotics. For the latter treatment, mice received *ad libitum* in drinking water either norfloxacin (500 mg/kg body weight/d) or a mixture of gentamycin (124 mg/kg body weight/d)

Address for correspondence: Sophie Pecquet, Ph.D., Food Immunology, Nestlé Research Center, BP44, CH 1000 Lausanne 26, Switzerland. Voice: +41-21-785-86-84; fax: +41-21-785-85-44.

sophie.pecquet@rdls.nestle.com

Ann. N.Y. Acad. Sci. 1029: 374–378 (2004). © 2004 New York Academy of Sciences.
doi: 10.1196/annals.1309.021

plus vancomycin (500 mg/kg body weight/d). To induce oral tolerance during these medicinal treatments, mice received by gavage whey proteins (WP) containing BLG (experimental mice) or saline (control mice) five days after the beginning of ibuprofen or antibiotic treatments (referred to as day 1). The mice were intraperitoneally challenged four days after gavage (day 5), with 80 mg BLG diluted in aluminum hydroxide $(Al(OH)_3)$. In the group of mice administered ibuprofen, a first subgroup and their controls (whey protein and saline) were sacrificed at day 5 prior to the systemic challenge in order to assess the effect of ibuprofen on PGE_2 production. For antibiotic- and NSAID-treated mice, a group of animals and their respective untreated controls were sacrificed three weeks (day 28) after the systemic challenge to test the induction of oral tolerance. The maintenance of the response was monitored subsequently only in mice receiving antibiotic treatment and their untreated controls. All these mice received additional booster injections on day 25, with subsequent sacrifice at day 35, or at both days 25 and 45 if sacrificed on day 60.

Quantitative Analysis of the PGE_2 Production

Isolated splenocytes were stimulated with BLG (2.5 mg/mL). Nonstimulated cells were used to determine baseline values. PGE_2 levels in the culture media, from splenocytes cultured for 12 h, were determined by an enzyme immunoassay.

Quantitative and Qualitative Analysis of the Intestinal Flora

The composition of the fecal microflora was measured in controls and in mice treated with the antibiotics. During antibiotic treatment, the flora were analyzed every two days; fecal samples were subsequently collected and analyzed weekly after completion of treatment.

Oral Tolerance Readouts

BLG-specific serum IgE levels were titered by ELISA. Splenocyte and mesenteric lymph node (MLN) cell proliferation were measured following *in vitro* BLG (2.5 mg/mL) restimulation. A stimulation index (whey protein-fed groups/control saline-fed groups) was then calculated.

RESULTS

Both of the drug protocols, antibiotics, and a typical nonsteroidal anti-inflammatory drug (ibuprofen), altered the processes of oral tolerance. Oral tolerance to BLG failed in ibuprofen-treated mice. Additionally, in antibiotic-treated mice, the more the gut microbiota was affected by the administration of antibiotics, the less oral tolerance was maintained.

Effect of Ibuprofen Treatment in Mice Treated at an Early Stage of Oral Tolerance Induction

We have previously shown that when splenocytes are isolated from mice that have been previously exposed to BLG and challenged *in vitro*, PGE_2 production by these

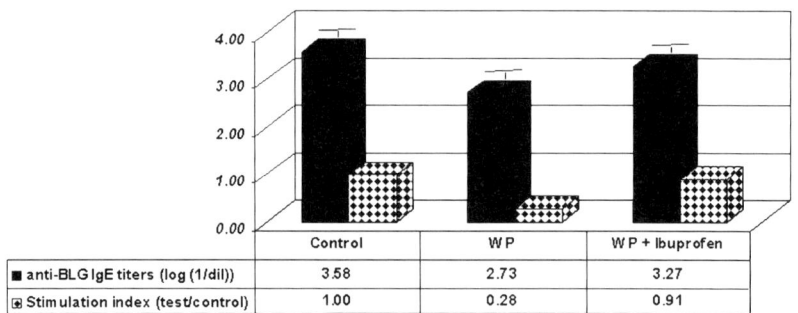

FIGURE 1.

splenocytes rises dramatically relative to splenocytes isolated from mice that have not been exposed to BLG.[8]

The increased production of PGE_2 observed in BLG-stimulated splenocytes from whey protein-fed mice (4449 pg/mL) was completely inhibited by ibuprofen; PGE_2 levels were statistically the same for mice fed ibuprofen plus whey protein (3182 pg/mL) and for the nontolerized saline control mice (2812 pg/mL).

Immunological data show that NSAID treatment impaired oral tolerance induction. In whey protein-fed mice that were treated with ibuprofen, anti-BLG IgE titers were statistically the same as the anti-BLG IgE titers observed in the nontolerized control group fed with saline ($P > .2$), both groups being significantly different from the whey protein fed (tolerized) mice ($P < .05$).

Further analyses revealed the same results as those observed for the specific humoral response. Ibuprofen treatment impaired the specific proliferative response of isolated splenocytes. At day 28, the hyporesponsiveness of the BLG-specific splenocyte proliferation typically observed in whey protein-fed mice was not seen. Instead, the immune response observed in the ibuprofen-treated group was similar to that seen in the nontolerized control group (FIG. 1).

Effect of Antibiotic Treatment in Mice Treated at the Early Stage of Oral Tolerance Induction

During treatment and at the time of induction of oral tolerance (day 1), the combination of gentamycin/vancomycin ostensibly cleared from the gut the detectable bacteria normally present in fecal flora, and none of the cultivatable bacterial species remained during treatment. In contrast, treatment with the antibiotic norfloxacin simply reduced the numbers of the different bacterial populations. In both cases, the microflora were re-established shortly after treatment. The flora remained stable up to end of the experiment.

Specific humoral hyporesponsiveness was obtained in mice orally treated with antibiotics. The antibiotic-induced impairment of the gut flora did not affect the oral tolerance at the humoral level, both for the induction and the maintenance phases (FIG. 2). The serum anti-BLG IgE titers from mice treated with either norfloxacin

(Nor-WP) or with the gentamycin-vancomycin mixture (Gen-Van-WP) were not significantly different from the IgE titers observed in tolerized whey protein-fed mice (Control-WP) ($P > .3$), and all three groups differed significantly from the saline-fed control group (Control-saline). This result was observed during both the induction (day 28) and the maintenance phases (day 35 and day 60).

This analysis was pursued, and FIGURE 3 shows that specific cellular tolerance in MLNs was induced even in the presence of antibiotics administered at the time of induction. Interestingly, this cellular tolerance was not maintained over time. Compared with the control group, untreated with antibiotics and with a normal microbiota, the more the intestinal flora were impaired by the antibiotic treatment at

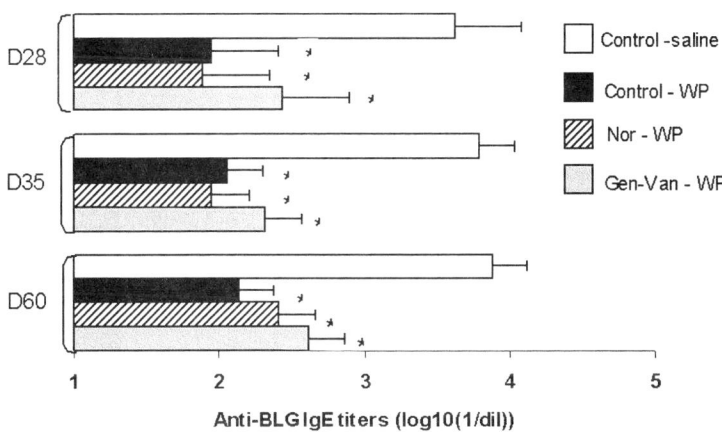

FIGURE 2. *Open bar*: control-saline; *black bar*: control-WP; *striped bar*: Nor-WP; *gray bar*: Gen-Van-WP.

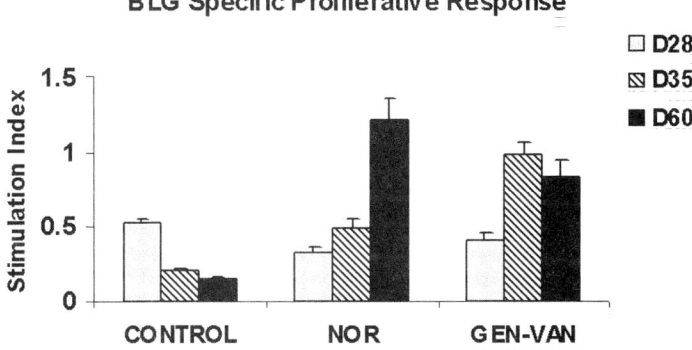

FIGURE 3. BLG-specific proliferative response. *Gray bar*: D28; *striped bar*: D35; *black bar*: D60.

the time of tolerogen exposure (Gen-Van), the less the tolerant state persisted (D35, D60; stimulation index higher than or close to 1).

CONCLUSION

During the very early stages of the induction of oral tolerance, compromising the normal state of the intestinal environment, either by inhibiting the PGE_2 pathway with ibuprofen or by depleting the gut microbiota with oral antibiotics, resulted in a weakening of either the induction or the maintenance of oral tolerance to cow's milk proteins. Links between both treatment types and certain atopic diseases have already been suggested.[9–13] However, no link has previously been made between the administration of NSAIDs or antibiotics and an increased risk of food allergy. Taken together, our data suggest that the coadministration of antibiotics and NSAIDs, routinely prescribed in pediatric practice during childhood infections, should be carefully supervised as it might be a particularly deleterious mixture in infants at risk of allergy. At the very least, a logical solution would be to avoid the introduction of new foods while the ability of the immune system to produce an effective tolerogenic response is compromised, for example, during infection. The same precaution should be taken in those infants when they are treated with NSAIDs for discomfort associated with teething, particularly during the weaning period.

REFERENCES

1. WHITACRE, C. 2000. New insights into oral tolerance. Gastroenterol. **119**: 260–263.
2. BJORKSTEN, B., E. SEPP, K. JULGE, et al. 2001. Allergy development and the intestinal microflora during the first year of life. J. Allergy Clin. Immunol. **108**: 516–520.
3. NEWBERRY, R., W. STENSON & G. LORENZ. 1999. Cyclooxygenase-2-dependent arachidonic acid metabolites are essential modulators of the intestinal immune response to dietary antigen. Nat. Med. **5**: 900–906.
4. PECQUET, S., A. PFEIFER, S. GAULDIE & R. FRITSCHÉ. 1999. Immunoglobulin E suppression and cytokine modulation in mice orally tolerized to β-lactoglobulin. Immunology **96**: 278–285.
5. BERGUS, G., B. LEVY, S. LEVY, et al. 1996. Antibiotic use during the first 200 days of life. Arch. Fam. Med. **5**: 523–526.
6. COENEN, S., P. VAN ROYEN, E. VERMEIRE, et al. 2000. Antibiotics are being overprescribed especially for respiratory tract infections. Fam. Pract. **17**: 210.
7. MORRIS, J.L., D.A. ROSEN & K.R. ROSEN. 2003. Nonsteroidal anti-inflammatory agents in neonates Paediatr. Drugs **5**: 385–405.
8. PECQUET, S. et al. 2003. Unpublished data.
9. WICKENS, K., N. PEARCE, J. CRANE & R. BEASLEY. 1999. Antibiotic use in early childhood and the development of asthma. Clin. Exp. Allergy **29**: 766–771.
10. MATTES, J. & W. KARMAUS. 1999. The use of antibiotics in the first year of life and development of asthma: Which comes first? Clin. Exp. Allergy **29**: 729–732.
11. HOPKIN, J.M. 1999. Early life receipt of antibiotics and atopic disorder. Clin. Exp. Allergy **29**: 733–734.
12. PAUL, E., G. GALL, I. MULLER & R. MOLLER. 2000. Dramatic augmentation of a food allergy by acetylsalicylic acid. J. Allergy Clin. Immunol. **105**: 844.
13. MORISSET, M. & D. MONERET-VAUTRIN. 2001. Food anaphylaxis induced by aspirin. Allerg. Immunol. **33**: 147–149.

Intestinal Myofibroblasts and Immune Tolerance

J. I. SAADA,[a] C. A. BARRERA,[a,e] V. E. REYES,[d,e] P. A. ADEGBOYEGA,[c]
G. SUAREZ,[e] R. A. TAMERISA,[a] K. F. PANG,[c] D. A. BLAND,[e] R. C. MIFFLIN,[a]
J. F. DI MARI,[a] AND D. W. POWELL[a,b]

[a]*Department of Internal Medicine,* [b]*Department of Cellular Physiology and Molecular Biophysics,* [c]*Department of Pathology,* [d]*Department of Microbiology and Immunology,* [e]*Department of Pediatrics, University of Texas Medical Branch, Galveston, Texas 77555-1058*

> ABSTRACT: Stromal cells, such as myofibroblasts and fibroblasts, represent a significant fraction of MHC class II–positive cells in the normal human colonic lamina propria, suggesting they may play an important role in $CD4^+$ T cell regulation in a tolerogenic environment. The aim of this study was to examine whether human colonic myofibroblasts (CMFs) phenotypically and functionally resemble conventional antigen-presenting cells (APCs). Our results support the hypothesis that intestinal myofibroblasts are a novel, nonprofessional APC phenotype important in modulating mucosal T cell responses. Given their strategic location, we propose that intestinal myofibroblasts play a critical role in mediating tolerance to luminal antigens.
>
> KEYWORDS: mucosal immunity; immune tolerance; antigen-presenting cell; HLA-DR; fibroblastic sheath

INTRODUCTION

Autoimmune, hypersensitivity, and idiopathic chronic inflammatory diseases of the intestine result from defects in immune tolerance to autoantigens, dietary antigens, or commensal microbes in the gastrointestinal tract.[1] Although much is known about mechanisms of oral tolerance in mice, the nature and spectrum of antigen-presenting cells (APCs) in the human gut that mediate oral tolerance are not well understood.[2] We have recently observed that stromal cells such as myofibroblasts and fibroblasts represent a significant fraction of MHC class II–positive cells in the normal human colonic lamina propria, suggesting that they may play a critical role in $CD4^+$ T cell regulation in what is considered to be a tolerogenic environment.

The aim of this study was to examine whether human colonic myofibroblasts (CMFs) phenotypically and functionally resemble conventional APCs. Myofibroblasts are fibroblast-like mesenchymal (stromal) cells that have smooth muscle

---

Address for correspondence: J.I. Saada, Department of Internal Medicine, Division of Gastroenterology, 301 University Boulevard, Route 1058, Galveston, TX 77555-1058. Voice: 409-772-7070; fax: 409-747-0692.
    jsaada@utmb.edu

properties, such as the expression of α-smooth muscle actin (α-SMA), and belong to a family of functionally related cells, such as hepatic stellate cells, glomerular mesangial cells, and synovial fibroblasts.[3] These cells are located just below the basement membrane and are thus positioned to sample antigens before conventional APCs (macrophages, dendritic cells, and B cells) in the intestine. Furthermore, activated myofibroblasts produce chemokines, cytokines, prostaglandins, and adhesion molecules that are capable of driving immune processes.[3]

RESULTS

In normal and inflamed colonic sections, CMFs constitutively expressed class II MHC *in situ* as determined by double immunohistochemical labeling with antibodies to HLA-DR and α-SMA. However, immunohistochemical staining *in situ* of myofibroblasts in archived normal colonic sections and FACS analysis of cultured myofibroblasts were negative for macrophage, dendritic cell, and B cell markers. CMFs freshly isolated from normal tissue constitutively expressed MHC class II as determined by FACS. When cultured and serially passed, they lost MHC class II expression. MHC class II and invariant chain expression in primary CMF cultures were highly induced by IFN-γ in a time-dependent fashion (FIG. 1). Cultured CMFs also expressed important accessory molecules such as ICOS and PD-1 ligands as well as B7-H3. Cultured CMFs induced allogeneic CD4$^+$ T cell proliferation in a class II–dependent manner.

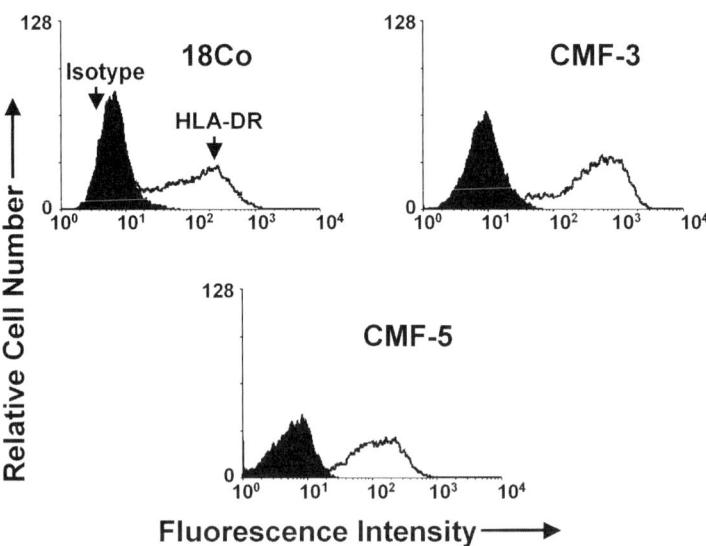

FIGURE 1. FACS analysis of three primary colonic myofibroblast cultures treated with IFN-γ for seven days shows significant increases in expression of MHC class II.

CONCLUSIONS

MHC class II (HLA-DR > DP > DQ)–expressing cells exist in the intestinal lamina propria as macrophages, dendritic cells, and occasional B cells. Intestinal epithelial cells are also capable of expressing MHC class II molecules, although the role of these nonspecialized APCs remains unclear.[4] We report here that α-smooth muscle actin-positive myofibroblasts, which exist as a syncytium under the basement membrane and are also connected to fibroblasts in the core of the lamina propria, express MHC class II *in situ*. MHC class II, invariant chain, and costimulatory molecules are expressed in cultured myofibroblasts after stimulation with IFN-γ. These results support the hypothesis that intestinal myofibroblasts represent a novel, nonspecialized APC phenotype that may be important in modulating mucosal T cell responses. Given their strategic location, we propose that intestinal myofibroblasts play a critical role in intestinal tolerance and/or immunity.

ACKNOWLEDGMENTS

This work was supported by grants from the National Institute of Diabetes & Digestive & Kidney Diseases (RO1 DK55783 and RO1 DK50669) and the Gulf Coast Digestive Disease Center (1 P30 DK56338), a Senior Collaborative Grant from the University of Texas Medical Branch Gastrointestinal Research Interdisciplinary Program (GRIP), and a John Sealy Memorial Endowment Fund Research Development Grant.

REFERENCES

1. MOWAT, A.M. 2003. Anatomical basis of tolerance and immunity to intestinal antigens. Nat. Rev. Immunol. **3:** 331–341.
2. BRANDTZAEG, P. 2001. Nature and function of gastrointestinal antigen-presenting cells. Allergy **56**(Suppl. 67)**:** 16–20.
3. POWELL, D.W., R.C. MIFFLIN, J.D. VALENTICH, *et al.* 1999. Myofibroblasts: II. Intestinal subepithelial myofibroblasts. Am. J. Physiol. Cell Physiol. **277:** C183–C201.
4. MAYER, L., D. EISENHARDT, P. SALOMON, *et al.* 1991. Expression of class II molecules on intestinal epithelial cells in humans: differences between normal and inflammatory bowel disease. Gastroenterology **100:** 3–12.

Transforming Growth Factor–β Regulates Susceptibility of Epithelial Apoptosis in Murine Model of Colitis

HIROTAKE SAKURABA,[a] YOH ISHIGURO,[a] KAZUFUMI YAMAGATA,[a] YOH-ICHI TAGAWA,[b] YOICHIRO IWAKURA,[c] KENJI SEKIKAWA,[d] AKIHIRO MUNAKATA,[a] AND AKIO NAKANE[e]

[a]*First Department of Internal Medicine and* [e]*Department of Bacteriology, Hirosaki University School of Medicine, Hirosaki, Japan*

[b]*Institute of Experimental Animals, Shinshu University School of Medicine, Matsumoto, Japan*

[c]*Center for Experimental Medicine, Institute of Medical Science, University of Tokyo, Tokyo, Japan*

[d]*Department of Molecular Biology and Immunology, National Institute of Agrobiological Sciences, Tsukuba, Japan*

ABSTRACT: Transforming growth factor (TGF)-beta has a key role in intestinal homeostasis. Our present data suggest that TGF-beta, which was constitutively expressed by lamina propria mononuclear cells and epithelium, affected epithelial cells. Abnormal suppression of TGF-beta could enhance the sensitivity of epithelial cells to apoptosis associated with interferon-gamma in DSS-induced colitis.

KEYWORDS: epithelial apoptosis; TGF-β; inflammatory bowel disease

INTRODUCTION

The development of various murine models of inflammatory bowel disease (IBD) has provided new insights into pathogenesis and therapy for human IBD.[1,2] However, mechanisms of the onset of mucosal injury, in particular, destruction of intestinal epithelial cells (IECs) are still poorly understood. Transforming growth factor–β (TGF-β) is a multifunctional cytokine capable of regulating growth, differentiation, and functions of immune and nonimmune cells.[3] Previous *in vitro* studies have shown that TGF-β plays an important role in intestinal epithelial proliferation and reconstitution of epithelial integrity after epithelial injury.[4,5] As it is hypothesized that the intestinal epithelial monolayer is maintained by continuous cycles of proliferation and apoptosis,[6] physiologically expressed TGF-β in intestinal mucosa may

---

Address for correspondence: Hirotake Sakuraba, First Department of Internal Medicine, Hirosaki University School of Medicine, 5 Zaifu-cho, Hirosaki, Aomori, 036-8562, Japan. Voice: +81-172-39-5053; fax: +81-172-39-5946.

hirotake@infoaomori.ne.jp

be involved in determining susceptibility to epithelial destruction, and dysregulation of TGF-β could be implicated in the onset of colitis in the presence of a trigger event(s).

TGF-β ACTION AGAINST IECs ATTENUATES DEXTRAN SULFATE SODIUM-INDUCED MUCOSAL INJURY

Several cell types found in intestinal mucosa, including T cells, dendritic cells, IECs, macrophages, and stromal cells, produce TGF-β. Herein, the analysis of TGF-β–producing cells showed that most TGF-β was constitutively produced by both epithelial cells and lamina propria macrophages/dendritic cells, rather than by lymphocytes. In addition, Sma- and Mad-related protein (Smad)4 mRNA, which acts in direct signal transduction after activation of TGF-β–superfamily receptors, was detected in IECs isolated from normal or dextran sulfate sodium (DSS)-treated mice. Anti–TGF-β monoclonal antibody (mAb) treatment reduced Smad4 mRNA expression in IECs and induced early mucosal destruction. These results indicate that TGF-β may act against IECs to attenuate DSS-induced mucosal injury.

TGF-β INHIBITS IFN-γ/STAT1–MEDIATED MUCOSAL DESTRUCTION

In this study, we demonstrated that intensive expression of IFN-γ and apparent IFN-γ mRNA expression was observed in the intestinal epithelia of anti–TGF-β mAb-treated mice. STAT1 mRNA level was also upregulated in IECs of anti–TGF-β mAb-treated mice. Thus, we hypothesized that IECs might produce IFN-γ in the absence of TGF-β. It is possible that the IEC is a novel IFN-γ–producing machinery. STAT1 plays a major role in mediating the immune and proinflammatory actions of IFN-γ. IFN-γ is known to activate STAT1, and the activated transcription factor up-regulates its own gene expression. These results suggest that the IFN-γ /STAT-1 pathway is upregulated in epithelia by blocking TGF-β in DSS-induced colitis. On the other hand, the injection of anti-IFN-γ mAb in the early phase of DSS treatment completely suppressed the augmented mucosal injury caused by anti–TGF-β, and no significant effect of administration with anti–TGF-β mAb was observed in IFN-γ$^{-/-}$ mice, suggesting that abnormal loss of the TGF-β signal would induce mucosal destruction through the IFN-γ/STAT-1 signal pathway. The imbalance between IFN-γ and TGF-β may be a key factor in epithelial destruction. The dysregulation between physiological TGF-β and "target" epithelial cells in the presence of a trigger event(s) would be a new clue to understanding the pathogenesis of inflammatory bowel disease.

REFERENCES

1. Fiocchi, C. 1998. Inflammatory bowel disease: etiology and pathogenesis. Gastroenterology **115:** 182–205.
2. Elson, C.O., R.B. Strober, G.S. Tennyson, *et al.* 1995. Experimental models of inflammatory bowel disease. Gastroenterology **109:** 1344–1367.

3. KITANI, A., I.J. FUSS, W. STROBER, *et al.* 2000. Treatment of experimental (trinitrobenzene sulfonic acid) colitis by intranasal administration of transforming growth factor (TGF)-β1 plasmid: TGF-β1-mediated suppression of T helper cell type 1 response occurs by interleukin (IL)-10 induction and IL-12 receptor β2 chain downregulation. J. Exp. Med. **192:** 41–52.
4. LETTERIO, J.J. & A.B. ROBERTS. 1998. Regulation of immune responses by TGF-β. Annu. Rev. Immunol. **16:** 137–161.
5. DIGNASS, A.U. & D.K. PODOLSKY. 1993. Cytokine modulation of intestinal cell restitution: central role of transforming growth factor β. Gastroenterology **105:** 1323–1332.
6. CIACCI, C., S.E. LIND & D.K. PODOLSKY. 1993. Transforming growth factor β regulation of migration in wounded rat intestinal epithelial monolayers. Gastroenterology **105:** 93–101.
7. POTTEN, C.S. 1997. Epithelial cell growth and differentiation. II. Intestinal apoptosis. Am. J. Physiol. **273:** G253–257.

Early Events in Antigen-Specific Regulatory T Cell Induction via Nasal and Oral Mucosa

JANNEKE N. SAMSOM, FEMKE HAUET-BROERE,[a] WENDY W. J. UNGER,[a] LISETTE A. van BERKEL, AND GEORG KRAAL

Department of Molecular Cell Biology and Immunology, VUMC, Amsterdam, the Netherlands

> ABSTRACT: Mucosal Tr prevent harmful immune responses to innocuous antigens that are encountered at the mucosae. This unique subset of Tr is adaptive, antigen specific, and suppresses irrespective of cytokine polarization. Here we study the earliest events of mucosal Tr induction and factors that control their differentiation from naive T cells.
>
> KEYWORDS: mucosa; tolerance; suppression; regulatory T cells

INTRODUCTION

Application of soluble proteins via mucosal surfaces induces a state of immunological unresponsiveness to subsequent challenge with the same antigen, also termed tolerance. In contrast, the application of antigen at a nonmucosal site results in T cell priming and the development of a productive immune response. In mice, oral or nasal application of ovalbumin (OVA) leads to antigen-specific suppression of both delayed-type hypersensitivity (DTH) and IgE responses. This tolerance can be transferred to naive recipients by $CD4^+$ regulatory T cells (Tr) from the spleen,[1,2] which exert their function irrespective of cytokine polarization, and propagate systemic suppression through "infectious" tolerance by passing their tolerizing capacity on to naive T cells.[3] Functional analysis of these $CD4^+$ Tr cells during induction of nasal tolerance revealed that they are present in both $CD25^+$ and $CD25^-$ T cell subsets, although, in contrast with the $CD25^+$ T cell subset, suppression by the $CD25^-$ Tr population is antigen-specific.[3] The mechanism underlying suppression by these mucosal Tr cells remains debated, but may include secretion of TGF-β (Th3 cells),[4] IL-10 (Tr1),[5] or cellular interaction via Notch-Notch ligands.[6]

Little is known about the earliest events in the induction of mucosal Tr cells *in vivo* and the factors that control their differentiation from naive T cells. To unravel where naive $CD4^+$ T cells differentiate into these specialized Tr cells during

---

Address for correspondence: Janneke N. Samsom, Ph.D., Department of Molecular Cell Biology and Immunology, VUMC, FdG, P.O. Box 7057, 1007 MB, Amsterdam, the Netherlands. Voice: +31-20-4448077; fax: +31-20-4448081.
jn.samsom@vumc.nl
[a]These authors contributed equally to this work.

TABLE 1. Cytokine profile of dividing T cells in mucosal versus nonmucosal responses

Cytokine[a]	OVA Intranasally	OVA Intragastrically		OVA Intramuscularly
	CV-LN	MLN	PP	ILN
IFN-γ	+/+	+/+	+/nd[b]	+/+
IL-4	–/–	–/–	–/nd	+/+
IL-2	+/+	+/+	+/nd	+/+
IL-10	+/+	+/–	+/nd	+/+

[a]o/n (overnight) release by draining LN cells/detection of cytokine-secreting OVA-specific DO11.10 T cells.
[b]Not determined.

induction of oral and nasal tolerance, we followed the fate of transferred OVA T cell receptor transgenic DO11.10 cells *in vivo*.[7,8]

COMPARISON OF Tr INDUCTION VIA THE NASAL AND ORAL MUCOSA

Within 72 h after nasal OVA application, CD4$^+$ DO11.10 T cells divided in the draining cervical lymph nodes (CV-LNs), but not in peripheral lymph nodes (PLNs). Similarly, the first detectable division during oral tolerance induction occurred in Peyer's patches (PPs) within 24 h after OVA feeding and was followed by multiple divisions in mesenteric lymph nodes (MLNs) during the 24 h thereafter. By comparison, nonmucosal intramuscular (i.m.) OVA injection induced CD4$^+$ DO11.10 T cells to proliferate in the draining inguinal lymph nodes (ILN), albeit more vigorously and with different kinetics than seen in MLNs, PPs, and CV-LNs (FIG. 1A).

In spite of this delayed T cell division after antigen application via a mucosal compared with a nonmucosal route, the differentiating mucosal T cells exhibited striking similarities to effector T cells in the ILNs in terms of surface marker expression (data not shown) and cytokine secretion (TABLE 1). IL-10, a cytokine often associated with mucosal immunity, was observed in all three types of responses and was only partially DO11.10 cell–derived (TABLE 1). Remarkably, mucosally induced Tr did not avidly release IL-4 within the first seven divisions, whereas effector T cells, generated by i.m. OVA treatment did (TABLE 1). Despite the great similarity between developing T cells in mucosal and nonmucosal draining LNs, adoptive transfer experiments revealed that only proliferating CD4$^+$ DO11.10 T

FIGURE 1. Difference in kinetics of division of antigen-specific T cells in CV-LN, MLN, and ILN. BALB/c mice received 1×10^7 CD4$^+$ KJ1-26$^+$ cells intravenously. One day later, mice received either 400 μg OVA i.n., 70 mg OVA i.g., or 400 μg OVA i.m. At 72 h after OVA administration, CV-LNs, MLNs, and ILNs were isolated and single cell suspensions were stained for CD4$^+$ KJ1-26$^+$ cells. (**A**) CFSE profiles of CD4$^+$ KJ1-26$^+$ T cells as determined by flow cytometry. (**B**) Expression of CD25$^+$ in each peak of division as determined by staining cell suspensions with anti–CD25-PE (clone PC61); data are representative for $n = 3$.

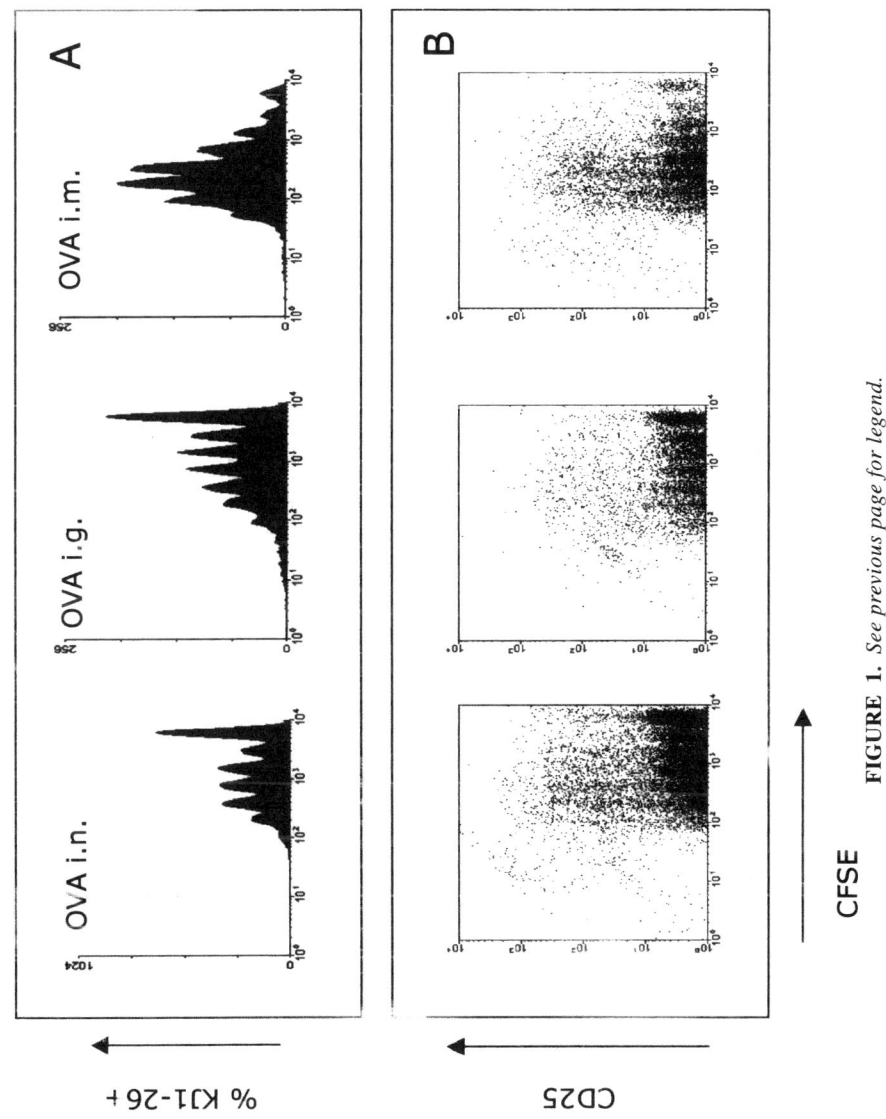

FIGURE 1. See previous page for legend.

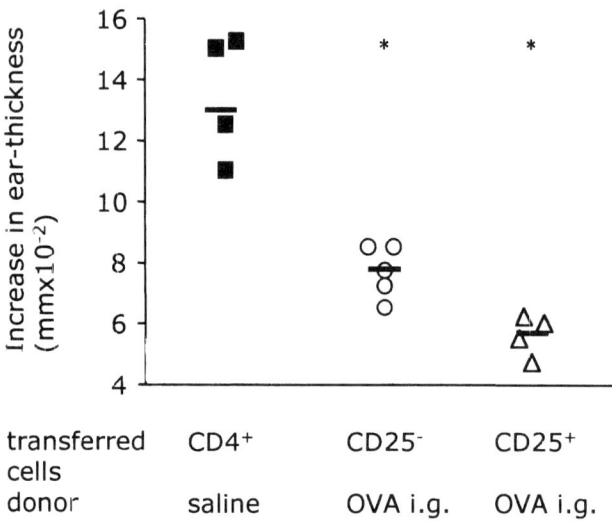

FIGURE 2. Both $CD25^+$ and $CD25^-$ dividing T cells in MLNs are regulatory T cells. BALB/c mice received $CD4^+$ KJ1-26$^+$ cells i.v., as described in FIGURE 1, and were tolerized by administration of 70 mg OVA i.g. or received 200 µL saline as control. MLNs were isolated 48 h later, enriched for $CD4^+$ T cells, and sorted into $CD25^+$ and $CD25^-$ dividing T cells by flow cytometry. Naive acceptor BALB/c mice received either 5×10^4 $CD25^-$ or 5×10^4 $CD25^+$ dividing antigen-specific T cells i.v. or 5×10^5 enriched $CD4^+$ cells isolated from MLNs of saline-treated mice as a DTH control. The next day, the acceptor mice were sensitized with OVA in IFA s.c. in the tail base, and after 5 d mice were challenged in both ears with 10 µg OVA in 10 µL saline per ear. DTH responses are expressed as the mean differences in ear thickness per mouse before and 24 h after OVA challenge in the ears. *Statistically significant ($P < .01$).

cells from mucosa-draining LNs and PPs, but not ILNs, could transfer tolerance to naive recipients.

Because it seemed unlikely that all developing T cells in the mucosa-draining LNs would differentiate into Tr cells, we assessed whether differential expression of surface markers could be detected within each peak of division. Indeed, CD25 expression was heterogeneous among the dividing cells in CV-LNs, MLNs, and PPs, but was also found in ILNs (FIG. 1B). Again, as observed for splenic Tr cells, the segregated expression of CD25 did not discriminate suppressive activity, as both dividing $CD25^+$ and $CD25^-$ T cell subsets in CV-LNs (data not shown) and MLNs were shown to possess regulatory capacity in adoptive transfer experiments (FIG. 2).

CONCLUDING REMARKS

In conclusion, mucosal Tr cells differentiate in the mucosa-draining LNs within a few days after OVA application and acquire their suppressive capacity at this time. The precise mechanisms underlying Tr cell differentiation in the mucosa-draining

LNs are unclear. As recently demonstrated, whether OVA is carried to the LN by migrating mucosal DCs or is ingested by DCs that reside in the LN may have direct consequences for the developing T cell response.[9] Furthermore, intrinsic capacities of the mucosa-draining lymphoid tissue likely govern the conditions under which antigen is presented to naive T cells, directing differentiation toward Tr cells. This is supported by our findings that the presence of the CV-LN was required for nasal tolerance induction and could not be replaced by any other lymph node when transplanted to the cervical site.[10] These intrinsic capacities can seemingly be overruled by treatment with proinflammatory adjuvant because, similar to i.m. treatment, mucosal priming induced by intranasal coadministration of OVA with lipopolysaccharide (LPS) enhanced the kinetics of division, was associated with loss of Tr function, and inhibited subsequent tolerance.[8] Such adjuvants, also including cholera toxin or IL-1, may activate DCs, alter the conditions of antigen presentation, and, as a result, abrogate the induction of tolerance.[11–13]

REFERENCES

1. VAN HALTEREN, A.G., M.J. VAN DER CAMMEN, D. COOPER, et al. 1997. Regulation of antigen-specific IgE, IgG1, and mast cell responses to ingested allergen by mucosal tolerance induction. J. Immunol. **159:** 3009–3015.
2. WOLVERS, D.A., M.J. VAN DER CAMMEN & G. KRAAL. 1997. Mucosal tolerance is associated with, but independent of, up-regulation Th2 responses. Immunology **92:** 328–333.
3. UNGER, W.W., W. JANSEN, D.A. WOLVERS, et al. 2003. Nasal tolerance induces antigen-specific CD4+CD25- regulatory T cells that can transfer their regulatory capacity to naive CD4+ T cells. Int. Immunol. **15:** 731–739.
4. WEINER, H.L. 2001. Induction and mechanism of action of transforming growth factor-beta-secreting Th3 regulatory cells. Immunol. Rev. **182:** 207–214.
5. RONCAROLO, M.G., R. BACCHETTA, C. BORDIGNON, et al. 2001. Type 1 T regulatory cells. Immunol. Rev. **182:** 68–79.
6. HOYNE, G.F., M.J. DALLMAN & J.R. LAMB. 2000. T-cell regulation of peripheral tolerance and immunity: the potential role for Notch signalling. Immunology **100:** 281–288.
7. HAUET-BROERE, F., W.W. UNGER, J. GARSSEN, et al. 2003. Functional CD25- and CD25+ mucosal regulatory T cells are induced in gut-draining lymphoid tissue within 48 h after oral antigen application. Eur. J. Immunol. **33:** 2801–2810.
8. UNGER, W.W. J., F. HAUET-BROERE, W. JANSEN, et al. 2003. Early events in peripheral regulatory T cell induction via the nasal mucosa. J. Immunology **171:** 4592–4603.
9. ITANO, A.A. & M.K. JENKINS. 2003. Antigen presentation to naive CD4 T cells in the lymph node. Nat. Immunol. **4:** 733–739.
10. WOLVERS, D.A., C.J. COENEN-DE ROO, R.E. MEBIUS, et al. 1999. Intranasally induced immunological tolerance is determined by characteristics of the draining lymph nodes: studies with OVA and human cartilage gp-39. J. Immunol. **162:** 1994–1998.
11. WILLIAMSON, E., G.M. WESTRICH & J.L. VINEY. 1999. Modulating dendritic cells to optimize mucosal immunization protocols. J. Immunol. **163:** 3668–3675.
12. SMITH, K.M., F. MCASKILL & P. GARSIDE. 2002. Orally tolerized T cells are only able to enter B cell follicles following challenge with antigen in adjuvant, but they remain unable to provide B cell help. J. Immunol. **168:** 4318–4325.
13. GRDIC, D., R. SMITH, A. DONACHIE, et al. 1999. The mucosal adjuvant effects of cholera toxin and immune-stimulating complexes differ in their requirement for IL-12, indicating different pathways of action. Eur. J. Immunol. **29:** 1774–1784.

Stochastic Resonance-Like Phenomena in the Context of the Alimentary Tract

PABLO SÁNCHEZ,[a] MÁXIMO LORENZO,[a] AND ENRIQUE REWALD[b]

[a]*Facultad de Ciencias Exactas y Naturales,
Universidad Nacional de Mar del Plata, Mar del Plata, Argentina*

[b]*Hipolito Yrigoyen 2184, 7600 Mar del Plata, Argentina*

> ABSTRACT: External noisy stimulation induces Ca^{2+} binding protein dynamics synchronization. Cell coupling chain fluctuation may lead to internal order facilitating information (generation and propagation). Body rhythms require cellular synchronization by interaction between nonlinear biological systems in a fluctuating environment. Could stochastic resonance add or subtract efficacy in digestive tolerogenic selection or disease?
>
> KEYWORDS: noise; stochastic process; calcium signaling; synchronization; signal transduction; temperature

Evolution has placed the bulk of a host's tolerogenic selection in the digestive tract, in which ingested material is subjected to degradation/absorption/transit supported by abundant secretions of a diverse nature, variably stirred by peristalsis. It is associated with relatively settled microflora and defenses from the host. Altogether, signal effects range from so far unnoticed to stimulatory or even to deletional. In addition, ambiguous invaders at the doorstep of the "virtual" intestinal barrier depend on multiple influences. Ubiquitous noise, specifically stochastic resonance (SR), might be expected to emerge as an influence as well. A role for SR is now accepted at the neuronal level, and behavioral SR has been demonstrated to be an important tool, for example, in the capture of food by paddlefish. We postulate that it cannot simply be dismissed as a nonfactor. Recent insight into cytosolic calcium oscillations reveals that they play a significant role in communication, both intracellularly and between adjacent cells.

Omnipresent complex body rhythms require synchronization of cellular mechanisms. They result from the interaction between nonlinear biological systems and a fluctuating environment (such as intestinal content). Could SR add or subtract functional efficacy in the development of immune response or tolerance? Whether SR may be significant in defining disease propensity also remains to be elucidated.

Evolution tends to take advantage of whatever is available. Biology has managed to propel noise phenomena from its place in the background to complex heights. Ubiquitous noise must be seen this way. In fact, it contributes to the main properties

---

Address for correspondence: Enrique Rewald, M.D., Hipolito Yrigoyen 2184, 7600 Mar del Plata, Argentina. Voice: +54-223-4948478; fax: +54-11-4756-2245.
  e.rewald@speedy.com.ar

in the thriving of living systems, energy input, and communications included. As a building block in biology, noise influences series of molecular pathways, for example, distortion-free signal transmission. It may also elicit changes in immune response, such as cytokine secretion modality. Like a double-edged sword, effects range from optimal to harmful.

Formerly seen as a "nuisance," the "functional window" of noise is of rather recent appreciation. A seemingly counterintuitive fact is that noise plays a role by SR effect, optimizing nonlinear system responses to weak periodic signals that, of course, depend on many factors (e.g., timing and quantities). Although ratios are thought to change continuously, the outcome is often still binary, as with an on/off switch. Promissory appears to be noise-induced hypersensitivity to small signals that arise in stochastic systems with on–off intermittency.[1] Complex spatiotemporal patterns of calcium waves and oscillations belong to a dynamic signaling pathway that controls many cellular processes.[2] Rhythms essential for life are generated from physiological functions derived from interactions between cells and with external inputs. This result may be fundamental in living cell systems in which information is critical.

Noise may belong to the toolkit for the events we are looking for. When singled out, it is revealed to be notably resilient. Many questions remain open: data about the absence of noise are not available and the precise panorama of additionally required parameters remains inconclusive. There is also uncertainty in predicting whether noise will become engaged as a promoter or as an impediment. Temperature is known to effect noise and is assumed to have a modulatory influence, but noise-induced hypersensitivity to ultrasmall signals (arising in stochastic systems with on–off intermittency) often is robust to additive thermal noise.[1] It deserves further analysis, in particular, in the setting of vulnerable extremes of human life conditions. At least clinically, tropical heat per se has not been demonstrated to have immunologic effects on humans, infants included,[3] and, as far as we are aware, does not induce changes in oral tolerance. It does not necessarily contradict the possibility that a physical parameter, such as temperature, can be a kind of initial condition. Potentially, by significantly surpassing body standards, some environmental temperature may cause an array of so far subclinical repercussions.

In cells that use Ca^{2+} as second messenger, signals play a vital role in communication, both intracellularly and intercellularly. Marhl et al.[4] and Haberichter et al.[5] have developed a stochastic dynamic model. They demonstrate that both mitochondria and Ca^{2+} binding proteins (CaPr) play important roles in the formation of cytosolic complex calcium oscillations. A more detailed analysis was made by Zhang et al.,[6] whose model extended to a linear array of a two-way coupled system of cells. The transfer of calcium ions between cells is known to occur through gap junctions by passive diffusion-like calcium transfer.

The dynamic characteristics of synchronous oscillations in such models have been studied when only the first cell of the chain system is subjected to external noise. The model predicts that the dynamics of the calcium-binding protein modulated by external stimulation leads to synchronization phenomena that can also be observed in the other cell chain system. Fluctuation from either end of a cell-coupling chain can lead to internal order. It suggests that this process in living cells may play an important role in generating and propagating information.

To investigate the effects of noise on the dynamics of CaPr in the coupled system, a perturbation is introduced in the control parameter k_- (the off rate of CaPr, in the reaction of dissociation/binding) with the form of Gaussian noise:

$$k_- = k_-^0(1 + \beta \cdot \xi(t)),$$

with

$$\langle \xi(t) \rangle = 0$$
$$\langle \xi(t)(\xi(t)) \rangle = \delta(t - t')$$

The noise intensity, β, is an adjustable parameter, and the noise-induced synchronization of oscillations is produced when the noise intensity equals, for example, 0.005.

High organization in space-time is other property of calcium signals and waves. To explain this behavior, a quantity is introduced:

$$\eta = \frac{\sum_{i=1}^{N} t_i}{NT} \cdot 100,$$

where N and T represent the number of cells and the total experimental time respectively; t_i denotes the time interval during which i-th cell can oscillate synchronously with the first cell.

With no noise present ($\beta=0$), the subsystems evolve like independent systems, and $t_1 = t_2 = \ldots = t_N = 0$; so $\eta = 0$. Thus only when all the other cells oscillate synchronously with the first one (i.e., $t_1 = t_2 = \ldots = t_N = T$) does $\eta = 1$. In other cases $t_i < T$, and $\eta < 1$.

The increment of noise level (β) produces the factor η and moves upward and then goes through a maximum plateau and descends at a higher noise level. The occurrence of SR is evident from this conduct. Although the extent of synchronous oscillation changes with noise, when the intensity of noise is appropriate ($\beta = 0.005$), all the subsystems oscillate together.

The plateau exists because the off-rate constant of CaPr has a saturation point. When noise increases and makes the reaction reach the saturation point, the CaPr does not dissociate any longer; so in this region the factor η does not increase with noise intensity. This defines a window within which the fluctuations do not have remarkable effect, and once more "the need for order has led to the proposal that robustness is an intrinsic property of intracellular networks."[7] For greater values of β, the noise will stimulate passive effects and put the coupled system into disorder, and the factor η falls.

The balance of immunogenic and tolerogenic signals affect immune cell responses. The results of antigen exposure represent a complex combination of the timing of antigen binding with signals from many other immunogenic and tolerogenic costimulatory pathways in which the calcium signals are included. A road map of these signaling pathways is, in fact, beginning to be charted, revealing possible mechanisms of action of SR and calcium oscillations.

ACKNOWLEDGMENTS

This work was sponsored by Dr. Lazar y Cía, S.A.Q.e I., Buenos Aires, Argentina.

REFERENCES

1. GERASHCHENKO, O.V., S.L. GINZBURG & M.A. PUSTOVOIT. 2003. Noise-induced hypersensitivity and stochastic resonance: can living systems use them at a molecular level? AIP Conf. Proc. **665:** 67–73.
2. BERRIDGE, M.J. 1993. Inositol triphosphate and calcium signaling. Nature **361:** 315–325.
3. LIEKE, T. 2003. (Bernhard-Nocht-Institut für Topenmedizin-Hamburg, personal communication.)
4. MARHL, M., T. HABERICHTER, M. BRUMEN & H. HEINRICH. 2000. Complex calcium oscillation and the role of mitochondria and cytosolic proteins. BioSystems **57:** 75–86.
5. HABERICHTER, T., M. MARHL & R. HEINRICH. 2001. Birhythmicity, trirhythmicity and chaos in bursting calcium oscillations. Biophys. Chem. **90:** 17–30.
6. ZHANG, J., F. QI & H. XIN. 2001. Effects of noise on the off rate of calcium binding proteins in a coupled biochemical cell system. Biophys. Chem. **94:** 201–207.
7. BARCAI, N. & S. LEIBLER. 1997. Robustness in simple biochemical networks. Nature **387:** 913–917.

Is Oral Tolerance Correlated with IgE Levels and Mast Cell Numbers?

ANTONIO CARLOS DA SILVA,[a] MARIA F. S. SILVA,[b]
CRISTINA BIANCHI,[a] RICARDO C. RIBEIRO,[a] ALBERTO NÓBREGA,[b]
AND OSVALDO SANT'ANNA[c]

[a]*Departamento de Biologia Celular e Genética,
Universidade do Estado do Rio de Janeiro, Rio de Janeiro, Brasil*

[b]*Departamento de Imunologia, Universidade Federal do Rio de Janeiro,
Rio de Janeiro, Brasil*

[c]*Laboratório Especial de Microbiologia, Instituto Butantan, São Paulo, Brasil*

> ABSTRACT: A triple genetic association between serum IgE levels, mast cell numbers, and susceptibility to oral tolerance was observed in mice genetically selected to extreme phenotypes of oral tolerance (susceptibility and resistance), suggesting a coadaptation of genes controlling these traits.
>
> KEYWORDS: IgE; mast cell; oral tolerance; mice; polygenic regulation

The gastrointestinal mucosa is the most important natural route for contact with foreign antigens, a route through which either tolerance or immunity to the antigen can result. Oral tolerance is a special case of immunological tolerance resulting from complex interactions between antigen intake, absorption, and immunoregulatory mechanisms. Loss of tolerance to food antigens can be manifested as food allergies.[1,2] IgE and mast cells play a central role in allergic phenomena, and it is interesting to note that IgE serum levels and mast cell numbers are both sensitive to immunoregulatory mechanisms of tolerance induced by the ingested antigens.[3,4] IgE production is the isotype most tightly regulated by oral tolerance induction.[5,6] Several reports have shown that intestinal mast cells are located in close proximity to T lymphocytes distributed all along the lamina propria and the intraepithelial space, influencing the T cell activation phenotype.[7,8]

We have developed a genetic selection process with the objective of accumulating genes of several independent loci, the additive effect of which are able to induce extreme phenotypes of oral tolerance to ovalbumin (OVA), as measured by antibody response (resistance and susceptibility to oral tolerance, TR and TS strains, respec-

---

Address for correspondence: Maria de Fátima Sarro da Silva, Laboratório de Imunobiologia, Departamento Biologia Celular e Genética, Instituto de Biologia, UERJ, Rua S. Francisco Xavier, 524, PHLC, Maracanã, Rio de Janeiro, RJ, Brasil, CEP 20.559-900. Voice: +55-21-2587-7567; fax: +55-21-2587-7377.
  dasilva@uerj.br and mf-sarro@uol.com.br

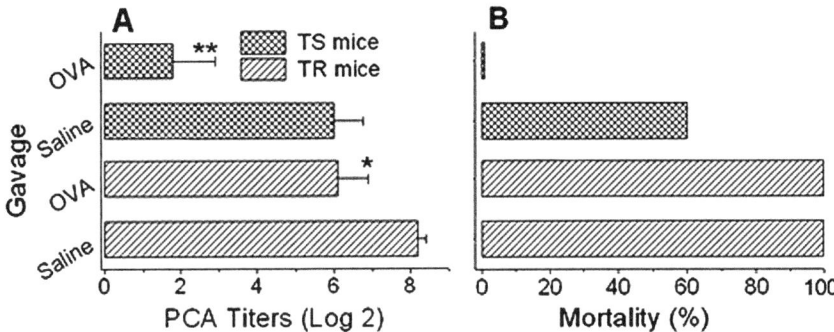

FIGURE 1. Oral tolerance inhibits OVA-specific IgE and protects oral tolerance–susceptible mice (TS) from systemic anaphylaxis. TS and TR mice (both sexes; $n = 8$ mice per group) were subjected to an antigen-dependent (OVA), systemic anaphylactic shock protocol. Death was observed within 30 min of antigenic challenge in both strains. Another group of animals was orally pretreated with 5 mg of soluble OVA in a single intragastric (i.g.) dose 7 d before i.p. immunization with OVA. In orally pretreated animals only TR mice died; all TS animals that were orally pretreated with OVA survived.

TABLE 1. Basal IgE level, mast cell numbers, and oral tolerance correlation in TS and TR mice

Strains of Mice	Basal IgE Mean Values (μg/mL)	Mesentery mast cells/mm^2
TS	0.11 ± 0.07	8.6 ± 3.2
TR	2.35 ± 0.22	18.0 ± 1.5

NOTE: Naive TS and TR mice were assayed for serum IgE levels by ELISA, and a representative experiment of each strain is shown ($n = 5$ for each strain). Mast cell number was counted in mesentery according Mota and Osler.[13]

tively).[9] This approach has the advantage of allowing the full interplay of genes to contribute to the generation of the phenotype. It may allow a more reliable evaluation of the relevance of a given gene to that phenotype in a physiological manner, as a selection process can be said to mimic natural selection when the selected trait adds to the fitness of the animal.

Knowing the central role of tolerance mechanisms in the IgE antibody synthesis, in the present study we investigated the influence of the accumulated *tr* and *ts* alleles on the IgE responsiveness and the physiological distribution of mast cells. Naive TS mice produced lower basal serum IgE and exhibited diminished mast cell numbers (TABLE 1) in all mucosal sites studied. No difference was found in skin (data not shown). Both strains developed severe anaphylactic shock when challenged 21 d after intraperitoneal sensitization (100% mortality in TR and 60% in TS within 30 min), showing that mast cells are fully functional in both strains. Intragastric OVA before immunization significantly reduced the IgE OVA specific response (FIG. 1A) and totally protected TS mice from anaphylactic shock. In TR mice the oral

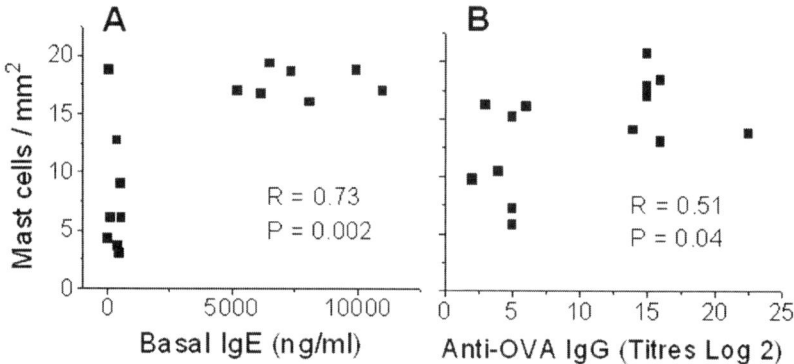

FIGURE 2. Phenotypic correlation between mast cell numbers, serum IgE level, and oral tolerance in F2 segregant populations. (**A**) Scatter plot of mast cell number versus serum IgE levels. The eight naive mice chosen based on low IgE levels had a mean IgE level of 0.00636 ± 0.0043 µg/mL and a mean mast cell count of 7.92 ± 5.38 cells/mm^2. The eight mice with higher IgE levels had a mean IgE level of 1.564 ± 0.443 µg/mL and a mean mast cell count of 17.62 ± 1.24 cells/mm^2. The mean IgE value and standard error of the F2 population was 0.514 ± 0.497 µg/mL. Correlation of phenotypes was not observed with total serum IgG (data not shown). (**B**) Scatter plot of the mast cell number versus serum-specific IgG from mice gavaged with OVA before i.p. immunization with 100 µg OVA + 1 mg Al(OH)$_3$. Serum anti-OVA IgG titers were determined by passive agglutination of OVA-coated erythrocytes. The animals on both extremes of the distribution were selected for mast cell count. The eight mice chosen based on low IgG anti-OVA serum levels had a mean titer of 4.00 ± 1.51 log2 and a mean mast cell count of 11.29 ± 4.07 cells/mm^2. The eight mice with higher IgG anti-OVA serum levels had a mean titer of 16.25 ± 2.81 µg/mL and a mean mast cell count of 16.00 ± 2.89 cells/mm^2.

ingestion of OVA seems to prime for a more severe anaphylaxis, as TR mice die earlier with this treatment (100% mortality within 15 min) (FIG. 1B). In an intestinal inflammatory model both strains had augmented number of mesenteric mast cells, but only TR showed leukocyte infiltration within the mucosa and throughout the length of the villus (TS = 1.5 ± 0.5 and TR = 3.8 ± 1.3 per villus). It is of note that the mast cell number was always twofold higher in TR mice. In the asthma model only TR mice developed allergic inflammation. The eosinophil numbers in the bronchoalveolar lavage fluid (BALF) were 12-fold higher in TR mice (TS = 1.32 ± 1.18 and TR = $16.01 \pm 3.93 \times 10^5$).

The biological significance of the mast cell numbers and basal IgE level was determined by the correlation between both traits through the individual analysis of segregant [TR × TS]F$_2$ populations of naive mice expressing extreme serum IgE level phenotypes. The correlation and respective distribution can be seen in FIGURE 2A. Individuals with lower levels of serum IgE had reduced mast cell numbers, whereas those with higher levels of serum IgE had higher mast cell counts. Thus, genes controlling basal IgE concentration may also contribute to or control basal mast cells number. Moreover, analysis of the [TR × TS]F$_2$ population showed that reduced mast cell numbers correlate with susceptibility to oral tolerance (FIG. 2B). It is also possible that the number of mastocytes could have an effect on T cell activation, especially on those lymphocytes residing in the gastrointestinal tract. Mastocytes are a known source of cytokines, such as IL–4 and IL–5, that are involved in the control of Th1/Th2 differentiation, transient expression, and activation of naive T lymphocytes.[10–12]

The results obtained indicate that the selective pressure for resistance or susceptibility to oral tolerance acted on the phenotypes for both traits, mast cell numbers and IgE production, and their effector functions in anaphylaxis. Altogether, the results suggest the relevant biological coadaptation and pleiotropy of *tr* and *ts* genes controlling these characters. Comparative genome scanning of TR and TS chromosomes will certainly reveal important genes controlling susceptibility to oral tolerance and their relevance to the immunobiological process.

ACKNOWLEDGMENTS

Financial support for this work was provided by grants from CAPES, CNPq, FAPERJ, and FUJB.

REFERENCES

1. MOWAT, A.M. 1994. Oral tolerance and regulation of immunity to dietary antigens. *In* Handbook of Mucosal Immunology. P.L. Ogra, Ed.: 185–210. Academic Press. London.
2. GARSIDE, P., A.M. MOWAT & A. KHORUTS. 1999. Oral tolerance in disease. Gut **44:** 137–142.
3. VAN HALTEREN, A.G., M.J. VAN DER CAMMEN, J. BIEWENGA, *et al.* 1997. IgE and mast cell response on intestinal allergen exposure: a murine model to study the onset of food allergy. J. Allergy Clin. Immunol. **99:** 94–99.
4. DAHLMAN-HOGLUND, A., L.A. HANSON & S. AHLSTEDT. 1997. Induction of oral tolerance with effects on numbers of IgE-carrying mast cells and on bystander suppression in young rats. Clin. Exp. Immunol. **108:** 128–137.
5. VAZ, N.M., L.C. MAIA, D.G. HANSON & J.M. LYNCH. 1977. Inhibition of homocytotropic antibody responses in adult inbred mice by previous feeding of the specific antigen. J. Allergy Clin. Immunol. **60:** 110–115.
6. JARRETT, E.E. 1984. Immunoregulation of IgE responses: the role of the gut in perspective. Ann. Allergy **53:** 550–556.
7. SMITH, T.J. & J.H. WEIS. 1996. Mucosal T cells and mast cells share common adhesion receptors. Immunol. Today **17:** 60–63.
8. YU, L.C., & M.H. PERDUE. 2001. Role of mast cells in intestinal mucosal function: studies in models of hypersensitivity and stress. Immunol. Rev. **179:** 61–73.
9. DA SILVA, A.C., K.W. DE SOUZA, R.C. MACHADO, *et al.* 1998. Genetics of immunological tolerance: I. Bidirectional selective breeding of mice for oral tolerance. Res. Immunol. **149:** 151–161.
10. LORENTZ, A., S. SCHWENGBERG, G. SELLGE, *et al.* 2000. Human intestinal mast cells are capable of producing different cytokine profiles: role of IgE receptor cross-linking and IL-4. J. Immunol. **164:** 43–48.
11. GAUCHAT, J.F., S. HENCHOZ, G. MAZZEI, *et al.* 1993. Induction of human IgE synthesis in B cells by mast cells and basophils. Nature **365:** 340–343.
12. FRANDJI, P., C. TKACZYK, C. OSKERITZIAN, *et al.* 1996. Exogenous and endogenous antigens are differentially presented by mast cells to CD4+ T lymphocytes. Eur. J. Immunol. **26:** 2517–2528.
13. MOTA, I. & A.G. OSLER. 1964. Mast cell degranulation. *In* Methods in Medical Research. H.N. Eisen, Ed.: 168–169. Year Book Medical Publishers. Chicago, IL.

Genetic Selection for Susceptibility to Oral Tolerance Leads to a Profound Reduction of the Acute Inflammatory Response

MARIA DE FÁTIMA SARRO DA SILVA,[a] ALBERTO DA NÓBREGA,[a] TEREZA CRISTINA BARJA-FIDALGO,[b] ALINE C. BRANDO-LIMA,[b] FERNANDO CUNHA,[c] AND ANTONIO CARLOS DA SILVA[b]

[a]*Departamento de Imunologia, Universidade Federal do Rio de Janeiro, Rio de Janeiro, Brasil*

[b]*Departamento de Biologia Celular e Genética, Universidade do Estado do Rio de Janeiro, Rio de Janeiro, Brasil*

[c]*Faculdade de Medicina de Ribeirão Preto, Universidade de São Paulo, São Paulo, Brasil*

ABSTRACT: Strains of mice obtained by genetic selection to extremes of phenotype for susceptibility or resistance to oral tolerance were investigated for possible genetic correlations with acute inflammatory response using different models of inflammation. The results show a strong genetic association.

KEYWORDS: oral tolerance; genetic selection; ovalbumin; acute inflammation; neutrophils; IL-1; IL-10; IL-12; TNF; LPS; corticoid; prostaglandin

We genetically selected two strains of mice for susceptibility or resistance to oral tolerance to ovalbumin (OVA) and for extremes of phenotype of these immunological characters. The strains were obtained by bidirectional genetic selection through assortative mating giving the best phenotypes for susceptibility (TS-Ab strain) and resistance (TR-Ab strain) to oral tolerance to ovalbumin humoral response.[1] The selection was started from a genetically heterogeneous population produced by intercrossing of eight inbred mouse strains, and carried out for eighteen generations of consecutive breeding. These studies showed that several independently segregating genes/loci (quantitative trait loci) interact and regulate oral tolerance.

Oral tolerance is a long-recognized process for inducing peripheral immunological tolerance, leading to suppression of the systemic specific immune response to parenteral administration of immunogens that have previously been ingested; induction of oral tolerance is being tested as a therapy for systemic inflammation.[2] Loss of tolerance to food antigens can manifest as food allergy, and loss of tolerance to commensal flora may manifest as inflammatory bowel disease.[3] Inflammatory

Address for correspondence: Antonio Carlos da Silva, Laboratório de Imunobiologia, Dept. Biol. Cel. e Genética, Instituto de Biologia, UERJ, Rua S. Francisco Xavier, 524, PHLC, Maracanã, Rio de Janeiro, RJ, Brasil, CEP 20.559-900. Voice: +55-21-2587-7567; fax: +55-21-2587-7377.

dasilva@uerj.br; ac-dasilva@uol.com.br

TABLE 1. Quantification of neutrophil migration in acute AIR induced by LPS and polyacrylamide

		TS Mice		TR Mice	
Inflammatory Treatment	Cavities	Neutrophils per cavity $\times 10^6 \pm SD$	Proteins mg/mL ± SD	Neutrophils per cavity $\times 10^6 \pm SD$	Proteins mg/mL ± SD
LPS	Pleural	1.50 ± 0.10***	1.66 ± 0.36	6.06 ± 1.32	3.9 ± 0.32
Polyacrylamide (P-100)	Subcutaneous	5.32 ± 2.73***	2.77 ± 0.94	24.25 ± 4.52	6.00 ± 0.38

Note: Asterisks show statistically significant interstrain differences in neutrophil number and protein concentration.

responses induced by commensal and pathogenic bacteria seem to be under the control of regulatory T cells,[4] which respond directly to bacterial products through Toll receptors.[5] Regulatory T cells secrete anti-inflammatory cytokines TGF-β and IL-10 that can play a critical role in controlling inflammatory processes. In preliminary experiments, we observed that the inflammatory component of the *in vivo* cellular response (DTH test)[6] to experimental infection with fungus[7] or *Leishmania amazonensis* (unpublished results) was lower in TS than in TR mice. These observations originated the supposition that the oral tolerance regulatory genes accumulated by a selective process could also be acting in the inflammatory response.

Here, we investigate the possible genetic correlations of oral tolerance with acute inflammatory response (AIR) using several different models of acute inflammation: systemic, and intraperitoneal or intrapleural injection, using such inflammatory agents as lipopolysaccharide (LPS) or carragenin, subcutaneous injection of polyacrylamide microbeads, and sepsis induced by cecal ligation and puncture (CLP). We show that the TS strain selected for susceptibility to oral tolerance has a significantly diminished acute inflammatory response (TABLE 1). The neutrophil migration in TS was always lower than in TR mice (two- to fivefold). The lower neutrophil migration in TS mice is also consistent with lower ICAM levels (not shown).

The production of several cytokines and other inflammatory mediators was evaluated in both strains. LPS treatment of TS mice induced higher serum corticosterone levels as compared with TR mice. Interestingly, dexamethasone administered before induction of inflammation by LPS or polyacrylamide microbeads inflammation was not able to reduce neutrophil migration in TS mice (FIG. 1). Proinflammatory cytokines such as TNF-α and IL-12 were higher in TR animals, and IL-10 was higher in TS mice (FIG. 2). Early PGE_2 levels were higher in the TS strain, as well as NO production (FIG. 3). The comparison of neutrophil migration between TS, TR, and a segregant F_1 population obtained from crosses of F_1 (TS × TR) and F_1 (TP × TS) shows that TS animals are indeed in the extreme of the distribution, with the lowest numbers of migrating neutrophils (FIG. 4).

Overall, we found that the AIR in TS mice was diminished, suggesting an influence of genes selected for susceptibility to oral tolerance on acute inflammatory response. The inflammatory process could be seen as a danger signal and could interfere with natural tolerance to dietary antigens. We propose that susceptibility to oral tolerance is dependent on regulatory mechanisms reducing inflammatory responses.

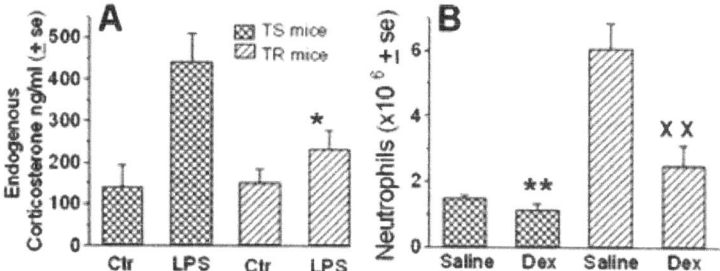

FIGURE 1. Quantification of (**A**) endogenous corticosterone in the plasma from normal and LPS-treated mice. (**B**) Effect of dexamethasone (4 mg/kg) on neutrophil migration 2 h before LPS. Results are expressed as mean ± SEM nanograms per milliliter of corticosterone and number of neutrophils (10^6 SE) per cavity in 10 mice per group. *$P=.05$ and **$P=.01$ for interstrain comparison of LPS-treated mice.

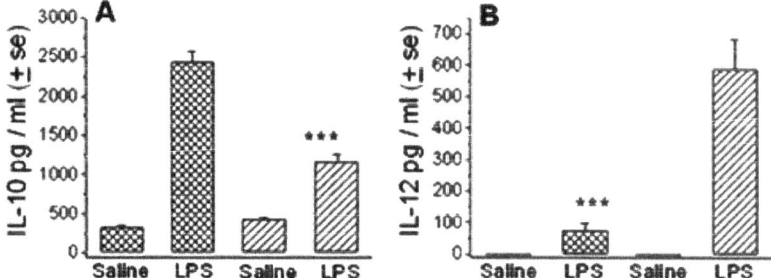

FIGURE 2. Quantification of IL-12 and IL-10 levels in serum at 90 min after intravenous LPS (3 mg/kg). Results are expressed as mean ± SEM picograms per milliliter ($n=6$ mice). *** $P=.001$ for interstrain comparison of LPS-treated mice.

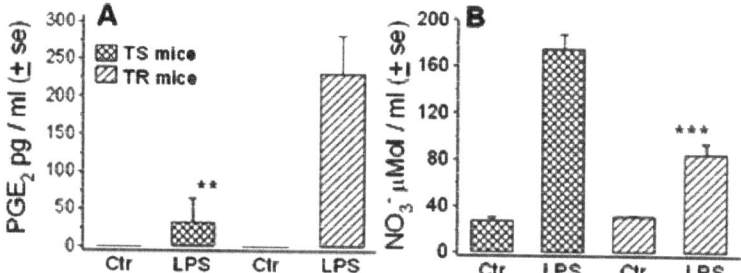

FIGURE 3. Quantification of (**A**) PGE_2 in the pleural wash at 2 h after LPS (250 ng/pleural cavity), and (**B**) nitrate in the plasma at 12 h after i.p. LPS (3 mg/kg). Nitrate results are expressed as mean ± SEM mmol per milliliter ($n=4$ mice). **$P=.01$ and *** $P=.001$ for interstrain comparison of LPS-treated mice. PGE_2 results are expressed as mean ± SEM picograms per milliliter ($n=4$ mice).

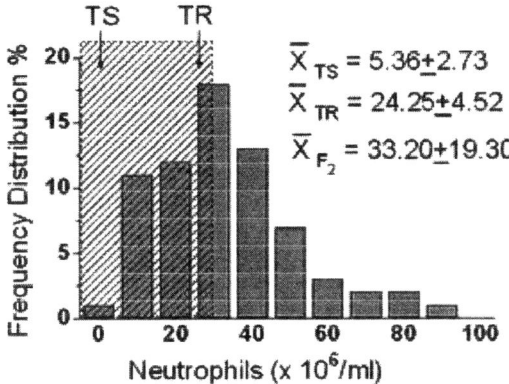

FIGURE 4. Polyacrylamide microbead subcutaneous inflammation induced in 70 mice of an F_2 population [F_1 (TS × TR) × F_1 (TR × TS)]. Polyacrylamide microbead suspension was injected subcutaneously into the shaved dorsal region. The exudate was collected 24 h after injecting 1 mL PBS containing 10 U/mL heparin into the site of the inflammatory swelling. The neutrophil migration to the subcutaneous cavity was evaluated. The *area with diagonal lines* situates the inflammatory response of TS and TR mice into the F_2 population frequency distribution.

ACKNOWLEDGMENTS

Support for this work was provided by grants from CAPES, CNPq, FAPERJ, and FUJB.

REFERENCES

1. DA SILVA, A.C., K.W. DE SOUZA, R.C. MACHADO, *et al.* 1998. Genetics of immunological tolerance: I. Bidirectional selective breeding of mice for oral tolerance. Res. Immunol. **149:** 151–161.
2. GARSIDE, P., A.M. MOWAT & A. KHORUTS. 1999. Oral tolerance in disease. Gut **44:** 137–142.
3. BILSBOROUGH, J. & J.L. VINEY. 2002. Getting to the guts of immune regulation. [comment]. Immunology **106:** 139–143.
4. SINGH, B., S. READ, C. ASSEMAN, *et al.* 2001. Control of intestinal inflammation by regulatory T cells. Immunol. Rev. **182:** 190–200.
5. CARAMALHO, I., T. LOPES-CARVALHO, D. OSTLER, *et al.* 2003. Regulatory T cells selectively express Toll-like receptors and are activated by lipopolysaccharide. [comment]. J. Exp. Med. **197:** 403–411.
6. DA SILVA, M.F., S.C. DA COSTA, R.C. RIBEIRO, *et al.* 2001. Independent genetic control of B- and T-cell tolerance in strains of mouse selected for extreme phenotypes of oral tolerance. Scand. J. Immunol. **53:** 148–154.
7. DA SILVA, A.C., L.M. BEZERRA, T.S. AGUIAR, *et al.* 2001. Effect of genetic modifications by selection for immunological tolerance on fungus infection in mice. Microbes Infect. **3:** 215–222.

The Thymus Plays a Role in Oral Tolerance Induction in Experimental Autoimmune Encephalomyelitis

FEI SONG, INGRID E. GIENAPP, TODD SHAWLER, ZHEN GUAN, AND CAROLINE C. WHITACRE

Department of Molecular Virology, Immunology, and Medical Genetics, The Ohio State University College of Medicine and Public Health, Columbus, Ohio 43210, USA

ABSTRACT: Mice are protected from experimental autoimmune encephalomyelitis (EAE) when fed myelin basic protein (MBP). Thymectomized mice do not exhibit oral tolerance. We found evidence for two mechanisms to explain the role of the thymus in oral tolerance: a site for deletion of autoreactive T cells and a source of regulatory T cells.

KEYWORDS: autoimmunity; EAE/MS; thymus; oral tolerance; T cell receptor

INTRODUCTION

Multiple sclerosis (MS) is a chronic demyelinating disease affecting the human central nervous system (CNS) and often first diagnosed between the ages of 20 and 40. It has been noted that 2.7 to 5% of all cases of MS are diagnosed before the age of 15. It has been reported that most of the putative antigens involved in MS are expressed in the human thymus,[1] suggesting a possible role for the thymus in the development of MS. Experimental autoimmune encephalomyelitis (EAE) shares many features with MS, and nearly all therapies tested in MS clinical trials were first tested in EAE. The oral administration of protein antigens induces a state of systemic immunologic nonresponsiveness specific for the fed antigen. The two major mechanisms to explain oral tolerance are deletion/anergy of antigen-reactive lymphocytes[2] and active suppression involving suppressive cytokines (i.e., TGF-β, IL-4, IL-10) and regulatory T cells such as $CD4^+CD25^+$ T cells.[3] It has been reported that $CD4^+CD25^+$ T cells originate in the thymus, and then migrate to the periphery.[4] However, Thorstenson *et al.* described a subpopulation of naturally occurring polyclonal immunoregulatory $CD4^+CD25^+$ T cells induced by specific antigen that originates in the periphery.[5] Here we explore the role played by the thymus in oral tolerance induction in EAE.

Address for correspondence: Dr. Fei Song, Dept. of Molecular Virology, Immunology, and Medical Genetics, The Ohio State University, 2078 Graves Hall, 333 West 10th Avenue, Columbus, OH 43210. Voice: 614-292-0373; fax: 614-292-9605.
song.89@osu.edu

TABLE 1. Euthymic MBP TCR Tg mice are protected from EAE when fed MBP, while adult thymectomized Tg mice are not

	Euthymic	Thymectomized
Vehicle fed	EAE	EAE
MBP fed	Protection	No protection

TABLE 2. Increased TCR downregulation correlates with an increase of $CD4^+CD25^+$ regulatory T cells in euthymic MBP-fed MBP TCR Tg mice

	Thymus	Peripheral LNs
Transgenic TCR	↓	↓
Apoptosis of Tg cells	↑	↑
$CD4^+CD25^+$ T cells	No change	↑
mRNA of cytokines	Not done	↑IL-4, ↑TGF-β
Proliferative response to MBP and MBP peptide	↓	↑

RESULTS AND DISCUSSION

To determine the role of the thymus in tolerance induction in EAE, euthymic and thymectomized myelin basic protein (MBP) T cell receptor (TCR) transgenic (Tg) mice were fed MBP or vehicle prior to MBP immunization. Euthymic MBP TCR Tg mice are protected from EAE when fed MBP, whereas adult thymectomized Tg mice are not (TABLE 1). The thymus appears to be an important site for deletion, as we observed a decrease in expression of the Tg TCR accompanied by an increase in apoptosis of Tg T cells in the thymus after MBP feeding (TABLE 2). Furthermore, the thymus is also reported to be an important site for generation of regulatory T cells.[4] We observed an increase in $CD4^+CD25^+$ regulatory T cells in the peripheral lymph nodes (pLNs) one day after MBP feeding, which coincided with elevated gene expression for IL-4 and TGF-β (TABLE 2). To determine whether CD25 expression represented activation or suppression, we also examined the proliferative response of thymocytes and LN cells to MBP and NAc1-11. Suppression of the proliferative response in the thymus was noted with MBP feeding relative to vehicle control, whereas T cell activation was observed in the pLNs (TABLE 2). Future experiments will be performed to determine the contribution of the thymus to $CD4^+CD25^+$ T cell generation in the periphery and the source of the oral antigen–induced $CD4^+CD25^+$ T cells. The mucosal administration of MBP has a profound effect on thymic selection, thymic deletion of autoreactive T cells, and generation of $CD4^+CD25^+$ regulatory T cells that cooperate to prevent or suppress the development of experimental autoimmune encephalomyelitis.

REFERENCES

1. BRUNO, R. *et al.* 2002. Multiple sclerosis candidate autoantigens except myelin oligodendrocyte glycoprotein are transcribed in human thymus. Eur. J. Immunol. **32:** 2737–2747.
2. BENSON, J.M. *et al.* 2000. T-cell activation and receptor downmodulation precede deletion induced by mucosally administered antigen. J. Clin. Invest. **106:** 1031–1038.
3. ZHANG, X. *et al.* 2001. Activation of CD25(+)CD4(+) regulatory T cells by oral antigen administration. J. Immunol. **167:** 4245–4253.
4. PAPIERNIK, M. *et al.* 1998. Regulatory CD4 T cells: expression of IL-2R alpha chain, resistance to clonal deletion and IL-2 dependency. Int. Immunol. **10:** 371–378.
5. THORSTENSON, K.M. & A. KHORUTS. 2001. Generation of anergic and potentially immunoregulatory CD25+CD4 T cells in vivo after induction of peripheral tolerance with intravenous or oral antigen. J. Immunol. **167:** 188–195.

Selective Generation of Gut-Tropic T Cells in Gut-Associated Lymphoid Tissues

Requirement for GALT Dendritic Cells and Adjuvant

MARCUS SVENSSON,[a,d] BENGT JOHANSSON-LINDBOM,[a,d]
MARC-ANDRÉ WURBEL,[b] BERNARD MALISSEN,[b]
GABRIEL MÁRQUEZ,[c] AND WILLIAM AGACE[a]

[a]*Immunology Section, Lund University, BMC I-13, S-22184 Lund, Sweden*

[b]*Centre d'Imunnologie de Marseille-Luminy, INSERN-CNRS-Université de la Méditerranée, Case 906, 13288 Marseille Cedex 9, France*

[c]*Departamento de Inmunologia y Oncologia, Centro Nacional de Biotecnologia/Consejo Superior de Investigaciones Cientificas, Universidad Autonoma de Madrid, Cantoblanco, 28040-Madrid, Spain*

> ABSTRACT: To gain entry into peripheral tissues, effector T lymphocytes express specific combinations of adhesion molecules and chemokine receptors. Expression of these are induced during activation in regional secondary lymphoid organs. Herein, we describe a role for GALT DCs in the generation of $CCR9^+$ $\alpha_4\beta_7^+$ gut tropic lymphocytes.
>
> KEYWORDS: lymphocytes; antigen-presenting cell; inflammation; chemokines; intestinal mucosa

INTRODUCTION

Adaptive immune responses start when antigen reaching local draining lymph nodes is processed and presented by antigen-presenting cells (APC), such as dendritic cells (DCs), to naive T lymphocytes. Upon activation, naive T lymphocytes initiate a program to become effector T cells. During this process the cells divide and acquire effector functions necessary for antigen eradication. As part of this program, T cells gain expression of adhesion molecules and chemokine receptors required for entry into tissue effector sites.[1–3]

The integrin $\alpha_4\beta_7$[4] and the chemokine receptor CCR9[5] are expressed on gut-homing effector T cells, and recent data have shown that these molecules are selectively induced on lymphocytes during their activation in mesenteric lymph nodes (MLN).[6,7] Here we determine the requirement for induction of $\alpha_4\beta_7$ and CCR9 on

---

Address for correspondence: Marcus Svensson, Immunology Section, Lund University, BMC I-13, S-22184 Lund, Sweden. Voice: +46-46-222-04-34; fax: +46-46-222-42-18.
Marcus.Svensson@immuno.lu.se

[d]These authors contributed equally to this work.

lymphocytes during antigen-driven activation, and the requirement for CCR9 in localization of lymphocytes to the small intestinal epithelium.

RESULTS

Ovalbumin (OVA) peptide-loaded MLN DCs, but not splenic DCs or non-DC APC, are sufficient and necessary for induction of CCR9 and $\alpha_4\beta_7$ expression on OT-1 TCR transgenic T cells *in vitro*.

Efficient induction of CCR9 and $\alpha_4\beta_7$ on adoptively transferred OT-1 lymphocytes requires immunization with OVA in the context of adjuvant and occurs selectively in MLN, but not in peripheral lymph nodes (PLN) or spleen.

In competitive adoptive transfers, CCR9$^{-/-}$ OT-1 cells were greatly inferior to wild type OT-1 cells in their ability to localize to the small intestinal epithelium following activation in gut-associated lymphoid tissue.

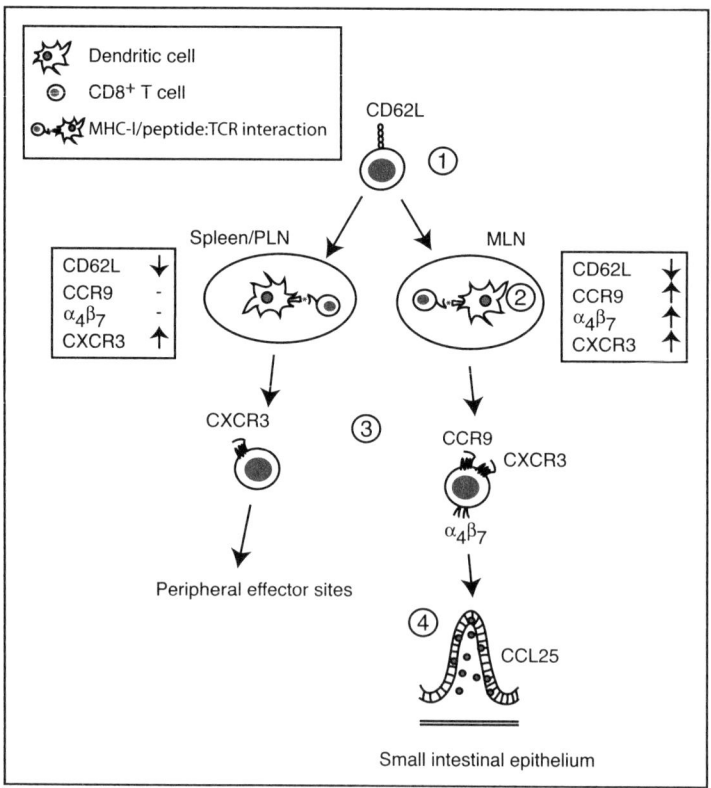

FIGURE 1. Model of acquisition of gut tropism by effector T cells.

SUMMARY

Together these data demonstrate a critical role for GALT DCs as inducers of gut-tropic T cells, and an important role for CCR9 in the recruitment of CD8$^+$ lymphocytes to small intestinal epithelium.

Based on these results we propose the following model for generation and recruitment of gut-tropic T cells to the intestinal epithelium (FIG. 1): (1) Naive T lymphocytes enter secondary lymphoid organs (Note: In the mouse, naive CD8$^+$ lymphocytes are CCR9^{+7}). (2) Upon interaction with antigen-loaded DCs in MLN, naive CD8$^+$ T cells proliferate, downregulate CD62L, and a large proportion acquire a CCR9$^+$ and $\alpha_4\beta_7^+$ phenotype. In the spleen/PLN, CD8$^+$ T cells lose expression of CCR9 and fail to upregulate $\alpha_4\beta_7$. (3) The activated lymphocytes exit lymph nodes via efferent lymphatics and enter into blood circulation. (4) Circulating CCR9$^+$ $\alpha_4\beta_7^+$ CD62L^{lo} CD8$^+$ effector T cells are selectively recruited into the small intestinal epithelium by the CCR9 ligand CCL25 expressed by small intestinal epithelial cells.

REFERENCES

1. SPRINGER, T.A. 1994. Traffic signals for lymphocyte recirculation and leukocyte emigration: the multistep paradigm. Cell **76:** 301.
2. BUTCHER, E.C. & L.J. PICKER. 1996. Lymphocyte homing and homeostasis. Science **272:** 60.
3. KIM, C.H. & H.E. BROXMEYER. 1999. Chemokines: signal lamps for trafficking of T and B cells for development and effector function. J. Leukocyte Biol. **65:** 6.
4. BERLIN, C. et al. 1995. Alpha 4 integrins mediate lymphocyte attachment and rolling under physiologic flow. Cell **80:** 413.
5. ZABEL, B.A. et al. 1999. Human G protein-coupled receptor GPR-9-6/CC chemokine receptor 9 is selectively expressed on intestinal homing T lymphocytes, mucosal lymphocytes, and thymocytes and is required for thymus-expressed chemokine-mediated chemotaxis. J. Exp. Med. **190:** 1241.
6. CAMPBELL, D.J. & E.C. BUTCHER. 2002. Rapid acquisition of tissue-specific homing phenotypes by CD4(+) T cells activated in cutaneous or mucosal lymphoid tissues. J. Exp. Med. **195:** 135.
7. SVENSSON, M. et al. 2002. CCL25 mediates the localization of recently activated CD8alphabeta(+) lymphocytes to the small-intestinal mucosa. J. Clin. Invest. **110:** 1113.

Long-Term Follow-Up of Oral Tolerance Induction with HLA-Peptide B27PD in Patients with Uveitis

STEPHAN R. THURAU,[a] HARALD FRICKE,[b] CHRISTIAN BURCHARDI,[b] MARIA DIEDRICHS-MÖHRING,[a] AND GERHILD WILDNER[a]

[a]*Department of Ophthalmology,* [b]*Department of Internal Medicine, Ludwig-Maximilians-University, Munich, Germany*

ABSTRACT: Oral tolerance induction with peptide B27PD had an ameliorating effect in uveitis patients, which was also observed in the five-year follow-up period. Repeated treatments with peptide B27PD were also effective. Side effects did not occur in this patient group, not even in patients receiving peptide for up to 42 weeks.

KEYWORDS: autoimmune disease; uveitis; tolerance induction; patient trial; peptide; mimicry

INTRODUCTION

Autoreactive CD4$^+$ T cells recognizing retinal autoantigens (i.e., interphotoreceptor retinoid-binding protein (IRBP), S-antigen (S-Ag), and peptides thereof)[1] play an important role in uveitis. Recently, we described a mechanism that could explain the association of certain HLA class I antigens with uveitis;[2] a cross-reactive T cell response to a peptide from the sequence of disease-associated HLA class I antigens (peptide B27PD, amino acids 125–138 of HLA-B: ALNEDLSSWTAADT). Peptide B27PD mimics a dominant epitope from retinal S-Ag (PDSAg, amino acids 342–355 of S-Ag: FLGELTSSEVATEV) and directs a systemic immune response to the antigens in the eye.

The apparent lack of side effects of oral tolerance induction offers the prospect of unlimited therapy to control intraocular inflammation.[3,4] In the rat model, oral administration of B27PD effectively downregulates experimental autoimmune uveitis (EAU). We therefore transferred this approach to uveitis patients.[5,6] Nine patients with endogenous uveitis and an average disease duration of 13 years (range 2 to 33 years) were treated orally with 4 mg of peptide B27PD three times per week for 12 weeks and followed for five years.[7,8] Here, we report on the long-term effects in this patient group, and the reinduction of oral tolerance in selected patients.

Address for correspondence: Stephan R. Thurau, M.D., Section of Immunobiology, Dept. of Ophthalmology, Ludwig-Maximilians-University, Mathildenstr. 8, 80336 Munich, Germany. Voice: +49-89-51603888; fax: +49-89-51603045.
Stephan.Thurau@med.uni-muenchen.de

METHODS

The first year of therapy is extensively described elsewhere.[8] Here, we describe the five-year follow-up of eight of the initially treated patients (one patient did not finish the first three months of peptide therapy[8]). Visual acuity and intraocular inflammation were recorded in a standardized fashion by one investigator (S.R.T.). Four patients were retreated with oral peptide. The local ethics committee approved the reinduction of oral tolerance in selected patients and all patients gave their informed consent.

FINDINGS

A summary of the course of disease for all patients is given in FIGURE 1.

Patient 1 required pars plana vitrectomy for vitreal opacities affecting visual acuity (month 14). Postoperative inflammation was not sufficiently controlled with systemic corticosteroids. She was offered a second course of oral peptide, and subsequently intraocular inflammation subsided quickly. A relapse at month 32 was successfully treated with oral peptide, and a further relapse (month 56) was treated with corticosteroids due to lack of availability of oral peptide.

At the end of year one, patient 2 developed cystoid macular edema, which required increasing doses of corticosteroids. At month 15, retreatment with oral peptide was initiated, visual acuity improved, and corticosteroids were discontinued. At month 20, cystoid macular edema developed and was treated with an average of 7 mg prednisone daily for 8 weeks. Since then, the patient has had no further relapses and has not received any further therapy for more than six years.

Uveitis in patient 3, who needed combined immunosuppressive therapy (azathioprine plus corticosteroids) before oral tolerance induction, subsided after the first peptide treatment without any further need for therapy for five years.

Patient 4 developed progressive disease, which was alleviated for a limited time by treatment with oral peptide B27PD. During follow-up, corticosteroids could not sufficiently control inflammation and, therefore, he received peptide B27PD through months 12 to 19, which partially downregulated inflammation, but additional steroids were required. Later he was treated with a combination of oral steroids and methotrexate, because inflammation became chronic and progressive, and peptide was not available.

After initial oral tolerance induction, uveitis in patient 5 remitted for two years until a secondary cataract required surgery. In order to prevent postoperative inflammation, the patient was given oral peptide prior to surgery. Despite this preventive approach, the patient required systemic corticosteroid therapy for eight months to control inflammation. Later he developed secondary glaucoma. Several surgical and laser procedures led to severe inflammation, which could only be controlled by systemic corticosteroids and mycophenolate mofetil treatment (oral peptide was no longer available).

Inflammation in patient 6 subsided after oral tolerance induction. Corticosteroids were only required to treat peri- and postoperative inflammation after cataract surgery for a period of eight months.

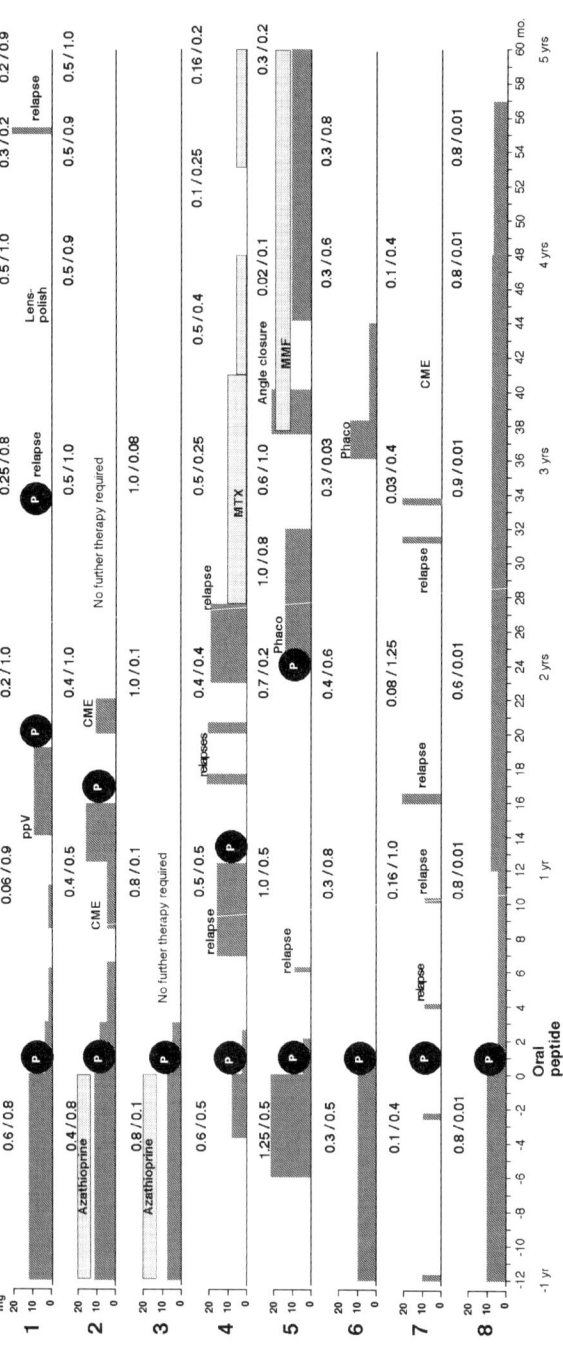

FIGURE 1. Long-term follow-up of uveitis patients after oral tolerance induction. *Black-filled circle* with **P** indicates oral peptide treatment. Hatched areas indicate corticosteroid use (in mg prednisone). *Gray areas* show treatment with immunosuppressive agents (MMF: mycophenolate mofetil; MTX: methotrexate). Paired numbers (e.g., 0.6/0.8 before treatment for patient 1) represent visual acuity (European decimals) of right and left eyes, respectively; CME: cystoid macular edema; Phaco: cataract extraction by phacoemulsification; Lens polish: surgical removal of inflammatory deposits on intraocular lens; ppV: pars plana vitrectomy; angel closure: type of secondary glaucoma.

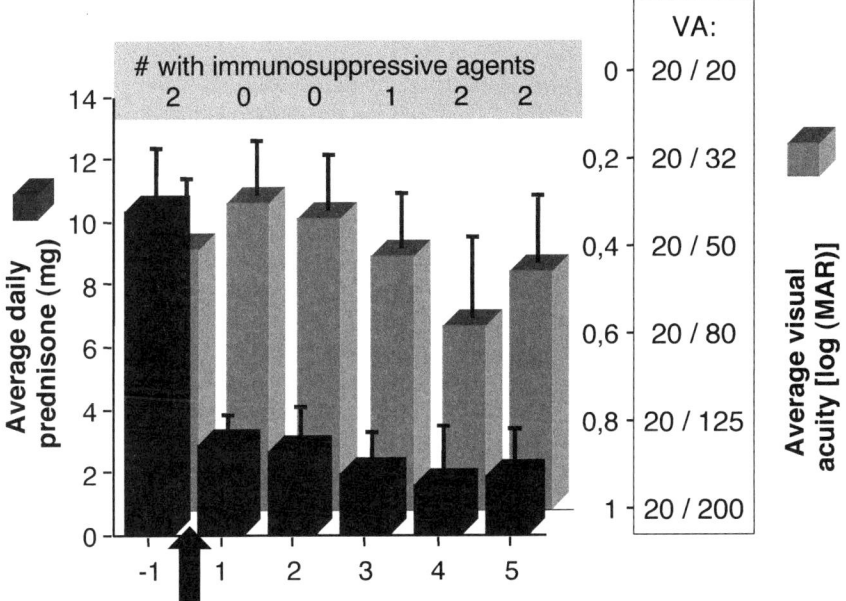

FIGURE 2. Summary of visual acuity [log (MAR)] and steroid use for all eight patients. Although conventional immunosuppressive therapy was reduced significantly, visual acuity remained stable during the 4-year follow-up. Log (MAR) is the log of the minimum angle of resolution. Small values indicate good visual acuity.

Patient 7 initially received oral peptide to treat acute relapses. In follow-up, relapses occurred almost as often as before oral peptide therapy and were treated with short courses of corticosteroids.

Patient 8 with chronic uveitis showed therapeutic response to oral peptide, as indicated by reduced doses of corticosteroids. After the first year, the patient's steroid requirement increased slightly, but remained below that prior to oral tolerance induction, without relapses.

In all patients the average use of corticosteroids was 10.4 mg per day of prednisone prior to oral tolerance induction, and two patients had additional immunosuppressive therapy (azathioprine) (FIG. 2). After tolerance induction, the average daily corticosteroid dose decreased to 2.9 mg (year 2) and 1.9 mg (year 5), while the average visual acuity remained stabile. During the third and fourth year after oral tolerance induction two patients had to be treated with immunosuppressive agents. No side effects that could be related to the repeated use of oral peptide were observed within this patient group.

CONCLUSION

Oral tolerance induced with the 14-mer peptide B27PD had an ameliorating effect on disease activity in patients with chronic autoimmune uveitis, even for an extended period of time. Although relapses occurred during follow-up, most patients required less immunosuppressive and anti-inflammatory drugs than before oral tolerance induction.

Some patients were retreated with oral peptide for recurrences of uveitis. All retreated patients responded with a decrease of inflammation, suggesting that oral tolerance can be reinduced. During this long-term follow-up we did not observe any side effects, not even in patients who were retreated with the peptide. Patients 1, 2, and 3 had suffered from severe side effects of conventional immunosuppressive therapy before oral tolerance induction, which was one of the reasons this new therapy was offered. Treatment with peptide B27PD allowed reductions in conventional medications and their side effects. During the five years post oral treatment with B27PD, the average corticosteroid dose of all patients remained low, while the average maximum visual acuity was unchanged; however, two of eight patients were on immunosuppressive therapy four years after onset of the oral peptide trial.

ACKNOWLEDGMENTS

This work was supported by the Sandoz-Stiftung für Therapeutische Forschung, preceding research projects by the Deutsche Forschungsgemeinschaft (Th 392/2-1, Wi 1382/1-1, and SFB 217), the Friedrich-Baur-Foundation, Münchener Medizinische Wochenschrift, Basotherm-Förderkreis, and the Fritz-Bender-Foundation.

REFERENCES

1. DE-SMET, M.D. *et al.* 2001. Human S-antigen determinant recognition in uveitis. Invest. Ophthalmol. Vis. Sci. **42:** 3233–3238.
2. WILDNER, G. & S.R. THURAU. 1994. Cross-reactivity between an HLA-B27-derived peptide and a retinal autoantigen peptide: a clue to major histocompatibility complex association with autoimmune disease. Eur. J. Immunol. **24:** 2579–2585.
3. WEINER, H.L. 2000. Oral tolerance, an active immunologic process mediated by multiple mechanisms. J. Clin. Invest. **106:** 935–937.
4. NUSSENBLATT, R.B. *et al.* 1997. Treatment of uveitis by oral administration of retinal antigens: results of a phase I/II randomized masked trial. Am. J. Ophthalmol. **123:** 583–592.
5. THURAU, S.R. & G. WILDNER. 2002. Oral tolerance for treating uveitis—new hope for an old immunological mechanism. Prog. Ret. Eye. Res. **21:** 577–589.
6. THURAU, S.R. & G. WILDNER. 2003. An HLA-peptide mimics organ-specific antigen in autoimmune uveitis: its role in pathogenesis and therapeutic induction of oral tolerance. Autoimm. Rev. **2:** 171–176.
7. THURAU, S.R. *et al.* 1997. Molecular mimicry as a therapeutic approach for an autoimmune disease: oral treatment of uveitis-patients with an MHC-peptide crossreactive with autoantigen--first results. Immunol. Lett. **57:** 193–201.
8. THURAU, S.R. *et al.* 1999. Oral tolerance with an HLA-peptide mimicking retinal autoantigen as a treatment of autoimmune uveitis. Immunol. Lett. **68:** 205–512.

IL-18 and Antigen-Specific CD4$^+$ Regulatory T Cells in Peyer's Patches

NORIKO M. TSUJI AND BERNADETA NOWAK

Department of Molecular Biology and Immunology,
National Institute of Agrobiological Sciences, Ibaraki, Japan

ABSTRACT: A study using gene-deficient mice revealed that IL-18 is essential for inducing antigen-specific regulatory T cells and oral tolerance. It is also suggested that IL-18 is a functional downregulator for immunogenic dendritic cells, contributing to the maintenance of homeostasis for intestinal immunity.

KEYWORDS: regulatory T cell; IL-18; Peyer's patch; oral tolerance

The intestinal mucosa covers an area 200 times greater than that of skin. Thus, food components and commensal bacteria are major sources of external antigens and environmental factors for humans. Although the immune system is able to cope with environmental factors, inflammation against beneficial components, such as food, must be avoided. Thus, the intestinal immune system may have developed ways to induce tolerance to environmental factors more efficiently than other organs. Regarding these aspects, we propose that the intestinal immune system, in particular, Peyer's patches (PPs), play an important role in inducing specific regulatory T (Tr) cells against fed antigens. Antigen-specific CD4$^+$ Tr clones that we established from PPs of mice fed high doses of β-lactoglobulin (BLG) exhibited anergic and CD25$^+$ phenotypes and produced TGF-β. When transferred *in vivo*, these Tr clones significantly regulated antigen-specific antibody production.[1]

In order to examine the responsiveness of intestinal Tr cells against external stimulation, PP Tr clones were cultured with various cytokines. Interestingly, PP Tr clones were highly responsive to inflammatory cytokines, especially to IL-18, when stimulated with antigen-presenting cells (APCs) plus BLG, or with plate-bound anti-CD3 antibodies. PP Tr clones also responded to IL-2, to which, in many cases, anergic cells respond and proliferate.

Thus, we tested whether IL-18 plays any role in the maintenance of PP Tr cells *in vivo*. To wild-type and IL-18$^{-/-}$ mice with a C57BL/6 background (kindly provided by Dr. S. Akira, Osaka University), we fed 100 mg of BLG or saline five times over two weeks by gastric intubation. PP cells were harvested seven days after the last BLG feeding. These primary PP cells were analyzed for their suppressive effects on antibody production when cocultured with an *in vitro* antibody production system

---

Address for correspondence: Noriko M. Tsuji, Department of Molecular Biology and Immunology, National Institute of Agrobiological Sciences, 2-1-2 Kannondai, Tsukuba, Ibaraki, Japan 305-8602. Voice: +81-29-838-7741; fax: +81-29-838-7802.
ten@affrc.go.jp

TABLE 1. Lack of oral tolerance induction in IL-18$^{-/-}$ mice

		Fed	
	Mouse Strain	Saline	BLG
T cell proliferative response (c.p.m.)	WT	12,406 ± 997	7,262 ± 339*
	IL-18 KO	19,218 ± 1,809	19,317 ± 1,950
BLG-specific antibody titer (units)	WT	32.58 ± 6.86	7.75 ± 2.29**
	IL-18 KO	53.32 ± 10.01	28.80 ± 7.96

*$P<.05$.
**$P<.01$.

consisting of Th clone cells and primed spleen B cells. In wild-type mice, PP cells showed significant suppressive activity after feeding 5 × 100 mg BLG, as we have observed previously.[1] However, the antigen-specific induction of regulatory effects was not observed in IL-18$^{-/-}$ PP cells. It is likely that IL-18 plays an important role in the induction and/or maintenance of PP Tr cells.

The next question is whether these PP Tr cells are physiologically important in the induction of oral tolerance. We tested the T cell proliferative response and BLG-specific antibody titer in serum after feeding wild-type or IL-18$^{-/-}$ mice 5 × 100 mg of BLG and immunizing them. As shown in TABLE 1, we found that the ability to induce oral tolerance was impaired in IL-18$^{-/-}$ mice. Thus, antigen-specific PP Tr cells seem to contribute to inducing systemic tolerance. It has been reported that antigen-specific Tr cells (Th3 and Tr1-like) are induced in low-dose oral tolerance.[2,3] Here, we propose that antigen-specific Tr cells (anergic type and IL-18–responding) were induced in PPs upon induction of high-dose oral tolerance and they are relevant to the mechanism for systemic tolerance.

The maturation of PPs and induction of oral tolerance are impaired in germ-free mice, suggesting that innate immune signals from commensal bacteria are important for the induction of oral tolerance. Thus, we consider it reasonable that IL-18, an inflammatory cytokine, is one of the key molecules for the maturation of the intestinal immune system. Interestingly, immune response of T cells from spleens and lymph nodes are normal in IL-18$^{-/-}$ mice. The impairment of antigen-specific PP Tr cells in IL-18$^{-/-}$ mice may be closely related to the unique intestinal environment with abundant innate immune signals.

Given that intestinal APCs constantly see the innate immune signals, we tested whether dendritic cells (DCs) derived from IL-18$^{-/-}$ mice function normally. We examined CD11c$^+$ cells and found that IL-10 production induced by microbial stimulation was partially but significantly impaired in IL-18–deficient bone marrow-derived DCs (BMDCs). Moreover, the expression of costimulatory molecules and the ability to support antigen-specific T cell proliferation were higher in IL-18$^{-/-}$ BMDCs after microbial stimulation. These data suggest that IL-18 may be a functional downregulator for immunogenic DCs.

Collectively, oral tolerance is a physiological way to generate antigen-specific Tr cells, and IL-18 seems to play important roles in maintaining PP-derived Tr and DC populations to support the functional maturation of such T cells. Because the active form of IL-18 is produced by APCs via an inflammatory response, innate immune signals from the intestinal environment should be considered significant in maintaining intestinal antigen-specific Tr cells.

REFERENCES

1. TSUJI, N.M., K. MIZUMACHI & J. KURISAKI. 2003. Antigen-specific, CD4$^+$CD25$^+$ regulatory T cell clones induced in Peyer's patches. Int. Immunol. **15:** 525–534.
2. TSUJI, N.M., K. MIZUMACHI & J. KURISAKI. 2001. Interleukin-10-secreting Peyer's patch cells are responsible for active suppression in low-dose oral tolerance. Immunology **103:** 458–464.
3. CHEN, Y., V.K. KUCHROO, J. INOBE, *et al.* 1994. Regulatory T cell clones induced by oral tolerance: suppression of autoimmune encephalomyelitis. Science **265:** 1237–1240.

Gamma-Delta T Cells as Orally Induced Suppressor Cells in Rats: *In Vitro* Characterization

GERHILD WILDNER, STEPHAN R. THURAU, AND MARIA DIEDRICHS-MÖHRING

Section of Immunobiology, Department of Ophthalmology, Ludwig-Maximilians-University, Munich, Germany

ABSTRACT: Gamma-delta T cells from orally tolerized rats adoptively transfer suppression of experimental autoimmune uveitis. *In vivo* and *in vitro* these regulatory cells specifically recognize retinal autoantigen peptide PDSAg and its mimotope B27PD, but not other mimicry peptides. Proliferation of γ/δ T cells was MHC class II and CD8 dependent.

KEYWORDS: experimental autoimmune uveitis; Lewis rat; peptide; antigenic mimicry; tolerance induction

INTRODUCTION

Experimental autoimmune uveitis (EAU) in Lewis rats can be induced by immunization with retinal proteins, peptides, or peptides from nonocular proteins that mimic retinal autoantigen. Furthermore, EAU can be prevented by feeding said antigens or even peptides prior to disease induction with whole autoantigen proteins. Oral tolerization with HLA-peptide B27PD, which mimics retinal S-antigen peptide PDSAg, efficiently suppresses EAU in rats induced with S-antigen (S-Ag) or interphotoreceptor retinoid–binding protein (IRBP).[1] However, specific amino acid residues from PDSAg or B27PD responsible for pathogenicity or oral tolerogenicity could not be defined.[2] A therapeutic trial with oral application of peptide B27PD for uveitis patients refractive to conventional therapy was performed successfully.[1] Other peptides, such as Rota or Cas, that mimic retinal peptide PDSAg and are pathogenic in rats do not function as oral tolerogens.[3] Bystander suppression in the eye was not effective in the acute and monophasic disease course of rat EAU, but was demonstrated to act in the peripheral lymph nodes by targeting the afferent immune response. Oral tolerance can be adoptively transferred with γ/δ T cells isolated from spleens of HLA- or S-Ag peptide–fed rats.[4] These T cells are CD8$^+$ and proliferate *in vitro* in coculture with their respective antigen peptide and antigen-specific α/β T

Address for correspondence: Dr. Gerhild Wildner, Section of Immunobiology, Dept. of Ophthalmology, Ludwig-Maximilians-University, Mathildenstr. 8, 80336 Munich, Germany. Voice: +49-89-5160-3888; fax: +49-89-5160-3045.
Gerhild.Wildner@med.uni-muenchen.de

cells. Here, we further characterize the peptide recognition and the role of antigen-presenting α/β T cells with respect to proliferation of γ/δ TCR$^+$ cells *in vitro*.

MATERIAL AND METHODS

Lewis rats were fed three or four times with 200 μg peptide (B27PD: ALNEDLSSWTAADT, HLA-B amino acids 125–138, Saxon, Hannover, Germany; B7PD: ALNEDLRSWTAADT, HLA-B7 amino acids 125–138; PDSAg: FLGELTSSWTAADT, retinal S-Ag amino acids 341–354; Rota: WTEVSEVATEV, Rotavirus vp4, amino acids 591–601; Cas: SEESAEVATEEV, bovine αs2-casein, amino acids 73–84; Biotrend, Cologne, Germany) or 1 mg protein (αs2-casein, Sigma, Deisenhofen, Germany). Two days after the last gavage, rats were either immunized with PDSAg in CFA to induce EAU, or spleens were removed to isolate γ/δ TCR$^+$ cells by MACS-separation, using antibody V65 (gift from T. Hünig) and magnetic bead-coupled rat anti–mouse-IgG1 (Miltenyi, Berg. Gladbach, Germany). α/β TCR$^+$ cells from peptide-specific rat T cell lines were isolated by MACS, using primary antibody R73 (gift from T. Hünig). Purity of the populations was analyzed by a FACScan.

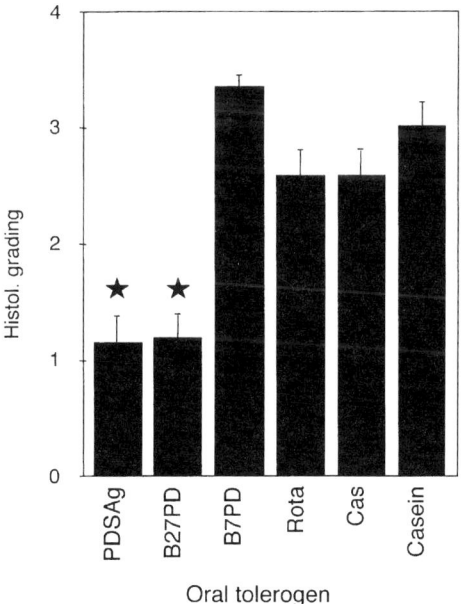

FIGURE 1. Feeding retinal autoantigens or peptides mimicking ocular peptides can prevent experimental autoimmune uveitis (EAU) in Lewis rats. HLA peptide B27PD prevented uveitis in Lewis rats as effectively as the retinal peptide PDSAg itself, although B27PD is only poorly pathogenic. Other pathogenic peptides that mimic PDSAg (Rota or Cas) are not effective as oral tolerogens. Asterisks mark significant reduction of uveitis compared to groups fed B7PD.

Irradiated α/β cells (6 × 10⁴) (10 Gy) and 3 × 10⁴ γ/δ cells were cocultured in round-bottom microtiter plates in RPMI 1640 with 10 μg/mL peptide and 2% rat serum for 3 days and labeled with [³H]thymidine for the last 16 to 20 hours. Dilutions of inhibitory antibodies (CD8α: Ox8, CD8β: 341, RT1.B: Ox6, RT1.D: Ox17, all from Pharmingen/BD, Wiesbaden, Germany) were added in the beginning of the cultures. Spleen-conditioned medium (SCM) was obtained by 40 h stimulation of rat splenocytes in RPMI containing 5% fetal calf serum and Concanavalin A (Con A) with final inactivation of Con A.

RESULTS AND DISCUSSION

HLA peptide B27PD with sequence homologies to peptide PDSAg from retinal S-Ag can induce oral tolerance in Lewis rats at least as effectively as the retinal peptide itself (FIG. 1). Two other peptides mimicking PDSAg, Rota and Cas, are not effective as oral tolerogens, although they are pathogenic in Lewis rats.[3] This indicates that effector T cells and orally induced regulatory T cells in rats are different cell populations with distinct antigen recognition. Not all antigens causing an autoimmune response are also capable of inducing therapeutic tolerance induction.

Gamma-delta T cells from spleens of rats orally tolerized with retinal peptide PDSAg or mimicry peptide B27PD, but not with control peptide B7PD, can transfer protection to naive animals.[4] These γ/δ T cells can proliferate *in vitro* upon stimulation with medium containing 10% SCM. Here, we tested the *in vitro* response of freshly isolated γ/δ T cells (purity greater than 90%) from rats fed with either peptide B27PD (FIG. 2a) or PDSAg (FIG. 2b) in response to various α/β T cell lines and different peptide antigens. Gamma-delta T cells from rats fed B27PD were able to proliferate *in vitro* in response to peptides B27PD and PDSAg and activated PDSAg-specific α/β T cells. Despite their amino acid similarities with peptides B27PD (B7PD) or PDSAg (Rota, Cas), peptides Rota, Cas or B7PD did not induce proliferation of B27PD-specific γ/δ T cells (FIG. 2a). Activated α/β T cells with an antigen specificity differing from that of the γ/δ T cells (peptide Ker333 from cytokeratin 5, amino acids 333–354; Ref. 5) were less sufficient in presenting specific peptides to the γ/δ T cells (FIG. 2b). Our findings point to peptide specificity of these γ/δ T cells, and in addition the need for cell–cell contact with α/β T cells, indicating the direct recognition of the effector T cells that ought to be suppressed.

The mode of antigen and α/β T cell recognition by γ/δ T cells is still unknown. In order to determine surface antigens important for induction of *in vitro* proliferation, we added antibodies specific for MHC class II (RT1.B, Ox6, and RT1.D, Ox17) as well as specific for CD8α (Ox8) and CD8β (341) chain to the cultures. The suppression mediated by Ox8, 341, and Ox6 (FIG. 3) indicated a role for CD8α/β and RT1.B. Peptides PDSAg and B27PD are both RT1.B-binding.[2] Up to 90% of freshly isolated γ/δ T cells are CD8α/β positive,[4] a minority of only 4% were CD4⁺, and about 14% were RT1.B⁺ (data not shown), whereas most activated CD4⁺αβ rat T cells express MHC class II antigens. These experiments did not clarify whether the inhibitory antibodies target surface MHC class II on α/β or γ/δ T cells.

The γ/δ T cells used here were a heterogeneous population, of which probably only a minor subpopulation responded to peptides and α/β T cells. In mice, γ/δ T cells were described that recognize peptide presented on MHC class II molecules

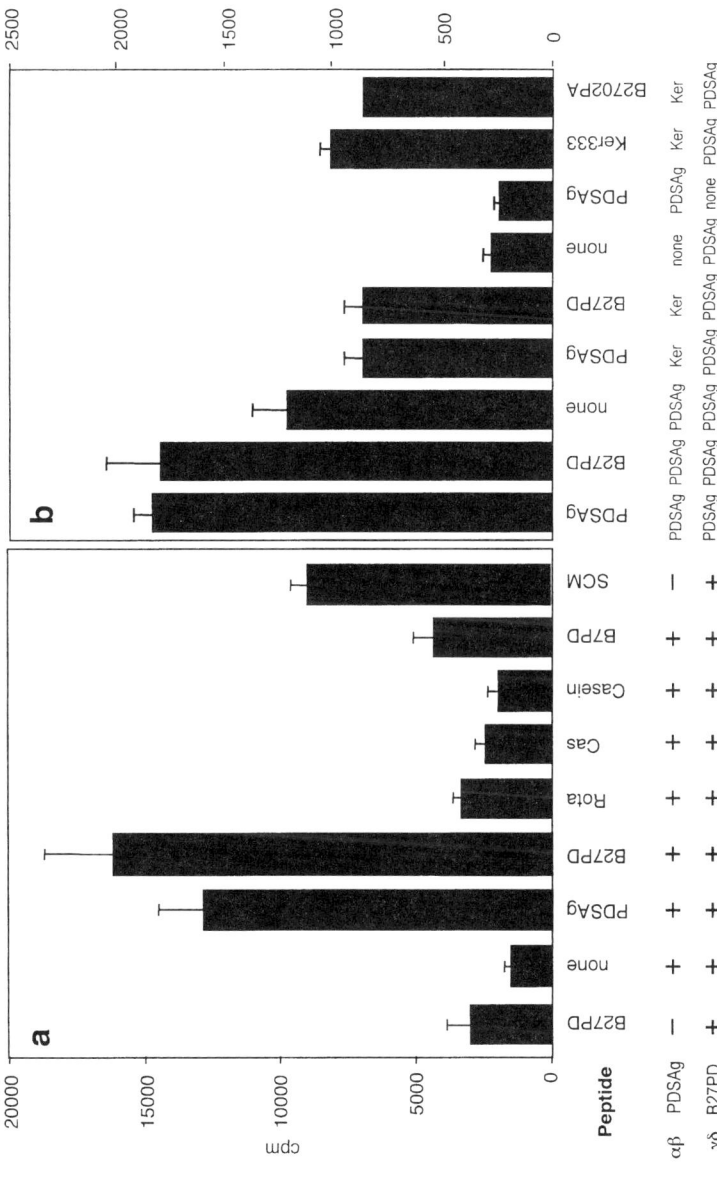

FIGURE 2. (a) MACS-separated γ/δ T cells from spleens of B27PD-fed rats were cocultured with or without a PDSAg-specific α/β T cell line and various peptides. Only SCM or a combination of PDSAg-specific α/β T cells and the specific peptide B27PD or the mimicry peptide PDSAg induced proliferation. (b) MACS-separated γ/δ T cells from spleens of PDSAg-fed rats were cocultured with a PDSAg- or a Ker333-specific α/β T cell line and various peptides. Again, only coculture with the respective α/β T cell line and the specific (here, PDSAg) or mimicry peptide B27PD stimulated the proliferation of γ/δ T cells.

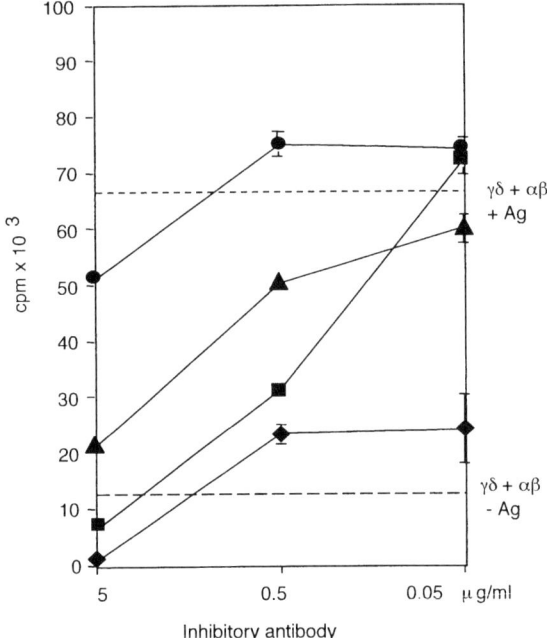

FIGURE 3. Inhibitory antibodies were added to cultures of freshly isolated PDSAg-induced γ/δ T cells with PDSAg-specific α/β T cell line and PDSAg. Antibody Ox6 (RT1.B-specific) as well as CD8α- and β-chain–specific monoclonal antibodies were able to efficiently block γ/δ T cell proliferation. ■, Ox6 (MHC class II, RT1.B); ●, Ox 17 (MHC class II, RT1.D); ▲, CD8 alpha; ◆, CD8 beta.

and differentiate between peptide variants.[6] This is similar to the γ/δ T cells described here that also differentiated between peptides and did not recognize the Rota and Cas peptides, which are mimotopes for α/β T cells. Murine γ/δ T cells can also recognize I-E molecules irrespective of the bound peptide,[6] but the majority of γ/δ T cells is thought to recognize nonclassical MHC class I molecules such as CD1 or T10/T22.

SUMMARY

In rat EAU we have described several peptides mimicking retinal peptide PDSAg that are either pathogenic (Rota, Cas) or tolerogenic (B27PD). Here we show that γ/δ T cells from spleens of rats orally tolerized with peptides PDSAg or B27PD proliferated specifically in response to certain peptides and α/β T cells, preferring those α/β T cell lines that are specific for the respective tolerizing peptides. The mode of peptide recognition by orally induced γ/δ T cells is still unclear, although antibodies specific for CD8 and MHC class II inhibited *in vitro* proliferation. Nevertheless, orally induced γ/δ T cells share certain antigen cross-reactivities with α/β T cells, but are also able to distinctively ignore variant peptides, pointing to the fact that not all antigens that are immunogenic on the level of α/β T cells are orally tolerogenic with respect to γ/δ T cell recognition.

ACKNOWLEDGMENTS

We thank I. Rädler-Angeli for excellent technical assistance. This work was supported by the Deutsche Forschungsgemeinschaft, SFB 571.

REFERENCES

1. WILDNER, G. & S.R. THURAU. 1994. Crossreactivity between an HLA-B27 derived peptide and a retinal autoantigen peptide: a clue to MHC-association with autoimmune disease. Eur. J. Immunol. **24:** 2579–2585.
2. WILDNER, G. & M. DIEDRICHS-MÖHRING. 2003. Differential recognition of a retinal autoantigen peptide and its variants by rat T cells in vitro and in vivo. Int. Immunol. **15:** 927–935.
3. WILDNER, G. & M. DIEDRICHS-MÖHRING. 2003. Autoimmune uveitis induced by molecular mimicry of rotavirus, bovine casein and retinal S-antigen. Eur. J. Immunol. **33:** 2577–2587.
4. WILDNER, G., T. HÜNIG & S.R. THURAU. 1996. Orally induced, peptide specific γ/δ TCR[+] cells suppress experimental autoimmune uveitis. Eur. J. Immunol. **26:** 2140–2148.
5. WILDNER, G., M. DIEDRICHS-MÖHRING & S.R. THURAU. 2002. Induction of arthritis and uveitis in Lewis rats by antigenic mimicry of peptides from HLA-B27 and cytokeratin. Eur. J. Immunol. **32:** 299–306.
6. CHIEN, Y.H. & J. HAMPL. 2000. Antigen recognition properties of murine γ/δ T cells. Springer Semin. Immunopathol. **22:** 239–250.

Index of Contributors

Adegboyega, P.A., 313–318, 379–381
Agace, W., 334–336, 405–407
Aharoni, R., 239–249
Ali, N., 250–259
Allavena, P., 66–74
Allez, M., 22–35
Anderle, P., 16–21
Anderton, S., 180–192
Arnon, R., 239–249
Arya, A., 334–336
Asai, K., 344–345

Barja-Fidalgo, T.C., 398–401
Barrera, C.A., 313–318, 379–381
Barrett, T.A., 94–100
Battaglia, M., 142–153
Beacock-Sharp, H., 1–8
Benson, J., 172–179
Beswick, E., 313–318
Bianchi, C., 394–397
Bilsborough, J., 83–87
Bland, D.A., 313–318, 379–381
Blumberg, R.S., 154–168
Bode, B., 260–277
Boesteanu, A., 101–114
Boirivant, M., 115–131
Brando-Lima, A.C., 398–401
Brimnes, J., 22–35
Burchardi, C., 408–412

Campbell, J., 374–378
Campbell, K., 172–179
Carvalho, C.R., 321–327, 350–354
Caton, A.J., 101–114
Chan, L., 225–238
Cheifetz, A., 225–238
Chieppa, M., 66–74
Childs, J., 225–238
Chirdo, F., 1–8
Colgan, S., 154–168
Cong, Y., 319–320
Contractor, N., 60–65
Cousins, L., 75–82
Cozzo, C., 101–114

Cunha, F., 398–401

da Cunha, A.P., 321–327
da Nóbrega, A., 398–401
da Silva, A.C., 350–354, 394–397, 398–401
da Silva, M.F.S., 350–354, 394–397, 398–401
Davies, D.H., 250–259
de Faria, A.M.C., 361–365
Debard, N., 16–21
DeKruyff, R.H., 88–93
Dermody, T., 60–65
Derry, C.J., 250–259
Devendra, D., 328–330, 331–333
Di Mari, J.F., 379–381
Didierlaurent, A., 16–21
Diedrichs-Möhring, M., 408–412, 416–421
Dotan, I., 22–35

Eisenbarth, G., 328–330, 331–333
Elson, C.O., 299–309, 319–320
Ergun-Longmire, B., 260–277
Ericsson, A., 334–336

Faria, A.M.C., 350–354
Finke, D., 16–21
Fleeton, M., 60–65
Fricke, H., 408–412
Fuss, I., 115–131, 154–168

Garside, P., 9–15
Gebbers, J.-O., 337–343
German, B., 374–378
Gianfrani, C., 142–153
Gienapp, I., 172–179, 402–404
Gomes, E., 361–365
Gregori, S., 142–153
Guan, Z., 172–179, 402–404

Hachimura, S., 344–345

Hauet-Broere, F., 385–389
He, J., 60–65
Holmes, N., 355–357
Huang, F.-P., 75–82

Ilan, Y., 286–298
Ise, W., 344–345
Ishiguro, Y., 346–347, 348–349, 382–384
Iwakura, Y., 382–384
Iwasaki, A., 60–65

Johansson-Lindbom, B., 405–407
Jordan, M.S., 101–114

Kaji, T., 344–345
Kaminogawa, S., 344–345
Kamphorst, A.O., 350–354
Kaser, A., 154–168
Keller, A.C., 361–365
Kelsall, B., 60–65
Kitani, A., 115–131
Klinger, E., 239–249
Komagata, Y., 366–370
Kraal, G., 385–389
Kraehenbuhl, J.-P., 16–21
Kraus, T.A., 225–238
Kreitman, R., 239–249
Krischer, J., 260–277
Kronenberg, M., 209–210

Laissue, J.-A., 337–343
Larkin III, J., 101–114
Leon, F., 60–65
Lerman, M.A., 101–114
Liu, C., 319–320
Liu, E., 328–330, 331–333
López, M.C., 355–357, 371–373
Lorenz, R.G., 44–57
Lorenzo, M., 358–360, 390–393
Lycke, N., 193–208

Maclaren, N.K., 260–277
Macpherson, A.J., 36–43
MacPherson, G., 75–82
Malissen, B., 405–407
Malley, A., 239–249
Malone, J., 260–277

Marinova-Mutafchieva, L., 250–259
Marker, J., 260–277
Márquez, G., 405–407
Marquez, M.G., 371–373
Mayer, L., xi, 22–35, 154–168, 225–238
Mazza, G., 180–192
McClain, M., 172–179
McI. Mowat, A., 1–8
Menezes, J.S., 361–365
Mestecky, J., 58–59, 299–309
Miao, D., 328–330, 331–333
Mifflin, R.C., 313–318, 379–381
Milling, S., 75–82
Millington, O., 1–8, 9–15
Moldoveanu, Z., 299–309
Morita, T., 348–349
Moriyama, H., 328–330, 331–333
Mucida, D.S., 361–365
Munakata, A., 346–347, 348–349, 382–384
Murphy, J.J., 250–259

Nagatani, K., 366–370
Nagler-Anderson, C., 169–171
Nakane, A., 348–349, 382–384
Nakayama, T., 344–345
Nakazawa, A., 22–35
Newberry, R.D., 44–57
Nicolson, K.S., 180–192
Nieuwenhuis, E.E.S., 154–168
Nishihira, J., 348–349
Nóbrega, A., 394–397
Nowak, B., 413–415
Nussenblatt, R., 278–285

O'Neill, E.J., 180–192
Oliver, F., 299–309
Olmos, S., 371–373

Pang, K.F., 379–381
Parker, L.A., 1–8
Paronen, J., 328–330, 331–333
Pecquet, S., 374–378
Pinchuk, I.V., 313–318
Ponsford, M., 180–192
Powell, D.W., 313–318, 379–381
Powrie, F., 132–141
Prioult, G., 374–378

INDEX OF CONTRIBUTORS

Rapaport, R., 260–277
Raskin, P., 260–277
Raymond, E., 239–249
Rescigno, M., 66–74
Rewald, E., 358–360, 390–393
Reyes, V.E., 313–318, 379–381
Ribeiro, R.C., 394–397
Rimoldi, M., 66–74
Rodríguez, D., 361–365
Rogers, D., 260–277
Roncarolo, M.-G., 142–153
Roux, M.E., 371–373
Rumbo, M., 16–21
Russo, M., 361–365

Saada, J.I., 313–318, 379–381
Sagawa, K., 366–370
Sakuraba, H., 346–347, 348–349, 382–384
Samsom, J.N., 385–389
Sánchez, P., 358–360, 390–393
Sant'Anna, O., 394–397
Saurer, L., 180–192
Schatz, D., 260–277
Schwartz, S., 260–277
Sekikawa, K., 382–384
Sela, M., 239–249
Shao, L., 22–35
Shawler, T., 402–404
Shofti, R., 239–249
Sierro, F., 16–21
Sirard, J.-C., 16–21
Smith, K.M., 9–15
Song, F., 172–179, 402–404
Staines, N.A., 250–259
Streeter, H., 180–192
Strober, W., 115–131, 154–168, 169–171, 310–312
Suarez, G., 313–318, 379–381
Sundstedt, A., 180–192
Svensson, M., 405–407

Tagawa, Y.-I., 382–384
Tamerisa, R.A., 379–381
Taylor, R., 331–333
Teitelbaum, D., 239–249
Thurau, S.R., 408–412, 416–421
Toy, L., 225–238
Tsuji, N.M., 413–415
Turini, M., 374–378
Turnbull, E., 75–82

Uhr, T., 36–43
Umetsu, D.T., 88–93
Unger, W.W.J., 385–389

Van Berkel, L.A., 385–389
Vargas, A., 260–277
Vaz, N.M., 321–327
Viney, J.L., 83–87
Vulcano, M., 66–74

Wardrop III, R.M., 172–179
Weaver, C.T., 319–320
Weiner, H.L., 211–224
Wetzel, D., 60–65
Whitacre, C.C., 172–179, 402–404
Wildner, G., 408–412, 416–421
Wraith, D.C., 180–192
Wurbel, M.-A., 405–407

Yamagata, K., 346–347, 348–349, 382–384
Yamamoto, K., 366–370
Yrlid, U., 75–82
Yu, L., 328–330, 331–333

Zeidler, A., 260–277

OHIO UNIVERSITY LIBRARY

Please return this book as soon as you have finished with it. In order to avoid a fine it must be returned by the latest date stamped below. All books are subject to recall after two weeks or immediately if needed for reserve.

CF

ANNALS OF THE NEW YORK ACADEMY OF SCIENCES

Volume 1029

EDITORIAL STAFF

Director, Publishing and New Media
SARAH GREENE

Managing Editor
JUSTINE CULLINAN

Associate Editor
STEVEN E. BOHALL

The New York Academy of Sciences
2 East 63rd Street
New York, New York 10021

THE NEW YORK ACADEMY OF SCIENCES
(Founded in 1817)

BOARD OF GOVERNORS, September 2004 – September 2005

TORSTEN N. WIESEL, *Chairman of the Board*
GERALD D. FISCHBACH, *Vice Chairman*
MICHAEL SCHMERTZLER, *Treasurer*
ELLIS RUBINSTEIN, *Chief Executive Officer* [ex officio]

Honorary Life Governors
WILLIAM T. GOLDEN   JOSHUA LEDERBERG

Governors

KAREN E. BURKE	VIRGINIA W. CORNISH	PETER B. CORR
R. BRIAN FERGUSON	RONALD L. GRAHAM	MARNIE IMHOFF
WENDY EVANS JOSEPH	JACQUELINE LEO	RODERT W. LUCKY
PAUL MARKS	BRUCE McEWEN	RONAY MENSCHEL
JOHN T. MORGAN	JOHN F. NIBLACK	SANDRA PANEM
PETER RINGROSE	DAVID D. SABATINI	JOHN SEXTON
	DEBORAH WILEY	

VICTORIA BJORKLUND, *Counsel* [ex officio]   LARRY R. SMITH, *Secretary* [ex officio]